Series in BioEngineering

Series Editor

Magdalena Stoeva, Medical Imaging Department, Medical University Plovdiv, Plovdiv, Bulgaria

The Series in Bioengineering serves as an information source for a professional audience in science and technology as well as for advanced students. It covers all applications of the physical sciences and technology to medicine and the life sciences. Its scope ranges from bioengineering, biomedical and clinical engineering to biophysics, biomechanics, biomaterials, and bioinformatics.

Indexed by WTI Frankfurt eG, zbMATH.

Mariam Adeoba • Thanyani Pandelani

Application of Biomaterials in Biomedical Engineering

Springer

Mariam Adeoba
Department of Mechanical, Bioresources and Biomedical Engineering
University of South Africa
Johannesburg, South Africa

Thanyani Pandelani
UNISA Biomedical Engineering Research Group, Department of Mechanical Bioresources and Biomedical Engineering
University of South Africa
Johannesburg, South Africa

ISSN 2196-8861 ISSN 2196-887X (electronic)
Series in BioEngineering
ISBN 978-3-032-34476-2 ISBN 978-3-032-34477-9 (eBook)
https://doi.org/10.1007/978-3-032-34477-9

This Springer imprint is published by the registered company Springer Nature Switzerland AG, part of Springer Nature.
The registered company address is: Gewerbestrasse 11, 6330 Cham, Switzerland

Foreword

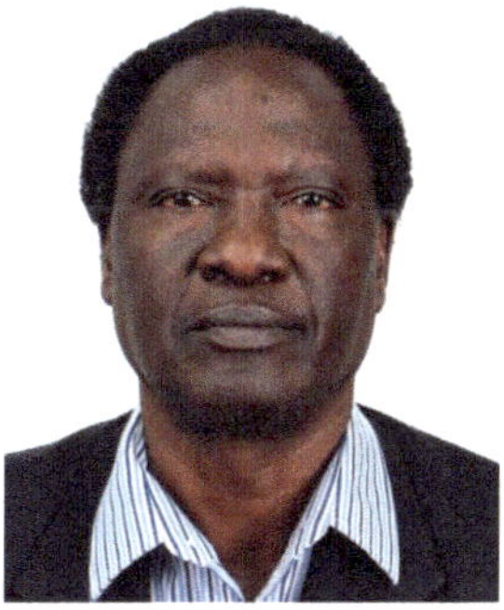

The field of biomaterials has progressed from a minor interdisciplinary interest to a fundamental component of contemporary biomedical engineering. In just a few decades, advancements in materials science, medicine, chemistry, information and communication technologies, and engineering have united to develop revolutionary solutions capable of repairing tissues, replacing malfunctioning organs, restoring physiological functions, and significantly improving human quality of life in previously unimagined ways. Currently, biomaterials not only sustain life but also engage, communicate, and integrate with biological systems, redefining the limits of healthcare capabilities. This book, *Application of Biomaterials in Biomedical Engineering*, provides a thorough and progressive examination of this swiftly evolving field based on facts, evidence, and research. Structured into ten informative chapters, it directs researchers, physicians, experts, and innovators through the essential ideas, technical aspects, and practical applications that underpin biomaterials science. The volume integrates foundational information and high-level scientific and technological advancements, encompassing molecular mechanisms of biocompatibility, the construction of intricate tissue scaffolds, intelligent drug-delivery systems, and therapies facilitated by nanomaterials.

This study is distinguished by its balance, as it encapsulates the precision of scientific detail while elucidating the wider context in which biomaterials influence clinical research, innovation, practice, and public health. It confronts the significant challenges within the field—ethical considerations, regulatory pathways, long-term stability, and host responses—while also anticipating the vast opportunities that lie ahead, such as regenerative medicine, neural interfaces, additive manufacturing, and novel immunomodulatory materials.

In an age of increasing chronic disease prevalence, evolving healthcare systems, and the prioritization of individualized medicine, comprehending biomaterials has become imperative. This book provides readers with research-, evidence-, and fact-based knowledge, imagination, and critical thinking essential for meaningful contributions to future biological discoveries and biomedical applications.

This research book offers a comprehensive, organized, and progressive foundation for both emerging, established, and leading researchers in biomaterials and biomedical engineering to extend the existing and current research frontiers in the field. This is an invitation to investigate, inquire, innovate, and guide at the convergence of biology, medicine, and engineering.

It is with full confidence that I believe the work herein will cultivate a profound respect for the materials that heal, support, and transform human existence and will enable readers to expand the limits of what is scientifically and medically achievable today and in the future.

Industrial Engineering, College of Science,
Engineering and Technology
Pretoria, South Africa
11 February 2026

Charles Mbohwa

Preface

Biomaterials are pivotal and more significant in contemporary biomedical engineering, fostering breakthroughs that impact diagnosis, treatment, rehabilitation, and overall patient quality of life. With the convergence of advancements in materials science, clinical practice, and engineering design, there is a critical need for comprehensive and accessible resources that connect basic ideas with emerging technologies and translational applications. The utilization of biomaterials in biomedical engineering was developed to address this necessity.

This book provides a comprehensive analysis of biomaterials, encompassing their physicochemical characteristics, biological interactions, and efficacy in many clinical applications. Although numerous texts discuss specific facets of biomaterials, few offer a comprehensive review encompassing classical notions, contemporary research trajectories, regulatory considerations, and practical applications. Our objective is to create a book that is both scientifically rigorous and practically pertinent, appropriate for researchers, physicians, engineers, educators, and students aiming to comprehend not just the nature of biomaterials but also their functionality and rationale within biomedical contexts.

The ten chapters of this book exhibit a balance between profundity and scope. They advance from foundational frameworks and biocompatibility principles to specific applications, including tissue engineering, medication delivery, biosensing, brain interfaces, nanomaterials, and additive manufacturing. Each chapter integrates conceptual foundations with contemporary accomplishments, problems, and future outlooks, allowing readers to follow the field's progress while recognizing its swiftly transforming terrain. This work possesses a distinctive multidisciplinary viewpoint. Biomedical engineering is fundamentally collaborative, necessitating contributions from biology, chemistry, physics, engineering, medicine, and regulatory science. We have thereby highlighted the interrelationship of these areas, portraying biomaterials not as discrete entities but as dynamic instruments influenced by design limitations, biological reactions, and societal demands. Furthermore, we emphasize emerging research within African contexts—an area sometimes overlooked in mainstream literature, yet abundant in innovation rooted in local health concerns and resource-appropriate solutions. This work results from continuous academic involvement, research experience, and collaborative discourse within the scientific community. We recognize the assistance of the UNISA Biomedical Engineering Group, University of South Africa, in cultivating a conducive research environment.

Johannesburg, South Africa — Mariam Adeoba
Johannesburg, South Africa — Thanyani Pandelani

Acknowledgments

We extend our deepest appreciation to all those whose support, expertise, and encouragement made this book, *Application of Biomaterials in Biomedical Engineering*, possible.

Our sincere gratitude goes to the University of South Africa (UNISA), particularly the Department of Mechanical, Bioresources, and Biomedical Engineering and the College of Science, Engineering and Technology (CSET), for providing an enabling environment for research, knowledge exchange, and interdisciplinary collaboration. We are especially thankful to the UNISA Biomedical Engineering Research Group for their continuous support, insightful discussions, and commitment to advancing biomedical innovation.

We acknowledge our colleagues, mentors, and collaborators whose scientific contributions, critical feedback, and shared expertise enriched the depth and quality of this work. Their input strengthened our perspectives and helped refine the multidisciplinary narratives presented in this book.

We are grateful to the students and emerging researchers whose curiosity, dedication, and enthusiasm continually inspire the advancement of biomedical engineering. Their passion reinforces the importance of creating accessible and impactful academic resources.

Special thanks go to Almighty God and to our families and loved ones, whose patience, encouragement, and unwavering support sustained us throughout the writing and editorial process. Their belief in our work made this journey fulfilling.

Finally, we recognize the broader scientific community, researchers, clinicians, engineers, and innovators, whose collective efforts continue to shape the evolving landscape of biomaterials and their transformative role in improving human health. It is our hope that this book contributes meaningfully to that ongoing endeavor.

Competing Interests The authors have no competing interests to declare that are relevant to the content of this manuscript.

Contents

About the Authors

Mariam Adeoba is an accomplished researcher and academic specializing in zoology, water resources, and environmental sustainability. She holds a Ph.D. in zoology from the University of Johannesburg, South Africa, where her doctoral research focused on the extinction patterns of African fish species in an area that underscores her deep commitment to biodiversity conservation and aquatic ecosystem health. She obtained her M.Sc. and B.Sc. degrees in animal physiology and animal production and health, respectively, from the University of Agriculture, Abeokuta, Nigeria. Building on her multidisciplinary background, Dr. Adeoba's research intersects animal science, animal physiology, ecology, and sustainable resource management, with a growing focus on the food-water-energy nexus. Currently, Dr. Adeoba serves as a Postdoctoral Research Fellow at the UNISA Biomedical Research Group, Department of Mechanical, Bioresources and Biomedical Engineering, College of Science, Engineering and Technology (CSET), University of South Africa. Her postdoctoral work integrates data-driven and systems-based approaches to optimize the use of natural resources in support of sustainability and resilience in African communities. Dr. Adeoba is also a Section Editor for *Marine Systems and Environment* (marine and environment), where she contributes to advancing scholarly communication in marine and environmental sciences. She has also coedited two books, including *Marine Microbial Products: Applications and Opportunities*, a multi-editor volume on marine microbes and their biotechnological applications, coedited with Sesan Abiodun Aransiola and Naga Raju Maddela. And *Water 4.0: Concepts and Application*, a book on the integration of Fourth Industrial Revolution technologies into water supply and water systems management, co-authored with Nnamdi Ikechi Nwulu. Her professional interests encompass biodiversity conservation, sustainable aquatic ecosystems, climate adaptation, and the circular economy in environmental management. Through her research, teaching, and advocacy, Dr. Adeoba continues to contribute meaningfully to the pursuit of sustainable development and environmental resilience across Africa and beyond.

Thanyani Pandelani is an Associate Professor in the Department of Mechanical, Bioresources, and Biomedical Engineering at the University of South Africa (UNISA). He holds a Ph.D. in bioengineering from Imperial College London, where his research focused on the biomechanics of the pelvis under underbody blast conditions. He also earned his M.Sc. and B.Sc. degrees in mechanical engineering from the University of Cape Town, specializing in injury mechanics and soft-tissue biomechanics.

Prof. Pandelani's research interests span biomechanics, computational biomedical engineering, soft-tissue mechanics, and injury modeling. He has contributed extensively to peer-reviewed journals and book chapters on topics such as blast loading effects on the human body, characterization of biological tissues, and the mechanical response of human extremities under impact. He is also a co-editor of the *Handbook of Physical and Mechanical Testing of Soft Tissues* (CRC Press/Taylor & Francis, 2024).

At UNISA, he leads innovative projects at the Centre for Biomedical Engineering and Healthcare Innovation (CBEHI), advancing interdisciplinary research in tissue mechanics, additive manufacturing, and biomedical device design. His work bridges engineering, biology, and trauma science, contributing to advances in prosthetics, human protection systems, and healthcare innovation.

Prof. Pandelani is recognized for his collaborative leadership in national and international research initiatives and continues to mentor emerging scholars and engineers across Africa and beyond.

Chapter 1
Introduction to Biomaterials in Biomedical Engineering

Abstract A fundamental review of the concepts, categories, and uses of biomaterials in the larger framework of biomedical innovation and clinical practice is given in Chap. 1, Introduction to Biomaterials in Biomedical Engineering. Biomaterials are defined as natural or artificial substances designed to interact with biological systems for diagnostic or therapeutic purposes. The interdisciplinary aspect of biomaterials science is highlighted in this chapter, which combines ideas from biology, chemistry, materials engineering, and medicine to create materials that preserve, enhance, or repair physiological capabilities. From early inert implants to modern smart and bioactive materials that may dynamically interact with live tissues, the evolution of biomaterials is traced from a historical viewpoint. The structural and functional characteristics of biomaterials that are pertinent to biomedical applications are described in this chapter, which divides them into metals, ceramics, polymers, and composites. It talks about important performance standards such mechanical integrity, sterilizability, biocompatibility, and biodegradability, emphasizing how crucial it is to match material characteristics with biological contexts. Focus is placed on the mechanisms of tissue response, immunological compatibility, and degradation behavior that affect the safety and long-term success of implants or devices. The chapter also examines new developments that support precision healthcare and regenerative medicine, such as tissue engineering scaffolds, nano biomaterials, and bioresorbable polymers. Also covered are ethical and legal issues, with a focus on sustainable development, patient safety, and responsible innovation. In Chap. 1, biomaterials are positioned as a fundamental component of contemporary biomedical engineering, bridging the gap between material science and clinical application, by laying a conceptual and technical basis. It emphasizes how diverse research and innovation are still needed to create next-generation materials that meet strict therapeutic criteria and mimic biological complexity. Thus, the foundation for a more thorough examination of biomaterial design, production, characterisation, and translational application in later text sections is laid forth in this introductory chapter.

M. Adeoba, T. Pandelani, *Application of Biomaterials in Biomedical Engineering*, Series in BioEngineering,
https://doi.org/10.1007/978-3-032-34477-9_1

1.1 Introduction

Biomedical engineering is a dynamic and interdisciplinary field that integrates engineering, life sciences, and medical principles to build and advance products that improve human health and quality of life. It encompasses various subfields, including prosthetics, tissue engineering, biomechanics, medical imaging, and biomaterials science. Fundamentally, biomedical engineering aims to solve problems in diagnosis, monitoring, treatment, and rehabilitation by bridging the gap between biological complexity and technology innovation. Biomedical engineers develop devices and systems that safely and effectively interact with living tissues by combining engineering techniques with physiological knowledge.

Biomedical engineering has a wide range of applications, from digital health systems and nanomedicine to implantable devices and artificial organs. It emphasizes the transfer of research from the lab bench to the clinical bedside and is by its very nature translational. To guarantee that technological solutions are not only practical but also biocompatible and morally sound, biomedical engineers work closely with doctors, biologists, and material scientists [1, 2]. Given that the materials used in medical devices have a significant impact on their longevity, performance, and safety, materials science is a fundamental component of biomedical innovation.

Materials science has a significant impact on medical innovation. It offers the basis for comprehending the mechanical, chemical, and physical characteristics of substances that interact with biological systems. Materials scientists investigate the ways in which metals, ceramics, polymers, and composites might be designed to satisfy medical needs, like controlled degradation in drug delivery systems, strength in orthopedic implants, or flexibility in vascular stents. The design of biofunctional materials that can trigger biological reactions, encourage tissue regeneration, or deliver medicinal compounds precisely where needed is made possible by the fusion of materials engineering and biology. Therefore, materials science not only drives technical progress in healthcare but also establishes the boundaries of what biomedical engineering can accomplish in terms of sustainability, safety, and efficacy.

1.1.1 Definition and Scope of Biomaterials

Natural or artificial materials created especially to interact with biological systems to assess, treat, enhance, or replace any tissue, organ, or bodily function are known as biomaterials. Biomaterials, in contrast to conventional engineering materials, are created with two goals in mind: they must be compatible with living things while meeting mechanical and structural specifications. A biomaterial must be able to interact harmoniously with physiological surroundings without causing toxicity, inflammation, or immunological rejection to achieve its intended therapeutic or diagnostic goal.

Biomaterials are used in more than just basic implants or gadgets. It includes the design of materials that can actively engage in biological processes, surface modification methods, degradation behavior, and the study of material–tissue interactions. Biomaterials, for instance, act as scaffolds in tissue engineering, directing the regeneration of new tissues and offering structural support for cell proliferation. Biodegradable polymers are employed in medication delivery to regulate the release of therapeutic substances over time, improving effectiveness and reducing adverse effects. Likewise, biomaterials in biosensors make it easier to identify biological signals, allowing for accurate medical diagnosis.

The design goals and assessment standards of biomaterials and conventional engineered materials differ significantly. Mechanical strength, thermal stability, or resistance to corrosion are the main criteria used to choose traditional materials like metals, polymers, or ceramics. On the other hand, biomaterials need to meet extra biological requirements such biocompatibility, bio functionality, and bioactivity. If resorption is necessary, they must safely disintegrate, promote cell adhesion or proliferation when necessary, and blend in perfectly with tissues. Furthermore, biomaterials function in the human body's extremely sensitive and variable environment, where variables like pH, enzyme activity, and immunological response have a big impact on performance. Therefore, to guarantee usefulness, safety, and long-term stability in vivo, biomaterial development necessitates a multidisciplinary approach combining materials engineering, cell biology, chemistry, and clinical sciences.

1.1.2 Importance of Biomaterials in Healthcare

By facilitating the development of innovative medical gadgets, prosthetics, and regenerative therapies, biomaterials have completely transformed contemporary healthcare. From functional restorations like cardiovascular stents and brain interfaces to structural replacements like orthopedic implants and dental restorations, their uses are numerous. Through the restoration of mobility, eyesight, heart function, and other vital physiological processes, biomaterials are critical to improve the quality of life for millions of patients worldwide [3, 4].

Biomaterials are essential to the development of lab-on-a-chip systems, biosensors, and diagnostic assays. These technologies make it possible to diagnose diseases including infections, malignancies, and metabolic abnormalities quickly, accurately, and with little invasiveness. Through hydrogels, nanoparticles, and encapsulating systems, biomaterials allow for regulated drug delivery in therapeutic contexts, guaranteeing localized treatment with fewer systemic side effects. They assist the formation of synthetic skin, bone, cartilage, and even entire organs by providing the structural and biochemical cues required for tissue healing and organ reconstruction in regenerative medicine.

Biomaterials technology has a huge social and economic influence outside of medicinal applications. The prevalence of chronic diseases, aging populations, and technical advancements have all contributed to the recent exponential growth of the worldwide biomaterials industry. This expansion has stimulated innovation in the clinical, industrial, and academic domains, opening new avenues for healthcare delivery, entrepreneurship, and research. Furthermore, by creating ecologically friendly and bioresorbable materials that lessen surgical problems and long-term waste, biomaterials support sustainable medicine. In order to guarantee that cutting-edge medical innovations benefit a variety of populations globally, the ethical aspect of biomaterials innovation additionally emphasizes the significance of safety, accessibility, and equity [5, 6].

Thus, biomaterials not only underpin modern medical practice but also shape the future trajectory of healthcare systems through their contributions to preventive, personalized, and regenerative medicine.

1.1.3 Chapter Objectives

This chapter's main goal is to give readers a basic understanding of biomaterial science in the context of biomedical engineering. Its goal is to present the rules that regulate the choice, creation, and use of materials that have an impact on living systems. This chapter allows readers to delve into more intricate subjects including material characterization, tissue compatibility, surface modification, and fabrication technologies in subsequent sections by providing the theoretical and practical foundation for the use of biomaterials.

The chapter specifically aims to clarify the basic ideas, categories, and functions of biomaterials in healthcare. Give examples of how materials science uses creativity and interdisciplinary cooperation to help address biomedical problems. Talk about the crucial mechanical, chemical, and biological requirements that determine effective biomaterial performance. Describe the development of biomaterials and how they have been incorporated into clinical practice from a historical and modern standpoint. In the next chapters, lay forth a conceptual framework for comprehending the design, testing, and regulatory assessment of biomaterials.

Biomaterials are the structural and functional cornerstone of biomedical engineering, as this introduction concludes. They represent the meeting point of clinical necessity and scientific innovation, when atomic or molecular-level material manipulation results in observable enhancements in patient care. This chapter helps readers grasp the importance of biomaterials in influencing the direction of medicine in the future, in addition to their complexity and promise.

1.2 Key Concepts and Definitions

Several fundamental ideas that specify how materials interact with biological systems form the basis of the scientific study of biomaterials. The most important ones are biocompatibility, biofunctionality, bioactivity, and biodegradability, each of which represents a distinct aspect of the behavior of materials in living things. The fundamental idea guiding the use of any biomaterial in medical applications is biocompatibility. It describes a material's capacity to carry out its intended purpose without causing unfavorable reactions in the host organism. According to Kyriakides et al. [7] and Bapat et al. [8], a biocompatible material should support proper cellular and tissue functioning without causing toxic, immunogenic, or carcinogenic reactions. Degradation products, surface chemistry, material composition, and the physiological milieu of the host all affect how biocompatible a material is. Crucially, biocompatibility is context-dependent rather than absolute; because of differences in vascularization, mechanical strain, and metabolic circumstances, what is biocompatible in one tissue type could not be in another.

The ability of a material to perform its intended mechanical, structural, or physiological function within the body is known as biofunctionality. Biofunctionality guarantees that the material carries out its intended purpose efficiently, whereas biocompatibility guarantees that it does not cause harm to the host. For instance, a prosthetic heart valve needs to be dependable when opening and closing under repeated hemodynamic pressures in addition to being biocompatible. Strength, fatigue resistance, and wear behavior are examples of biofunctionality in orthopedic implants that are essential for long-term performance. Therefore, biofunctionality emphasizes that successful biomaterials must preserve their functional integrity in complex biological environments by fusing biological performance with engineering design.

Beyond passive compatibility, bioactivity refers to substances that actively engage with biological systems to stimulate tissue or cellular reactions. Bioactive substances can promote mineralization, differentiation, and cell adhesion. One well-known example is bioactive glass, which creates hydroxycarbonate apatite on the surface of bone to establish a direct chemical link. Similarly, by presenting biochemical signals that resemble the extracellular matrix, surface-modified polymers and nanostructured coatings can promote tissue integration and increase bioactivity. The transition from inert to "smart" biomaterials which can interact with their biological environment is known as bioactivity, and it paves the way for tissue engineering and regenerative medicine.

Conversely, biodegradability describes the regulated hydrolysis or enzymatic breakdown of materials in the biological environment. After serving their purpose, biodegradable materials are made to slowly dissolve or disintegrate, removing the need for surgical removal. In applications like controlled drug delivery systems, temporary scaffolds, and resorbable sutures, this feature is especially advantageous. Environmental circumstances (e.g., pH, temperature, enzymatic presence), molecular weight, crystallinity, and polymer composition all affect biodegradability. For instance, biodegradable polymers like polylactic acid (PLA) and polyglycolic acid (PGA) are frequently utilized in surgical procedures. Degradation products must be kept non-toxic and safely digested or eliminated while degradation rates must be adjusted to correspond with the healing or regeneration process.

The basic standards for assessing and creating materials meant for biomedical applications are defined by these four ideas taken together: biocompatibility, biofunctionality, bioactivity, and biodegradability. They capture the multifaceted character of biomaterials, wherein within the physiological milieu, mechanical, chemical, and biological performance must be balanced.

1.2.1 Classification of Biomaterials

Although there are many ways to categorize biomaterials, two of the most popular methods are based on their functionality (permanent or temporary implants) and place of origin (natural or synthetic) as shown in Fig. 1.1. The vast range of materials used in biomedical engineering are arranged according to these classifications, which also help choose the best ones for certain uses.

Natural biomaterials come directly from biological sources and, because of their biological makeup, frequently have greater biocompatibility and biofunctionality. Collagen, hyaluronic acid, chitosan, silk fibroin, and alginate are a few examples. They can encourage cell adhesion, proliferation, and differentiation because they resemble the extracellular matrix. However, natural materials may encounter difficulties such enzymatic degradation susceptibility, low mechanical strength, and source variability. Conversely, synthetic biomaterials are manufactured to have specific mechanical, chemical, and physical characteristics. Typical examples include ceramics (like hydroxyapatite and alumina), metals (like stainless steel and titanium), and polymers (like polyethylene, polyurethane, and polylactic acid). Synthetic materials are perfect for applications needing mechanical or structural properties since they are reproducible and customizable. Nevertheless, they may require surface modification to enhance biocompatibility or bioactivity.

Biomaterials can be roughly classified as either temporary or permanent implants based on their functionality. Long-term or lifetime use is intended for permanent implants, which preserve stability and mechanical integrity without suffering appreciable deterioration. Dental implants, cardiac pacemaker housings, and hip

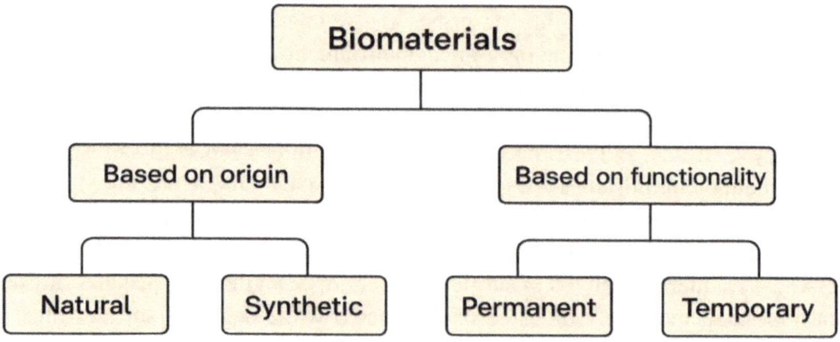

Fig. 1.1 Classification of biomaterials based on origin (natural vs. synthetic) and functional properties, illustrating the major categories used in biomedical engineering applications

prosthesis are a few examples. These materials need to be mechanically compatible with the surrounding tissues, have outstanding fatigue resistance, and be corrosion stable. Conversely, temporary implants are designed to break down or resorb after their intended use, which is consistent with the previously mentioned biodegradability principles. Applications for temporary materials include orthopedic fixation devices, sutures, and tissue scaffolds. For the best healing results, their pace of deterioration needs to be in rhythm with the rate of tissue regeneration.

The two categories, origin and functionality showcase the variety and adaptability of biomaterials in contemporary medicine. Because both natural and synthetic materials can be tuned for either short-term or long-term biomedical uses, it also emphasizes how crucial it is to balance material qualities with clinical requirements.

1.2.2 Material–Biological Interface

The crucial area where a biomaterial directly interacts with biological tissues, cells, and fluids is known as the material–biological interface. The quality of this interface has a major impact on how well any implant or biomedical device performs. The host reaction, tissue integration, and long-term functionality are all influenced by a confluence of physical, chemical, and biological elements that govern interactions at this level.

Interactions between cells and materials start as soon as the cell is implanted. The way proteins from body fluids adsorb to a biomaterial's surface depend on its surface characteristics, including its roughness, charge, hydrophilicity, and chemical makeup. Cell adhesion, proliferation, and differentiation are subsequently influenced by this protein layer. For instance, micro- or nanoscale roughness that resembles bone structure improves osteoblast attachment to titanium surfaces. Likewise, adding bioactive peptides (such RGD sequences) to polymeric surfaces can facilitate tissue regeneration and cell attachment.

The creation of a stable, functional contact between the implant and surrounding tissue is referred to as tissue integration, which may also be called osseointegration or biointegration, depending on the type of tissue [9, 10]. Effective tissue integration encourages direct bonding between artificial and biological components and reduces fibrous encapsulation. Enhancing tissue ingrowth using porous or textured surfaces can improve stability and mechanical coupling. In dental and orthopedic implants, where close tissue contact is necessary for mechanical load transfer, this procedure is particularly important.

Since the immune system always keeps an eye on foreign substances that are ingested into the body, immune reactions at the material biological interface are equally significant. Depending on the chemistry and degrading behavior of the substance, the reaction can range from mild inflammation to chronic rejection. Instead of causing fibrosis or rejection, biomaterials should ideally elicit a modest, temporary immune response that promotes healing. Designing surfaces that can control macrophage polarization and encourage regenerative rather than inflammatory effects is the goal of developments in immunomodulatory biomaterials. In general, the logical design of biomaterials depends on an understanding of the material–biological interface. It connects clinical performance with molecular-level interactions, guaranteeing that components actively aid in healing and restoration in addition to surviving in the body.

1.3 Historical Background

One of the most revolutionary developments in medical science is the creation of biomaterials, which have progressed from simple applications in antiquity to intricate, interdisciplinary inventions in the current biomedical era. The history of biomaterials tells the story of humanity's tenacious attempts to replace, repair, and regenerate biological functions in addition to documenting advances in material science as shown in Fig. 1.2. Changes in scientific knowledge, technological prowess, and ethical obligation are reflected in this progression.

1.3.1 Early Uses of Biomaterials

Biomaterials were first used thousands of years ago when people tried to employ naturally occurring materials to heal wounds or restore lost bodily functions. Gold, ivory, wood, and bone were all used in primitive medicinal practices by ancient

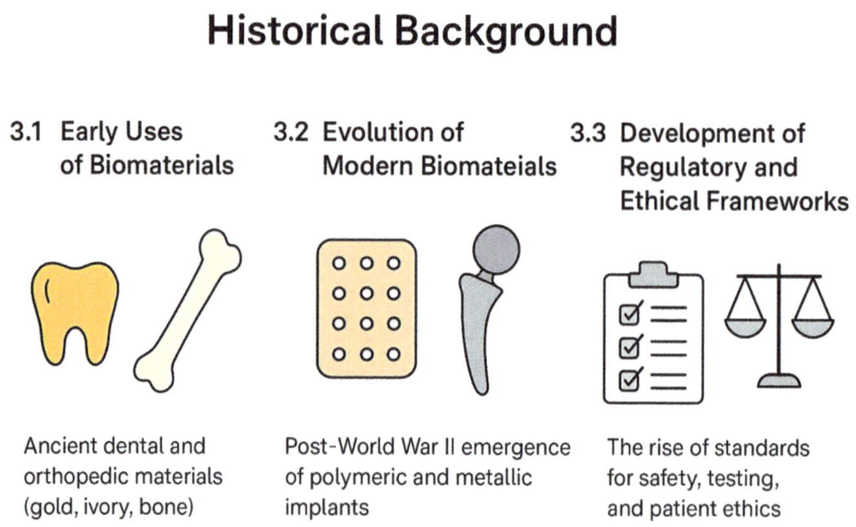

Fig. 1.2 Historical timeline illustrating the evolution of biomaterials from early natural materials used in ancient medical practices to modern bioactive, biodegradable, and smart materials integrated into contemporary biomedical engineering

societies, according to archeological data. As early as 2000 BCE, ancient Egyptian and Etruscan dentists utilized gold, which is prized for its noncorrosive and malleable qualities, to replace or stabilize teeth. A crude but efficient example of what is now known as biocompatibility, its chemical inertness guaranteed little biological reaction.

Likewise, pre-Columbian South America, ancient China, and Rome often utilized bone and ivory as substitutes for skeletal or dental repairs. Although these naturally occurring materials lack the structural and mechanical optimization of modern biomaterials, they demonstrated some compatibility with human tissues. To seal wounds and encourage healing, ancient surgeons also used linen, silk, and animal sinew as sutures, exhibiting an innate understanding of the relationship between biological material and body.

Interventions in orthopedics were equally noteworthy. Early attempts to regain movement and function following amputation are demonstrated by the employment of wooden prosthetics, such as the ancient Egyptian "Cairo toe," a wooden and leather prosthesis found on a mummy dated to approximately 1000 BCE. Despite their basic nature, these gadgets demonstrated a developing grasp of biofunctionality, which is the notion that a material or device should have a structural or mechanical purpose that is compatible with the body.

Despite the lack of empirical proof, these age-old methods serve as the cornerstone of biomaterial research. Even if empirical knowledge of tissue compatibility or immune response was centuries distant, they show that human societies have long sought materials that might interact with biological systems in a safe and efficient manner [11, 12].

1.3.2 Evolution of Modern Biomaterials

The development of polymer science, chemistry, and metallurgy during and after World War II sparked the modern era of biomaterials in the middle of the twentieth century. The industrial demands of the war sparked the development of synthetic materials including titanium, stainless steel, polymers, and cobalt-chromium alloys, which were later modified for use in medicine. Orthopedic, cardiovascular, and dental applications could benefit from these materials' advantageous mechanical strength, corrosion resistance, and manufacturability.

The advent of polyethylene and polymethylmethacrylate (PMMA), which were initially applied for dental restoration and joint replacement in the 1940s and 1950s, was one of the major advancements. Because of its moldability and implant-anchoring capabilities, PMMA, also marketed as acrylic, became the industry standard for bone cement. In a similar manner, silicone rubber, initially produced by Dow Corning in the 1950s, revolutionized reconstructive surgery and soft tissue prostheses, encompassing breast implants and facial reconstruction.

During this time, metallic biomaterials advanced quickly. Because of its great tensile strength and resistance to corrosion, stainless steel (316 L) has emerged as the main material for orthopedic fixation devices. Because of their exceptional biocompatibility and capacity to create persistent oxide layers that promote osseointegration the direct structural and functional bond between living bone and the implant surface titanium and its alloys later became preferable substitutes. Numerous lives were saved in the cardiovascular area thanks to the discovery of Teflon (PTFE) and Dacron (polyethylene terephthalate), which made it possible to produce prosthetic heart valves and vascular grafts.

A paradigm shifts toward bioactive and biodegradable materials also occurred in the postwar decades. Bioactive materials like hydroxyapatite and bioglass were created to interact favorably with biological tissues, encouraging cell adhesion, differentiation, and integration, in contrast to inert implants that simply replaced tissue function. To avoid the necessity for surgical removal, biodegradable polymers such as polylactic acid (PLA) and polyglycolic acid (PGA) were launched at the same time for temporary implants. These polymers allow for slow decomposition and absorption by the body.

The development of tissue engineering and regenerative medicine in the late twentieth century considerably broadened the field's scope by fusing materials science with biotechnology and cellular biology. Biomaterials were developed to direct tissue regeneration or precisely administer medications in both space and time, transforming them from passive supports into active players in the healing process. This progression from gold fillings to bioengineered scaffolds demonstrates how biomaterials have significantly evolved into a vital component of contemporary medicine.

1.3.3 Development of Regulatory and Ethical Frameworks

Regulatory and ethical frameworks arose to protect patient safety and guarantee responsible innovation as biomaterials grew in complexity and usage. Medical device testing was informal and unregulated in the early twentieth century, frequently depending on surgeon expertise or anecdotal evidence. However, instances of infection, toxicity, and material failure highlighted how urgent thorough supervision is needed.

The Federal Food, Drug, and Cosmetic Act (FD&C Act) of 1938, which established safety testing for medical products, was the first major step toward regulation in the United States. Later, the Medical Device Amendments of 1976 created the need for premarket evaluation, performance criteria, and post-market surveillance, and they legally classified devices according to risk. International organizations like the World Health Organization (WHO), International Organization for Standardization (ISO), and European Medicines Agency (EMA) adopted similar frameworks, which resulted in the creation of standards like ISO 10993, which regulates the biological evaluation of medical devices.

As regulatory frameworks changed, so did ethical considerations. The development of concepts like informed permission, risk-benefit analysis, and patient autonomy was spurred by the historical context of unethical research, including unconsented implant trials and the opaqueness of early surgical discoveries. These ethical requirements were codified in documents like the Belmont Report (1979) and the Declaration of Helsinki (1964), which placed a strong emphasis on protecting human beings in biomedical research.

Furthermore, institutional review boards (IRBs) and ethical review committees have become essential to biomaterials research, guaranteeing that clinical studies adhere to moral and scientific norms. Since then, it has become expected that biomaterial development will incorporate ethical design principles, such as limiting harm, guaranteeing fair access, and maintaining transparency.

Since nanomaterials, smart biomaterials, and hybrid bioengineered systems present novel safety and long-term evaluation concerns, regulatory oversight has broadened in the twenty-first century. Modern frameworks provide an emphasis on biological performance, immunogenicity, and sustainability in addition to physical and chemical testing. Beyond clinical safety, ethical considerations increasingly include environmental impact, bioinformatics data privacy, and global equity in access to cutting-edge biomaterial technologies [13, 14].

From prehistoric gold and ivory restorations to contemporary bioactive, biodegradable, and legally compliant implants, the development of biomaterials demonstrates humanity's persistent pursuit of combining biology and technology for medical applications. Every age added a crucial layer of knowledge: the postwar industrial revolution offered the materials and engineering know-how; the modern era institutionalized safety, ethics, and patient-centered regulation; and early civilizations provided the empirical underpinnings of biocompatibility. Together, these advancements have turned biomaterials from crude stand-ins into ethically guided, scientifically advanced instruments that support and improve life, representing the union of creativity, empathy, and accountability in contemporary medicine.

1.4 Material Types and Properties

Biomaterials are a broad category of materials that have been specially designed to interact with biological systems to perform diagnostic, therapeutic, or regenerative functions. Combining advantageous mechanical, physical, chemical, and biological qualities is essential to their success in biomedical applications. Biomaterials can be generically categorized as metallic, ceramic, polymeric, or composite materials based on their composition and functional properties as shown in Table 1.1. Each category has unique benefits and drawbacks that dictate which medical applications it is appropriate for. Optimizing performance, biocompatibility, and long-term stability in physiological conditions requires a deep understanding of various material types and their inherent characteristics as shown in Fig. 1.3.

Table 1.1 Biomaterial types and properties

Biomaterial type	Representative materials	Key features	Primary advantages	Typical applications
Metallic Biomaterials	Titanium (Ti, Ti-6Al-4 V), Cobalt–Chromium alloys, Stainless steel (316 L)	High tensile & fatigue strength; load-bearing ability; corrosion resistance	Superior mechanical performance; high biocompatibility	Orthopedic & dental implants, cardiovascular stents, fixation devices
Ceramic Biomaterials	Alumina, Zirconia, Hydroxyapatite (HA), Bioglass	High compressive strength; brittle; wear resistance	Excellent corrosion resistance; strong bone bonding	Dental crowns, bone grafts, implant coatings
Polymeric Biomaterials	Collagen, Chitosan, Alginate, PE, PLA, PEG	Low density; tunable flexibility; biodegradability	Versatile degradation profiles; biocompatible	Soft tissue scaffolds, wound dressings, drug delivery
Composite Materials	PLA/HA, Ti–HA, polymer–metal hybrids	Combined mechanical + biological advantages	Balanced strength, toughness, and bioactivity	Bone scaffolds, dental restorations, load-sharing implants
Key Material Properties (General Overview)	Mechanical: Strength, elasticity, fatigue resistance; Thermal: Conductivity, expansion; Chemical: Corrosion, oxidation, hydrolysis; Surface: Roughness, wettability, charge	Optimized properties improve tissue response, osseointegration, implant longevity	Enhanced stability, biological integration, predictable performance	Foundational across all biomaterial selection & design

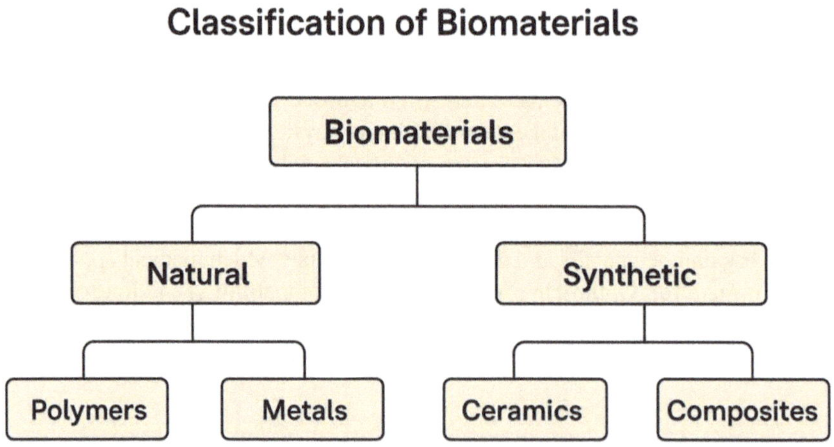

Fig. 1.3 Classification chart of biomaterials organized by origin (natural vs. synthetic) and composition (metals, polymers, ceramics, and composites), illustrating the major categories used in biomedical engineering applications

1.4.1 Metallic Biomaterials

Recent advances in biomedical implant materials including surface-modified metallic alloys, ceramics, and polymers have further refined the balance between mechanical performance, corrosion resistance, and biocompatibility essential for modern implant design [15]. Among the earliest and most popular materials in biomedical engineering are metallic biomaterials, especially for load-bearing applications such implants for the heart, teeth, and joints. They are perfect for providing structural support in dynamic bodily situations because of their great mechanical strength, durability, and resistance to fatigue. Cobalt-chromium (Co-Cr) alloys, stainless steels, and titanium (Ti) and its alloys are examples of common metallic biomaterials.

The most biocompatible metals used in medicine are titanium and its alloys, particularly Ti-6Al-4V, because of their superior strength-to-weight ratio, resistance to corrosion, and capacity to produce a stable oxide layer (TiO_2) on their surface. Titanium is the material of choice for orthopedic and dental implants because of this passive oxide coating, which reduces ion leakage and encourages osseointegration. Compared to other metals, its modulus of elasticity is more like that of bone, which lessens stress shielding and the resorption of bone implants.

Because of their remarkable hardness and wear resistance, cobalt-chromium (Co–Cr) alloys are especially well-suited for joint replacement parts such knee joint surfaces and femoral heads in hip prosthesis. While the cobalt matrix offers mechanical durability under cyclic stress, the chromium concentration improves corrosion resistance by forming a protective CrO_3 layer. Ongoing enhancements in alloy composition and surface treatments are necessary, nevertheless, as the possible release of Co and Cr ions in vivo may cause systemic effects or local tissue irritation.

Magnesium and its alloys have emerged as promising biodegradable metallic biomaterials for orthopedic and cardiovascular applications, offering bio-corrosiveness and tissue stimulation properties that reduce the need for secondary surgeries and mitigate long-term complications associated with permanent metallic implants [16].

Stainless steel, particularly the 316 L surgical grade, is another commonly used metal for temporary fixation devices such as screws, plates, and wires. It offers good strength and ductility at relatively low cost [17, 18]. The presence of chromium enhances corrosion resistance, while molybdenum improves pitting resistance in chloride-containing body fluids. However, stainless steel's higher elastic modulus and susceptibility to corrosion fatigue limit its long-term use compared to titanium or Co–Cr alloys.

Superior mechanical strength, ductility, and fatigue endurance are the main benefits of metallic biomaterials; nevertheless, possible ion release, corrosion in physiological fluids, and stiffness mismatch with biological tissues are some of its drawbacks. To increase the biofunctionality of metallic implants, research is still being done on creating new alloys, surface coatings (such titanium nitride or hydroxyapatite), and additive manufacturing processes.

1.4.2 Ceramic Biomaterials

High hardness, chemical inertness, and superior wear resistance define ceramic biomaterials as a special class of inorganic, non-metallic materials. Depending on their tissue-bonding capabilities, ceramics are employed in biomedical applications in both bioinert and bioactive forms.

Ceramics that are bioinert, like zirconia (ZrO_2) and alumina (AlO_3), are chemically stable and don't interact much with biological tissues. Because of its great compressive strength, hardness, and resistance to corrosion and wear, alumina has long been utilized in dental prosthesis and orthopedic joint replacements. Similar to this, zirconia, especially yttria-stabilized zirconia (YSZ), is appropriate for load-bearing implants because it provides improved fracture toughness by phase change toughening. The primary benefit of bioinert ceramics is their low wear rates and durability; nevertheless, they are unable to establish direct chemical bonds with tissues and frequently rely on cementation or mechanical interlocking for fixing.

Bioactive ceramics, on the other hand, actively engage with biological surroundings to encourage tissue regeneration and attachment. The two most well-known examples are bioglass and hydroxyapatite ($Ca_{10}(PO_4)_6(OH)_2$). Because of its exceptional osteoconductivity and chemical resemblance to the mineral component of bone, hydroxyapatite enables bone cells to adhere and multiply directly on its surface. It is frequently used in reconstructive surgery as a bone graft substitute or as a covering substance on metallic implants to improve osseointegration. Silica (SiO_2), calcium oxide (CaO), sodium oxide (NaO), and phosphorus pentoxide (P_2O_5) combine to make bioglass, which in vivo forms a hydroxycarbonate apatite layer that promotes a robust connection to soft tissues and bone. Its adaptable composition allows for customized ion release profiles and breakdown rates, which can promote cellular activity and angiogenesis.

Ceramics' low tensile strength and brittleness restrict their usage in high-load applications, but their wear resistance, chemical stability, and possible bioactivity make them essential for maxillofacial, dental, and orthopedic reconstruction. Their durability and functional integration with living tissues are being further improved by developments in nanoceramics and composite reinforcing techniques.

1.4.3 Polymeric Biomaterials

A vast array of mechanical, physical, and chemical properties can be created into polymeric biomaterials, which are adaptable organic materials. They are widely employed in biomedical applications, from scaffolds for tissue engineering and drug delivery systems to sutures and catheters. Polymers are categorized as either natural or synthetic based on their place of origin.

Natural polymers with inherent biocompatibility and biodegradability, including collagen and chitosan, come from biological sources. The primary structural protein in the extracellular matrix, collagen, finds extensive application in soft tissue repair, wound dressings, and as a scaffold for tissue regeneration. Because of its inherent bioactivity, it promotes cell adhesion and proliferation. Because of its superior hemostatic qualities, antibacterial activity, and biocompatibility, chitosan, which is derived from chitin, a polysaccharide present in crab shells is useful in medication delivery and wound healing systems. However, depending on the source, natural polymers might vary in purity, have limited mechanical strength, and even be immunogenic.

Advances in biodegradable biobased polymers including PLA, PHAs, and succinate-based systems have expanded their biomedical applications in sutures, implants, and drug delivery while addressing sustainability challenges through circular economy frameworks [19]. More consistent characteristics and tunability are provided by synthetic polymers like polyethylene (PE), polylactic acid (PLA), and polyethylene glycol (PEG). Because of its superior wear resistance and low coefficient of friction, polyethylene in particular, ultra-high molecular weight polyethylene, or UHMWPE is utilized in joint prosthesis. Biodegradable, polylactic acid (PLA) and its copolymers (PLGA) are utilized as medication carriers, fixation devices, and resorbable sutures. Because it is non-immunogenic and hydrophilic, polyethylene glycol (PEG) is frequently used in drug delivery formulations and hydrogels. Through copolymerization and chemical modification, synthetic polymers' flexibility enables customisation in terms of mechanical strength, surface functionality, and rate of degradation.

The main benefits of polymers are their processability, flexibility, and light weight; nevertheless, their drawbacks include the possibility of creeping, instability in breakdown, and the buildup of acidic byproducts in biodegradable forms. Current developments center on bioresorbable polymers intended for regulated therapeutic release and tissue regeneration, as well as smart polymers that react to stimuli (pH, temperature, and enzymes).

1.4.4 Composite Materials

Composite biomaterials are formed by combining two or more distinct material phases to achieve synergistic mechanical and biological properties unattainable by individual materials alone. Composites typically merge the pliability and manufacturability of polymers with the durability of metals or ceramics.

Fiber-reinforced polymer composites, in which glass or carbon fibers are incorporated in a polymer matrix to improve stiffness and fatigue resistance, are a typical example. In biomedical applications, hydroxyapatite–polymer composites provide scaffolds that are appropriate for bone regeneration by fusing the bioactivity of hydroxyapatite with the durability of biodegradable polymers. In a similar vein, ceramic–metal composites, or Cermets, combine enhanced toughness and wear resistance in dental and orthopedic applications.

By changing the type, volume percentage, and distribution of constituent phases, composites have the benefit of property tailoring, allowing for the adjustment of mechanical, biological, and degrading characteristics. This adaptability makes it possible to create scaffolds and implants tailored to each patient that replicate the hierarchical structure of natural tissues like bone, which is a naturally occurring mixture of hydroxyapatite and collagen. There are still issues with preserving biocompatibility throughout long-term implantation, minimizing interfacial delamination, and guaranteeing uniform phase distribution.

1.4.5 Key Material Properties

A variety of mechanical, thermal, chemical, and surface characteristics affect how well biomaterials function in vivo and how they interact with the physiological environment.

A biomaterial's capacity to tolerate physiological loads is determined by its mechanical characteristics, including strength, toughness, fatigue resistance, and modulus of elasticity. Materials for load-bearing implants must strike a balance between stiffness and flexibility to avoid stress shielding. On the other hand, elastomeric materials that can withstand deformation without experiencing mechanical failure are necessary for soft tissues.

For materials subjected to temperature changes during sterilization or operation, thermal characteristics such as thermal conductivity and expansion coefficient are essential. Microcracks and delamination are avoided by aligning the thermal expansion of implants with the surrounding tissues, particularly at ceramic–metal interactions.

Biocompatibility and endurance are influenced by chemical characteristics, including chemical stability, corrosion resistance, and rate of deterioration. While excessive polymer degradation can result in the buildup of acidic byproducts, corrosion of metallic implants might release ions that cause toxicity or irritation. For safe clinical performance, chemical inertness or regulated reactivity is therefore essential. Lastly, at the material–biological interface, surface characteristics such as charge, wettability, roughness, and chemical activity control protein adsorption, cell attachment, and immunological responses. To improve surface compatibility without changing bulk properties, surface modification procedures such coating deposition, plasma treatment, and functionalization with bioactive compounds are frequently used.

For biomaterials to be designed rationally and to be successful in clinical settings, it is crucial to comprehend their types and characteristics. Each of the biomaterials metal, ceramic, polymeric, and composite offers distinct benefits, and their ongoing development via sophisticated fabrication, nanotechnology, and biofunctionalization is influencing the development of the next wave of safer, more efficient biomedical devices [20, 21].

1.5 Mechanisms and Processes

Complex biological, chemical, and physical processes that control how materials behave inside the body and interact with surrounding tissues control how well biomaterials operate in therapeutic settings. For implants and gadgets to remain safe, functioning, and integrated over the long term, it is essential to comprehend these mechanisms. A biomaterial's behavior is influenced by its surface chemistry, degradation kinetics, and biological interface dynamics in addition to its bulk characteristics, such as composition or mechanical strength. The life cycle of a biomaterial in vivo is defined by three key processes: surface modification and sterilization, degradation and resorption, and biological interactions. These factors work together to determine the material's lifespan, biocompatibility, and ability to support functional replacement or healing.

1.5.1 Biological Interactions

When a biomaterial is implanted into the human body, the first and most immediate response occurs at the interface between the material's surface and biological fluids. This interface is dynamic and determines subsequent cellular and tissue-level reactions.

The first and most important thing that happens after implantation is protein adsorption. A biological layer that mediates future cell responses is formed when plasma proteins, including albumin, fibrinogen, fibronectin, and immunoglobulins, adsorb onto the material's surface in a matter of seconds. The surface energy, charge, topography, and hydrophilicity of the material influence the morphology and composition of the adsorbed protein layer. Hydrophobic surfaces tend to denature adsorbed proteins, exposing novel epitopes that may either promote or hinder immunological activation and cell adhesion.

The competitive displacement of proteins according to their concentration and affinity is known as the Vroman effect, and it is a well-established phenomenon that causes the adsorbed layer to dynamically remodel over time.

Cell adhesion proceeds after protein adsorption, mainly through the action of integrin receptors, which identify amino acid sequences in adsorbed extracellular matrix (ECM) proteins, such as the arginine–glycine–aspartic acid (RGD) motif found in vitronectin and fibronectin. Cellular behavior, including differentiation, apoptosis, and proliferation, is influenced by the quality and strength of this adhesion. For example, endothelial cell attachment on vascular grafts supports antithrombogenicity, whereas osteoblast adherence on titanium surfaces encourages bone formation. Fibrous encapsulation is a condition in which the body isolates the implant in a collagenous sheath, so rendering it inert and non-functional can result from materials that are unable to promote persistent cell attachment.

Immune regulation is another essential element of the host response. Implanted biomaterials are seen by the immune system as alien substances, which sets off a chain of inflammatory responses. To break down or change the implant surface, neutrophils and macrophages are first drawn to the area and release cytokines and reactive oxygen species. The development of multinucleated giant cells and fibrotic tissue surrounding the implant are hallmarks of a foreign body reaction (FBR), which can be brought on by chronic activation. By using immunomodulatory surface coatings (such as heparin, polyethylene glycol, or bioactive peptides) that lessen protein denaturation and macrophage activation, modern biomaterial design aims to regulate this immunological response. An important area of regenerative medicine is the developing discipline of immunoengineering, which seeks to create materials that actively direct immune cell behavior toward pro-healing phenotypes as opposed to chronic inflammation. The success or failure of an implant is determined by molecular-scale events that control the biological interactions between biomaterials and host tissues. A biocompatible substance must provide sustained cell adhesion, advantageous protein adsorption, and regulated immune responses that encourage healing and integration rather than rejection.

1.5.2 Degradation and Resorption

Both permanent and temporary implants' lifetime and functioning are largely determined by the basic processes of biomaterial breakdown and resorption. While uncontrolled degradation might jeopardize structural integrity, produce harmful byproducts, or cause inflammation, controlled degradation can be advantageous because it permits a steady transfer of mechanical strain to regenerated tissue.

The backbone bonds of polymeric biomaterials are frequently hydrolyzed or cleaved by enzymes. Water molecules enter the polymer matrix and break ester, amide or anhydride bonds during hydrolytic breakdown. Lactic and glycolic acids are produced by hydrolyzing common biodegradable polymers like polylactic acid (PLA), polyglycolic acid (PGA), and its copolymer PLGA. These acids are then degraded by natural metabolic pathways. Surface area, molecular weight, and polymer crystallinity are some of the variables that affect the rate of degradation. In contrast, enzymes such as lipases or proteases that target certain bonds mediate enzymatic breakdown; this mechanism is predominant in natural polymers including collagen, chitosan, and fibrin [22].

Corrosion, an electrochemical process that involves metal atom oxidation and reduction reactions in surrounding fluids, is the main mechanism of degradation in metallic biomaterials. For instance, titanium naturally generates a stable titanium dioxide (TiO_2) layer, which confers outstanding biostability, whereas cobalt-chromium alloys and stainless-steel form protective passive oxide layers that resist corrosion. However, these passive films can be broken down by micro-motion, pH changes, or chloride ions under physiological settings, which can result in ion release or localized corrosion. Surface coating or alloy optimization are necessary because corrosion products like nickel, chromium, or cobalt ions can cause cytotoxicity or allergic reactions. New corrosion-resistant materials like nitinol and tantalum are made to strike a balance between electrochemical stability and mechanical toughness.

Despite being mostly inert, ceramic biomaterials may dissolve or change phases based on their makeup. Bioactive ceramics, such as bioglass and hydroxyapatite (HA), are designed to partially dissolve in bodily fluids, releasing phosphate and calcium ions that promote osteogenesis. By creating a layer of hydroxycarbonate apatite, this regulated dissolution promotes chemical connection between the implant and bone. Alumina and zirconia, on the other hand, are bioinert ceramics that dissolve very little, guaranteeing long-term durability for load-bearing applications like joint replacements.

Biodegradable polymers and bioactive ceramics are the main examples of materials that can be biologically assimilated, or resorption. The best resorbable materials retain structural support until native tissue has fully matured by degrading at a rate that corresponds with tissue regeneration. The necessity for exact control through material chemistry and architecture is highlighted by the fact that misaligned degradation rates might result in chronic inflammation or early mechanical failure.

1.5.3 Sterilization and Surface Modification

A biomaterial's sterility and surface properties are also critical to its success because they have a direct impact on clinical performance and biocompatibility. Surfaces that are contaminated or not properly prepared may cause inflammation, infection, or inadequate tissue integration. Thus, surface modification and sterilization are crucial last stages in the processing of biomaterials.

The goal of sterilization methods is to get rid of microbiological contamination without changing the characteristics of the material. The most widely used of these are steam autoclaving, ethylene oxide (EtO) gas, and gamma irradiation. By shattering microbial DNA strands, gamma irradiation, which uses high-energy photons from cobalt-60, efficiently sterilizes metals and polymers. But too much exposure can weaken polymer chains, which lowers their mechanical strength. Low-temperature EtO sterilization works well for materials that are sensitive to heat, but it needs to be aerated to get rid of any harmful residues. For metals and ceramics, steam sterilization (autoclaving) offers dependable sterilization; however, it is not appropriate for temperature-sensitive polymers. For sensitive bioengineered structures, more sophisticated techniques such plasma sterilization with reactive oxygen or hydrogen peroxide species provide low-temperature options with little material modification.

Techniques for surface modification are used to customize a material's biological response without changing its bulk characteristics. These consist of surface coating, ion implantation, chemical etching, and plasma treatment. Functional groups (-OH, -COOH, -NH_2) are added to polymer surfaces by plasma treatment, which improves hydrophilicity and cell adhesion. Thin coatings of bioactive materials, including titanium nitride or hydroxyapatite, can be applied via physical vapor deposition (PVD) and chemical vapor deposition (CVD), which enhance osseointegration and corrosion resistance. Certain biochemical cues can be presented by peptide coatings and self-assembled monolayers (SAMs) to alter cell behavior and lower immune activation.

Nanostructured surface engineering, which mimics the extracellular matrix and influences stem cell development by optimizing surface topography and roughness at the nanoscale scale, is a rapidly expanding field of study. Like this, antimicrobial coatings that contain antibiotic-releasing polymers or silver nanoparticles are used to stop bacterial colonization, which is a leading cause of implant failure. Together, surface modification and sterilization mark the nexus of nanotechnology, microbiology, and materials science, allowing biomaterials to be tailored for certain biological processes and clinical settings.

Degradation dynamics, surface engineering techniques, and biological interactions are only a few of the intricately linked systems and processes that control the performance of biomaterials. Initial compatibility is determined by immune modulation and protein adsorption; lifetime and integration are governed by degradation and resorption; and safety and functionality are guaranteed by surface modification and sterilization. By controlling these processes, biomaterials have evolved from inert substitutes into intelligent, active systems that may regulate immune responses, promote tissue regeneration, and lower infection [23]. The future of biomaterials, as research progresses, rests in creating intelligent, adaptable materials that react dynamically to physiological stimuli, resulting in both structural restoration and functional harmony with the human body.

1.6 Design Considerations

A crucial stage in biomedical engineering is the design of biomaterials, which connects scientific advancement with practical application. To ensure their efficient and responsible usage in humans, it necessitates not only the optimization of material qualities but also adherence to safety, mechanical, ethical, and regulatory criteria. Throughout its service life or degradation period, a biomaterial must be structurally and chemically stable, function as intended, and blend in smoothly with the biological environment. As a result, the design process considers a number of factors, such as safety and biocompatibility, structural and mechanical compatibility, manufacturing and fabrication, and ethical and legal considerations. The total effectiveness and sustainability of biomaterials in medical applications are influenced by each parameter.

1.6.1 Biocompatibility and Safety

Since they establish whether a material can work well in interaction with live tissues without producing negative reactions, biocompatibility and safety are the cornerstones of biomaterial design. Beyond just not being hazardous, biocompatibility also refers to a material's capacity to trigger the right biological reactions at the cellular, tissue, and systemic levels. Contrarily, safety guarantees that the biomaterial and the byproducts of its breakdown do not cause negative side effects such immunological rejection, thrombosis, inflammation, or cancer.

Strict testing guidelines and evaluation techniques are necessary for determining biocompatibility, and many of these are outlined in global regulatory frameworks like the U.S. Food and Drug Administration (FDA) and the International Organization for Standardization (ISO). Comprehensive guidelines for the biological evaluation of medical devices are provided by the ISO 10993 series of standards, which provide a step-by-step procedure that includes testing for cytotoxicity, sensitization, irritation, systemic toxicity, genotoxicity, implantation, and hemocompatibility. While in vivo implantation studies assess tissue responses and integration, in vitro assays like hemolysis analysis and cell viability (MTT or Live/Dead tests) function as initial screening techniques.

Additionally, toxicological profiling and risk assessment are essential components of safety evaluation. To evaluate long-term impacts, materials meant for long-term implantation are subjected to analyses of chronic toxicity, carcinogenicity, and biodegradation products. Immunological tests and histopathological analysis aid in detecting fibrotic or inflammatory reactions at the material–tissue contact. Furthermore, improvements in computational modeling have made it possible to simulate host-material interactions and do predictive toxicology, which lessens the need for animal testing and speeds up design optimization.

To decrease immunological reactions and maximize biointegration, materials must be modified through surface treatment, coating, or chemical adjustment. This iterative design approach is ultimately necessary to achieve biocompatibility and safety.

1.6.2 Mechanical and Structural Compatibility

A biomaterial must be structurally and mechanically compatible with the tissue it is meant to support, replace, or interact with to function well. The mechanical properties of human tissues differ greatly; blood vessels are flexible and dynamic, cartilage is elastic and shock-absorbing, and bone is stiff and load bearing. To avoid failure or physiological imbalance, biomaterials must be made to replicate or enhance these tissue-specific mechanical characteristics.

In orthopedic and cardiovascular applications, matching tissue mechanics is especially important. For example, stress shielding in bone implants, where the implant carries most of the load, can result from a mismatch in the stiffness of the implant and the surrounding bone. This can promote bone resorption and implant loosening. In contrast to stainless steel or cobalt-chromium alloys, materials like titanium and its alloys are favored because their elastic modulus (about 100 GPa) is more like that of cortical bone (10–30 GPa). The viscoelastic and compressive characteristics of native cartilage must also be replicated by bioresorbable scaffolds used in cartilage repair to promote tissue remodeling and cell differentiation.

The biomaterial used in soft tissue engineering, such as cardiac patches or vascular grafts, must be able to withstand cyclic deformation and retain its flexibility without deteriorating or rupturing. Because of their compliance and fatigue resistance, polymeric materials such as polyurethane and poly (ethylene terephthalate) (PET) are frequently used. Furthermore, directional variation in mechanical characteristics, or anisotropy, is an important factor to consider, particularly in tissues that encounter multidirectional stresses like the heart and musculoskeletal system.

Porosity, surface topology, and microarchitecture are further components of biomaterial structural design that affect tissue ingrowth, nutrition delivery, and cell adhesion. For example, bone scaffolds interconnected porous networks promote vascularization and osteointegration. Finite element analysis (FEA) and other computational modeling techniques are being utilized more to optimize design prior to production and simulate mechanical performance. As a result, precise design and microstructural engineering that is adapted to the physiological environment produce mechanical and structural compatibility rather than only being a function of material composition.

1.6.3 Manufacturing and Fabrication

Advanced manufacturing and fabrication technologies that enable exact control of structure, content, and functioning are essential for converting biomaterial design concepts into useful medical devices or scaffolds. Among these, surface engineering, electrospinning, and 3D printing have become revolutionary methods for the manufacturing of contemporary biomaterials.

Using computer-aided design (CAD) models, 3D printing, sometimes referred to as additive manufacturing, allows complicated shapes to be built layer by layer. Unmatched personalization is possible with this method, enabling implants to be tailored to each patient's unique anatomical characteristics. Porous scaffolds with regulated architecture and mechanical characteristics can be produced using 3D printing from materials such hydroxyapatite composites, polycaprolactone (PCL), and titanium alloys. Furthermore, tissue and organ engineering is made easier by 3D bioprinting, which integrates bioinks and living cells into the creation process. Personalized therapy is made possible by 3D bioprinting, which places cells and biomaterials precisely.

Another essential method for creating nanofibrous scaffolds that resemble the extracellular matrix (ECM) of natural tissues is electrospinning. A polymer solution is drawn into ultrafine fibers by a high-voltage electric field in this technique, and the fibers are gathered into a porous mat. High surface area-to-volume ratios found in electrospun scaffolds facilitate medication delivery, nutrition transport, and cell adhesion. Collagen, poly (lactic-co-glycolic acid) (PLGA), and silk fibroin are materials that are frequently utilized for vascular grafts, nerve guiding, and skin regeneration. Electrospinning's versatility in creating composite fibers and adding bioactive compounds increases its usefulness in the construction of functional biomaterials.

Without changing the bulk qualities, surface engineering techniques enhance the biomaterials' topmost layer to increase biocompatibility and functionality. Methods such as plasma treatment, chemical etching, anodization, and thin-film deposition can tailor surface chemistry, topography, and wettability. Coating metallic implants with bioactive ceramics (e.g., hydroxyapatite) or polymeric films can enhance osseointegration and reduce corrosion. Functionalization with peptides, growth factors, or antimicrobial compounds, on the other hand, encourages cellular reactions or lowers the chance of infection.

When combined, these production techniques allow for exact control over the biological and physical properties of biomaterials. As 3D printing, nanotechnology, and biofabrication continue to advance design, next-generation biomaterials that are adaptable to biological environments, multipurpose, and customizable are made possible.

1.6.4 Ethical and Regulatory Aspects

Biomaterials must be incorporated into clinical practice in accordance with legal and ethical frameworks intended to guarantee patient safety, product dependability, and social responsibility. These frameworks cover both more general ethical concepts like informed consent, environmental sustainability, and fair access to biomedical innovations, as well as regulatory standards like those set forth by the FDA (U.S. Food and Drug Administration) and ISO (International Organization for Standardization).

Class I (low risk), Class II (moderate risk), and Class III (high risk) are the risk classifications used by the FDA to regulate biomaterials and medical devices. Before being approved for clinical use, each class must pass varying testing and documentation requirements. For example, in compliance with ISO 10993, Class III products, including heart valves or joint prostheses, must pass rigorous clinical studies and biocompatibility testing before obtaining premarket approval (PMA). In contrast, the ISO standards offer internationally standardized norms for environmental responsibility, quality control, and material testing in the production of biomaterials.

Beyond merely adhering to regulations, ethical issues also include respecting patient autonomy, being open and honest about clinical trials, and using developing technologies responsibly. By ensuring that patients are aware of the possible dangers and advantages of getting implants or experimental biomaterials, informed consent helps to preserve public confidence in biomedical research and healthcare delivery. In order to ensure that the values of beneficence, justice, and non-maleficence are followed when doing research utilizing innovative biomaterials, ethical review boards are essential.

Sustainability is an increasingly important aspect of biomaterial ethics. Environmental effects result from the manufacture and disposal of medical products, particularly given the growing use of metals and synthetic polymers. Energy-efficient manufacturing techniques and components that are recyclable, non-toxic, and biodegradable are key components of sustainable biomaterial design. In biomedical innovation, the idea of a circular bioeconomy where materials are made for reuse and have little effect on the environment is becoming increasingly popular.

The long-term sustainability of biomaterial technologies depends on striking a balance between ethical responsibility, environmental stewardship, and regulatory compliance. Innovation is ensured to develop responsibly by an open and accountable design framework, which synchronizes scientific advancement with ecological sustainability and public trust.

A comprehensive grasp of the biological, mechanical, technological, and ethical aspects is necessary for the design of biomaterials. Advanced fabrication techniques convert design thoughts into practical solutions, mechanical and structural compatibility offer functional stability, and biocompatibility and safety guarantee physiological harmony. In the meantime, patient welfare is protected, and sustainability is encouraged by ethical and regulatory control. Integrating these design concerns will be essential as biomedical technologies advance to create biomaterials that are safe, effective, and morally and environmentally acceptable [24].

1.7 Applications and Case Studies

The applications of biomaterials span nearly every branch of medicine, reflecting their capacity to restore structure, function, and biological activity within the human body. Over the past century, advances in material science, engineering, and biotechnology have enabled biomaterials to evolve from inert mechanical supports into dynamic, bioactive, and multifunctional systems. These materials are now integral to orthopedic, cardiovascular, dental, regenerative, and pharmaceutical innovations, improving millions of lives worldwide. This section explores key clinical applications and case studies that highlight the transformative impact of biomaterials in modern healthcare.

1.7.1 Orthopedic Implants

With joint replacements, bone transplants, and fixation devices intended to restore mobility and structural integrity, orthopedics continues to be the largest and most well-established application of biomaterials. Among the most effective biomedical procedures of the twentieth century were joint replacements, especially those for the hip and knee. Industry standards now include materials like ultra-high molecular weight polyethylene (UHMWPE), cobalt-chromium (Co-Cr) alloys, and titanium alloys. Because of its corrosion resistance, biocompatibility, and modulus of elasticity that is like that of natural bone which reduces stress shielding titanium and its alloys are preferred. Because of its low friction coefficient, UHMWPE is used as the bearing material in joint prosthesis, whereas Co-Cr alloys offer greater wear resistance in articulating surfaces.

The Charnley hip replacement, which was originally used in the 1960s and involved a polyethylene acetabular cup, a PMMA bone cement interface, and a stainless steel femoral stem, is a prime example of a case study. This tri-material approach laid the groundwork for contemporary prosthetic design by significantly lowering postoperative pain and restoring function in arthritic patients. Both natural and artificial bone grafts are utilized to encourage bone growth in areas of damage or deformity. Bioactive ceramics like hydroxyapatite (HA), tricalcium phosphate (TCP), and bioglass are synthetic alternatives that fuse with bone by forming a layer of hydroxycarbonate apatite. Osteoconductivity and mechanical robustness are further improved by composite scaffolds that combine HA with biodegradable polymers like PLGA.

Although titanium or stainless steel are commonly used to make fixation devices like screws, plates, and rods, more recent developments have focused on biodegradable substitutes such magnesium alloys and polymer composites. After healing, these materials progressively resorb, minimizing long-term consequences and removing the need for subsequent removal operations.

1.7.2 Cardiovascular Devices

Cardiovascular biomaterials have revolutionized the management of heart and vascular diseases through stents, artificial heart valves, and vascular grafts. Each application demands materials that balance mechanical durability, hemocompatibility, and biofunctionality.

316 L stainless steel, cobalt-chromium alloys, or nitinol (nickel–titanium shape-memory alloy) are frequently used to create stents, which are tiny tubular scaffolds used to preserve vessel patency. These metals offer the flexibility and radial strength needed for vascular deployment. But bare-metal stents frequently cause neointimal hyperplasia, which results in restenosis. Drug-eluting stents (DES), which have polymer coatings that gradually release antiproliferative medications like paclitaxel

or sirolimus, were created to solve this issue. By preventing the growth of smooth muscle cells, this regulated release lowers restenosis rates by more than 70%. Recent studies investigate bioresorbable stents composed of poly-L-lactic acid (PLLA), which dissolve as the vessel remodels and restores normal vasomotion.

Another significant development in cardiovascular biomaterials is artificial heart valves. Titanium and pyrolytic carbon mechanical valves are incredibly durable, although they need lifetime anticoagulation treatment. On the other hand, bioprosthetic valves made from pig or cow tissue and treated with glutaraldehyde offer improved hemodynamics and decreased thrombogenicity, but they deteriorate with time because of calcification. Using flexible materials such expanded PTFE or polyurethane, polymeric heart valve innovations seek to combine the biocompatibility of biological tissues with the mechanical strength of synthetic valves [25].

Expanded polytetrafluoroethylene (ePTFE) and polyethylene terephthalate (Dacron) are essential components of vascular grafts, which are used to replace or circumvent damaged arteries. These artificial polymers give large-diameter arteries the tensile strength and thrombosis resistance they require. However, endothelialized graft biomaterial scaffolds seeded with endothelial cells to reproduce natural vascular linings are being researched because of their poor efficacy in small-diameter grafts (<6 mm) due to clot formation. Nanofiber electrospun grafts, which imitate the extracellular matrix and improve endothelial cell adhesion, are also highlighted in recent research as having potential for next-generation vascular repair.

1.7.3 Dental and Craniofacial Applications

In dental and craniofacial reconstruction, biomaterials are essential because they restore biomechanics, function, and aesthetics. Applications include tissue scaffolds for maxillofacial repair, dental implants, and restorative materials. To support a prosthetic crown, dental implants usually consist of a titanium or titanium alloy screw that is placed into the jawbone. The formation of a persistent titanium oxide layer by titanium promotes osseointegration, which enables direct bone-implant connection without fibrous encapsulation. Surface treatments like plasma spraying, acid etching, or sandblasting improve bone-implant contact and speed up the healing process. One of the most dependable procedures in restorative dentistry is the use of titanium dental implants, which have a success rate of 95%.

Materials such as glass ionomer cements, composite resins, and ceramics are utilized for crowns and fillings in dental restorations. Composite resins provide great wear resistance and beautiful translucency since they are made of a polymer matrix supplemented with glass or silica fillers. Dental ceramics that closely resemble natural enamel, such zirconia and alumina, offer exceptional strength and stability in color.

Bioresorbable scaffolds made of collagen-hydroxyapatite composites or polycaprolactone (PCL) are used in craniofacial reconstruction to restore bone following damage or tumor excision. Successful bone growth and defect closure are demonstrated in case studies of orbital floor and mandibular restorations using 3D-printed PCL scaffolds seeded with stem cells, minimizing the requirement for autologous transplants. These developments demonstrate how biomaterials combine regenerative potential and functional restoration intricate craniofacial architecture.

1.7.4 Tissue Engineering and Regenerative Medicine

Tissue engineering represents the convergence of biomaterials, cellular biology, and bioactive signaling, aiming to regenerate functional tissues and organs rather than merely replacing them. Central to this field are scaffolds, which provide structural and biochemical cues for cell attachment, proliferation, and differentiation.

Usually, scaffolds are made of natural biopolymers (collagen, gelatin, alginate, and chitosan) or biodegradable polymers (PLA, PGA, and PCL). By imitating the extracellular matrix (ECM), these materials provide bioactive signals in addition to mechanical support. Two important factors that affect nutrition delivery and cell infiltration are porosity and surface chemistry. The construction of scaffolds and their rates of degradation can be precisely controlled thanks to methods like 3D printing, electrospinning, and freeze-drying.

Collagen and hydroxyapatite composites aid in the osteogenic differentiation of mesenchymal stem cells in bone tissue engineering, which promotes bone regeneration in non-union fractures and deformities. Hydrogels composed of hyaluronic acid and PEG give cartilage restoration the elasticity required to resemble natural cartilage, while bilayered scaffolds containing fibroblasts and keratinocytes are utilized to heal severe burns in skin regeneration. One noteworthy example is the bioengineered trachea, in which patient-derived stem cells were used to seed a decellularized scaffold, which was then successfully implanted to restore airway function. Similarly, studies on bioartificial liver and pancreas constructs seek to produce functional tissue with the ability to regulate metabolism, demonstrating the enormous promise of regenerative medicine based on biomaterials to treat chronic illnesses and organ shortages.

1.7.5 Drug Delivery Systems

Beyond structural repair, biomaterials play a pivotal role in drug delivery, offering platforms for controlled, localized, and sustained therapeutic release. The goal is to optimize drug bioavailability while minimizing systemic side effects.

Therapeutic compounds are encapsulated in controlled release matrices, which are composed of biodegradable polymers like PCL, PEG, and PLGA. The chemicals are released gradually by polymer degradation and diffusion. Applications for these systems include hormone therapy (e.g., Lupron Depot®) and chemotherapy (e.g., Gliadel® wafers releasing carmustine). Systems based on nanoparticles provide targeted drug delivery at the molecular or cellular level. It is possible to create lipid nanoparticles (LNPs) and polymeric nanoparticles to deliver medications to certain organs while overcoming biological barriers like the blood–brain barrier. PEGylated liposomes, such as Doxil®, have greatly enhanced the pharmacokinetics and decreased the toxicity of chemotherapeutic drugs in oncology. Precision medicine techniques are improved by the active targeting of sick cells made possible by functionalized nanoparticles containing ligands or antibodies.

Another adaptable medium for the transport of drugs and cells is hydrogel. They can encapsulate cells or biomolecules for on-demand release because of their high-water content and adjustable crosslinking. Angiogenesis and bone regeneration have been shown to be effectively promoted by injectable hydrogels loaded with growth factors like bone morphogenetic protein-2 (BMP-2) or vascular endothelial growth factor (VEGF). Furthermore, dynamic and adaptable therapeutic administration is made possible by stimuli-responsive hydrogels, which change their structure in response to pH, temperature, or enzymes.

Biomaterials are the cornerstone of contemporary biomedicine, from orthopaedic implants that restore mobility to nanoparticle carriers that deliver life-saving medications. Their uses demonstrate a range of biological, chemical, and mechanical capabilities designed to work in harmony with living systems. In the fields of orthopedics, cardiovascular therapy, dentistry, regenerative medicine, and pharmacology, clinical case studies highlight how customized biomaterials have transformed patient outcomes [26]. A new era of personalized healthcare is promised by the integration of bioactive, intelligent, and patient-specific biomaterials as innovative advances. In this era, materials will actively contribute to cellular healing, communication, and regeneration rather than just replacing damaged tissue.

1.8 Recent Advances and Innovations

Beyond its initial emphasis on inert materials intended only for structural replacement, biomaterials science has advanced significantly. The creation of intelligent, responsive, and biomimetic systems that dynamically interact with biological environments is what defines the field in the current day. Advances in materials science, nanotechnology, bioengineering, and computer modeling are driving these developments, which are coming together to produce materials that can sense, adapt, regenerate, and even communicate with cells and tissues. Biofabrication and 3D bioprinting, nanobiomaterials and biointerfaces, bioinspired and sustainable biomaterials, and smart and responsive biomaterials are the most revolutionary fields. Every one of these fields helps to develop biological systems of the future that are more precise, functional, and environmentally conscious.

1.8.1 Smart and Responsive Biomaterials

Smart and responsive biomaterials represent a paradigm shift from passive medical materials toward adaptive systems that respond intelligently to environmental cues. These materials can sense changes in pH, temperature, ionic strength, mechanical stress, or biochemical signals, and subsequently alter their physical or chemical properties to produce a desired therapeutic effect. The convergence of smart and biodegradable polymer technologies has produced bioresponsive and transient biomedical devices including shape-memory stents, pH-sensitive hydrogels, and cardiovascular occluders that combine stimuli-responsiveness with controlled degradation to meet the evolving demands of regenerative medicine [27].

A significant subset of this class consists of stimuli-responsive polymers, also known as "smart polymers." In reaction to stimuli, these materials experience reversible changes, such as swelling, sol-gel transitions, or deterioration. For example, temperature-sensitive polymers such as poly(N-isopropylacrylamide) (PNIPAAm) have a lower critical solution temperature (LCST) that is close to body temperature, which allows for on-demand tissue adherence or regulated drug release. Similarly, to improve site-specific treatment efficacy, pH-responsive hydrogels are made to release medications in reaction to inflammatory tissues or acidic tumor microenvironments.

The creation of biomaterials that can cure themselves, motivated by biological repair processes, is another developing field. The durability and dependability of implants or scaffolds can be increased by these materials' ability to self-repair their integrity following mechanical damage. Dynamic covalent connections (like disulfide, imine, or Diels-Alder linkages) or supramolecular interactions (like hydrogen bonding and metal–ligand coordination) are frequently the basis of self-healing mechanisms. Hydrogels with reversible crosslinking networks, for instance, can self-heal by following a fracture, which qualifies them for use in soft tissue healing, wound dressings, and cartilage regeneration. Smart biomaterials have demonstrated breakthroughs across tissue engineering, immunomodulation, patient-specific therapies, and biosensor applications, representing a transition from inert to actively responsive biomedical materials [28].

Biosensing technologies are also being used with smart materials to produce therapeutic systems that are controlled by feedback. Shape-memory polymers that alter their structure in response to physiological changes for minimally invasive administration are two examples, as are glucose-responsive insulin delivery systems that only release insulin when blood glucose levels surpass a certain threshold. These developments represent the trend in biomaterials toward functional intelligence, in which materials actively contribute to the regulation of biological processes in addition to supporting them. A comprehensive synthesis of these advances, including stimuli-responsive hydrogels and their classification by stimulus type, tissue application, and response mechanism, has recently been published [29].

1.8.2 Nanobiomaterials and Biointerfaces

The scale and accuracy of the interaction between biomaterials and tissues have been redefined by nanobiomaterials. Materials can imitate the extracellular matrix's (ECM) structure at the nanoscale (1–100 nm), affecting biological functions as adhesion, proliferation, and differentiation. Improved biointerfaces that provide regulated interaction between synthetic materials and biological systems have been made possible by the combination of nanotechnology and biomaterials [30].

By adjusting cellular reactions and protein adsorption, nanoscale surface changes enhance biointegration. For instance, when compared to traditional micro-textured surfaces, titanium implants with nanostructured oxide layers exhibit better osteoblast adhesion and quicker bone growth. Similarly, via improving cellular signaling, nanorough surfaces on polymeric scaffolds encourage angiogenesis and brain regeneration.

Additionally, tailored medicine and gene delivery is facilitated by nanobiomaterials. Therapeutic compounds can be encapsulated in nanoparticles consisting of lipids, biodegradable polymers (like PLGA and PEG), or inorganic materials (like silica, gold, and iron oxide) and released at precise locations in response to physiological or external stimuli. Nanoparticles' high surface area-to-volume ratio makes it easier for them to conjugate with peptides, antibodies, or targeting ligands, enabling targeted delivery to sick tissues like tumors or inflammatory organs.

Furthermore, hybrids that include nanoparticles into polymeric or ceramic matrices, known as nanocomposite biomaterials, combine improved biological function with mechanical strength. For example, because of their structural resemblance to real bone mineral, hydroxyapatite–polymer nanocomposites enhance bone regeneration. Because of their electrical conductivity, mechanical reinforcement, and capacity to connect with neural tissues, carbon-based nanomaterials like graphene and carbon nanotubes are also becoming increasingly well-known.

The goal of recent developments in biointerface engineering is to create surfaces that actively interact with cells. Certain cellular actions are guided by functional coatings that contain growth hormones, extracellular vesicles, or peptides (such as RGD sequences). By focusing immune responses on tissue repair rather than inflammation, the newly developed idea of "immuno-instructive materials" expands the utility of nanobiomaterials. To achieve smooth, molecular-level integration between artificial structures and live systems, nanobiomaterials and designed biointerfaces are therefore essential.

1.8.3 Biofabrication and 3D Bioprinting

The field of biomaterials has undergone a revolution with the introduction of biofabrication and 3D bioprinting technologies, which allow for the incredibly precise construction of intricate, patient-specific tissues and organs. In contrast to conventional scaffold production, bioprinting replicates native tissue architecture by enabling the digitally controlled layer-by-layer deposition of cells, biomaterials, and bioactive compounds. Depending on the requirements for viscosity, resolution, and cell viability, 3D bioprinting techniques can be divided into extrusion-based, inkjet-based, and laser-assisted approaches, each of which offers unique benefits. The most popular method, extrusion bioprinting, uses hydrogel-based bioinks to encapsulate living cells in biocompatible matrices like collagen, alginate, or gelatin methacrylate (GelMA). After printing, these bioinks can be crosslinked to create stable three-dimensional structures that promote cell division and growth.

To replicate the variety of biological tissues, recent innovations have concentrated on multi-material and multi-cellular printing, which entails the deposition of many cell types and biomaterials in spatially designated regions. Co-printing endothelial cells and supporting matrices generates vascularized constructs, enabling the formation of perfusable microvasculature essential for tissue viability. 4D bioprinting, an advancement of 3D printing, incorporates time as a dimension, allowing things to change in composition, shape, or function in reaction to external stimuli. This invention possesses potential applications in self-assembling tissue constructs and dynamic implants.

To increase accuracy and repeatability, biofabrication systems also incorporate computational modeling and real-time imaging. The quality of printed tissues is improved by using digital twins, which are virtual representations of biological features that direct print routes and material distribution. Applications of 3D bioprinting include drug screening, illness modeling, and regenerative medicine (e.g., cartilage, bone, skin, and heart tissues). Drug discovery is accelerated and customized medicine is made possible by bioprinted tissue models, which offer morally sound and physiologically relevant substitutes for animal experimentation. Recent innovations in 3D bioactive scaffold design incorporating multiscale porosity, oxygen-generating nanoparticles, and multi-material co-printing have significantly advanced vascularization and functional organ fabrication for regenerative medicine and transdermal therapeutics [31].

The combination of biofabrication technologies with smart and nanostructured materials is propelling the field toward fully functional, implantable tissues that can integrate, remodel, and regenerate within the human body.

1.8.4 Bioinspired and Sustainable Biomaterials

Modern biomaterial innovation increasingly draws inspiration from nature's design strategies giving rise to bioinspired and sustainable materials that emulate the structure, function, and adaptability of biological systems. These biomaterials not only enhance performance but also address environmental and ethical challenges associated with synthetic materials and medical waste. The application of bio-based and biodegradable green polymers in medical devices and packaging is reshaping the biomedical sector toward a more sustainable, circular economy, with biodegradability and bioconversion emerging as central design criteria [32].

Replicating dynamic qualities, hierarchical structure, and natural architectures of living things is the goal of biomimetic design. For load-bearing implants, for example, nacre-inspired composites combine toughness and lightness to mimic the "brick-and-mortar" structure of seashells. Similarly, to create strong, moist adherence for wound closure and surgical applications, mussel-inspired adhesives employ chemistries based on catechols. For use in neurological, ophthalmic, and cardiovascular applications, hydrogels that replicate the viscoelastic characteristics of soft tissues are being created to give cells a realistic mechanical and biochemical environment.

Simultaneously, environmentally sustainable biomaterials are developed using green chemistry concepts. Energy-efficient procedures, biodegradable polymers, renewable resources, and non-toxic solvents are all highlighted in this strategy. Natural polymers including cellulose, silk fibroin, alginate, and chitosan are becoming more popular as environmentally friendly substitutes for plastics made from petroleum. These biopolymers can be chemically modified to adjust their functionality and are naturally biocompatible and biodegradable.

To reduce the environmental impact, medical polymers and device components should be recycled and upcycled. Closed-loop systems that collect and reuse solvents, water, and byproducts are being used more in biomanufacturing processes. Furthermore, to make sure that biomedical innovation is in line with international sustainability standards, life-cycle assessment (LCA) technologies are being used to assess the environmental impact of biomaterials from synthesis to disposal.

Combining sustainability and biomimicry is not just a technological breakthrough but also a moral requirement. It represents an increasing understanding that to support the circular bioeconomy and the long-term health of the earth, biomedical materials of the future must be both highly effective and ecologically conscious.

Biomedical engineering is changing from passive support systems to active, intelligent, and sustainable technologies due to recent developments and advancements in biomaterials [33]. Biofabrication makes it possible to create living tissues with anatomical accuracy; nanobiomaterials improve biointegration and therapeutic precision; bioinspired, sustainable designs balance medical advancement with environmental stewardship; and smart and responsive materials bring flexibility and self-regulation. When taken as a whole, these developments herald the emergence of a new class of biomaterials that not only renew and restore life but also work in harmony with the laws of nature.

1.9 Challenges and Limitations

Biomaterial research has made tremendous strides, but several obstacles still stand in the way of its broad and sustained clinical success. When biomaterials interact with extremely complicated biological systems, even slight changes in their chemistry, structure, or mechanical properties can have negative effects like rejection, failure, or inflammation. Additionally, there are significant manufacturing, legal, ethical, and financial obstacles in the way of a medical device's transition from laboratory innovation to market readiness. A interdisciplinary strategy combining material science, immunology, engineering, ethical, and sustainability principles is needed to address these issues.

1.9.1 Biocompatibility and Immune Reactions

Although it is one of the most enduring and complex issues, biocompatibility continues to be the key to the success of biomaterials. Inflammation, infection, or immune-mediated rejection are examples of negative local or systemic effects that a biomaterial must avoid in order to fulfill its intended purpose. When a foreign substance enters the body, it sets off a series of biological reactions that include immunological modulation, cell activation, and protein adsorption [34]. If left unchecked, these reactions may result in implant failure or material encapsulation.

When the immune system views the biomaterial as alien, inflammatory responses take place. Pro-inflammatory cytokines and reactive oxygen species are released after neutrophils, macrophages, and lymphocytes are first recruited. Chronic inflammation may result in tissue necrosis, fibrosis, or sustained inflammation surrounding the implant. This often results in chronic complications associated with orthopedic implants and vascular grafts.

The foreign body reaction (FBR), which is a prominent example of an unfavorable immune response, is typified by the development of multinucleated giant cells and a fibrotic capsule that separates the implant from the surrounding tissue. Although this might shield the body from foreign objects, it hinders the integration of functional implants, which lowers their lifespan and performance. For example, fibrous encapsulation of brain electrodes reduces signal transmission, and encapsulation of glucose sensors in diabetic patients might impede accurate monitoring.

In hybrid or tissue-engineered structures with biological components, rejection is especially important. Minor contaminants or results of scaffold breakdown can cause immunological sensitization even when autologous cells are used. Surface modification using inert polymers like polyethylene glycol (PEG) or biofunctional coatings that release anti-inflammatory chemicals or foster immunological tolerance are two ways to lessen these effects. Complete immunological acceptance is still an open question, though, particularly for regenerative materials and long-term implants.

Biocompatibility evaluations are further complicated by individual variability, which results from genetic variables, pre-existing diseases, and microbiota composition. In one patient, something that is stable and non-toxic could trigger hypersensitivity or deterioration in another. Personalized methods to biomaterial design are becoming essential for tailoring surface chemistry and degradation profiles to the specific physiological conditions of the patient.

1.9.2 Mechanical and Structural Failures

The mechanical and chemical strains of the physiological environment can cause even the most biocompatible materials to fail. A significant drawback is mechanical failure, which includes wear, corrosion, fatigue, and fracture. This is especially true for load-bearing applications like orthopedic and cardiovascular implants. Repetitive cyclic loading causes fatigue failure, which eventually results in microcracks and fracture. Micro-motion at the bone–implant interface and manufacturing flaws in the material aggravate fatigue in metallic implants, such as hip prosthesis. Early models of cobalt-chromium and stainless steel implants, for example, experienced fatigue-related fractures when subjected to prolonged physiological stresses.

Structural integrity is further jeopardized by corrosion and deterioration. When metals meet electrolytic bodily fluids, they oxidize and release ions that may cause allergic reactions or be cytotoxic. Under stress or mechanical wear, titanium's stable oxide layer that protects against corrosion may disintegrate, resulting in fretting corrosion. Similar to this, polymeric materials deteriorate over time due to oxidation or hydrolysis, losing strength and developing erratic mechanical behavior.

Another important problem is wearing debris. Micro-sized metal or polyethylene particles produced by frictional wear in joint replacements can cause osteolysis, a bone-resorption process that causes implant failure and loosening. This occurrence highlights the need for wear-resistant materials or sophisticated surface coatings, like diamond-like carbon or ceramic composites, and needs expensive revision surgeries.

Structural instability during deterioration poses additional challenges for tissue-engineered products. Although early deterioration might result in collapse or non-union, biodegradable scaffolds must continue to provide mechanical support until the host tissue regenerates enough. On the other hand, excessively sluggish breakdown may impede the natural remodeling of tissue. When designing resorbable biomaterials, striking the ideal balance between mechanical strength and degradation kinetics is still a difficult task.

1.9.3 Manufacturing and Cost Barriers

There are significant manufacturing and financial obstacles in moving biomaterials from research to clinical use. Scalability frequently proves challenging without sacrificing quality, repeatability, or safety, even when laboratory-scale synthesis may show promising qualities. Strict standards for cleanliness, sterility, and structural accuracy lead to manufacturing complexity. Advanced biomaterial synthesis requires specialized tools and carefully regulated conditions, especially for nano-structured surfaces, smart polymers, and hybrid composites. Clinical dependability may be impacted by irregularities resulting from variations in the sourcing of raw materials, batch processing, and sterilization. Development schedules and expenses are further prolonged by regulatory bodies like the European Medicines Agency (EMA) and the U.S. Food and Drug Administration (FDA), which set stringent testing and documentation requirements for validation and approval.

Cost obstacles are substantial, particularly for nations with low and moderate incomes. Costly raw materials (like titanium or bioactive ceramics), advanced manufacturing techniques (like 3D printing or atomic-layer deposition), and stringent clinical studies are all necessary for the creation and upkeep of biomaterial implants. High-performance implants are frequently only available to more affluent healthcare systems due to these financial constraints. Custom 3D-printed bone scaffolds and bioresorbable stents, for instance, are scientific advances, but widespread clinical acceptance is hampered by their high production costs.

Tissue engineering and regenerative medicine are equally impacted by scalability concerns. Bioreactor systems are expensive and resource-intensive for preserving sterility over extended periods of time, cultivating huge numbers of cells, and guaranteeing consistent seeding within scaffolds. Furthermore, preserving reproducibility between biological construct batches continues to be a significant technical and legal problem. Green chemical techniques, which lessen waste and the environmental impact, and additive manufacturing (3D printing), which provides cost-effective prototype and customized design, are the main focuses of efforts to address these issues. However, creating an egalitarian and sustainable biomaterials production pipeline is still a long-term objective that calls for international policy coordination and industry-academia cooperation.

1.9.4 Ethical, Environmental, and Regulatory Constraints

Beyond technical challenges, the development and application of biomaterials raise important ethical, environmental, and regulatory issues that influence research, approval, and post-market surveillance.

Patient safety, informed consent, and the use of synthetic or biological materials in human systems are the main ethical concerns [35]. Human testing of new biomaterials entails weighing the unknown long-term dangers against any potential therapeutic benefits. To ensure respect for autonomy, beneficence, and justice, clinical trials must abide by ethical frameworks like the Belmont Report and the Declaration of Helsinki. The use of stem cells, particularly those from embryonic sources, in tissue engineering continues to raise ethical questions about permission and the morality of biological resources.

The speed at which biomaterials are being developed exacerbates regulatory challenges. Approval procedures become unclear when hybrid devices that include synthetic and biological components fall into one of the existing regulatory categories. Guidelines must be updated frequently by regulatory bodies to consider new materials like gene-activated scaffolds and nanocomposites. Even materials that are initially thought to be biocompatible may have late-stage problems like carcinogenicity, immunogenicity, or environmental toxicity as they degrade, therefore long-term safety monitoring is equally important.

In the assessment of biomaterials, environmental sustainability has become a new frontier. Non-biodegradable medical disposables add to environmental contamination, and the manufacturing of metals and polymers uses a lot of energy and produces waste. Furthermore, some sterilizing techniques, like the use of ethylene oxide gas, leave behind hazardous residues that have an impact on the environment. Green biomaterials, which are made from renewable resources and processed with eco-friendly methods, are becoming increasingly important as the healthcare sector works toward sustainability to lessen the environmental impact of biomedical manufacturing.

Additionally, fair access and data transparency provide new moral and legal issues. Control of expensive biomaterial technology by a private company has the risk of making healthcare disparities worse, especially in underdeveloped nations. Policymakers support fair pricing mechanisms, open innovation frameworks, and technology transfer partnerships that democratize access to life-saving biomaterial advances to ensure global health parity.

At the nexus of science, ethics, and society is the field of biomaterials. Even with remarkable advancements, there are still major obstacles in the way of perfect biocompatibility, mechanical dependability, production scalability, and ethical accountability. The long-term success of implants and devices is still constrained by inflammation, structural failure, and cost limitations, but new environmental and regulatory demands call for more transparent and sustainable innovation routes. Creating biomaterials that are adaptable, patient-specific, and ecologically conscious under strict ethical supervision and international cooperation will be essential to future advancement. Resolving these issues not only guarantees safer and more efficient medical procedures, but it also reaffirms biomedical science's ethical and environmental obligation to improve human health.

1.10 Future Directions

Biomaterials are about to enter a revolutionary phase that is defined by sustainability, personalization, and technology convergence. The next generation of biomaterials will be intelligent, adaptable, data-informed, and environmentally conscious, going beyond the conventional emphasis on mechanical performance and biocompatibility. Advances in regenerative medicine, artificial intelligence (AI), computational modeling, and systems-level cooperation among scientists, engineers, and clinicians are what are propelling this development. Furthermore, the design, production, and application of biomaterials are changing because of global imperatives including resource conservation and sustainable development. This outlines four major trajectories defining the future of biomaterials: integration of artificial intelligence and predictive modeling, personalized and regenerative approaches, cross-disciplinary and global collaboration, and sustainability through circular bio-economy frameworks.

1.10.1 Integration of Artificial Intelligence and Predictive Modeling

One of the most exciting areas in biomaterials research is the combination of predictive modeling and artificial intelligence (AI). AI-powered technologies are transforming the design, characterization, and optimization of materials and making it possible to quickly find new biomaterials with specialized qualities. Biomaterial development has historically depended on laborious experimental iterations. However, researchers can now simulate intricate biological-material interactions and forecast performance outcomes prior to physical testing because of the development of machine learning (ML), computer simulations, and data-driven design [36].

Large datasets from material chemistry, structure, and biological response can be processed by machine learning algorithms to find hidden correlations between variables. For instance, ML models can forecast the effects of minute modifications to surface shape or polymer composition on immunological compatibility, cell attachment, or protein adsorption. Researchers can create materials with regulated degradation rates or targeted biocompatibility that are best suited for medicinal applications because of their predictive capabilities.

Furthermore, multiscale modeling, which combines computational fluid dynamics (CFD), molecular dynamics (MD), and finite element analysis (FEA), sheds light on the behavior of biomaterials at many length scales, ranging from molecular interactions to organ-level performance. Given the simultaneous interaction of mechanical, chemical, and biological elements in implanted devices, this feature is very beneficial. Predictive modeling, for example, can describe the behavior of bone-implant interfaces under cyclic loading, predicting the dynamics of fatigue, corrosion, or tissue remodeling.

AI is also being utilized to create "digital twins," which are virtual versions of biological tissues or biomaterials that change in real time based on clinical or experimental data. Based on patient-specific information, these digital twins enable ongoing adjustment of scaffold construction, drug delivery kinetics, or implant design. Furthermore, AI systems can facilitate precision biomaterial design, the process of creating materials that are customized to each person's unique genetic or physiological profile by combining omics data (genomics, proteomics, and metabolomics) with material performance metrics. An AI-driven closed-loop framework integrating reverse material design, ML-based property prediction, and biological response forecasting has recently been proposed to systematically accelerate biomaterial translation from computational design to clinical application [37].

Autonomous labs with robotic synthesis equipment controlled by AI algorithms will soon speed up the discovery of biomaterials and lower experimental errors. By replicating long-term safety and performance, predictive modeling will help improve regulatory evaluation and reduce the need for extensive testing on humans or animals. Finally, a paradigm shifts toward computationally intelligent materials where design, synthesis, and validation create an integrated digital ecosystem is embodied by AI-guided biomaterials research. The integration of AI with smart biomaterial design including ML-guided discovery, synthesis automation, and property prediction has been reviewed with particular focus on bridging experimental and computational workflows [38].

1.10.2 Personalized and Regenerative Approaches

Next-generation biomedical solutions are increasingly built on the twin pillars of personalization and regeneration. The way biomaterials are conceived and applied in therapeutic settings is changing because of the combination of biological self-repair processes, sophisticated manufacturing, and patient-specific data. Utilizing patient-derived information, including genetic, biomechanical, and imaging profiles, personalized biomaterials create scaffolds or implants that correspond to unique anatomical and physiological traits. Custom implants that fit patient-specific geometries can be precisely fabricated thanks to additive manufacturing technologies, especially 3D and 4D printing. For instance, titanium or bioceramic composites can be used to print cranial or maxillofacial implants using CT scan data, guaranteeing a precise anatomical fit and enhanced integration.

By adding time-dependent modifications, 4D biomaterials increase the potential of conventional 3D structures. When exposed to stimuli like light, temperature, or biological signals, these materials can alter their stiffness, shape, or functionality. 4D scaffolds in regenerative medicine enable smooth integration and repair by dynamically adjusting to tissue growth or physiological stress. For example, pH-sensitive hydrogels can release medications in reaction to inflammatory conditions, while shape-memory polymers can expand after implantation to fill uneven flaws.

Regenerative biomaterials, on the other hand, are made to promote natural regeneration through biological signals rather than just replacing damaged tissues. To encourage angiogenesis, osteogenesis, or neurogenesis, these materials frequently contain bioactive compounds, growth factors, or stem cells. To direct tissue-specific differentiation and remodeling, hybrid scaffolds which blend artificial frameworks with naturally occurring extracellular matrix components are being investigated. By seeding patient-derived stem cells onto specially designed biomaterial scaffolds, personalized regenerative medicine holds promise for achieving genuinely customized treatments and eradicating immunological rejection. For example, patient-specific cardiac patches are being bioprinted for post-infarction recovery, while hydrogel structures seeded with autologous stem cells are being produced for cartilage regeneration. Smart biomaterials have demonstrated breakthroughs across tissue engineering, immunomodulation, patient-specific therapies, and biosensor applications, representing a transition from inert to actively responsive biomedical materials [39].

Developments in tissue maturation, organoid engineering, and bioprinting will make it possible to fabricate functional tissues and organs on demand in the ensuing decades. Personalized and regenerative biomaterials, in conjunction with real-time physiological monitoring and AI-based feedback, will usher in a new era of precision medicine, where scaffolds and implants are not only customized for each patient but can also change as they do.

1.10.3 Cross-Disciplinary Research and Global Collaboration

Cross-disciplinary integration and international cooperation between the academic, business, and healthcare sectors are essential for the next generation of biomaterial innovation. By its very nature, biomaterials research lies in the nexus of data science, biology, materials engineering, and medicine. Addressing medical issues, which range from organ failure to chronic diseases, calls for a coordinated strategy that brings together knowledge from various fields and geographical areas.

Cross-disciplinary research makes it easier to jointly build biological models and materials. For example, immunologists and chemists have worked together to develop immune-modulatory materials that actively influence healing responses, while engineers and physicians have collaborated to develop implant technologies tailored to individual patients. Another developing field is the fusion of synthetic biology with biomaterials engineering, which makes it possible to create “living materials” that can interact with biological tissues to communicate, self-regulate, and repair.

International cooperation is equally important for fair advancement in the study of biomaterials. Standardized testing procedures, open-access platforms, and shared databases can all be established to guarantee reproducibility and spur innovation. Global efforts to standardize biomaterials development and regulation are exemplified by international programs like the European Materials Modelling Council, the U.S. National Nanotechnology Initiative, and WHO-led health technology networks. Collaborative consortia help facilitate translation from lab to clinic, overcoming the “valley of death” that frequently prevents innovative biomaterials from being commercialized. Resources can be combined through public-private partnerships to assist sustainable manufacturing, regulatory approval, and clinical trials. Additionally, international cooperation promotes inclusivity by employing context-appropriate biomaterial advances to address region-specific health issues (such as diabetic ulcers, infectious disease-related tissue loss, or orthopedic injuries in elderly populations).

Ultimately, the fusion of multidisciplinary expertise and international cooperation will define the next chapter of biomaterials science, ensuring that innovation translates efficiently into accessible, safe, and equitable healthcare solutions.

1.10.4 Sustainability and Circular Economy in Biomaterials

Sustainability is becoming more of a scientific and moral necessity as biomaterials develop. Medical materials' environmental impact, from resource extraction to disposal, necessitates the development of novel strategies based on the circular economy, biodegradability, and green chemistry.

Renewable feedstocks, such as plant-derived polymers (cellulose, alginate, chitosan) and bio-based polyesters (PLA, PHA), are given priority in the creation of sustainable biomaterials. These materials minimize biological waste by decomposing spontaneously and reducing reliance on petroleum resources. Energy usage and harmful emissions are further decreased by advancements in solvent-free processing and enzymatic synthesis.

The life-cycle assessment (LCA), which assesses the economic and environmental effects of biomaterials from manufacture to end-of-life, is a key idea in this direction. Designers can optimize materials for minimal carbon footprint, reusability, and recycling with the help of life cycle assessment (LCA) technologies. For instance, surgical removal is not necessary with biodegradable implants that dissolve once tissue heals, lowering patient risk and medical waste.

Additionally, the concept of a circular bioeconomy, in which resources and waste are continuously recycled, is consistent with international sustainability objectives. This technology closes the gap between environmental preservation and healthcare innovation by using biomedical polymers and composites that are made to be recovered and reused. This change is being aided by developments in biomanufacturing, which incorporate waste valorization procedures, water recycling systems, and energy-efficient fabrication techniques.

Social responsibility and sustainability in biomaterials are related. Future innovation in medical technology must be guided by equitable access to safe, reasonably priced, and environmentally friendly solutions. This comprises creating affordable biomaterials for environments with limited resources, fostering local production capacity, and guaranteeing adherence to global ethical and environmental norms. Biomaterials research can advance toward a regenerative and circular paradigm where advancements in medicine benefit not only human health but also the health of the earth by integrating sustainability into every phase, from molecular design to disposal.

Biomaterials' future will be characterized by sustainability, intelligence, personalization, and teamwork. Personalized and regenerative approaches will revolutionize patient care; cross-disciplinary and international collaboration will bring knowledge and practice together; sustainability will guarantee ethical stewardship of resources; and artificial intelligence and predictive modeling will speed up discovery and maximize safety [40, 41]. Together, these paths suggest a future in which biomaterials are essential parts of a networked, data-driven, and sustainable healthcare ecosystem, able to improve life while protecting the earth that supports it.

1.11 Conclusion

1.11.1 Summary of Key Points

The development of biomaterials has changed the field of biomedical engineering by expanding the potential for medicinal delivery systems, medical devices, and tissue regeneration. The area has advanced over the past few decades from passive implants to dynamic, responsive materials that can intelligently interact with biological settings. Along with the urgent issues and constraints that continue to influence the direction of biomaterial research, this scientific essay has examined the complex mechanisms governing biological interactions, material degradation, sterilization, and surface modification.

Fundamentally, the success of biomaterials depends on striking a careful balance between durability, functionality, and biocompatibility. Immunological modulation, cell adhesion, and protein adsorption are important factors that determine how a substance integrates with host tissues and prevents negative immunological responses. Analyzing the processes of deterioration, such as metal corrosion, polymer hydrolysis, or ceramic dissolution, is also essential for forecasting longevity and guaranteeing safety in physiological settings. Improved bioactivity, lower infection risks, and regulated degradation rates have been made possible by developments in surface modification techniques, such as plasma treatment, coating, and nanostructuring.

These scientific developments do, however, coexist with enduring challenges. Foreign body reaction, rejection, and inflammation are examples of biocompatibility problems that continue to be significant obstacles to long-term therapeutic success. In addition, structural fatigue and mechanical instability jeopardize the longevity of implants subjected to ongoing physiological loads. Accessibility is further restricted by manufacturing issues such as economic viability, scalability, and reproducibility, especially in environments with limited resources. Furthermore, biomaterial design and regulatory frameworks are increasingly influenced by ethical and environmental factors, such as sustainable production, patient safety, and responsible sourcing.

When taken as a whole, these talks confirm that biomaterials are essential components of biomedical innovation rather than discrete technological structures. From vascular grafts and prosthetic joints to regenerative scaffolds and drug-eluting stents, they make it possible to realize cutting-edge medical solutions that depend on the meticulous fusion of materials science, biological understanding, and engineering precision. Biomaterials will continue to be essential for bridging the gap between synthetic engineering and biological systems as healthcare moves toward precision and regenerative paradigms.

1.11.2 Reflection on Interdisciplinary Relevance

Biomaterials have an interdisciplinary future that necessitates ongoing integration of clinical practice, technical design, and scientific knowledge. It takes cooperation amongst chemists, material scientists, biomedical engineers, doctors, and regulatory specialists to fully capture the complexity of biological systems. Modern biomaterial innovation is defined by this interdisciplinary confluence, which also guarantees that scientific discoveries are not only technically possible but also morally and clinically sound.

At the scientific level, materials chemistry and nanotechnology offer instruments for modifying surface topographies, degradation kinetics, and molecular structures at previously unheard-of scales. For example, tissue integration and cell activity can be influenced by nanoscale patterning, and material–tissue interactions can be predicted using computer modeling prior to clinical trials. Through mechanical design, additive manufacturing, and process optimization, these scientific discoveries are converted into engineering applications that guarantee the production of materials with accuracy, repeatability, and scalability.

The clinical viewpoint, which grounds innovation in the requirements and results of human health, is equally important. Clinicians provide crucial input on patient variability, biocompatibility, and implant function, which directs ongoing material improvement. Translational biomaterials science dynamic process of turning basic findings into workable medicinal interventions was born out of this conversation between laboratory research and clinical application. For instance, cardiologists and polymer scientists work together to create bioresorbable vascular scaffolds that lower the risk of thrombosis, while orthopedic surgeons and materials engineers make titanium alloys that replicate the elasticity of bone.

Moreover, artificial intelligence and data science are emerging as significant accelerators for transdisciplinary progress. To develop materials with optimal biological responses and performance characteristics, predictive modeling, machine learning, and bioinformatics are being employed. By connecting clinical and experimental research in an integrated innovation cycle, these computational methods enable quicker screening of material candidates and more precise long-term outcome prediction.

To ensure that innovation is in line with safety, transparency, and societal values, the synergy between disciplines also extends to ethical and regulatory collaboration. Ethicists, legislators, and sustainability specialists are essential in evaluating the wider effects of using biomaterials, ranging from environmental stewardship to therapeutic risk management. In the end, this convergence of knowledge creates an innovative environment that is patient-centered, socially conscious, and scientifically sound.

1.11.3 Future Outlook

In the future, the biomaterials industry is set to usher in a new era characterized by patient-centered, innovation-driven development. Personalized medicine could undergo a revolution thanks to emerging technologies like regenerative scaffolds, biofabrication, and 4D biomaterials. 4D biomaterials, which may alter their characteristics or form in reaction to physiological inputs, serve as an example of how intelligent design can dynamically adjust to changing biological situations, facilitating better integration and healing. With these developments, static implants will give way to interactive, responsive devices that actively contribute to the healing process.

One of the key characteristics of upcoming biomaterial applications will be personalization. Researchers may create scaffolds and implants that are suited to each patient's biological profile by combining genetic, proteomic, and metabolic data. This reduces the possibility of rejection and maximizes the effectiveness of treatment. AI-driven design tools will enable quick prototype and predictive performance testing, while additive manufacturing (3D and 4D printing) will allow for the custom production of implants tailored to each patient. With this change, generic solutions give way to precision biomaterial engineering, which is entirely consistent with the more general objectives of regenerative and customized medicine.

Integrating sustainability and the circular economy into the development of biomaterials is another crucial frontier. Future innovations must reduce their negative effects on the environment by using eco-friendly production, waste reduction, and renewable sourcing. Natural biopolymers, such chitosan, collagen, and polylactic acid, are good substitutes for petroleum-based products since they are biodegradable and less harmful to the environment. The development of green biomaterials ensures that advancements in biomedical engineering do not jeopardize ethical or environmental integrity, bringing healthcare innovation into line with global sustainability goals.

From a systemic standpoint, the future also necessitates more fair access and robust international cooperation. Innovation in biomaterials should assist underprivileged people everywhere, not just in technologically developed countries. International research collaborations, standardized regulatory frameworks, and open science platforms may democratize innovation, cut down on redundancy, and speed up information transfer. Turning discoveries into scalable, reasonably priced medical treatments would require cooperative consortia involving academics, business, and healthcare organizations.

In the end, the future of biomaterials is a vision of humanity, adaptability, and integration. In addition to restoring lost functionalities, the upcoming generation of biomaterials will actively support sustainability, resilience, and regeneration.

Biomaterials will continue to be central to the goal of biomedical engineering, which is to improve quality of life via research guided by responsibility and compassion, through ongoing interdisciplinary collaboration, ethical governance, and patient-focused innovation.

Intelligent, sustainable, and patient-specific materials will serve as the cornerstone of sophisticated healthcare systems in the future, according to the trajectory of biomaterial research. Biomaterials will keep bridging the gap between artificial constructs and live tissues, supported by interdisciplinary collaboration and directed by ethical and environmental consciousness. Despite the rapid pace of invention, the field's long-term objective is still to use biological harmony and material science principles to promote human well-being, healing, and regeneration.

References

1. Dzobo, K., Adotey, S., Thomford, N.E., Dzobo, W.: Integrating artificial and human intelligence: a partnership for responsible innovation in biomedical engineering and medicine. Omics : a journal of integrative biology. **24**(5), 247–263 (2020)
2. Terzopoulou, Z., Zamboulis, A., Koumentakou, I., Michailidou, G., Noordam, M.J., Bikiaris, D.N.: Biocompatible synthetic polymers for tissue engineering purposes. Biomacromolecules. **23**(5), 1841–1863 (2022)
3. Dobrzański, L.A., Dobrzańska-Danikiewicz, A.D., Dobrzański, L.B.: Effect of biomedical materials in the implementation of a long and healthy life policy. PRO. **9**(5), 865 (2021)
4. Yaneva, A., Shopova, D., Bakova, D., Mihaylova, A., Kasnakova, P., Hristozova, M., Semerdjieva, M.: The progress in bioprinting and its potential impact on health-related quality of life. Bioengineering. **10**(8), 910 (2023)
5. Gera, R., Chadha, P., Banerjee, S.P., Sharma, M., Pandey, A.K., Kampani, S., Dixit, S., Tummala, S.K., Gatea, M.A.: A narrative review on use of biomaterials in achieving SDG 9: build resilient infrastructure, promote sustainable industrialization and foster innovation. In: E3S Web of Conferences, vol. 391, p. 01180. EDP Sciences (2023)
6. Hunckler, M.D., Levine, A.D.: Navigating ethical challenges in the development and translation of biomaterials research. Front. Bioeng. Biotechnol. **10**, 949280 (2022)
7. Kyriakides, T.R., Raj, A., Tseng, T.H., Xiao, H., Nguyen, R., Mohammed, F.S., Halder, S., Xu, M., Wu, M.J., Bao, S., Sheu, W.C.: Biocompatibility of nanomaterials and their immunological properties. Biomed. Mater. **16**(4), 042005 (2021)
8. Bapat, R.A., Parolia, A., Chaubal, T., Dharamadhikari, S., Abdulla, A.M., Sakkir, N., Arora, S., Bapat, P., Sindi, A.M., Kesharwani, P.: Recent update on potential cytotoxicity, biocompatibility and preventive measures of biomaterials used in dentistry. Biomater. Sci. **9**(9), 3244–3283 (2021)
9. Forna, N.: Osseointegration of dental implants: a review. Rom. J. Med. Dent. Educ. **9**(4), 6–17 (2020)
10. Pandey, C., Rokaya, D., Bhattarai, B.P.: Contemporary concepts in osseointegration of dental implants: a review. Biomed. Res. Int. **1**, p.6170452 (2022)
11. Marin, E., Boschetto, F., Pezzotti, G.: Biomaterials and biocompatibility: an historical overview. J. Biomed. Mater. Res. A. **108**(8), 1617–1633 (2020)
12. Nicholson, J.W.: The Chemistry of Medical and Dental Materials, vol. 7. Royal Society of Chemistry (2020)
13. Raab, C.D.: Information privacy, impact assessment, and the place of ethics. Comput. Law Secur. Rev. **37**, 105404 (2020)

14. Safarlou, C.W., Jongsma, K.R., Vermeulen, R., Bredenoord, A.L.: The ethical aspects of exposome research: a systematic review. Exposome. **3**(1), osad004 (2023)
15. Ashish Daniel, S., Suya Prem Anand, P., Naveen, J., Khan, T., Khahro, S.H.: Advancement in biomedical implant materials—a mini review. Front. Bioeng. Biotechnol. **12**, 1400918 (2024). https://doi.org/10.3389/fbioe.2024.1400918
16. Mubeen, B., Anwar, M.J., Menaa, F., Ikram, R., Jan, B., Khan, R.: Advancements in magnesium applications, biocompatible implants to nanoparticles in medicine and biomedical innovations. MetalMat, e70003 (2025). https://doi.org/10.1002/metm.70003
17. Bazaka, O., Bazaka, K., Kingshott, P., Crawford, R. J., Ivanova, E. P.: Metallic implants for biomedical applications. In C. Spicer (Ed.), The chemistry of inorganic biomaterials (pp. 1–98) (2021). Royal Society of Chemistry. https://doi.org/10.1039/9781788019828-00001
18. Nouri, A., Wen, C.: Stainless steels in orthopedics. In: Structural Biomaterials, pp. 67–101. Woodhead Publishing (2021)
19. Garrison, T.F., Smith, A.P., Mathers, R.T.: Biodegradable biobased polymers: a review of the state of the art, challenges, and future directions. Polymers. **16**(16), 2262 (2024). https://doi.org/10.3390/polym16162262
20. Nagabushanam, M., Devade, K., Reddy, G.A., Goud, B.N., Sayed, R.M., Sood, S., Sonia, P.: Advance biomedical engineering–a fundamental review of composite materials and its applications. Mater. Today Proc. (2023)
21. Nayak, G.S., Carradò, A., Masson, P., Pourroy, G., Mouillard, F., Migonney, V., Falentin-Daudre, C., Pereira, C., Palkowski, H.: Trends in metal-based composite biomaterials for hard tissue applications. JOM. **74**(1), 102–125 (2022)
22. Tournier, V., Duquesne, S., Guillamot, F., Cramail, H., Taton, D., Marty, A., André, I.: Enzymes' power for plastics degradation. Chem. Rev. **123**(9), 5612–5701 (2023)
23. Todros, S., Todesco, M., Bagno, A.: Biomaterials and their biomedical applications: from replacement to regeneration. PRO. **9**(11), 1949 (2021)
24. Jaime, F.J., Muñoz, A., Rodríguez-Gómez, F., Jerez-Calero, A.: Strengthening privacy and data security in biomedical microelectromechanical systems by IoT communication security and protection in smart healthcare. Sensors. **23**(21), 8944 (2023)
25. Ciolacu, D.E., Nicu, R., Ciolacu, F.: Natural polymers in heart valve tissue engineering: strategies, advances and challenges. Biomedicine. **10**(5), 1095 (2022)
26. Pathak, K., Saikia, R., Das, A., Das, D., Islam, M.A., Pramanik, P., Parasar, A., Borthakur, P.P., Sarmah, P., Saikia, M., Borthakur, B.: 3D printing in biomedicine: advancing personalized care through additive manufacturing. Explor. Med. **4**(6), 1135–1167 (2023)
27. Aziz, T., Akhtar, K., Habib, A., Rashid, B., Alharbi, A., Jamal, M.A.: Smart and biodegradable polymers in tissue engineering and interventional devices: a brief review. Polymers. **17**(14), 1950 (2025). https://doi.org/10.3390/polym17141950
28. John, J.V., Kim, H., Dokmeci, M.R., Popat, K.C., Zhu, Y., Manivasagam, G.: Smart biomaterials in healthcare: breakthroughs in tissue engineering, immunomodulation, patient-specific therapies, and biosensor applications. Appl. Phys. Rev. **12**(1), 011333 (2025). https://doi.org/10.1063/5.0238817
29. Sojdeh, S., Panjipour, A., Castillo, M., Arabpour, Z., Djalilian, A.R.: Emerging smart and adaptive hydrogels for next-generation tissue engineering. Bioengineering. **13**(1), 50 (2025). https://doi.org/10.3390/bioengineering13010050
30. Zhao, H., Wang, Y., Bao, L., Chen, C.: Engineering nano–bio interfaces from nanomaterials to nanomedicines. Acc. Mater. Res. **3**(8), 812–829 (2022)
31. Yücer, R., Kemal Ener, R., Tekin, E., Türk, M.: Bioprinting revolution: innovative design of 3D bioactive scaffolds for living organs and transdermal tissues. Bioeng. Transl. Med. **10**(6), e70080 (2025). https://doi.org/10.1002/btm2.70080
32. Rydz, J., Musioł, M., Zawidlak-Węgrzyńska, B., Molnar, K.: Advanced green polymers for medical purpose—trends and challenges in the circular economy. Front. Bioeng. Biotechnol. **12**, 1511632 (2024). https://doi.org/10.3389/fbioe.2024.1511632

33. Hosseini, E.S., Dervin, S., Ganguly, P.a., Dahiya, R.: Biodegradable materials for sustainable health monitoring devices. ACS Appl. Bio Mater. **4**(1), 163–194 (2020)
34. Pinals, R.L., Chio, L., Ledesma, F., Landry, M.P.: Engineering at the nano-bio interface: harnessing the protein corona towards nanoparticle design and function. Analyst. **145**(15), 5090–5112 (2020)
35. Ou, Y., Guo, S.: Safety risks and ethical governance of biomedical applications of synthetic biology. Front. Bioeng. Biotechnol. **11**, 1292029 (2023)
36. Zhai, C., Li, T., Shi, H., Yeo, J.: Discovery and design of soft polymeric bio-inspired materials with multiscale simulations and artificial intelligence. J. Mater. Chem. B. **8**(31), 6562–6587 (2020)
37. Liu, M., Zhou, Y., Mei, X., Yu, Z., Guan, B., Xiao, Y., Liu, S., Wang, H., Qin, Y.: AI-driven biomaterial design: an intelligent closed loop from reverse design to biological response. Front. Cell Dev. Biol. **13**, 1755565 (2025). https://doi.org/10.3389/fcell.2025.1755565
38. Jiang, Y., Liu, Y., Zheng, Y., Chen, X.: Artificial intelligence-assisted design, synthesis and analysis of smart biomaterials. BMEMat. **3**(2), e70004 (2025). https://doi.org/10.1002/bmm2.70004
39. Raheem, A., Mandal, K., Biswas, S., Ahari, A., Hassani Najafabadi, A., Farhadi, N., et al.: Smart biomaterials in healthcare: breakthroughs in tissue engineering, immunomodulation, patient-specific therapies, and biosensor applications. Appl. Phys. Rev. **12**(1) (2025)
40. Ali, H.: Artificial intelligence in multi-omics data integration: advancing precision medicine, biomarker discovery and genomic-driven disease interventions. Int. J. Sci. Res. Arch. **8**(1), 1012–1030 (2023)
41. Gregory, F.D., Trump, B.D.: The Evolving Landscape of Biotechnology Research: Challenges and Opportunities in Acquisitions, Funding, Education, and Workforce Development for a Productive Bioeconomy, pp. 25–50. Advanced Study Institute on NATO ASI on Quantum Nano-Photonics (2023)

Chapter 2
Biocompatibility and Host Response and Immunomodulation

Abstract A key characteristic of biomaterials is their biocompatibility, which refers to their capacity to interact with living tissues in a safe and efficient manner without causing unfavorable biological reactions. The host response, which includes the series of cellular and molecular processes brought on by material implantation, such as protein adsorption, immune cell recruitment, inflammation, and tissue remodeling, is at the heart of this idea. Long-term results are determined by the first interactions between biomaterial surfaces and the biological environment, which affect integration, functionality, and overall therapeutic success. Therefore, it is essential to comprehend these mechanisms in order to rationally develop next-generation biomaterials. With both innate and adaptive immune mechanisms involved, the host response is intrinsically complex. Macrophage polarization and subsequent foreign body reactions can be influenced by early processes such complement activation and protein adsorption. While dysregulated inflammation can result in fibrosis, implant encapsulation, or rejection, a coordinated immune response promotes tissue healing and integration. Therefore, a material's ability to evoke suitable, positive host reactions is what defines its biocompatibility rather than just its inertness. In biomaterials science, immunomodulation has become a key tactic with the goal of actively controlling the immune response to promote tissue regeneration and lessen negative effects. Methods include adding cytokines or immunoregulatory molecules, surface functionalization with anti-inflammatory drugs, and bioactive coatings that affect macrophage polarization. By promoting integration and long-term functionality, materials with immunomodulatory qualities can change the host response from one that is pro-inflammatory to one that is pro-regenerative. Recent developments that combine materials science, cell biology, and immunology demonstrate the multidisciplinary character of biocompatibility research. Biomaterials can be designed to affect particular immunological pathways by modifying their mechanics, surface chemical, and topography, striking a fine balance between tolerance and immune activation. This confluence makes it possible to create medication delivery systems, scaffolds, and implants of the future that actively promote healing and regeneration in addition to being tolerant by the host. The success of biomedical devices is determined by the interaction of immu-

M. Adeoba, T. Pandelani, *Application of Biomaterials in Biomedical Engineering*, Series in BioEngineering,
https://doi.org/10.1007/978-3-032-34477-9_2

nomodulation, host response, and biocompatibility. By using this knowledge, materials that are safe and therapeutically active can be logically designed, signaling a paradigm change away from passive compatibility and toward immune-informed, regenerative biomaterials.

2.1 Introduction

A fundamental idea in the field of biomaterials, biocompatibility refers to a material's capacity to interact with biological systems while preserving intended functioning and avoiding adverse reactions. Because it controls how the material integrates with tissues, maintains mechanical and chemical stability, and promotes therapeutic results, this feature is critical to the success of medical devices, implants, scaffolds, and drug delivery systems. Biocompatibility goes beyond inertness to include the dynamic interaction of materials with biological systems, where clinical performance is determined by host reactions, immunological modulation, and cellular interactions [1, 2]. Any biomaterial meant for implantation or long-term usage in the human body must take biocompatibility into account; it is not an optional factor.

2.1.1 Overview of Biocompatibility as a Determinant of Biomaterial Success

The biocompatibility characteristic of biomaterials directly affects their clinical effectiveness and durability. A biocompatible substance promotes desired cellular processes like adhesion, proliferation, and differentiation while reducing cytotoxicity and preventing inflammatory or fibrotic reactions. Its crucial role in medical applications is highlighted by the fact that failure to achieve biocompatibility can lead to implant failure, infection, or device rejection. In practice, biocompatibility is evaluated by analyzing tissue integration, immunological activation, protein adsorption patterns, and cellular viability using a combination of in vitro, in vivo, and computational analyses. These evaluations guarantee that the substance functions predictably under physiological conditions by offering insight into both short-term reactions and long-term results.

Mechanical and chemical stability, which affect how well a material performs under physiological stress, are also included in biocompatibility. For instance, cardiovascular stents need corrosion-resistant surfaces to avoid thrombosis, whereas orthopedic implants must tolerate cyclic loads without releasing hazardous degradation products. Therefore, a material's overall compatibility with its intended biological and mechanical environment is a component of biocompatibility, which goes beyond simple cytocompatibility.

2.1.2 Role of Host Response in Material Performance, Integration, and Longevity

Immediately following implantation, the host response is a dynamic biological process that includes tissue remodeling, immune cell recruitment, protein adsorption, and inflammation. This reaction impacts a material's long-term functionality and establishes how well it integrates into host tissue. Proteins first adsorb onto the surface of the biomaterial to create a "biological interface" that facilitates further cellular interactions. Depending on its structure and makeup, this protein layer can either help or hurt cell adhesion.

The polarization state of macrophages affects tissue outcomes, making them essential to the host response. While M2 macrophages aid in tissue repair and regeneration, M1 macrophages promote pro-inflammatory reactions that might result in fibrosis or chronic inflammation. For steady integration and long-term device success, a material's ability to regulate this equilibrium is consequently essential. Careful material design and surface engineering are essential because improper host response management can lead to foreign body responses, fibrotic encapsulation, or implant rejection.

2.1.3 Importance of Immunomodulation in Controlling Adverse Reactions and Promoting Tissue Regeneration

In biomaterials research, immunomodulation is a cutting-edge tactic that actively controls the host immune response to encourage healing and lessen negative effects. Immunomodulatory biomaterials engage in dynamic interactions with immune cells, directing their behavior to promote tissue repair, as opposed to only concentrating on inertness. Methods that have shown great promise in regulating immune activation and boosting regenerative responses include surface functionalization with anti-inflammatory chemicals, bioactive coatings that affect macrophage polarization, and the addition of cytokines or growth factors.

The efficient integration of implants and scaffolds depends on angiogenesis, extracellular matrix deposition, and tissue remodeling, all of which are facilitated by immunomodulatory materials that foster a pro-regenerative immunological milieu. These tactics are especially pertinent in intricate clinical situations where dysregulated inflammation frequently restricts the effectiveness of treatment, such as chronic wounds, orthopedic reconstruction, cardiovascular implants, and scaffolds tailored to particular organs. By bridging the gap between biological function and material design, immunomodulation positions biomaterials as active players in healing and regeneration rather than merely passive structures [3, 4].

2.1.4 Scope of the Chapter

The goal of this chapter is to give a thorough review of immunomodulation, host response, and biocompatibility in relation to biomaterials. The basic ideas and terminologies will be discussed, along with the main ways that materials interact with the biological environment. The topic will cover a variety of material types, such as metals, ceramics, composites, and polymers, emphasizing how surface changes and inherent characteristics affect host interactions. In addition to design tactics for improving biocompatibility and guiding beneficial host outcomes, mechanistic insights into cellular and immunological responses will be investigated.

The chapter will also look at translational applications, showing how biocompatible and immunomodulatory materials are used in drug delivery, tissue engineering, regenerative medicine, and implanted devices. The importance of multidisciplinary integration combining materials science, immunology, and bioengineering to maximize biomaterial performance will be highlighted through case studies and new developments. After reading this chapter, readers will have a comprehensive grasp of how host response and biocompatibility affect biomaterial performance and how deliberate immunomodulation can improve safety, integration, and regenerative results.

Together, host response, immunomodulation, and biocompatibility establish the biological interface of biomaterials, impacting their lifetime, integration, and therapeutic effectiveness. Designing materials that are not only absorbed by the body but also actively support tissue regeneration and repair requires an understanding of how they interact. The knowledge provided in this chapter lays the groundwork for comprehending the ways in which materials interact with biological systems and outlines methods for creating safe, functionally instructive biomaterials of the future.

2.2 Key Concepts and Definitions

The logical design, assessment, and clinical use of implants and devices depend on an understanding of the fundamental ideas and terminology in biomaterials research. The effectiveness of biomaterials depends on their interactions with the host environment, which include intricate cellular, molecular, and immunological processes. This clarifies the language used in current biomaterials research by offering a thorough summary of the terminologies and important ideas pertaining to immunomodulation, host response, biocompatibility, and evaluation metrics.

2.2.1 Definition of Biocompatibility, Biofunctionality and Bioinertness

The capacity of a material to carry out its intended function without producing undesired local or systemic consequences while evoking an adequate host response is known as biocompatibility. This idea includes encouraging tissue integration and functional recovery in addition to the lack of toxicity or inflammation. A biocompatible substance minimizes negative effects like fibrosis, necrosis, or chronic inflammation while promoting cellular adhesion, proliferation, and differentiation through predictable interactions with the biological environment [5, 6].

Beyond just providing structural support, a material's ability to actively engage in biological processes is referred to as biofunctionality. Biofunctional materials have the potential to release therapeutic compounds, guide tissue regeneration, control host immunological responses, and drive cell signaling. A vascular graft that promotes endothelialization or a scaffold that delivers osteogenic growth factors, for instance, exhibit biofunctional performance by actively supporting tissue integration and healing.

On the other hand, bioinertness refers to materials that are made to interact with biological tissues as little as possible. These substances cause little cellular activation or protein adsorption and are chemically and physically stable. Examples include some noble metals (like platinum and gold) and ceramics (like alumina and zirconia) utilized in orthopedic and cardiovascular applications where low reactivity and long-term structural stability are important. The difference between passive compatibility and active functionality is highlighted by the fact that whereas bioinert materials lessen unpleasant reactions, they might not actively encourage tissue regeneration.

2.2.2 Definitions of Host Response: Acute, Chronic and Foreign Body Reaction

The range of biological processes brought on by a biomaterial during implantation is known as the host response. These reactions are multi-phase, dynamic processes that involve short-, medium-, and long-term interactions. Hemostasis, temporary inflammation, and innate immune activation are the hallmarks of the acute response, which happens right after implantation. Monocytes and neutrophils invade the implant site in a matter of hours to days, generating chemokines, reactive oxygen species, and cytokines. Usually temporary and protective, acute inflammation removes debris from the tissue and gets it ready for further repair. Necrosis or poor integration may result from materials that worsen acute inflammation.

Prolonged inflammation that lasts longer than the acute phase often weeks to months is referred to as a chronic response. Prolonged cytokine production, lymphocyte recruitment, and macrophage activation are all components of chronic inflammation, which may cause fibrosis or delayed healing. Tissue integration and device function may be hampered by materials that are not completely biodegradable or cause persistent discomfort.

A specific, long-term reaction to biomaterials that are non-biodegradable or slowly resorbing is known as a foreign body reaction (FBR). Multinucleated giant cells (also known as foreign body giant cells), continuous macrophage activity, and the development of fibrous capsules surrounding the implant are all involved. A certain amount of FBR is inevitable, but too much fibrous encapsulation can impair functional integration, mass transport, and cell penetration. Designing materials that limit negative effects while encouraging desired tissue outcomes requires an understanding of the cellular and temporal dynamics of host responses.

2.2.3 Immunomodulation: Active and Passive Strategies for Influencing Immune Response

Strategies that change, direct, or regulate the host immune response to a biomaterial in order to improve compatibility, lessen negative reactions, or encourage tissue regeneration are referred to as immunomodulation. These tactics fall into one of two categories: aggressive or passive.

Deliberately presenting biological cues to guide immune cell behavior is known as active immunomodulation. Examples include stimulating anti-inflammatory macrophages (M2 polarization) or regulatory T cells by immobilizing cytokines, chemokines, or immunoregulatory chemicals on the scaffold surface. Controlled drug delivery from biomaterials to locally alter immune activity is another active strategy that may be used to enhance targeted responses while lowering systemic exposure.

Without the use of exogenous drugs, passive immunomodulation shapes immunological interactions via material-intrinsic characteristics. Protein adsorption, complement activation, and macrophage polarization are influenced by surface chemistry, charge, hydrophilicity, stiffness, and nanotopography. Smooth and hydrophilic surfaces, for instance, tend to decrease macrophage activation and non-specific protein fouling, but nanotextured surfaces can encourage M2 phenotypic polarization, which is advantageous for tissue repair. By utilizing the material's natural properties, passive techniques produce immunological results that are predictable.

2.2.4 *Parameters for Evaluation: Cytotoxicity, Hemocompatibility, Inflammatory Markers and Tissue Integration*

Both quantitative and qualitative evaluation of biomaterials' interactions with cells, tissues, and the immune system are necessary for evaluation. Typical parameters consist of Cytotoxicity evaluates whether a substance or the byproducts of its breakdown cause cell death or hindered growth. Assays include live/dead staining, MTT, and LDH release measure the viability of various cell types. A criterion for biocompatibility is low cytotoxicity. Platelet adhesion, coagulation activation, hemolysis, and other interactions with blood components are all assessed by hemocompatibility. Hemocompatible materials reduce inflammation and thrombosis, which is crucial for cardiovascular devices. Measurements of cytokines (such as TNF-α and IL-6), chemokines, complement activation, and inflammatory markers offer information about immune activation and inflammatory potential. Increased markers could be a sign of a foreign body reaction or chronic inflammation risk. Tissue integration evaluates the degree to which the material integrates with the host tissue, taking into account angiogenesis, extracellular matrix deposition, cellular infiltration, and functional recovery. Common methods include imaging, biomechanical testing, and histological examination. A synergistic balance between material qualities and host reaction is reflected in effective integration. Together, these factors offer a comprehensive evaluation of immunomodulatory potential, biocompatibility, and biofunctionality that directs surface design and material choice.

2.2.5 *Terminology: Bioactivity, Immunoengineering, Cytokine Modulation and Immune Tolerance*

In biomaterials research, precise language is crucial for clarity. Bioactivity is the material's capacity to trigger particular biological responses, such as promoting osteogenesis, angiogenesis, or antimicrobial effects. Through interactions with cells and tissues, bioactive surfaces facilitate functional integration. The multidisciplinary topic of immunoengineering modifies immune responses by using engineering concepts. In order to achieve regulated immunological outcomes, such decreased inflammation or improved tissue healing, it includes scaffold design, drug delivery, and surface functionalization. The deliberate control of pro- and anti-inflammatory cytokines to influence the immune system surrounding a biomaterial is known as cytokine modulation. Surface coatings, localized therapeutic administration, or material chemistry can all be used to modulate cytokines. Immunological tolerance, which preserves homeostasis by allowing the host to accept the biomaterial without triggering an unfavorable immunological reaction. A major goal of long-term implant success is immunological tolerance, which reduces fibrotic encapsulation and persistent inflammation. Understanding this jargon is essential for developing, testing, and translating biomaterials that interact with the host in a predictable, secure, and therapeutically advantageous manner.

Modern biomaterials science is built on a solid understanding of immunomodulation, host response, and biocompatibility. While biofunctionality stresses active biological involvement, biocompatibility refers to the capacity to carry out desired functions without experiencing negative repercussions. The success and long-term integration of implants are influenced by host reactions, which include acute, chronic, and foreign body reactions. Both active and passive immunomodulation offer methods for guiding immune responses, maximizing tissue healing and reducing inflammation. Measurable standards for evaluating material performance are provided by standardized evaluation parameters, such as tissue integration, inflammatory indicators, hemocompatibility, and cytotoxicity. Finally, using precise terms like immunoengineering, cytokine modulation, bioactivity, and immunological tolerance guarantee clear communication and directs the development of next-generation biomaterials. Researchers and engineers may logically create biomaterials that are safe, efficient, and able to work in harmony with the intricate biology of the human body by combining these ideas [7, 8].

2.3 Historical Background

Over the past century, the research of host response and biocompatibility has changed to reflect the convergence of clinical medicine, immunology, and materials science. The field has moved from trial-and-error methods to logically designed, immunomodulatory biomaterials throughout time, as early implant experiences demonstrated the significant impact of material–host interactions on device success. Understanding the historical evolution of biomaterials science is essential to comprehending current tactics meant to regulate immune responses and encourage tissue regeneration.

2.3.1 Early Observations of Implant Rejection and Inflammatory Complications

Researchers and physicians noticed that implanted materials frequently caused negative tissue reactions in the early decades of the twentieth century, such as inflammation, infection, and outright rejection. Early attempts using metals, ceramics, and natural materials like ivory or bone from animals showed varying degrees of success, frequently hindered by unchecked inflammatory and immunological reactions. There have been reported cases of foreign body reactions, in which fibrous tissue enclosed implanted objects, preventing mechanical integration and functional performance.

These first findings demonstrated how important the host reaction is in influencing implant results. Recurring failures highlighted the significance of material selection, surface characteristics, and chemical composition, despite the fact that the underlying mechanisms were not well understood at the time. Surgeons realized that whereas natural biomaterials frequently deteriorated randomly or triggered immunological activation, some metals, such stainless steel and cobalt-chromium alloys, caused less difficulties than other materials. These realizations paved the way for a methodical examination of biocompatibility as a key need for biomedical applications.

2.3.2 *Development of the Concept of Bioinert Vs. Bioactive Materials*

The distinction between bioinert and bioactive materials was created by researchers as their understanding of material–host interactions improved. Polished titanium and some ceramics are examples of bioinert materials that were created to reduce inflammatory reactions and immunological activation. In order to prevent rejection, their approach depended on passive integration and avoided chemical or biological reaction. Bioinert metals were used in early orthopedic and dental implants to guarantee mechanical stability and lower host problems.

Bioactive materials, on the other hand, were purposefully created to interact with the biological environment. Materials that can encourage osteoconduction and direct bonding with bone tissue include calcium phosphates, hydroxyapatite, and bioactive glasses [9, 10]. These developments signaled a paradigm shift by showing that effective biomaterials don't have to be inactive; rather, they can improve integration and functionality through controlled tissue interaction. The idea of bioactivity opened the door for materials designed to actively promote tissue regeneration in addition to preventing negative effects.

2.3.3 *Introduction of Synthetic Polymers and Metals with Controlled Host Responses*

Advanced metallic alloys and synthetic polymers emerged in the middle of the twentieth century, offering previously unheard-of control over mechanical characteristics, degradation kinetics, and host reaction. Polymers including polyesters, polyethylene, and polymethyl methacrylate (PMMA) made it possible to fabricate heart valves, joint replacements, and vascular grafts with consistent results. These substances were frequently used in conjunction with coatings or surface treatments to control inflammatory reactions, cellular adhesion, and protein adsorption.

Cobalt-chromium, titanium, and stainless steel alloys are examples of metallic biomaterials that were designed for their mechanical strength, biocompatibility, and resistance to corrosion. Their compatibility with host tissues was enhanced by oxide layer development, surface passivation, and electropolishing. Early research showed that immune activation might be decreased while preserving structural integrity by regulating alloying elements, surface roughness, and chemical composition. These developments laid the groundwork for logical biomaterial design, which moved away from empirical methods and toward materials designed to strike a compromise between functional performance and host tolerance.

2.3.4 Milestones in Immunomodulatory Biomaterials and Tissue Engineering

The development of immunomodulatory biomaterials in the late 20th and early 21st centuries reflected a greater comprehension of tissue regeneration and immunological systems. Researchers realized that host reactions may be used to aid in healing rather than only acting as barriers. Biomaterials were able to actively direct immune responses toward regeneration pathways through the use of strategies such surface functionalization with anti-inflammatory agents, cytokine and growth factor incorporation, and macrophage polarization regulation.

At the same time, tissue engineering became a revolutionary method that combined cells, scaffolds, and signaling molecules to generate functioning tissues. Surface characteristics were adjusted to regulate cell adhesion and differentiation, and biodegradable polymers, hydrogel matrices, and composite materials were created to break down in tandem with tissue regeneration. In order to achieve functional tissue integration, landmark research showed that scaffolds with regulated topography, biochemical signals, and mechanical qualities might coordinate host responses. These turning points marked a change from passively biocompatible materials to carefully crafted biomaterials that could control particular immunological and cellular responses.

2.3.5 Evolution Toward Patient-Specific and Adaptive Immunomodulatory Strategies

The focus of recent advances in biomaterials research is on tailored and flexible immunomodulation strategies. Nowadays, patient-specific implants and scaffolds that are adapted to anatomical and immunological traits can be made thanks to developments in computational modeling, additive manufacturing, and nanotechnology. Materials can react to changes in pH, enzyme activity, or mechanical stress thanks to surface modification techniques including nanostructuring, bioactive coatings, and stimuli-responsive materials, which enable dynamic interaction with the host environment.

Personalized responses are essential for intricate tissue healing in regenerative medicine, which makes these adaptive biomaterials more pertinent. For instance, in individuals who are at risk for chronic inflammation, immunomodulatory scaffolds can enhance integration and healing by promoting M2 macrophage polarization. By interacting with endothelial cells in a way that is unique to each patient, bioactive coatings on customized cardiovascular stents can also reduce the risk of restenosis. These approaches are the result of decades of research that combine contemporary developments in materials science, immunology, and bioengineering with historical understanding of rejection and inflammatory consequences.

The development of immunomodulation and biocompatibility throughout time shows a shift from empirical observation to logical, patient-centered design. Synthetic polymers, corrosion-resistant metals, and bioinert and bioactive materials were developed in response to early issues with implant rejection and inflammatory consequences. Recent developments in personalization and adaptive strategies promise dynamic control of host responses, while immunomodulatory biomaterials and tissue engineering milestones have changed implants from passive devices to active participants in tissue regeneration [11, 12]. To appreciate modern methods and direct the development of biomaterials that are safe, therapeutically effective, and able to communicate intelligently with intricate biological systems, it is imperative to comprehend this historical background.

2.4 Material Types and Properties

The way biomaterials interact with the biological environment and their bulk mechanical characteristics impact how well they perform in therapeutic settings. Protein adsorption, cellular adhesion, immunological activation, and tissue integration are all strongly influenced by the type of material and its inherent characteristics. Designing implants, scaffolds, and other devices that reduce negative immune responses and enhance therapeutic effectiveness requires an understanding of these features. The main biomaterial types polymeric, metallic, ceramic, and composite are thoroughly described here, along with the essential characteristics that control immunogenicity and host response as shown in Table 2.1.

2.4.1 Polymeric Biomaterials

Because of their mechanical flexibility, variable chemical composition, and capacity for surface functionalization, polymeric biomaterials are extensively utilized and adaptable. They might be natural hydrogels like collagen, chitosan, or alginate, or

Table 2.1 Summary of host responses to different biomaterials

Material type	Representative examples	Key material properties	Biological/host response mechanisms	Summary of immune and tissue reactions
Polymeric Biomaterials	Poly (ethylene glycol) (PEG), Polylactic acid (PLA), Polycaprolactone (PCL), Hydrogels	• Hydrophilicity and surface charge regulate protein adsorption. • Surface chemistry influences macrophage and fibroblast adhesion. • Degradation products (e.g., lactic acid) modulate local pH and inflammation	• Adsorbed protein layers mediate immune cell recognition. • Hydrophilic surfaces (PEG) reduce fouling and cell attachment. • Biodegradable polymers trigger transient inflammatory response as they degrade	• Generally good biocompatibility when degradation is controlled. • Excessive acid by-products may induce mild inflammation. • PEG and hydrogels often elicit minimal immune activation
Metallic Biomaterials	Titanium (Ti), Stainless Steel, Magnesium (Mg) Alloys	• High mechanical strength and corrosion resistance. • Surface oxide layers determine ion release and biostability. • Electrical conductivity can affect protein and cell interactions	• Ion release (Ni, Cr, or Mg) may activate macrophages and induce oxidative stress. • Titanium forms stable TiO_2 passivation layer, minimizing immune activation	• Excellent tissue integration (e.g., Ti). • Mg alloys promote transient inflammation during degradation. • Stainless steel may elicit chronic low-grade immune response due to ion leaching
Ceramic Biomaterials	Hydroxyapatite (HA), Bioactive Glasses	• Chemically stable, bioactive, and osteoconductive. • Ionic dissolution products (Ca^{2+}, Si^{4+}) promote osteogenesis and cell signaling. • Brittle but highly biocompatible	• Bioactive ion release enhances osteoblast differentiation. • Limited macrophage activation compared to polymers or metals	• Minimal inflammatory response. • Excellent bone integration due to bioactivity. • Often used as coatings to enhance implant–tissue bonding

(continued)

Table 2.1 (continued)

Material type	Representative examples	Key material properties	Biological/host response mechanisms	Summary of immune and tissue reactions
Composite and Hybrid Materials	Polymer–ceramic or metal–polymer composites, Nanocomposites	• Tunable interfacial chemistry and mechanical compliance. • Fillers and coatings regulate degradation and protein adsorption. • Synergistic properties for tailored immune modulation	• Interface between components dictates macrophage behavior. • Coatings (e.g., hydroxyapatite, graphene oxide) can reduce fibrotic encapsulation	• Controlled immune activation promoting healing rather than chronic inflammation. • Enhanced mechanical integrity with adaptive biological response
Key Material Properties Influencing Immunogenicity		• Surface chemistry (hydrophilicity, charge). • Topography and roughness affecting cell adhesion. • Degradation products influencing local pH. • Mechanical compliance matching native tissue	• Protein adsorption and macrophage polarization (M1/M2) are material-dependent. • Smooth, hydrophilic, and compliant surfaces favor M2-like, regenerative response	• Optimized design can reduce chronic inflammation and promote integration. • Misaligned mechanical or chemical properties may trigger fibrosis or rejection

they can be manufactured hydrogels like poly (lactic acid) (PLA), polycaprolactone (PCL), and polyethylene glycol (PEG).

Protein adsorption and immune cell interactions are significantly impacted by the surface chemistry of polymers, which includes hydrophilicity, charge, and functional groups. Immune tolerance is increased by hydrophilic surfaces, such as PEG-modified polymers, which inhibit nonspecific protein adsorption and lower macrophage activation. [13, 14] On the other hand, hydrophobic polymers like PLA and PCL have a tendency to adsorb plasma proteins more easily, which can cause complement activation and neutrophil recruitment, potentially causing a foreign body response.

Another important consideration is charge modulation. While negatively charged or zwitterionic surfaces can decrease inflammatory cell adhesion, positively charged polymers can increase cell adherence by electrostatically interacting with negatively charged cell membranes. By precisely controlling polymer–cell interactions, surface modification procedures including chemical grafting, plasma treatment, or the addition of bioactive ligands maximize immunological compatibility.

In particular, hydrogels high-water content and tissue-mimetic mechanical characteristics promote cell penetration and nutrient absorption. They are frequently used in wound healing, tissue engineering, and medication delivery. Hydrogels can be designed to modify tissue integration, cytokine release, and immune cell adherence by adjusting the crosslinking density, polymer composition, and functional groups. This highlights the significance of polymer chemistry in regulating host response.

2.4.2 Metallic Biomaterials

Metals are indispensable in load-bearing implants, cardiovascular stents, and orthopedic devices due to their high mechanical strength and fatigue resistance. Common metallic biomaterials include titanium, stainless steel, cobalt–chromium alloys, and magnesium-based biodegradable metals.

Because metal deterioration can produce ions that interact with the host immune system, corrosion resistance is an essential characteristic. Because of its passive oxide layer, which restricts ion release and lessens inflammatory responses, titanium has exceptional corrosion resistance. Despite its mechanical strength, stainless steel can corrode locally in situations with a lot of chloride, which can release chromium or nickel ions that cause persistent inflammation or hypersensitivity. Because magnesium alloys are biodegradable, they emit magnesium ions as they break down, which can affect the pH of local tissues and the behavior of immune cells. For temporary implants that resorb gradually and reduce foreign body reactions, controlled degradation of magnesium alloys has been investigated.

By improving corrosion resistance and lowering protein-mediated immune activation, metallic surfaces can be further enhanced through anodization, surface texturing, ion implantation, or coatings. Additionally, surface treatments can add bioactive signals that modulate the macrophage response and enhance osteointegration, such as calcium phosphate layers on titanium.

2.4.3 Ceramic Biomaterials

Because of their low immunogenicity, chemical stability, and bioactivity, ceramics provide special benefits for biomedical applications. They are frequently used in coatings for metallic substrates, dental implants, and bone grafts. Two such examples are bioactive glasses and hydroxyapatite (HA), which imitate natural bone minerals and promote tissue regeneration. Ceramic biomaterials use surface-mediated bioactivity and ionic dissolution to increase biocompatibility. The calcium and phosphate ions that HA releases have the ability to promote angiogenesis, improve matrix deposition, and drive osteoblast differentiation. Soluble ions (such as Si, Ca, and P) released by bioactive glasses alter cellular activity, promoting tissue healing and reducing inflammatory activation.

Under physiological conditions, ceramics typically show little deterioration, which lowers the possibility of foreign body reactions. Their surface roughness and chemistry can also be adjusted to maximize cell adhesion and protein adsorption. Ceramics can promote vascularization and cellular infiltration by regulating porosity and microstructure, which will help to reduce chronic inflammation and assist tissue integration [15, 16].

2.4.4 Composites and Hybrid Materials

Composites increase mechanical performance, bioactivity, and immunological compatibility by combining two or more material types, such as metals, polymers, or ceramics. Both host responsiveness and long-term stability are significantly impacted by the interface characteristics between the component materials. For instance, bone regeneration with little immune activation is made possible by polymer–ceramic composites, which preserve osteoconductive bioactivity from the ceramic phase while supplying mechanical flexibility from the polymer matrix. In a similar vein, metallic substrates covered in ceramic or polymeric layers might enhance tissue integration, lessen inflammation, and minimize ion release.

Composites can have immunomodulatory effects, such encouraging M2 macrophage polarization or regulating cytokine release, by adding fillers, nanoparticles, or bioactive coatings. To prevent delamination, uneven deterioration, or immune cell accumulation at the material junction, which could lead to chronic inflammatory reactions, interface design is essential. Hybrid approaches offer highly tailored solutions for complex clinical applications by concurrently modifying mechanical, chemical, and biological properties.

2.4.4.1 Key Material Properties Influencing Immunogenicity

Composites can have immunomodulatory effects, such encouraging M2 macrophage polarization or regulating cytokine release, by adding fillers, nanoparticles, or bioactive coatings. To avoid delamination, uneven degradation, or immune cell buildup at the material junctional of which could otherwise result in persistent inflammatory responses interface design is crucial. By simultaneously adjusting mechanical, chemical, and biological characteristics, hybrid techniques provide highly personalized solutions for intricate clinical applications. Non-toxic products that either break down naturally or actively alter the immune system must be released by biodegradable materials. Inflammation that is mechanically produced might be brought on by an uneven stiffness between the implant and the surrounding tissue. Stress-induced cytokine release and fibrotic encapsulation are lessened by materials whose mechanical characteristics are more like those of native tissues.

By carefully regulating these variables, biomaterials can balance with the host immune system, reducing negative reactions and encouraging functional integration.

The success of biomedical implants is determined by the interaction of surface features, intrinsic properties, and material type. The chemistry and hydrophilicity of polymeric biomaterials can be adjusted to modify immune cell adherence, whereas metallic biomaterials give mechanical strength while taking corrosion and ion release into account. Ceramics are biocompatible due to their limited inflammatory response and dissolution of bioactive ions, while composites and hybrid materials allow for the synergistic enhancement of biological and mechanical performance [17, 18]. Critical factors influencing immunogenicity in all classes include surface chemistry, roughness, degradation products, and mechanical compliance. The development of next-generation implants and regenerative scaffolds that can coexist with their host environment is advanced by an understanding of these material qualities, which makes it possible to rationally design biomaterials that balance immunomodulation, biofunctionality, and structural integrity.

2.5 Mechanisms and Processes

Designing scaffolds, drug delivery systems, and implants that are safe, effective, and long-lasting requires an understanding of the mechanisms via which biomaterials interact with the host as shown in Fig. 2.1. Acute immune activation, persistent inflammation, and tissue remodeling are all components of the dynamic, multistage host response to biomaterials, which starts as soon as the materials are implanted and changes over time. The local tissue environment, surface characteristics, degradation behavior, and material chemistry all affect these interactions. Targeted immunomodulation can improve integration, reduce problems, and encourage tissue

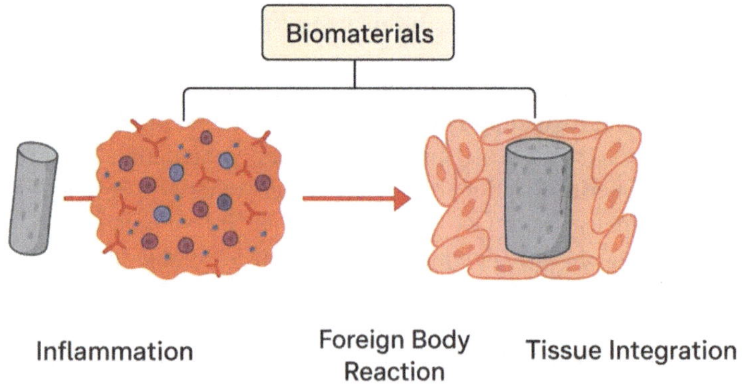

Fig. 2.1 Schematic representation of the host immune response to biomaterial implants, highlighting inflammation, foreign body reaction and tissue integration

regeneration thanks to mechanistic discoveries that serve as the basis for logical biomaterial design.

2.5.1 *Acute Host Response*

The first stage of biological interaction with an implanted biomaterial is known as the acute host response, and it usually happens in a matter of minutes to days. Protein adsorption onto the material surface is among the first things that happen. Proteins including albumin, immunoglobulins, and fibrinogen quickly cover the biomaterial to provide a temporary coating that facilitates further cellular interactions. Because they affect cell adhesion, activation, and inflammatory signaling, the density, content, and shape of this adsorbed protein layer are crucial. Proteins are variably adsorbed by hydrophilic, hydrophobic, charged, or chemically functionalized surfaces, which alters subsequent biological reactions.

Another essential element of the acute response is complementing activation. Opsonins and membrane assault complexes are produced by the complement cascade, specifically through the conventional and alternative pathways. These molecules mark biomaterials for immune recognition and initiate the recruitment of neutrophils and monocytes. Early neutrophil infiltration creates an inflammatory milieu that determines the course of the host response by removing debris, releasing proteolytic enzymes, and secreting reactive oxygen species. The biological interface that controls long-term material integration is created by the combined effects of protein adsorption, complement activation, and the recruitment of first immune cells.

2.5.2 *Chronic Response and Foreign Body Reaction*

A chronic host response, which is marked by continuous inflammation and tissue remodeling, may arise if the acute reaction lasts or if the substance is not biodegradable. During this phase, macrophages continue to play a key role, and extended activation may result in fusion into foreign body giant cells (FBGCs). These multinucleated cells release cytokines, growth factors, and reactive species that influence tissue healing and fibrosis in an effort to phagocytose materials too big for individual macrophages.

The development of a fibrous capsule around the implant is a defining feature of chronic response. The capsule may hinder nutrient transport, integration, and functional performance, especially in tissue-engineered scaffolds or drug delivery systems, even if it can offer mechanical isolation. Prolonged recruitment of lymphocytes, fibroblasts, and endothelial cells is another aspect of chronic inflammation that results in a complicated interaction between tissue remodeling and immune control. Long-term foreign body reactions emphasize how crucial surface modification, material selection, and degradation control are to reducing unfavorable effects. Although the FBR has historically been viewed as a detrimental process requiring mitigation, emerging immunoengineering approaches have reframed the fibrotic capsule as a resource that can be actively harnessed for tissue engineering and disease monitoring, representing a paradigm shift in how biomaterial–host interaction is understood [19].

2.5.3 Cellular and Molecular Immunomodulation

Understanding cellular and molecular immunomodulation is used in the design of modern biomaterials to affect host response. A key factor in determining the outcome is macrophage polarization: M1 macrophages promote tissue-damaging, pro-inflammatory responses, while M2 macrophages aid in angiogenesis, tissue healing, and the deposition of extracellular matrix. Macrophage polarization can be influenced by material characteristics, such as stiffness, surface chemistry, topography, and the presence of bioactive compounds, to promote restorative results. Macrophage polarization represents a fundamental plasticity process in innate immunity, with M1/M2 balance governed by key signaling hubs including NF-κB and JAK–STAT pathways; therapeutic modulation of these pathways through biomaterial-based strategies is now recognised as a promising approach for breaking the cycle of chronic inflammation in non-healing conditions [20].

Cytokine signaling mediates immunological responses in a complementary manner. While anti-inflammatory cytokines like TGF-β and IL-10 promote tissue regeneration and scaffold integration, pro-inflammatory cytokines like TNF-α, IL-1β, and IL-6 enhance immune cell recruitment and fibrosis. Lymphocyte interactions impact humoral and cell-mediated responses, further regulating adaptive immunity and chronic inflammation [21, 22]. Biomaterials can actively control cellular behavior, lower fibrosis and fostering integration, by carefully adding immunomodulatory compounds or bioactive coatings.

2.5.4 Interaction Between Degradation Products and Host Response

Additional complexity is introduced by biodegradable compounds because the degradation products themselves alter the host's reaction. The hydrolysis of polymers including PLA, PLGA, and PCL produces monomers and oligomers that can change the pH of the surrounding area, affect protein adsorption, or stimulate immune cells. Biodegradable metals, such as magnesium alloys, also release ions that can influence osteogenesis, local inflammation, and macrophage polarization. Immobilized peptides or growth factors are examples of surface-modified compounds that can be released gradually and interact with nearby cells to provide controlled biological cues.

These interactions demonstrate how immune response and degradation kinetics are interdependent. While excessively slow degradation can prolong fiber encapsulation and foreign body reactions, rapid degradation may cause localized irritation due to the accumulation of acidic chemicals. Carefully adjusting the material composition, surface chemistry, and structural architecture is necessary for the rational design of degradable biomaterials in order to synchronize degradation with immune regulation and tissue repair.

2.5.5 Mechanistic Models for Predicting Tissue-Material Interactions

Researchers have created computational and mechanistic models of tissue-material interactions in order to forecast and maximize host responses. To replicate both acute and long-term reactions, these models include cytokine signaling, material properties, surface features, and immune cell behavior. To forecast the equilibrium between M1 and M2 phenotypes across time, for example, macrophage polarization models take into account pharmacological and biophysical inputs. The dispersion of degradation products, which affect local pH, ion concentrations, and cellular activity, can also be predicted using diffusion simulations and finite element models.

In order to optimize surface characteristics, degradation rates, and immunomodulatory tactics prior to in vivo testing, high-throughput and multiscale models that integrate molecular dynamics, cellular automata, and tissue-level simulations offer predictive insights for biomaterial design. These methods make it easier to create next-generation biomaterials that are more efficient, safer, and suited to certain tissue conditions.

Acute immune activation, chronic inflammation, cellular communication, and interactions with degradation products are all part of the intricate and multistage mechanisms that underlie immunomodulation, host response, and biocompatibility. Long-term integration is determined by chronic responses like fibrous encapsulation and FBGC development, whereas acute responses like complement activation and protein adsorption prepare the way for immune detection and macrophage recruitment. Actively directing tissue restoration is made possible by cellular and molecular immunomodulation, specifically cytokine signaling and macrophage polarization. Local immune activity is further influenced by degradation products, underscoring the necessity of coordinated material design. Predictive design is now possible because to mechanistic and computational models, which combine biological reactions and material characteristics to maximize results. To bridge the gap between laboratory research and clinical translation, biomaterials must be rationally engineered to attain safe, functional, and regenerative performance. This requires a complete understanding of these processes.

2.6 Design Considerations

Biomaterials must be carefully designed to balance mechanical, chemical, and biological aspects in order to successfully integrate into their host environment. Modern biomaterial design must put tissue-specific functionality, cytotoxicity reduction, and immunocompatibility above bulk characteristics like strength or flexibility. Because the host immune system is extremely sensitive to foreign substances, improper reactions may result in fibrosis, persistent inflammation, or implant failure. A comprehensive surgical perspective on the foreign body response highlights how the biomaterial surface, host physiology, and implantation technique collectively modulate inflammation and fibrous encapsulation, offering practical guidance for implant design and surgical protocol to reduce device-related morbidity [23]. The main design factors that affect biomaterial performance are examined in this part, with a focus on methods to maximize tissue integration and control host response.

2.6.1 Strategies to Minimize Immune Activation and Cytotoxicity

Reducing immune activation and cytotoxicity is a key design objective, making sure that implanted materials don't cause excessive inflammation or cellular damage. This goal can be accomplished in a number of ways; hydrophilic, neutral, or zwitterionic surfaces lessen complement activation and nonspecific protein adsorption, two important factors that stimulate the recruitment of immune cells. For instance, polyethylene glycol (PEG) coatings minimize macrophage activation by forming hydration layers that sterically prevent protein binding.

Processing and material purity: Cytotoxicity or hypersensitivity may be brought on by leftover monomers, catalysts, or impurities. Adverse reaction risk is decreased by ensuring high-purity synthesis and comprehensive post-processing washing. Overly rough nanoscale surfaces can promote the development of foreign body giant cells and macrophage activation. Designers can maintain desired tissue contacts while reducing pro-inflammatory signaling by carefully adjusting surface texture. Materials with a passive baseline of biocompatibility, such zirconia, titanium, or certain ceramics, are naturally resistant to immune activation. When combined, these tactics allow materials to keep a "stealth" profile in relation to the immune system, lowering both acute and long-term inflammatory reactions while maintaining functionality.

2.6.2 *Surface Functionalization to Promote Anti-Inflammatory Responses*

One direct way to affect immune cell activity and encourage anti-inflammatory reactions is through surface functionalization. A bioactive environment that directs host reactions can be created by designers by altering the chemical or physical characteristics of a biomaterial interface.

Interleukin-10 (IL-10) or transforming growth factor-beta (TGF-β) coatings have the ability to promote tissue-repairing M2 polarization and locally inhibit pro-inflammatory macrophage activation (M1). Certain peptides, including laminin-derived sequences or RGD (arginine–glycine–aspartic acid), improve cellular adherence while lowering the activation of inflammatory pathways. Macrophage morphology and function can be selectively influenced by patterns at the micro- and nanoscale. Aligned nanofibers, for instance, can improve fibroblast or endothelial integration and encourage anti-inflammatory phenotypes.

Functionalization allows materials to actively modulate the host environment, rather than simply avoiding immune detection. Such designs are particularly valuable for long-term implants, where persistent inflammation can compromise tissue integration.

2.6.3 *Material Selection Based on Intended Tissue Environment*

The target tissue's mechanical requirements and unique physiological milieu must guide the material selection. Biomaterials must be adapted to the significantly differing needs of soft tissue and bone; To prevent inflammation brought on by stress, materials for skin, vascular, or brain interfaces need to be flexible, have low stiffness, and have little mechanical mismatch. Because of their compliance and capacity to accept tissue deformation without causing foreign body reactions, hydrogels, elastomers, and soft polymer composites are recommended. High mechanical strength, stiffness, and osteoconductivity are required for orthopedic implants. Bioactive ceramics like hydroxyapatite and metals like titanium assist bone repair while maintaining structural integrity. Surface alterations can decrease macrophage-mediated fibrotic encapsulation and promote osteointegration even more [24, 25]. Surface chemistry should be compatible with the cellular and extracellular matrix milieu of the target tissue in addition to its mechanical characteristics. Surfaces rich in calcium and phosphate are advantageous for bone-targeting materials, whereas surfaces that are hemocompatible and anti-thrombogenic are necessary for vascular grafts. By ensuring compatibility with local tissue biomechanics, cellular populations, and regenerating capacity, appropriate material selection lowers the risk of immune-mediated problems.

Appropriate material selection ensures compatibility with local tissue biomechanics, cellular populations, and regenerative capacity, reducing the likelihood of immune-mediated complications.

2.6.4 Incorporation of Immunomodulatory Agents

Biologically active components found in biomaterials offer a controlled method of guiding immune responses and promoting tissue regeneration. These materials can be incorporated in the bulk material, covalently linked to the surface, or combined form degradable carriers. In addition to controlling inflammatory responses, fibroblast growth factor (FGF), vascular endothelial growth factor (VEGF), and bone morphogenetic proteins (BMPs) all encourage tissue-specific cellular proliferation and differentiation. Local delivery of anti-inflammatory cytokines such as TGF-β or IL-10 reduces chronic inflammation and promotes regeneration processes by reorienting macrophage polarization toward M2 phenotypes. Controlled releases of corticosteroids, immunosuppressive drugs, or non-steroidal anti-inflammatory drugs (NSAIDs) may be made to reduce the initial inflammatory reactions following implantation. By combining these substances, biomaterials become active players in immune regulation and tissue healing rather than passive scaffolds, improving integration and therapeutic results.

2.6.5 Design of Degradable Materials to Match Healing Kinetics

In tissue engineering and temporary implants, biodegradable biomaterials are being used more and more. A proper design must minimize potentially inflammatory byproducts while coordinating degradation kinetics with tissue healing. Polymers like poly (lactic-co-glycolic acid) (PLGA) or polycaprolactone can be designed to break down over a period of weeks to months, in accordance with the target tissue's regenerative timeline. Neutral or bioactive metabolites that don't cause undue inflammation must be produced via hydrolytic or enzymatic breakdown. For example, when properly managed, the lactic acid and caproic acid produced by PLA and PCL are often digested without triggering adverse immunological reactions. Advanced methods, such core-shell designs or multilayer coatings, enable staged degradation, revealing bioactive surfaces gradually to encourage tissue healing while initially offering mechanical support. Matching degradation profiles to tissue remodeling rates reduces the risk of chronic inflammation, fibrotic encapsulation, and implant failure.

2.6.6 Sterilization and Processing Considerations Affecting Immune Response

Because sterilization and processing techniques can change surface chemistry, roughness, and residual pollutants, they can have a substantial impact on immune compatibility; Gamma irradiation works well for sterilizing, but it can also cause polymers to oxidize or undergo chain scission, which could result in the production of breakdown products that promote inflammation. Gas sterilization of ethylene oxide (EtO) maintains bulk characteristics, but in order to avoid cytotoxicity, any remaining EtO must be completely removed. Heat-based techniques like autoclaving are good for metals and ceramics, but they can change the mechanical characteristics or surface topography of polymers. Immune activation may be triggered by surface contaminants, unreacted monomers, residual solvents, or processing endotoxins. To preserve immunological compatibility, thorough cleaning, washing, and quality monitoring are necessary.

Designers must integrate sterilization considerations early in the material selection and surface modification process to preserve biofunctionality while ensuring clinical safety. A multifaceted approach that takes into account tissue specificity, immunological compatibility, and functional performance is necessary when designing biomaterials for therapeutic success. One fundamental necessity is to optimize surface chemistry and material purity in order to minimize cytotoxicity and immunological activation. Active immunomodulation is made possible by surface functionalization with anti-inflammatory cues, and harmonious integration is ensured by material selection based on tissue mechanics. Immune control and regeneration potential are further improved by the addition of growth factors, cytokines, and other bioactive substances. Sterilization procedures must maintain surface integrity and biocompatibility, and biodegradable materials must minimize inflammatory byproducts while coordinating with tissue repair kinetics. Biomaterials can accomplish predictable, safe, and therapeutically effective interactions with the host by incorporating these factors, opening the door for next-generation implants and sophisticated regeneration therapies [26].

2.7 Applications and Case Studies

A thorough grasp of immunomodulation, host response, and biocompatibility is essential for transferring biomaterial science from the bench to the clinic. By combining these ideas, biomaterials can be created that actively promote healing, tissue regeneration, and functional restoration rather than just preventing negative reactions. Tissue engineering, orthopedic and dental implants, cardiovascular devices, drug delivery systems, and wound healing are just a few of the biomedical applications where deliberately built materials use immune regulation to maximize results. Case studies and comparative analyses illustrate the practical utility of these strategies and highlight the interplay between material properties, cellular responses, and therapeutic objectives.

2.7.1 *Tissue Engineering*

The combination of immunomodulation and biomaterial design is best demonstrated by tissue engineering scaffolds. In addition to provide structural support, scaffolds made of hydrogels, biodegradable polymers, or composite matrices are designed to actively guide macrophage polarization toward pro-regenerative (M2) phenotypes. For instance, vascularization, extracellular matrix deposition, and tissue integration can all be improved by surface functionalization with bioactive peptides or anti-inflammatory cytokines, which can decrease M1-driven inflammatory responses.

Scaffolds with particular surface chemistry and topology are shown to preferentially attract and polarize macrophages in in vitro experiments, which can impact subsequent osteogenesis, angiogenesis, or skin regeneration. These scaffolds reduce chronic inflammation and fibrosis and expedite tissue repair in vivo, underscoring the significance of immunomodulatory signals in scaffold design. Controlling local immune responses is a major improvement over conventional inert scaffolds and offers a foundation for regenerative therapies of the future.

2.7.2 *Orthopedic and Dental Implants*

Foreign body responses and osseointegration provide difficulties for dental and orthopedic implants. Fibrous encapsulation, inadequate bone integration, or persistent inflammation were frequently the causes of early implant failures. In order to maximize osteointegration and reduce immunological activation, contemporary methods use surface coatings and changes. For example, bioactive ceramics, polymeric layers functionalized with osteogenic peptides, or titanium implants covered with hydroxyapatite promote bone cell adhesion and proliferation while lowering inflammation mediated by macrophages.

It has been demonstrated that nanostructured surfaces, including titanium dioxide nanotubes, alter macrophage behavior, fostering a pro-healing milieu that supports long-term bone integration. In contrast to unaltered controls, immunomodulatory coating-coated implants show improved vascularization, decreased fibrous capsule development, and increased mechanical stability, according to comparative in vivo studies. These results highlight how important surface engineering is in orthopaedic and dental applications for striking a balance between host reaction and functional integration.

2.7.3 Cardiovascular Devices

Stents, grafts, and heart valves are examples of cardiovascular implants that must interact with extremely dynamic settings that are defined by blood flow, shear stress, and immune surveillance. Common side effects from improper host reactions include thrombosis, inflammation, and neointimal hyperplasia. The goal of immunomodulatory techniques is to minimize adverse outcomes by reducing platelet adhesion and promoting endothelialization.

It has been shown that surface coatings containing heparin, nitric oxide-releasing polymers, or peptides that attract endothelial cells are effective at guiding the host response. Studies conducted in vivo reveal decreased leukocyte recruitment, faster endothelium layer development, and inhibition of inflammatory cytokines. These materials actively interact with the immune system to improve patient outcomes and long-term graft patency while also lowering complications.

2.7.4 Drug Delivery Systems

In order to maximize treatment efficacy, immunomodulatory concepts have been increasingly integrated into drug delivery systems. It is possible to design hydrogel-based carriers, liposomes, polymers, and nanoparticles to release medications in a regulated, tissue-specific way while also influencing local immune responses. By delivering cytokines or checkpoint inhibitors to certain tissues, nanoparticle carriers in cancer immunotherapy can promote local immune regulation without causing systemic damage. Similar to this, polymeric carriers made for the long-term release of growth factors in skin or bone regeneration can strike a balance between tissue repair and inflammation. Such immunomodulatory delivery methods operate better than traditional carriers, resulting in improved tissue regeneration, less fibrosis, and regulated inflammatory responses, according to comparative in vitro and in vivo investigations [27].

2.7.5 Wound Healing Applications

Controlling the immune response over time is crucial for wound healing because it strikes a balance between the need for initial inflammation and later tissue restoration. Composite wound matrices, hydrogels, and nanofiber dressings have all been developed to actively alter immune cells, fostering an environment that promotes quicker healing. For instance, hydrophilic dressings containing immobilized anti-inflammatory cytokines promote M2-driven angiogenesis and extracellular matrix deposition while decreasing M1 macrophage dominance in chronic wounds.

Immunomodulatory hydrogels outperform passive dressings in studies utilizing diabetic wound models by improving vascularization, reducing scar formation, and enhancing epithelialization. Through customization of surface characteristics, degradation rate, and release kinetics, these materials offer a dynamic interface between the biomaterial and the host, maximizing cellular penetration and regenerative results. Surface properties of implants including topography, hydrophobicity, and surface charge establish a molecular fingerprint through differential protein adsorption that governs subsequent macrophage polarization, fibrosis, and capsular contracture, underscoring the importance of rational surface design in minimising adverse host responses [28].

2.7.6 Comparative Analysis of In Vivo and In Vitro Outcomes

The significance of assessing immune modulation techniques in both in vitro and in vivo settings is highlighted by translational research. Comprehensive mechanistic investigations, including protein adsorption patterns, cytokine production, and macrophage polarization, are made possible by in vitro tests. Although these findings shed important light on material-cell interactions, they might not adequately convey the intricacy of vascularization, mechanical stressors, or tissue-level immunological responses.

The combined effects of immunomodulatory biomaterials, such as immune cell recruitment, angiogenesis, extracellular matrix deposition, and overall tissue integration, are demonstrated in vivo in animal models or clinical settings. Comparative studies reveal that biomaterials that actively direct host responses regularly produce better results, such as less chronic inflammation, increased tissue regeneration, and longer implant life. These results emphasize the value of a multiscale assessment system that connects tissue and organ-level performance with cellular mechanisms.

Immunomodulation, host response comprehension, and biocompatibility are used in a wide range of biomedical devices and regenerative treatments. Materials that actively engage and modulate the immune system are useful for wound healing applications, cardiovascular devices, orthopedic and dental implants, tissue engineering scaffolds, and drug delivery systems. Case studies show how bioactive coatings, degradable matrices, and logically designed surfaces can influence macrophage polarization, lower chronic inflammation, and encourage regenerative healing converting mechanistic discoveries into practical applications. The production of next-generation biomaterials that are safe, functional, and regenerative is made possible by the integration of material science, immunology, and engineering concepts, as demonstrated by comparative in vitro and in vivo investigations. Combining immunomodulatory techniques with tailored and flexible design holds potential for improving treatment results and patient-specific biomaterial performance as the field develops.

2.8 Recent Advances and Innovations

Recent decades have seen a revolutionary development in the field of biomaterials, propelled by developments in surface engineering, nanotechnology, computer modeling, and regenerative medicine. Conventional biomaterials prioritized mechanical and chemical stability and were largely intended to be inert or minimally reactive. However, recent developments have a strong emphasis on actively modifying host responses, which makes it possible for biomaterials to direct immune behavior, encourage tissue regeneration, and improve therapeutic results [29]. These developments signal a move toward intelligent, patient-specific biomaterials that dynamically interact with biological systems and demonstrate the confluence of materials science, immunology, and bioengineering.

2.8.1 Nanotechnology and Surface Engineering

Emerging evidence demonstrates that physical cues from biomaterials including scaffold porosity, stiffness, topography, and fibre geometry are potent regulators of macrophage polarization in bone regeneration, with softer, aligned, or nanopatterned surfaces favouring M2-driven anti-inflammatory and osteogenic responses [30]. Protein adsorption, cell adhesion, and immune cell activation are all significantly impacted by the exact manipulation of surface topography made possible by nanotechnology, which has completely changed the design of biomaterials. By modifying macrophage behavior, nanopatterning techniques including nanopillars, nanogrooves, and nanotubes can increase M2 polarization and reduce pro-inflammatory reactions. Similarly, targeted bioactive cues can be delivered while preserving mechanical stability by incorporating nanoparticles into surfaces.

Nanoscale hydroxyapatite coatings and titanium dioxide nanotubes have been demonstrated to improve osteoblast adhesion and decrease macrophage-mediated inflammation in dental and orthopedic implants. Nanoscale surface roughness in cardiovascular devices can reduce complement activation and platelet adhesion, reducing the risk of thrombosis. These developments demonstrate how nanotechnology may precisely regulate host-material interactions, offering a platform for regenerative and immunomodulatory effects.

2.8.2 Bioactive and Immunomodulatory Coatings

Protein adsorption, cell adhesion, and immune cell activation are all significantly impacted by the exact manipulation of surface topography made possible by nanotechnology, which has completely changed the design of biomaterials. By modifying macrophage behavior, nanopatterning techniques including nanopillars, nanogrooves, and nanotubes can increase M2 polarization and reduce pro-inflammatory reactions. Similarly, targeted bioactive cues can be delivered while preserving mechanical stability by incorporating nanoparticles into surfaces.

Covalent immobilization, smart polymer matrices, and layer-by-layer assembly provide temporal and geographical control of bioactive release, guaranteeing that immune modulation takes place during crucial stages of tissue regeneration. While hydrogel dressings in wound healing offer both antimicrobial protection and immune-guiding signals, bioactive coatings in cardiovascular stents encourage endothelialization while reducing leukocyte adherence. These methods show how immunomodulation and surface engineering can work together to transform biomaterials from passive scaffolds into active players in tissue regeneration.

2.8.3 Personalized Immunomodulation

By creating scaffolds, implants, and coatings that are unique to each patient, personalized medicine has spread into the biomaterials industry. Implants that are customized to each patient's unique anatomical and immunological characteristics can be made because to developments in 3D printing, additive manufacturing, and computational imaging. These materials can anticipate changes in immune response by integrating patient-specific cellular and molecular cues, lowering the likelihood of rejection, fibrosis, or inflammation.

For instance, scaffold responses can be tested in vitro using patient-derived immune cells, which helps designers create coatings that maximize lymphocyte contacts and macrophage polarization. By functionalizing customized scaffolds with bioactive substances that correspond to the patient's ability for regeneration, tissue engineering can improve vascularization, matrix deposition, and functional integration. Immunomodulatory techniques are guaranteed to be efficient and customized to each patient's unique biological circumstances according to this precise approach.

2.8.4 Computational Modeling and Artificial Intelligence

The design of biomaterials now includes predictive capacities thanks to the combination of artificial intelligence (AI) and computer modeling. Based on material characteristics, surface chemistry, and shape, machine learning algorithms and multiscale models describe biological behavior, protein adsorption, and immunological responses. These techniques lessen the need for trial-and-error experimentation by enabling the logical optimization of immunomodulatory biomaterials before in vivo testing.

Likewise, bioactive compound release kinetics, tissue integration results, and degradation profiles can all be estimated by AI-driven simulations. By enabling quicker design cycles, these computational techniques provide light on the intricate, multifaceted relationships that exist between biomaterials and the host immune system. AI increases the effectiveness and efficiency of biomaterial creation by facilitating data-driven decision-making.

2.8.5 Integration with Regenerative Medicine

Regenerative medicine, which aims to restore biological activity and functional architecture rather than just replace tissue, is closely related to recent developments in biomaterials. In order to guide inflammation, angiogenesis, and extracellular matrix deposition in tandem with tissue regeneration, immunomodulatory materials are presently developed to coordinate host responses. In order to achieve functional tissue repair, scaffolds in bone and cartilage engineering, for instance, combine immunomodulatory coatings with breakdown kinetics to coordinate matrix deposition and cell infiltration.

Materials designed for organ-specific uses, such brain scaffolds or cardiac patches, are made to reduce pro-inflammatory signals and encourage the growth of regenerative cell populations. The host immune system actively engages in the healing process rather than impeding it thanks to the combination of nanotechnology, bioactive coatings, and customized design. Coordinated immunomodulation dramatically increases tissue regeneration, decreases fibrosis, and extends implant longevity, according to comparative studies.

Through the integration of nanotechnology, bioactive coatings, tailored design, computational modeling, and the concepts of regenerative medicine, recent developments in biomaterials have changed the paradigm from passive biocompatibility to active immunomodulation. Bioactive coatings allow for the regulated release of immunoregulatory drugs, whereas nano-engineered surfaces alter the polarization and adherence of immune cells. Personalized scaffolds and implants improve safety and efficacy by matching material design to patient-specific immune profiles.

Predictive insights provided by AI and computational tools speed up material development and improve host interactions. These developments facilitate coordinated host responses that support tissue regeneration, lessen adverse effects, and enhance long-term results when paired with regenerative medicine techniques [31]. When taken as a whole, these developments mark a revolutionary shift in biomaterial design, as materials actively interact with the body to promote therapeutic success rather than just being tolerated by it.

2.9 Challenges and Limitations

Many obstacles still stand in the way of the clinical translation and reliable performance of biocompatible and immunomodulatory biomaterials, despite tremendous advancements in their design as shown in Fig. 2.2. Both researchers and doctors

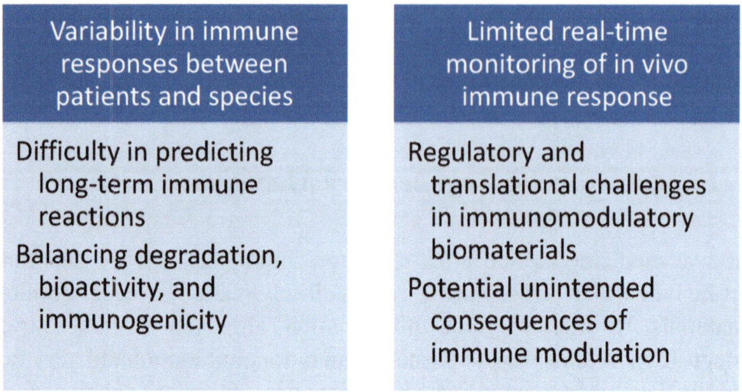

Fig. 2.2 Schematic illustration of the major challenges and limitations associated with biocompatibility, host response, and immunomodulation, including interpatient immune variability, difficulty in predicting long-term reactions, balancing degradation with bioactivity, limited real-time monitoring, regulatory constraints, and potential unintended immune effects

face challenges because to the intricacy of host-material interactions, interpatient variability, degradation dynamics, and regulatory barriers. Comprehending these constraints is crucial for directing forthcoming biomaterial advancements, enhancing security, and attaining consistent therapeutic results.

2.9.1 *Variability in Immune Responses Between Patients and Species*

The variability of immune responses among patients and species is one of the main obstacles in the field of immunomodulatory biomaterials. Although animal models are frequently used in preclinical research, immune systems vary greatly among species in terms of inflammatory signaling pathways, cytokine patterns, and cell populations. For example, T-cell activity and macrophage polarization dynamics shown in rodent models might not precisely represent human reactions, which could result in an overestimation or underestimating of biocompatibility and regeneration potential.

Genetic diversity, age, comorbidities, and previous antigen exposure can all lead to different immune responses to the same biomaterial, even in human patients. Because of these variations, it is challenging to predict both acute and chronic responses, which makes extrapolating results from one cohort to another challenging. Because of this, biomaterial design needs to take patient-specific immunological variability into consideration. This can be done by preclinical screening with human-derived cells and tissue models, customized coatings, or flexible materials.

2.9.2 Difficulty in Predicting Long-Term Immune Reactions

Long-term immune responses are still difficult to anticipate, despite the relative ease with which acute host responses may be tracked and described. Over the course of months or years, fibrous encapsulation, foreign body responses, and chronic inflammation may arise, endangering the longevity and functionality of implants [32]. Long-term forecasts are made more difficult by the possibility that degradation products, especially those derived from biodegradable metals or polymers, may build up and cause delayed immune activation. The temporal and dynamic characteristics of in vivo responses are frequently not captured by current in vitro models. Long-term replication of the human immunological milieu is impossible, even with highly advanced animal models. Due to this unpredictability, lengthy preclinical research, post-implantation monitoring, and backup design techniques are required, which lengthens the development period and raises costs.

2.9.3 Balancing Degradation, Bioactivity, and Immunogenicity

It is difficult to balance controlled degradation, functional bioactivity, and low immunogenicity when designing biomaterials. While slow-decaying materials may prolong foreign body reactions, rapidly degrading scaffolds may release bioactive or acidic byproducts too fast, causing tissue damage or inflammation. Likewise, surface alterations and bioactive coatings intended to improve tissue regeneration or cell adhesion may unintentionally cause immunological activation or hypersensitivity. A multifaceted adjustment of the material composition, surface chemistry, degradation kinetics, and structural architecture is necessary to achieve this equilibrium. The sensitive relationship between material design and host response is highlighted by the possibility of suboptimal healing, implant failure, or long-term problems if these elements are not appropriately integrated.

2.9.4 Limited Real-Time Monitoring of In Vivo Immune Response

The lack of real-time in vivo host response monitoring is a significant drawback of immunomodulatory biomaterials. The majority of evaluations rely on imaging, biomarker measurement, or histological analysis at specific times, which might not be able to detect fast immunological fluctuations or dynamic cellular function. Adjusting material qualities or therapeutic interventions in response to changing immune reactions is made more difficult by this lack of real-time understanding. Although they are still in the early stages of development, emerging techniques including wearable diagnostic platforms, biosensors, and molecular imaging provide possible solutions. The safety and efficacy of immunomodulatory biomaterials mostly depend on preclinical models and post-implantation observation until real-time monitoring is practical, which may overlook mild or delayed adverse effects.

2.9.5 *Regulatory and Translational Challenges in Immunomodulatory Biomaterials*

Since immunomodulatory biomaterials actively engage with the immune system rather than passively existing in the body, their regulatory routes are intricate and frequently unclear. For implants that produce cytokines, bioactive substances, or immunomodulatory coatings, conventional safety evaluations for inert implants might not be adequate. Regulatory bodies need thorough assessments of systemic toxicity, degradation byproducts, biocompatibility, and both immediate and long-term immunological effects. Manufacturing scalability, repeatability, and cost limitations further expand the translational gap between laboratory innovation and clinical application. It can be difficult to reliably generate customized coatings, nanopatterning, and advanced surface alterations at industrial scale, which could postpone clinical adoption. Researchers, physicians, regulators, and manufacturers must work together to create standards and expedite approval processes in order to overcome these obstacles.

2.9.6 *Potential Unintended Consequences of Immune Modulation*

Although immunomodulatory techniques have potential, there is a chance that they could have unforeseen repercussions. Suppressing pro-inflammatory pathways in an attempt to encourage tissue regeneration may unintentionally make people more vulnerable to infection or make it more difficult to get rid of pathogens. Likewise, excessive tissue development, fibrosis, or abnormal remodeling may result from overactivation of regenerative signals. Therefore, it's crucial to strike a balance between immune activation and repression, which calls for exact control over the dosage, time, and location of immunomodulatory drugs. In order to minimize systemic effects and respond dynamically to the host environment, advanced biomaterials must be engineered to provide cues only when necessary. This emphasizes the necessity of thorough preclinical testing and flexible design techniques to reduce the possibility of unfavorable results.

There are many obstacles and restrictions in the development and therapeutic application of immunomodulatory biomaterials. Material design is complicated by interpatient and interspecies diversity, erratic long-term immune responses, and the intricate interactions between immunogenicity, bioactivity, and degradation. Translation is further limited by real-time monitoring limitations, regulatory uncertainty, and possible unforeseen repercussions. A interdisciplinary strategy combining materials science, immunology, computer modeling, and clinical knowledge is needed to overcome these obstacles. Notwithstanding these challenges, the safe, efficient, and predictable use of next-generation immunomodulatory biomaterials that may actively direct tissue repair and regeneration is anticipated to be made possible by meticulous design, sophisticated monitoring methods, and iterative testing [33].

2.10 Future Directions

Rapid advancements in biomaterials are pushing the industry away from conventional biocompatibility paradigms and toward dynamic, intelligent, and immunomodulatory designs. Materials that can predictably react to environmental stimuli, actively engage with the host immune system, and smoothly integrate with tissue-specific healing processes are the focus of current study. With an emphasis on advancements in smart materials, computational modeling, immunoengineering, biomimicry, real-time monitoring, and sustainable development, this section examines important future directions in biomaterial design.

2.10.1 Development of Smart, Responsive, and Adaptive Biomaterials

Intelligent and flexible systems that can instantly alter immune responses are a key trend in next-generation biomaterials. Conventional biomaterials are mostly passive and reduce negative reactions by depending on intrinsic surface characteristics. Conversely, sensitive biomaterials react to local physiological cues such pH shifts, oxidative stress, or enzymatic activity by dynamically modifying their characteristics, such as stiffness, topography, or ligand presentation.

In response to macrophage-derived proteases, hydrogels embedded with enzyme-cleavable linkers, for instance, can release anti-inflammatory drugs, therefore encouraging an M2 phenotype and lowering chronic inflammation. In order to direct cell adherence and reduce fibrotic encapsulation, shape-memory polymers and stimuli-responsive coatings can change the wettability or surface geometry. These substances make it possible to regulate immunological interactions both spatially and temporally, coordinating material behavior with the host's healing process.

The development of such adaptive systems represents a shift toward "immune-aware" biomaterials, which do not merely avoid detection but actively participate in orchestrating favorable host responses.

2.10.2 Integration of AI and Machine Learning for Predictive Immune Response Modeling

Immunomodulatory biomaterials by offering forecasts about interactions between the material and its host [34]. The intricacy of immune responses, which include cellular signaling, tissue remodeling, and cytokine networks, makes empirical methods inadequate for material optimization. Immune activation, cytokine release, and tissue integration can all be predicted by machine learning models that have been trained on datasets of biomaterial characteristics, surface chemistry, topography, and in vivo results. These predictive frameworks enable the logical design of materials that minimize negative reactions while striking a balance between bioactivity and immunological tolerance. Optimization is accelerated through integration with high-throughput screening, which lessens the need for expensive and time-consuming animal research. AI-guided modeling also makes it easier to choose customized biomaterials, allowing for the creation of devices that are suited to the immunological profiles, genetic predispositions, or illness conditions of individual patients. This strategy aids in the creation of precise regeneration treatments that are safer and more effective.

2.10.3 Exploration of Immunoengineering for Personalized Regenerative Therapies

One of the main areas of regenerative medicine is immunoengineering, which is the intentional manipulation of immune responses through material design. The goal of immunoengineering is to direct the host response toward tissue healing rather than chronic inflammation by fusing materials science, cellular biology, and immunology. Future uses could involve patient-specific scaffolds designed to precisely administer growth factors, chemokines, or cytokines based on each patient's unique immunological profile. For instance, depending on the patient's immunological condition and potential for healing, a scaffold for bone regeneration may be created to encourage osteogenic differentiation and M2 macrophage polarization. Precision and effectiveness are further increased by combining immunoengineering with stem cell therapies and gene editing technologies. This allows for regenerative implants that are not only structurally supportive but also actively therapeutic, interacting with host immune signaling pathways.

2.10.4 Advanced Biomimetic Surfaces to Mimic Natural Tissue Interfaces

The key to improving tissue integration and immunological tolerance is biomimetic surface engineering. Biomaterials can direct cellular function and lessen foreign body reactions by mimicking the topography, architecture, and molecular cues of the extracellular matrix (ECM).

Natural tissue-inspired nanotopographies, including basement membrane structures or collagen fibers, enable protein adsorption patterns that support endothelialization and regenerative macrophage phenotypes. By modifying integrin clustering, cellular alignment, and mechanotransduction, hierarchical micro- and nanoscale features can enhance tissue-specific results. Additionally, bioactive ligands can be spatially presented thanks to advanced biomimetic coatings, which regulate immune cell activation and cell adhesion in a location-specific way. By facilitating the smooth integration of biomaterials with host tissue, these developments improve immunological and structural compatibility.

2.10.5 Long-Term In Vivo Monitoring and Feedback Systems

Embedded sensors and feedback systems will be used more frequently in future biomaterials to track host reactions in real time. Conventional assessment uses periodic imaging or ex vivo analysis, which offers little understanding of the dynamic tissue-material interaction. Biosensors that can measure pH, oxidative stress, mechanical strain, or local cytokine concentrations are part of emerging technologies that can continuously provide information on the host reaction. When combined with responsive material platforms, these systems can initiate structural modifications or the on-demand release of immunomodulatory drugs, preserve optimal integration and reducing negative reactions. These closed-loop technologies allow for adaptive implants that, over time, adjust to the biology of each patient, lowering problems and improving regenerative results. Instead of being passive structural supports, biomaterials become active players in patient care when monitoring and actuation are combined.

2.10.6 Sustainable and Biodegradable Immunomodulatory Materials

In the development of biomaterials, sustainability is becoming more and more important. Biodegradable, ecologically friendly, and minimally systemic-impact materials are prioritized in future designs. In order to decrease systemic exposure and long-term foreign body reactions, biodegradable polymers and composites can be designed to break down into non-toxic metabolites while also influencing local immune responses. Green synthesis methods that save energy and chemical waste, including solvent-free polymerization or biomimetic mineralization, let materials be designed with the environment and regulations in mind. Natural polymers like collagen, chitosan, or alginate can also be used to integrate intrinsic bioactivity while lowering synthetic byproducts that could trigger immunological response. Regenerative treatments are both efficient and environmentally friendly thanks to sustainable, immunomodulatory ingredients that combine clinical utility with environmental responsibility.

Sustainable, immunomodulatory materials combine environmental responsibility with clinical functionality, ensuring that regenerative therapies are both effective and ecologically compatible. Intelligent, flexible, and patient-centered designs that actively interact with the host immune system will characterize the future of biomaterials. Better integration and less chronic inflammation are promised by intelligent, responsive materials that can modulate immune responses both spatially and temporally. Predictive modeling of immunological interactions is made possible by the use of AI and machine learning, which speeds up logical design and allows for the customization of regenerative treatments [35]. Biomimetic surfaces mimic natural tissue interfaces to improve tolerance and functional results, whereas immunoengineering techniques enable precise control of immune cell behavior. Implants can become active, adaptive therapeutic devices thanks to materials that can dynamically react to in vivo signals thanks to real-time monitoring and feedback systems. Lastly, long-term ecological and clinical compatibility is guaranteed by sustainable and biodegradable biomaterials, which aid in the creation of next-generation regeneration solutions. When taken as a whole, these paths signify a paradigm change in precision regenerative medicine from passive biocompatibility to active, intelligent, and ecologically conscious biomaterial design.

2.11 Conclusion

The integration, performance, and durability of scaffolds, drug delivery systems, and medical implants are all influenced by biocompatibility and host reaction, which continue to be key factors in biomaterial success. The capacity of a material to interact with biological systems without causing negative reactions is a crucial prerequisite for therapeutic utility, not just a desired property. Tissue integration, fibrosis, and implant longevity are all directly impacted by the host response, which includes acute immune activation, persistent inflammation, and tissue remodeling. Comprehending these interplays offers crucial direction for the logical development of safe and efficient biomaterials. Therapeutic success is determined by the interaction between material qualities and host biology in a variety of applications, including tissue engineering, orthopedic, cardiovascular, and wound healing devices.

2.11.1 Central Role of Biocompatibility and Host Response

Beyond passive tolerance, biocompatibility includes dynamic interactions with immunological mediators, proteins, and cells. A biological interface is created by the first protein adsorption, immune cell recruitment, and complement activation, which determines the course for integration and healing. Long-term results are then determined by lymphocyte signaling, macrophage activity, and chronic reactions like fibrous encapsulation. Failure to take these processes into consideration may lead to implant rejection, fibrosis, or inflammation. Predictable host reactions are therefore given top priority in the development of contemporary biomaterials, which strike a balance between cellular compatibility and mechanical and chemical stability. Designers can predict possible issues and maximize biomaterial performance in a variety of physiological settings by combining knowledge from immunology, materials science, and tissue biology.

2.11.2 Immunomodulation as a Strategy for Regeneration

Immunomodulation is a potent tactic to actively reduce inflammation and encourage tissue regeneration, according to recent developments. Immunomodulatory biomaterials direct host responses to favor regeneration pathways rather than just avoiding immune activation. By using strategies including surface nanostructuring, cytokine delivery, bioactive coatings, and macrophage polarization, materials can balance pro-inflammatory and anti-inflammatory signals and coordinate local immune activity. These methods have shown promise in improving cellular infiltration, angiogenesis, and extracellular matrix deposition in tissue-engineered scaffolds, cardiovascular devices, wound healing applications, and drug delivery systems. Biomaterials that are passive implants can become dynamic, educational platforms that actively shape tissue healing and functional integration through immunomodulation.

2.11.3 Interdisciplinary Integration in Biomaterial Design

Engineering, materials science, and biology must work together harmoniously to create immunomodulatory biomaterials that work. While materials science gives control over chemistry, degradation, and surface characteristics, biological knowledge guides the selection of molecular cues, immunological targets, and regenerative techniques. The precise manufacture, structural integrity, and spatial-temporal control of bioactive release are made possible by engineering concepts. When combined, these fields make it easier to develop biomaterials that work consistently with intricate host systems, taking into account variations in tissue healing dynamics and immunological responses. Multidisciplinary cooperation is crucial for both innovation and converting lab results into treatments that may be used in clinical settings.

2.11.4 Outlook Toward Adaptive, Patient-Centered Biomaterials

In the future, the field is heading toward biomaterials that are regenerative, patient-centered, and adaptive. Developments in computer modeling, nanotechnology, and additive manufacturing enable the development of scaffolds and implants that are customized to each patient's unique immunological and anatomical characteristics. In order to maximize integration and healing, these materials can adapt their degradation rates, bioactive release, or surface cues in real time to changes in the host environment. Coordinated tissue repair is made possible by integration with regenerative medicine techniques, which guarantee that host responses are stimulated rather than inhibited. In order to bridge the gap between material design and patient-specific treatment outcomes, the next generation of biomaterials will be intelligent, responsive, and personalized.

Integrity, longevity, and therapeutic efficacy are all determined by biocompatibility and host reaction, which are essential to biomaterial performance and clinical success. A game-changing tactic that allows materials to actively regulate inflammation and direct regeneration is immunomodulation. In order to accomplish these goals, interdisciplinary cooperation is needed, integrating knowledge from engineering, materials science, and biology. Adaptive, patient-specific biomaterials that react dynamically to the host environment and balance regenerative and immunological processes are the way of the future. As these technologies advance, they have the potential to completely alter the field of regenerative therapies and medical implants by providing materials that are not only absorbed by the body but also actively contribute to the restoration of tissue health and function.

References

1. Crawford, L., Wyatt, M., Bryers, J., Ratner, B.: Biocompatibility evolves: phenomenology to toxicology to regeneration. Adv. Healthc. Mater. **10**(11), 2002153 (2021)
2. Shariati, K., Ling, A.S., Fuchs, S., Dillenburger, B., Liu, W., Ma, M.: Hylozoic by design: converging material and biological complexities for cell-driven living materials with 4D behaviors. Adv. Funct. Mater. **32**(7), 2108057 (2022)
3. Batool, F., Özçelik, H., Stutz, C., Gegout, P.Y., Benkirane-Jessel, N., Petit, C., Huck, O.: Modulation of immune-inflammatory responses through surface modifications of biomaterials to promote bone healing and regeneration. J. Tissue Eng. **12**, 20417314211041428 (2021)
4. Whitaker, R., Hernaez-Estrada, B., Hernandez, R.M., Santos-Vizcaino, E., Spiller, K.L.: Immunomodulatory biomaterials for tissue repair. Chem. Rev. **121**(18), 11305–11335 (2021)

5. Revete, A., Aparicio, A., Cisterna, B.A., Revete, J., Luis, L., Ibarra, E., Segura González, E.A., Molino, J., Reginensi, D.: Advancements in the use of hydrogels for regenerative medicine: properties and biomedical applications. Int. J. Biomater. **2022**(1), 3606765 (2022)
6. Williams, D.F.: Assessing the triad of biocompatibility, medical device functionality and biological safety. Med. Devices Sens. **4**(1), e10150 (2021)
7. Alshangiti, D.M., El-Damhougy, T.K., Zaher, A.a., Madani, M.: Revolutionizing biomedicine: advancements, applications, and prospects of nanocomposite macromolecular carbohydrate-based hydrogel biomaterials: a review. RSC Adv. **13**(50), 35251–35291 (2023)
8. Wang, B., Kostarelos, K., Nelson, B.J., Zhang, L.: Trends in micro−/nanorobotics: materials development, actuation, localization, and system integration for biomedical applications. Adv. Mater. **33**(4), 2002047 (2021)
9. Ferraz, M.P.: Bone grafts in dental medicine: an overview of autografts, allografts and synthetic materials. Materials. **16**(11), 4117 (2023)
10. Pupilli, F., Ruffini, A., Dapporto, M., Tavoni, M., Tampieri, A., Sprio, S.: Design strategies and biomimetic approaches for calcium phosphate scaffolds in bone tissue regeneration. Biomimetics. **7**(3), 112 (2022)
11. Kabirian, F., Mozafari, M., Mela, P., Heying, R.: Incorporation of controlled release systems improves the functionality of biodegradable 3D printed cardiovascular implants. ACS Biomater. Sci. Eng. **9**(11), 5953–5967 (2023)
12. Zhong, J.X., Raghavan, P., Desai, T.A.: Harnessing biomaterials for immunomodulatory-driven tissue engineering. Regen. Eng. Transl. Med. **9**(2), 224–239 (2023)
13. Drobota, M., Ursache, S., Aflori, M.: Surface functionalities of polymers for biomaterial applications. Polymers. **14**(12), 2307 (2022)
14. Panico, S., Capolla, S., Bozzer, S., Toffoli, G., Dal Bo, M., Macor, P.: Biological features of nanoparticles: protein corona formation and interaction with the immune system. Pharmaceutics. **14**(12), 2605 (2022)
15. Chen, Z., Xing, F., Zhou, Y., Yu, P., Xu, J., Luo, R., Zhou, C., Xiang, Z., Rommens, P.M., Liu, M., Ritz, U.: Integrated osteoimmunomodulatory strategies based on designing scaffold surface properties in bone regeneration. J. Mater. Chem. B. **11**(29), 6718–6745 (2023)
16. Hernandez, J.L., Woodrow, K.A.: Medical applications of porous biomaterials: features of porosity and tissue-specific implications for biocompatibility. Adv. Healthc. Mater. **11**(9), 2102087 (2022)
17. Barreto, M.E., Medeiros, R.P., Shearer, A., Fook, M.V., Montazerian, M., Mauro, J.C.: Gelatin and bioactive glass composites for tissue engineering: a review. J. Func. Biomater. **14**(1), 23 (2022)
18. Kumari, S., Katiyar, S., Darshna, Anand, A., Singh, D., Singh, B.N., Mallick, S.P., Mishra, A., Srivastava, P.: Design strategies for composite matrix and multifunctional polymeric scaffolds with enhanced bioactivity for bone tissue engineering. Front. Chem. **10**, 1051678 (2022)
19. Oakes, R.S., Morris, A.H.: Don't judge an implant by its cover: how the foreign body response and fibrotic capsule might be harnessed for good. Npj Biomed. Innov. **3**, 3 (2026). https://doi.org/10.1038/s44385-025-00053-7
20. Zhang, Y., Liu, R., Chen, M.: Macrophage polarization: molecular mechanisms, disease implications, and targeted therapeutic strategies. Front. Immunol. **16**, 1732718 (2025). https://doi.org/10.3389/fimmu.2025.1732718
21. Gray, K.J., Gibbs, J.E.: Adaptive immunity, chronic inflammation and the clock. In: Seminars in immunopathology (Vol. 44, No. 2), pp. 209–224. Springer Berlin Heidelberg, Berlin/Heidelberg (2022)
22. Sonnenberg, G.F., Hepworth, M.R.: Functional interactions between innate lymphoid cells and adaptive immunity. Nat. Rev. Immunol. **19**(10), 599–613 (2019)
23. Kalashnikov, A., Vorstenbosch, J.: Implantable medical devices, biomaterials, and the foreign body response: a surgical perspective. J. Biomed. Mater. Res. A. **113**(9), e37983 (2025). https://doi.org/10.1002/jbm.a.37983

24. Dong, J., Wang, W., Zhou, W., Zhang, S., Li, M., Li, N., Pan, G., Zhang, X., Bai, J., Zhu, C.: Immunomodulatory biomaterials for implant-associated infections: from conventional to advanced therapeutic strategies. Biomater. Res. **26**(1), 72 (2022)
25. Mofarrah, M., Jafari-Gharabaghlou, D., Farhoudi-Sefidan-Jadid, M., Zarghami, N.: Potential application of inorganic nano-materials in modulation of macrophage function: possible application in bone tissue engineering. Heliyon. **9**(6), e16309 (2023)
26. Bashor, C.J., Hilton, I.B., Bandukwala, H., Smith, D.M., Veiseh, O.: Engineering the next generation of cell-based therapeutics. Nat. Rev. Drug Discov. **21**(9), 655–675 (2022)
27. Kim, B., Pradhan, L., Hernandez, A., Yenurkar, D., Nethi, S.K., Mukherjee, S.: Current advances in immunomodulatory biomaterials for cell therapy and tissue engineering. Adv. Ther. **6**(8), 2300002 (2023)
28. Dzobo, K., Wilgus, T.A., Zamora Mora, V., Zoncsich, A., de Mezerville, R., Khumalo, N., Bayat, A.: Biomimetic optimization of silicone breast implant integration: insights into wound healing and the foreign body response. Front. Bioeng. Biotechnol. **13**, 1668930 (2025). https://doi.org/10.3389/fbioe.2025.1668930
29. Mariani, E., Lisignoli, G., Borzì, R.M., Pulsatelli, L.: Biomaterials: foreign bodies or tuners for the immune response? Int. J. Mol. Sci. **20**(3), 636 (2019)
30. Yang, T., Fang, Z., Zhang, J., Zheng, S.: Physical cues in biomaterials modulate macrophage polarization for bone regeneration: a review. Front. Bioeng. Biotechnol. **13**, 1640560 (2025). https://doi.org/10.3389/fbioe.2025.1640560
31. Vasconcelos, D.P., Águas, A.P., Barbosa, M.A., Pelegrín, P., Barbosa, J.N.: The inflammasome in host response to biomaterials: bridging inflammation and tissue regeneration. Acta Biomater. **83**, 1–12 (2019)
32. Capuani, S., Malgir, G., Chua, C.Y.X., Grattoni, A.: Advanced strategies to thwart foreign body response to implantable devices. Bioeng. Transl. Med. **7**(3), e10300 (2022)
33. Sánchez, C., Schneider, G., Ahrendt, W., Bartocci, E., Bianculli, D., Colombo, C., Falcone, Y., Francalanza, A., Krstić, S., Lourenço, J.M., Nickovic, D.: A survey of challenges for runtime verification from advanced application domains (beyond software). Form. Methods Syst. Des. **54**(3), 279–335 (2019)
34. Ana, G., Cockrella, C., Zamorab, R., Vodovotzb, Y.: Machine learning and mechanistic computational modeling of inflammation as tools for designing immunomodulatory biomaterials. In: Immunomodulatory Biomaterials: Regulating the Immune Response with Biomaterials to Affect Clinical Outcome, p. 251. Elsevier (2021)
35. Suwardi, A., Wang, F., Xue, K., Han, M.Y., Teo, P., Wang, P., Wang, S., Liu, Y., Ye, E., Li, Z., Loh, X.J.: Machine learning-driven biomaterials evolution. Adv. Mater. **34**(1), 2102703 (2022)

Chapter 3
Degradation and Stability of Biomaterials

Abstract The performance, safety, and long-term usefulness of biomaterials in biomedical applications are significantly influenced by their stability and rate of degradation. While stability refers to a material's ability to withstand these changes over time, degradation refers to the physical, chemical, and biological processes that gradually change a material's structure and characteristics within physiological settings. The success of drug delivery systems, scaffolds, implants, and other medical devices is determined by the balance between these two factors. Polymers, ceramics, and composites are examples of biodegradable materials that are designed to break down in a regulated way in accordance with therapeutic or tissue regeneration schedules. On the other hand, to guarantee extended compatibility and functionality without unfavorable reactions, permanent materials need to possess remarkable chemical and mechanical stability. The processes that cause degradation hydrolysis, oxidation, enzymatic attack, and mechanical fatigue are influenced by both extrinsic variables like pH, temperature, and enzyme activity as well as intrinsic variables like molecular structure, crystallinity, and crosslinking density. By comprehending these relationships, material design, surface modification, and composite engineering may precisely regulate the kinetics of degradation. Developments in analytical methods, including spectroscopy, microscopy, and computer modeling, have expanded our understanding of failure mechanisms and degradation processes at both the molecular and macroscopic levels. The goal of recent developments, such as intelligent and self-healing biomaterials, is to improve stability and functionality by incorporating responsiveness and adaptability into material systems. Accurately forecasting in vivo degradation, converting lab results into clinical performance, and guaranteeing consistency in various biological settings are still difficult tasks, nevertheless. Future research will concentrate on developing bioinspired, multi-responsive materials that integrate mechanical integrity with dynamic degradability to align material lifespans with therapeutic needs. Ultimately, the advancement of safe, efficient, and regenerative biomaterials for modern medicine is fundamentally reliant on optimizing the degradation-stability continuum.

M. Adeoba, T. Pandelani, *Application of Biomaterials in Biomedical Engineering*, Series in BioEngineering,
https://doi.org/10.1007/978-3-032-34477-9_3

3.1 Introduction

The goal of recent developments, such as intelligent and self-healing biomaterials, is to improve stability and functionality by incorporating responsiveness and adaptability into material systems. Accurately forecasting in vivo degradation, converting lab results into clinical performance, and guaranteeing consistency in various biological settings are still difficult tasks, nevertheless. To match material lifespans with therapeutic requirements, future research will focus on creating bioinspired, multi-responsive materials that combine mechanical integrity and dynamic degradability. In the end, developing safe, efficient, and regenerative biomaterials for contemporary medicine depends critically on maximizing the degradation–stability continuum. Therefore, the rate, mechanism, and byproducts of the degradation profile must be in line with the desired biological function. Inadequate degradation management can undermine therapeutic results by causing toxic by-product accumulation, inflammatory responses, or premature mechanical failure. Therefore, creating biomaterials that satisfy the intricate requirements of biomedical applications requires an awareness of the ability to manage deterioration.

3.1.1 Importance of Understanding Stability for Safety, Functionality and Clinical Success

The ability of a biomaterial to preserve its mechanical, chemical, and physical integrity throughout usage, storage, and sterilization is known as stability, and it is the inverse of deterioration. Stability in the physiological environment guarantees that a material fulfills its original purpose without releasing toxic compounds or causing unfavorable biological reactions. High stability is necessary for permanent implants, such as dental restorations, cardiovascular stents, and orthopedic prostheses, in order to guarantee dependability and minimize revision surgeries. Stability controls the predictability of mechanical support and degradation kinetics during tissue regeneration, even in resorbable systems.

Clinically speaking, insufficient stability can show up as calcification of synthetic scaffolds, hydrolysis of polymeric chains, or oxidation of metallic surfaces, which can result in toxicity, inflammation, or mechanical instability. Degradation and stability must therefore be carefully balanced. Biodegradable material should not break down too slowly to impede biological healing or too swiftly to lose structural integrity too soon. To guarantee the long-term safety of biomaterials, regulatory bodies like the European Medicines Agency (EMA) and the U.S. Food and Drug Administration (FDA) place a strong emphasis on thorough stability evaluations. This comprises computer modeling of degradation dynamics under physiologically simulated settings, in vitro degradation testing, and accelerated aging tests. To predict how materials would react in a variety of dynamic biological contexts, stability studies are essential as biomaterials become more multifunctional by integrating mechanical support, bioactivity, and controlled drug administration.

3.1.2 *Relationship Between Degradation Kinetics and Biological Response*

One of the most intricate and important facets of biomaterial research is the connection between biological response and degradation kinetics. While biological response refers to how tissues and cells respond to that process, degradation kinetics describe how quickly and by what mechanism a material breaks down. Degradation rates and the biological timescale for healing or regeneration are in harmony in an ideal biomaterial design. For instance, in scaffolds used in tissue engineering, breakdown should occur concurrently with the production of extracellular matrix, enabling the material to be gradually replaced by native tissue. If degradation happens too slowly, the remaining material may impede remodeling or cause chronic inflammation; if it happens too quickly, structural support is lost before enough tissue is formed.

Furthermore, byproducts of degradation, including metal ions from corrosion or acidic monomers from polymeric hydrolysis, might affect local pH, enzyme activity, and immune cell behavior. For example, although biodegradable, implants made of magnesium emit hydrogen gas and raise alkalinity, which need to be managed to avoid cytotoxic consequences. Crosslinking density can also be used to control the enzymatic breakdown of collagen-based materials to balance biocompatibility and mechanical performance. The requirement for predictive models that incorporate material chemistry, mechanical behavior, and cellular responses is highlighted by the dynamic interaction between biological processes and degradation kinetics. Real-time tracking of degradation and host interaction is now possible because to advanced imaging, molecular biology, and computational simulations, which makes it easier to develop materials with specific degradation–response profiles.

3.1.3 *Scope of the Chapter Covering Mechanisms, Influencing Factors and Emerging Stabilization Strategies*

This chapter examines the entire field of biomaterial stability and degradation, including the basic processes, determining variables, and new stabilization techniques that characterize next-generation biomedical materials. The material's composition, morphology, and processing history will all be taken into consideration when analyzing the degradation mechanisms, which include oxidation, hydrolysis, enzymatic catalysis, and mechanical wear. The synergistic effects of environmental factors like temperature, pH, enzymatic concentration, and mechanical stress on degradation pathways will receive particular emphasis. Autocatalytic hydrolysis and copolymer design strategies that control the rate of degradation will be discussed for polymeric systems, while corrosion resistance, surface passivation, and biofilm formation will be the main topics for metals and ceramics [1, 2].

The chapter will also discuss how material engineering and design can improve stability and control degradation. To fine-tune degradation kinetics, strategies such molecular blending, crosslinking optimization, surface coatings, and nanocomposite reinforcement will be examined. The use of clever stabilizing strategies, such as hydrogels that react to stimuli, coatings that release antioxidants, and self-healing polymers, demonstrates the trend toward biomaterials that are adaptive and can react to physiological changes.

Recent developments in characterisation methods and prediction modeling that connect in vitro and in vivo observations are also highlighted in the chapter. The use of computational models that combine biological data, kinetics, and thermodynamics to model long-term degradation behavior is growing. Degradation mechanisms at the molecular and nanoscale levels can now be thoroughly understood because of analytical methods like electrochemical impedance spectroscopy (EIS), atomic force microscopy (AFM), and Fourier-transform infrared spectroscopy (FTIR).

Lastly, the wider ramifications of stability and degradation studies will be examined in relation to sustainability, regulatory compliance, and the prospects for regenerative medicine. Understanding and managing degradation processes will continue to be essential to guaranteeing safety, functionality, and clinical success as biomaterials advance toward bioresorbable electronics, intelligent implants, and 4D-printed scaffolds. The scientific basis for future talks on environmental interactions, degradation mechanisms, and stabilization innovations is thus provided by this chapter, which outlines how biomaterials might attain both durability and dynamic flexibility within the human body.

3.2 Key Concepts and Definitions

In the context of biomaterials, degradation is the process through which a material gradually loses its mechanical, chemical, or structural integrity because of environmental influences. Physical forces, chemical interactions, or biological activities can all cause this change. The material's shape and functionality gradually deteriorate because of the process, which may include chain scission, oxidation, corrosion, or surface erosion. Degradation is a key factor in biomedical applications because it determines how long a material stays useful in the body and how safely it changes into byproducts that the organism can either tolerate or get rid of [3, 4].

The breakdown of materials mediated by biological systems, such as enzymes, microbes, or cellular activity, is known as biodegradation, which is a subset of degradation. Enzymatic or hydrolytic cleavage of polymer chains, which results in the formation of smaller oligomers or monomers that can be metabolized or eliminated, is the usual process of biodegradation for polymeric biomaterials. Examples of biodegradable biomaterials include polylactic acid (PLA), polycaprolactone (PCL), and natural polymers like collagen and chitosan. These materials are made to break down in tandem with the processes of tissue regeneration. Degradation by-products must be non-toxic and compatible with metabolic pathways for biodegradation to merge material science and biological dynamics.

The term "bioresorption" broadens the definition of "biodegradation" to encompass both the material's breakdown and its subsequent absorption or assimilation by the body. A bioresorbable material is one that can be fully digested and eliminated without the need for surgical retrieval once it has served its purpose. This is especially ideal for medicine delivery systems, bone fixation devices, and temporary implants. Bioresorption minimizes long-term foreign body reactions or chronic inflammatory reactions by ensuring that the material's residues are incorporated into normal physiological processes. Therefore, biodegradation suggests biologically induced breakdown, bioresorption indicates full biological assimilation, and degradation often refers to structural disintegration. This hierarchical relationship highlights the continuum of material transformation in biomedical situations.

3.2.1 Distinction Between Physical, Chemical and Biological Degradation

The three main categories of biomaterial degradation physical, chemical, and biological are each controlled by unique mechanisms and impacted by the characteristics of the material and the surrounding environment. When a substance deteriorates mechanically or morphologically without significantly changing its chemical composition, this is referred to as physical degradation. Physical deterioration is caused by several factors, including hydrostatic pressure, abrasion, swelling, temperature cycling, and mechanical fatigue. For instance, in watery settings, polymeric hydrogels may swell and then mechanically weaken, whereas cyclic stress may cause ceramics to microcrack. The porosity, roughness, and dimensional stability of a material can be changed by physical degradation, which can affect tissue integration and cellular adhesion.

On the other hand, chemical degradation describes alterations in the material's chemical structure at the molecular level. It includes processes that result in long-lasting changes to molecular bonds, such as hydrolysis, oxidation, reduction, or chain scission. Water molecules frequently cleave ester or amide bonds in polyesters, polyamides, and polyurethanes, causing hydrolytic degradation. In polymeric and metallic implants, oxidative deterioration frequently occurs because of an interaction with reactive oxygen species (ROS) generated by inflammatory cells. When corrosion occurs in metals like iron and magnesium, ions are released and the surface deteriorates because of chemical degradation. The physiological environment, which includes pH, temperature, and ionic concentration, has a significant impact on the rate and mechanism of chemical breakdown.

The breakdown of materials is catalyzed by cellular or enzymatic activity in biological degradation. Certain polymeric bonds can be broken by enzymes such lipases, proteases, and esterases, and degrading compounds can be encapsulated or phagocytosed by fibroblasts and macrophages. For natural polymers like collagen, fibrin, or chitosan, whose breakdown is controlled by enzymatic balance and tissue-specific factors, biological degradation is especially important. Crucially, chemical and physical degradation frequently coexist with biological degradation, creating a synergistic effect in vivo. For instance, mechanical stress promotes physical erosion, whereas reactive species produced during inflammation may hasten chemical degradation. These factors together may affect the overall kinetics of deterioration.

3.2.2 *Definition of Stability in the Context of Biomaterials Mechanical, Chemical and Biological Stability*

A biomaterial is said to be stable if it can sustain its intended composition, structure, and functional characteristics for a given period under predetermined circumstances. Stability guarantees a material's consistent performance in biomedical systems without causing negative reactions or losing mechanical support before its intended therapeutic effect is realized. There are mechanical, chemical, and biological aspects to stability.

The ability of a material to tolerate applied stresses and preserve structural integrity during physiological loading is known as mechanical stability. For load-bearing implants like vascular stents, dental prostheses, and orthopedic plates, this is essential. Fatigue, cracking, or creep can cause mechanical stability to deteriorate, which can result in tissue damage or device failure. As a result, materials are created with mechanical qualities that can tolerate cyclic biological stresses and match the modulus of the target tissue.

Resistance to chemical alterations like oxidation, hydrolysis, or ion exchange is known as chemical stability. The development of passive oxide layers that stop corrosion is essential to the chemical stability of metals like titanium and stainless steel. Chemical stability for polymers refers to their capacity to withstand oxidative or hydrolytic degradation while maintaining their molecular weight and functional groups. In order to decrease reactivity, chemically stable biomaterials are frequently designed with hydrophobic coatings, crosslinking agents, or antioxidant compounds.

The material's resistance to cellular or enzymatic breakdown and its capacity to preserve non-immunogenic contact with surrounding tissues are two aspects of biological stability. Protein adsorption, bacterial colonization, and inflammatory activation are all reduced by a physiologically stable substance. To allow for slow deterioration and tissue replacement, resorbable systems require a controlled loss of biological stability. Therefore, a key component of biomaterial design is striking the correct balance between stability in the mechanical, chemical, and biological domains, which affects both safety and therapeutic efficacy.

3.2.3 *Key Parameters: Degradation Rate, Half-Life, Molecular Weight Retention and Mechanical Integrity*

Several critical factors that characterize the rate and degree of deterioration of a material are essential to the quantitative evaluation of biomaterial degradation. The pace at which mass, molecular weight, or structural characteristics deteriorate over time is known as the degradation rate. Environmental circumstances, surface area, crystalline and material composition are some of the variables that affect it. How long a material retains mechanical strength before completely eroding is determined by the rate of degradation of biodegradable polymers. The amount of time needed for a material's properties (such as mass, molecular weight, or strength) to decrease by 50% is known as its half-life. This measure forecasts in vivo performance and enables material comparison. For drug delivery vehicles, a short half-life might be useful, but for load-bearing scaffolds, it is undesirable.

Another important sign of polymer degradation is molecular weight retention, since chain scission during oxidation or hydrolysis lowers the average molecular weight, which is correlated with a reduction in mechanical characteristics. Molecular-level degradation kinetics can be understood by tracking molecular weight retention with methods such as gel permeation chromatography (GPC). A material's ability to maintain enough strength and stiffness over time is reflected in its mechanical integrity. The material must continue to offer sufficient mechanical support until biological healing is finished, even as molecular breakdown occurs. Mechanical integrity is measured over time using common mechanical tests, including tensile, compressive, and fatigue testing. A quantitative framework for connecting material design to degradation behavior and functional longevity is provided by these parameters taken together.

3.2.4 *Metrics and Standards Used for Evaluating Degradation Behavior (e.g., ISO, ASTM)*

Standardized testing procedures are necessary for evaluating the stability and degradation of biomaterials to guarantee clinical dependability, regulatory compliance, and reproducibility. A thorough set of criteria guiding the evaluation of degrading behavior in biomaterials has been established by the American Society for Testing and Materials (ASTM) and the International Organization for Standardization (ISO). Procedures for in vitro degradation testing of absorbable polymers under physiologically simulated conditions are outlined in ASTM F1635 and ISO 13781 for polymeric materials. These include changes in mechanical characteristics, mass loss measurement, and molecular weight reduction. While ASTM F2129 offers standards for evaluating the corrosion susceptibility of metallic biomaterials using electrochemical techniques, ISO 15814 specifies tests for the degradation of ceramic biomaterials in simulated bodily fluids.

Biocompatibility testing, toxicity assessment, and degradation product characterisation are covered by other standards such ASTM F2450 and ISO 10993-13. Before being used in clinical settings, these standards guarantee that degradation by-products are both chemically and physiologically safe. To evaluate systemic safety, ISO 10993-9 also requires the identification and measurement of degradation products. To more accurately imitate physiological challenges, contemporary evaluation also uses dynamic flow systems, accelerated aging research, and computational modeling. To guarantee that biomaterials are functional, safe, stable, and predictable in their long-term performance, ISO and ASTM standards collaborate to establish the scientific and regulatory framework necessary for translating degradation data from laboratory settings to clinical applications [5, 6].

3.3 Historical Background

Growing knowledge of material–tissue interactions, therapeutic effects, and the mechanical and chemical behaviors of materials within biological systems is reflected in the historical development of biomaterial degradation and stability research. The development of smart, tunable systems for patient-specific applications and the early detection of implant failures due to uncontrolled degradation highlight the interdisciplinary nature of biomaterials science, which integrates engineering, chemistry, physics, and biology.

3.3.1 Early Recognition of Biomaterial Degradation in Implant Failures

Growing knowledge of material–tissue interactions, therapeutic effects, and the mechanical and chemical behaviors of materials within biological systems is reflected in the historical development of biomaterial degradation and stability research. The development of smart, tunable systems for patient-specific applications and the early detection of implant failures due to uncontrolled degradation highlight the interdisciplinary nature of biomaterials science, which integrates engineering, chemistry, physics, and biology.

By the 1940s and 1950s, methodical research started to show that degradation was a complicated process impacted by bodily fluids, mechanical stress, and electrochemical processes rather than just being a surface occurrence. For example, in physiological settings, the corrosion of nickel-based steels and cobalt-chromium alloys generated toxic ions that caused inflammation and tissue necrosis. The necessity for materials that could withstand both chemical attack and biological reactivity was brought to light by these failures. The field of biomaterial degradation science was founded on this early realization, which established the idea that stability and degradation control are just as important to implant success as mechanical strength and usefulness.

3.3.2 Evolution of Biodegradable Polymers and Bioresorbable Implants (e.g., PLA, PGA, PCL)

A paradigm change occurred in the 1960s and 1970s when biodegradable polymers were developed that could break down in vivo through enzymatic or hydrolysis processes, doing away with the necessity for surgical removal. Among the first synthetic polymers investigated for biomedical applications were polylactic acid (PLA) and polyglycolic acid (PGA), namely in tissue scaffolds and sutures. By manipulating the molecular weight and copolymer ratio, a controlled resorption profile was produced by the hydrolytic breakdown of these aliphatic polyesters into lactic and glycolic acids.

The design space for biodegradable polymers was considerably broadened with the advent of poly(ε-caprolactone) (PCL). PCL has slower degradation kinetics than PLA and PGA, which makes it appropriate for long-term tissue regeneration and drug delivery applications. As the host tissue remodels, these polymers showed that biodegradation might be used as a functional design element to provide short-term mechanical support. Copolymerization techniques, including PLA–PGA copolymers (PLGA), allowed degradation rates to be fine-tuned to correspond with tissue healing timeframes by the late twentieth century. The creation of these materials resulted in the introduction of cardiovascular stents, guided tissue regeneration membranes, and bioresorbable implants for orthopedic fixation [7, 8]. The concept of “designed degradation” became central to biomaterial innovation, aligning degradation kinetics with biological regeneration processes.

3.3.3 Milestones in Corrosion-Resistant Metallic Biomaterials (e.g., Titanium, Stainless Steel, Magnesium Alloys)

Although soft tissue applications were dominated by biodegradable polymers, metals were still essential for load-bearing implants. Significant progress was made in metallic biomaterials by the middle of the twentieth century, especially in terms of enhancing biocompatibility and corrosion resistance. Stainless steel (316 L) was the initial implant metal employed extensively due to its strength and corrosion resistance; nonetheless, issues with stress corrosion and ion leaching persisted.

A significant turning point was reached in the 1950s with the advent of titanium and its alloys. Because of its remarkable corrosion resistance and superior biocompatibility, titanium spontaneously formed a stable oxide layer (TiO_2), which promoted osseointegration with bone. Stress shielding was further lessened by its low elastic modulus, which is more like that of real bone than stainless steel. The groundwork for contemporary orthopedic and dental implants was laid by this shift.

At the same time, alloys based on magnesium showed promise as biodegradable metals. Magnesium was first written off because of its quick corrosion, but in the 1990s, surface modification and alloying techniques that permitted controlled degradation brought it back into favor. Magnesium alloys are attractive because they break down into physiologically innocuous compounds like magnesium ions and hydroxides and have a mechanical similarity to bone. As a result, the development of metallic biomaterials shows an ongoing attempt to strike a compromise between mechanical integrity, biological compatibility, and corrosion resistance.

3.3.4 Development of Surface Coatings and Stabilization Techniques through the Twentieth Century

Significant advancements in surface engineering were made in the twentieth century to reduce deterioration and increase implant longevity. Early methods for creating protective oxide layers on metals included passivation treatments and electroplating. Coatings changed from being merely protective barriers to being bioactive interfaces as our understanding of surface–tissue interactions improved.

A significant advancement was made in the 1980s with the introduction of hydroxyapatite (HA) coatings, which protected metallic substrates from corrosion and encouraged direct bone attachment. In a similar vein, titanium coatings applied by plasma enhanced joint prosthesis corrosion resistance and mechanical interlocking. The creation of polymeric coatings, including poly (ethylene glycol) (PEG) and polyurethane, made it possible to modify biological reactions and protein adsorption, which in turn decreased immunological responses and biofouling.

Incorporating antioxidants to prevent oxidative degradation and cross-linking polymers to improve mechanical and thermal stability were further developments in stabilization techniques. Grain-boundary engineering and sintering techniques enhanced the chemical durability of ceramics. When coupled, these methods made it possible to create multi-layered systems that integrated biological activity, controlled deterioration, and structural support.

3.3.5 Transition toward Smart and Tunable Degradation Systems in Modern Biomaterial Design

Research on biomaterials began to concentrate on "smart" materials that may degrade in response to stimuli as the twenty-first century progressed. Developments in polymer chemistry, nanotechnology, and computer modeling have made it easier to create materials that break down in response to physiological triggers like temperature, pH, enzyme activity, or oxidative stress.

For instance, hydrogels that are sensitive to pH are designed to release therapeutic compounds when they break down in acidic environments linked to tumors or inflammation. Scaffolds based on enzyme-degradable peptides enable cell-mediated and targeted resorption during tissue remodeling. Likewise, time-dependent degradation behavior is included into shape-memory and 4D biomaterials, allowing for dynamic interactions with the biological environment. Self-healing polymer coatings operating through intrinsic mechanisms such as dynamic covalent bonds (disulfide, imine, Diels–Alder linkages) and extrinsic microcapsule-based systems represent a transformative strategy for improving the durability and stimuli-responsiveness of biomaterial surfaces, enabling autonomous restoration of structural integrity following mechanical damage and extending implant longevity under physiological stress [9].

Degradation science has also changed because of machine learning and predictive modeling, which make it possible to simulate molecular breakdown and forecast lifetime under different physiological situations. These resources aid in the logical development of biomaterials with adjustable degradation profiles that correspond to the healing paths of individual patients. Furthermore, multipurpose platforms for drug delivery, biosensing, and regenerative medicine are now available thanks to hybrid systems that include metals, polymers, and ceramics.

A philosophical change from considering deterioration as a constraint to using it as an inherent and manageable aspect of biomaterial performance is reflected in the move toward smart degradation systems.

From the early difficulties of uncontrolled corrosion and mechanical failure to the complex control of bioresorbable, corrosion-resistant, and intelligent systems, the historical trajectory of biomaterial degradation research demonstrates a tremendous progression. Every significant advancement, from the first metallic implants to the most recent stimuli-responsive polymers, is the result of interdisciplinary cooperation and a deeper understanding of mechanisms.

Degradation and stability are now primary design considerations rather than secondary ones as biomaterial science develops. A new era when materials actively contribute to the healing process rather than just acting as inert supports is being ushered in by the modern vision, which places an emphasis on predictability, adaptability, and bio-integration [10]. This historical development emphasizes how materials engineering, biological systems, and clinical innovation interact dynamically to shape the future of biomedical technology and regenerative medicine.

3.4 Material Types and Properties

The material class of biomaterials whether polymeric, metallic, ceramic, or composite fundamentally determines their stability and rate of deterioration as shown in Table 3.1. The unique structural, chemical, and mechanical properties of each class

Table 3.1 Mechanical properties of biomaterials

Biomaterial class	Representative examples	Degradation mechanisms	Influencing factors	Mechanical characteristics	Key notes/biomedical implications
Polymeric Biomaterials	Polylactic acid (PLA), Polycaprolactone (PCL), Polyethylene glycol (PEG), Collagen, Chitosan	Hydrolytic degradation: cleavage of ester or amide bonds in aqueous environments. Enzymatic degradation: proteases, esterases, and lysozymes catalyze chain scission in natural polymers	Crystallinity: Higher crystallinity slows hydrolysis Molecular weight: Higher Mw delays degradation onset Copolymer composition: Hydrophilic segments accelerate breakdown	Low modulus (0.001–4 GPa); ductile or flexible; limited strength (10–100 MPa)	Degradation rate can be tailored via polymer chemistry; ideal for resorbable sutures, scaffolds, and drug delivery systems
Metallic Biomaterials	Titanium (Ti, Ti–6Al–4 V), stainless steel (316 L), cobalt–chromium (co–Cr), magnesium alloys	Electrochemical corrosion: Anodic dissolution and cathodic reactions in body fluids Passive film formation: TiO_2 and Cr_2O_3 layers provide corrosion resistance; breakdown leads to localized pitting and ion release	Alloy composition (Cr, Mo, Ni content) Surface finish and oxide stability Physiological pH, chloride concentration, and protein adsorption	High modulus (40–210 GPa); strong (200–1200 MPa); excellent fatigue and wear resistance	Corrosion affects ion release and biocompatibility; surface modification improves passivation and reduces immune activation
Ceramic Biomaterials	Alumina (Al_2O_3), zirconia (ZrO_2), hydroxyapatite (HA), bioglass	Dissolution: Ionic exchange and partial solubilization in body fluids Phase transformation: Tetragonal–monoclinic shifts (ZrO_2) reduce stability. • Mechanical instability: Microcracking under cyclic load	Grain size and porosity Phase composition and crystallinity pH and ionic strength of environment	Very stiff (50–400 GPa); high compressive strength (500–4000 MPa); brittle (K_IC = 2–10 MPa·m½)	Biodegradable ceramics (calcium phosphates, bioactive glasses) support bone regeneration via controlled resorption and ion release

Biomaterial class	Representative examples	Degradation mechanisms	Influencing factors	Mechanical characteristics	Key notes/biomedical implications
Composite Biomaterials	Polymer–ceramic (PLA/HA), Metal–ceramic (Ti/HA), fiber-reinforced polymers	Interface degradation: Differential swelling, hydrolysis, or corrosion at filler–matrix boundaries. • Synergistic effects: Degradation of one phase accelerates the other. • Environmental fatigue: Microcrack propagation at interfaces	• Filler–matrix interactions: Chemical bonding, interfacial adhesion. • Volume fraction and dispersion: Influence strength and degradation uniformity	Intermediate modulus (10–150 GPa); tunable strength (100–1200 MPa); improved toughness (5–30 $MPa \cdot m^{1/2}$)	Combined mechanical and biological performance; tailored degradation for bone and dental scaffolds; key for load-sharing implants

dictate how it interacts with the physiological environment and how it either retains or degrades over time. Selecting appropriate materials for certain biomedical applications, such as tissue scaffolds, orthopedic implants, cardiovascular devices, or drug delivery systems, requires an understanding of these interactions. The degradation characteristics of the four main types of biomaterials are compared at the end of this, which also examines their stability parameters, interfacial behaviors, and degradation mechanisms.

3.4.1 Polymeric Biomaterials

The customizable chemical structures, flexibility, and controlled degradation capabilities of polymeric biomaterials make them a flexible and commonly used category in medical applications. Polylactic acid [PLA], polyglycolic acid [PGA], and polycaprolactone [PCL] are examples of synthetic substances. Collagen, chitosan, and alginate are examples of natural substances. Molecular structure, shape, and environmental factors all have an impact on the hydrolytic and enzymatic pathways that are the main means by which polymers degrade.

Water molecules cleave vulnerable chemical bonds, usually urethane, amide, or ester connections, in a process known as hydrolytic breakdown. Chain scission and a decrease in molecular weight are the outcomes of this process, which ultimately causes erosion and a loss of mechanical strength. The hydrophilicity, crystallinity, and chain mobility of the polymer all have a significant impact on the rate of hydrolysis. For instance, PGA degrades more quickly than PLA due to its strong hydrophilicity, but PCL degrades more slowly due to its higher hydrophobicity and crystal structure. When acidic breakdown byproducts, such as lactic or glycolic acid, build up inside the material, autocatalysis may take place, speeding up the process.

Conversely, biological catalysts include lipases, proteases, and esterases aid in enzymatic breakdown. Collagen and fibrin are examples of natural polymers that are especially vulnerable to enzymatic degradation. Depending on the enzyme concentration, molecular recognition sites, and polymer chain accessibility, the degradation is site-specific [11, 12]. This mechanism enables spatially regulated degradation that is closely aligned with the processes of tissue remodeling.

The copolymer composition, molecular weight, and crystallinity all have a significant impact on polymer stability. In general, higher crystallinity decrease enzymatic accessibility and water penetration, improving stability while decreasing rates of bioresorption. On the other hand, because of their increased permeability, amorphous patches deteriorate more quickly. Chain entanglement and mechanical resilience are determined by molecular weight; polymers with lower molecular weights break down more quickly because of increased chain-end availability. Copolymerization, as in poly(lactic-co-glycolic acid) (PLGA), enables the fine-tuning of degradation kinetics: lactic acid increases mechanical strength and hydrophobicity, whereas a higher glycolic acid component speeds up hydrolysis. Because of their design-dependent degradation spectrum, polymeric biomaterials provide for individualized mechanical and temporal performance.

3.4.2 *Metallic Biomaterials*

The main use of metallic biomaterials, such as titanium and its alloys, cobalt-chromium alloys, stainless steels, and new magnesium-based systems, is in load-bearing applications that demand great mechanical strength, toughness, and fatigue resistance. However, a major degradation mechanism that can jeopardize mechanical integrity and biocompatibility is electrochemical corrosion, which metals are naturally prone to in physiological settings.

Redox processes at the metal–electrolyte contact are the source of electrochemical corrosion mechanisms. Proteins, dissolved oxygen, and chloride ions all function as aggressive substances in the body that promote the oxidation of metal atoms into ions. The ionic dissolution that results can cause local pH shifts, release cytotoxic species, and modify surface chemistry. Galvanic corrosion (between dissimilar metals in contact), pitting corrosion (localized attack in passive layers), and uniform corrosion (general surface assault) are common types of corrosion. For instance, titanium alloys may have rapid degradation due to galvanic interactions with other metals, whereas stainless steel implants may experience pitting due to localized breakdown of the passive chromium oxide layer.

The stability of metallic biomaterials over time is determined by the creation and breakdown of passive films. The spontaneous development of a nanometric titanium dioxide (TiO_2) coating, which serves as a protective barrier, is responsible for the biocompatibility and corrosion resistance of titanium and its alloys. Cobalt-chromium alloys form a chromium-rich oxide layer, whereas stainless steel forms a chromium oxide film. These films are not impervious, though; hostile ions, micromotion, or mechanical wear can all result in passive film disintegration, which can hasten corrosion in exposed regions. Although repassivation is possible after damage, metal ion release and inflammatory responses may result from repeated cycles of film rupture and reformation.

Anodization, plasma spraying, and hydroxyapatite coating are examples of recent advancements in surface modification that are intended to improve biological integration and corrosion resistance. As biodegradable metals, iron and magnesium alloys are made to corrode in a controlled manner, releasing ions that take part in organic metabolic processes. A comprehensive comparative review of magnesium, iron, and zinc as biodegradable metallic implants addressing their degradation mechanisms, corrosion kinetics, mechanical performance, and ongoing clinical trials has clarified the relative suitability of each metal for cardiovascular and orthopedic applications and identified remaining barriers to clinical translation [13] It is still difficult to prevent the quick evolution of hydrogen gas in magnesium-based systems and to strike a balance between mechanical stability and degradation rate.

Therefore, creating safe and long-lasting metallic biomaterials requires a grasp of passive film behavior and electrochemical dynamics.

3.4.3 Ceramic Biomaterials

Excellent hardness, wear resistance, and chemical inertness are characteristics of ceramic biomaterials, including alumina, zirconia, calcium phosphates, and bioactive glasses. They are widely used in orthopedic and dentistry applications. Nonetheless, their stability and degradation behavior are influenced by their brittleness and susceptibility to dissolution or phase shift in physiological settings.

The main ways that ceramics degrade include dissolution, phase change, and mechanical instability. Because of their strong ionic and covalent interactions, non-biodegradable ceramics like zirconia (ZrO_2) and alumina (AlO_3) have great chemical stability and are therefore perfect for permanent implants. However, zirconia may experience mechanical weakening and microcracking as well as low-temperature deterioration (LTD), which is a transition from the tetragonal to monoclinic phase, under physiological conditions. Like this, bioactive ceramics that dissolve over time may gradually lose their structural integrity, particularly if they are porous.

Bioactive glasses and biodegradable calcium phosphates belong to a unique family of ceramics made for tissue replacement and controlled resorption. Crystallinity, particle size, and the Ca/P ratio all affect the ionic dissolution and reprecipitation processes that break down calcium phosphates, such as hydroxyapatite (HA) and tricalcium phosphate (TCP). While TCP dissolves more quickly and promotes rapid bone regeneration, HA degrades more slowly and is appropriate for long-term stability. A hydroxycarbonate apatite layer is created by surface reactions in bioactive glasses (such 45S5 Bioglass®), which encourage chemical interaction with bone. By modifying their composition, their degradation can be regulated; a higher silica content improves stability, whereas a larger sodium or calcium content speeds up dissolution. These ceramics are essential in non-load-bearing regeneration applications because of their controlled deterioration, which promotes tissue mineralization and integration, even though they are brittle.

3.4.4 Composite Biomaterials

In order to obtain synergistic increases in mechanical, chemical, or biological performance, composite biomaterials integrate two or more unique material phases, usually a matrix and a filler. They are extensively utilized in soft tissue engineering, dental restorations, and bone scaffolds. However, the interactions between their constituent parts control their complex deterioration behavior.

Composite stability is largely dependent on synergistic effects and interface deterioration. A site of stress concentration and possible deterioration beginning is the interface between the polymeric matrix and the filler (such as ceramic fibers or particles). Delamination or the development of microcracks can result from the weakening of interfacial bonds caused by hydrolysis, mechanical wear, or differential swelling between phases. Water intrusion, for example, can lead to linked degradation events in polymer–ceramic composites used for bone regeneration by hydrolyzing the polymer phase and encouraging the dissolution of the ceramic filler. Depending on the material design, this synergistic degradation could either cause premature mechanical failure or beneficially speed bioresorption.

Surface treatment and interfacial chemistry determine how filler–matrix interactions affect stability. Strong chemical bonding improves load transfer and lessens interfacial degradation. This can be accomplished via surface functionalization or silane coupling agents. Poor adhesion, on the other hand, makes it possible for micro voids to form, which increases permeability and hydrolysis susceptibility. While nanocomposite designs enable the fine-tuning of both mechanical integrity and degradation kinetics, the addition of nanoparticles or fibers can enhance barrier qualities and postpone degradation. To attain dynamic stability, where the composite retains its usefulness even as one phase deteriorates, sophisticated hybrid composites such as metal–polymer systems or polymer-infiltrated ceramics are being developed.

3.4.5 *Comparative Degradation Characteristics Across Classes of Biomaterials*

Clinical appropriateness is determined by the inherent features of various biomaterial classes, as demonstrated by a comparison of their degradation behavior. The most tunable and controlled degradation is seen in polymeric biomaterials, which are controlled by the copolymer mix and molecular structure. Although they may produce acidic byproducts and have unpredictable autocatalytic effects, their primary advantages are biodegradability and compatibility to both soft-tissue and load-bearing settings. Despite their higher mechanical strength, metallic biomaterials are limited by their sensitivity to corrosion and the possible cytotoxicity of liberated ions. Biodegradable metals like magnesium and zinc offer the potential for temporary implants with precisely regulated corrosion rates, while non-biodegradable metals like titanium offer long-term durability.

Ceramic biomaterials are perfect for permanent or slow-resorbing applications because of their exceptional chemical inertness and biocompatibility. However, their usage in dynamic load-bearing situations is limited by their brittleness and vulnerability to dissolution or phase instability. A bioactive and biodegradable substitute that promotes tissue adhesion and mineralization is offered by calcium phosphates and bioactive glasses. Composite biomaterials provide a link between controlled degradation and mechanical resilience. Composites replicate the hierarchical structure of organic tissues by fusing metals, ceramics, and polymers to provide hybrid functioning. However, maintaining long-term predictability is still difficult due to the complexity of interfacial deterioration.

Metals and ceramics offer mechanical stability and chemical stability, respectively, whereas polymers offer the most design freedom for deterioration. By providing an integrative approach, composites allow for the customisation of mechanical properties and degradation dynamics for certain clinical settings. Thus, developing biomaterials that are stable and dynamically responsive in physiological settings continues to depend heavily on proficiency in material selection and interfacial engineering [14, 15].

3.5 Mechanisms and Processes

Degradation of biomaterials is a complex process that is impacted by environmental, mechanical, biological, and chemical variables. Predicting in-vivo performance, adjusting degradation rates, and creating materials that coordinate tissue regeneration and structural resorption all depend on an understanding of these systems as shown in Fig. 3.1. Local factors including pH, temperature, and moisture all influence the physicochemical changes, biological interactions, and mechanical stress that led to degradation [16, 17]. The way these processes interact influences the biomaterial's biocompatibility, clinical success, and functional longevity.

3.5.1 Physicochemical Degradation

The basic chemical processes that disassemble a biomaterial's molecular structure and frequently start the process of mechanical failure or resorption are referred to as physicochemical degradation. Environmental factors including pH, temperature, and moisture content have an impact on the three main processes of hydrolysis, oxidation, and photodegradation. The most common degradation method for biodegradable polymers, like polyesters (e.g., PLA, PGA, and PLGA), is hydrolysis. Water molecules break ester bonds in the polymer backbone during this process, which causes chain scission and a decrease in molecular weight. Water diffusion dominates the first induction phase of hydrolysis, which is followed by autocatalytic degradation sped up by acidic degradation products. Local pH (hydrolysis is catalyzed by acidic environments), temperature (higher temperatures increase molecular mobility and reaction rates), and water availability all have a significant impact on the rate of hydrolysis.

Another important degradation mechanism is oxidation, which is particularly pertinent to polymers like polyethylene and polyurethane that are utilized in long-term implants. Chain scission, embrittlement, and surface cracking are caused by

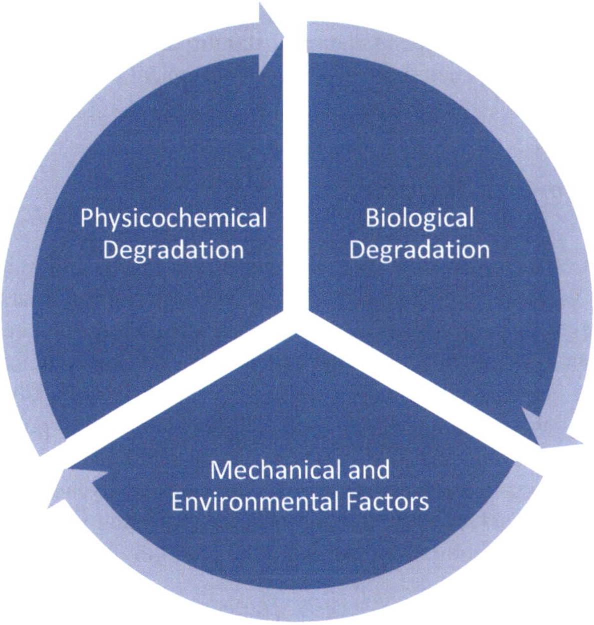

Fig. 3.1 Schematic representation of key degradation mechanisms in biomaterials, including physicochemical processes (hydrolysis, oxidation), biological degradation pathways (enzymatic and immune-mediated), and mechanical/environmental influences (fatigue, wear, and stress-assisted degradation)

reactive oxygen species (ROS) that are produced by inflammatory cells and damage the polymer surface. In a similar vein, metallic biomaterials like cobalt-chromium alloys and stainless-steel experience electrochemical oxidation, producing corrosion products that could jeopardize their structural stability and biocompatibility.

Despite being less important in vivo, photodegradation is crucial for polymer sterilization and pre-implantation aging. In polymeric chains, ultraviolet (UV) light causes bond cleavage and cross-linking, which alters degradation kinetics and mechanical performance. Because light exposure can start unintended oxidation events during manufacture and storage, this mechanism is very important. A key component of physicochemical degradation is the influence of environmental variables, particularly pH, temperature, and moisture. Elevated body temperatures in localized inflammation zones accelerate degradation rates, whereas changes in tissue pH brought on by infection or inflammation can speed up hydrolytic and oxidative processes. A detailed mechanistic review of the hydrolytic degradation of PLA and PLGA encompassing the effects of pH, crystallinity, molecular weight, stereoisomerism, and temperature on degradation rate, and addressing the limitations of in vitro–in vivo correlation provides an essential quantitative framework for predicting and controlling the degradation kinetics of these FDA-approved biodegradable polymers in clinical applications [18]. Moisture influences diffusion kinetics and promotes molecular rearrangements by acting as a plasticizer and a reactant. Therefore, the inherent chemical stability of biomaterials in intricate biological environments is determined by physicochemical degradation mechanisms.

3.5.2 *Biological Degradation*

Degradation of materials caused by living things, enzymes, or cellular activity is referred to as biological degradation. The two interrelated routes of immune-mediated degradation and enzymatic catalysis are how this process takes place. Certain enzymes released by cells that hydrolyze or oxidize chemical bonds in biomaterials are known as enzymatic catalysis. Particularly vulnerable to enzymatic breakdown by proteases, lysozymes, and cellulases are natural polymers including collagen, chitosan, and alginate. Certain lipases and esterases can catalyze the breaking of bonds in synthetic polymers, including polycaprolactone and poly (lactic-co-glycolic acid). Enzyme concentration, substrate accessibility, and local microenvironmental factors like pH and ionic strength all affect the rate of enzymatic degradation.

A systematic study of lipase-mediated enzymatic degradation in PCL composites blended with gelatin, collagen, and PLGA demonstrates that composite composition critically governs degradation rate constants with hydrophilic components accelerating enzymatic breakdown providing a practical basis for tailoring biodegradation kinetics in tissue-engineered scaffolds where rapid scaffold removal is needed to minimise immune reactions [19].

Degradation is also modulated by cellular contacts. For instance, extracellular matrix components and biomimetic scaffolds are broken down by matrix metalloproteinases (MMPs), which are secreted by osteoclasts and fibroblasts. This regulated enzymatic degradation is useful in tissue engineering because it permits slow scaffold resorption that is timed to extracellular matrix deposition and cell proliferation. When the host immune system perceives the biomaterial as alien, immune-mediated destruction occurs. During the inflammatory response, macrophagesthe primary effector cells produce proteolytic enzymes and oxidative species. This "foreign-body reaction" may cause fibrous tissue to enclose the implant or, in more extreme situations to accelerate material deterioration and surface erosion. While metals implants may be more susceptible to corrosion because of inflammatory microenvironments that are rich in hydrogen peroxide and chloride ions, polymers like polyurethanes have been demonstrated to degrade through macrophage-induced oxidation.

Therefore, biological degradation mechanisms embody the interface between biomaterial chemistry and host physiology balancing desirable resorption in regenerative systems with the need to prevent unwanted immune-driven degradation in permanent implants.

3.5.3 Mechanical and Environmental Factors

Rarely is in vivo degradation solely a chemical or biological process; wear, fatigue, and stress-assisted degradation are all major effects of mechanical stressors on material breakdown. In orthopaedic and cardiovascular implants, fatigue degradation is caused by cyclic loading, which increases surface area exposure and causes microcracks and chemical degradation. While fatigue in metals can result in localized corrosion known as stress corrosion cracking (SCC), mechanical deformation in polymers encourages molecular chain scission. One common mechanical deterioration mechanism in articulating implants, including hip and knee prosthesis, is wear. Wear debris particles that are micron or nanoscale in size causes inflammatory reactions that result in osteolysis and implant loosening. For instance, wear particles made of polyethylene pose a serious risk when replacing entire joints.

The combined action of chemical processes and mechanical loading leads to stress-assisted deterioration. Tensile stress, for example, can speed up hydrolysis in biodegradable polymers by increasing water intrusion and molecular chain mobility. Like this, fretting corrosion in metallic systems is encouraged by micro-motion at implant interfaces. This occurs when protective oxide layers are removed through repetitive contact, leaving new surfaces vulnerable to electrochemical attack.

Environmental factors that determine failure modes and the functional lifespan of biomaterials include mechanical stress, micro-motion, and tissue strain. These factors work together to build the degradation landscape.

3.5.4 Surface Vs. Bulk Degradation

Surface and bulk degradation differ in morphology and kinetics, which is a crucial difference in degradation behavior. Since water enters a material more quickly than bond cleavage, bulk deterioration takes place throughout the substance's full volume. This results in a consistent drop in molecular weight without an instantaneous mass loss until later stages. Polyesters that degrade in bulk include PLA, PGA, and PLGA. Their internal hydrolysis causes autocatalytic effects, which accelerate degradation from the inside out by accumulating acidic byproducts within the matrix. If bulk degradation is not adequately managed, it may result in unpredictably mechanical weakening and catastrophic failure.

In contrast, as the rate of bond cleavage surpasses the rate of water diffusion, surface degradation occurs layer by layer. Up until almost total resorption, the material steadily erodes from the outside while retaining its mechanical integrity and geometry. Surface-eroding biomaterials include polyanhydrides and poly(ortho esters). They are perfect for drug delivery systems that need regulated release because of their predictable, zero-order mass loss caused by their degradation kinetics. The morphological difference between surface and bulk degradation highlights design strategies in biomaterials engineering: bulk-degrading materials are appropriate for volumetric tissue scaffolds where internal porosity encourages cell infiltration, while surface-degrading systems are preferred when controlled erosion and dimensional stability are crucial.

3.5.5 Kinetic Modeling and Predictive Simulation of Degradation Processes

Clinical dependability and regulatory approval depend on the quantitative prediction of biomaterial degradation. A mathematical framework for describing the rate and degree of degradation as a function of time and environmental factors is provided by kinetic modeling. While diffusion-controlled models capture the dynamics of surface erosion, classical models use first-order or autocatalytic kinetics to describe hydrolysis in polyesters. Multi-physics simulations that combine chemical reactions, mechanical stress, and diffusion are integrated by sophisticated computer techniques. Molecular dynamics (MD) simulations and finite element modeling (FEM) are being utilized more to forecast the evolution of mechanical properties, depict degradation pathways, and optimize geometry for applications.

Stochastic components are also incorporated into predictive simulation to take into consideration biological variability and diverse in vivo circumstances. There are new data-driven methods that use machine learning to correlate observed degradation trends with compositional factors including hydrophobicity, molecular weight, and crystallinity. By speeding up biomaterial creation, these predictive models eliminate the need for drawn-out animal research and allow virtual testing.

A complex interaction between chemical reactions, biological activity, and mechanical forces, all of which are influenced by environmental factors defines the mechanisms and processes of biomaterial deterioration. Mechanical stressors affect lifetime under functional load, biological degradation promotes host–material compatibility, and physicochemical degradation establishes intrinsic stability. While kinetic modeling provides predictive insight into performance and safety, morphological control is defined by the balance between surface and bulk degradation.

The rational design of next generation biomaterials that can adapt to physiological conditions, degrade predictably, and promote regenerative healing requires a mechanistic knowledge of these processes [20, 21]. Modern biomaterial research is continuing to turn degradation from a failure mechanism into a finely tailored characteristic of biomedical functionality by fusing computational modeling and mechanistic science.

3.6 Design Considerations

Degradation kinetics, stability, biocompatibility, and mechanical performance must all be carefully balanced when designing biomaterials for use in biomedical applications. To achieve clinical success, materials must be engineered to deteriorate at predictable rates, retain enough integrity during their functioning duration, and interact well with biological surroundings. Therefore, design concerns encompass more than just material choice; they also include environmental response, surface treatments, production techniques, and molecular engineering. This examines the fundamental ideas that underpin the creation of stable and biodegradable biomaterials, highlighting how they integrate with mechanical performance, biological safety and tissue regeneration.

3.6.1 Tailoring Degradation Rates to Match Tissue Healing or Regeneration Timelines

In biomaterials engineering, coordinating degradation rates with the biological process of tissue regeneration or healing is one of the most important design ideas. While a substance that breaks down too slowly may obstruct cellular infiltration, remodeling, or nutrition exchange, one that breaks down too quickly may lose mechanical support before new tissue has sufficiently grown. To guarantee temporal compatibility between the material's lifespan and the target tissue's regenerative timeline, degradation kinetics must be tailored.

Designers use a variety of techniques, such as structural optimization, copolymerization, and alteration of polymer chemistry, to attain this equilibrium. For example, in polymeric scaffolds, such as poly(lactic-co-glycolic acid) (PLGA), the ratio of hydrophilic to hydrophobic monomers can be changed to modify the rate at which ester linkages hydrolyze. Higher lactic acid level delays degradation through increased hydrophobicity, while higher glycolic acid content speeds up degradation through improved water penetration. Likewise, adding crystalline domains or crosslinking decreases the water molecules' accessibility to polymer chains, prolonging the material's useful life.

Recent advances in biodegradable magnesium alloys for short-term orthopedic fixation demonstrate that alloy microstructure engineering combined with advanced surface modification strategies including micro-arc oxidation and biomimetic coatings can significantly slow corrosion, improve biofunctionality, and modulate osteogenesis and immune responses during degradation [22]. When it comes to biodegradable metals like magnesium or zinc alloys, surface coatings that regulate electrochemical activity and alloying elements like calcium, manganese, or rare earth metals regulate the pace of deterioration. By varying the porosity or calcium-to-phosphate ratio, the dissolution rate of ceramic biomaterials such as calcium phosphates can be controlled. Furthermore, in vitro–in vivo correlation studies and computational modeling are being used more to forecast deterioration timelines. This allows for the logical design of materials that dynamically adjust to the stages of bone, skin, or vascular tissue healing [23].

The ultimate objective is to create materials that break down in a way that corresponds with biological remodeling, providing support during the proliferative and inflammatory stages and progressively shifting mechanical loads to newly produced tissue during the maturation stage. A secondary surgical removal is not necessary thanks to its time-sensitive degrading design, which also improves regenerative efficiency and reduces complications.

3.6.2 Material Selection and Molecular Engineering for Predictable Stability

A key component of safe and dependable biomaterial design is predictable stability. Selecting the right type of material polymeric, metallic, ceramic, or composite is simply one step in the process; another is designing its molecular structure to withstand early deterioration and function reliably in physiological settings. It is necessary to guarantee stability in the mechanical, chemical, and biological domains.

At the molecular level, stereochemistry, crosslink density, and bond strength all affect stability. For example, compared to amorphous polyesters, polycaprolactone (PCL), which has a semicrystalline structure and strong C–C and C–O linkages, shows better hydrolytic stability. Degradation can be postponed by adding crosslinkers or stabilizing side groups, which increase the stiffness of the polymer network and decrease chain mobility. On the other hand, molecular tailoring in bioresorbable systems seeks to produce controlled instability by adding labile bonds, like imides or anhydrides, that encourage predictable disintegration in response to physiological stimuli.

Alloy design is essential for metallic biomaterials to achieve predictable stability and corrosion control. Passive oxide coatings provide titanium alloys with remarkable durability, but magnesium-based alloys need to be precisely tuned in terms of composition to avoid quick corrosion. Like this, phase composition and crystalline determine ceramic stability; for example, yttria stabilizes zirconia to avoid undesired phase transformation in physiological settings.

Alloy design is essential for metallic biomaterials to achieve predictable stability and corrosion control. Passive oxide coatings provide titanium alloys with remarkable durability, but magnesium-based alloys need to be precisely tuned in terms of composition to avoid quick corrosion. Similar to this, phase composition and crystallinity determine ceramic stability; for example, yttria stabilizes zirconia to avoid undesired phase transformation in physiological settings.

3.6.3 *Influence of Processing Parameters (Sterilization, Fabrication, Storage)*

Processing parameters have a significant impact on the stability and degrading behavior of biomaterials. Manufacturing, sterilizing, and storing can all change mechanical characteristics, surface chemistry, and molecular structure, which can impact in vivo performance.

Microstructure, porosity, and crystallinity are determined by fabrication techniques including solvent casting, electrospinning, 3D printing, or melt extrusion. These factors in turn regulate the kinetics of water uptake and degradation. For instance, solvent-based processing may leave behind leftover solvents that stimulate hydrolysis, whereas high-temperature extrusion may improve crystallinity in polymers, slowing the rate of breakdown. For tissue-specific applications, additive manufacturing (3D printing) enables fine control over scaffold architecture, pore size, and interconnectivity, adjusting mechanical characteristics and degradation profiles.

Significant chemical or structural changes can be brought about by sterilization methods such as autoclaving, ethylene oxide exposure, and gamma irradiation. Gamma irradiation can change the way polymers degrade by causing chain scission or crosslinking. While high-temperature steam sterilization may cause oxidation or hydrolysis in delicate materials, ethylene oxide sterilization may leave harmful residues. In order to preserve both sterility and material integrity, sterilization techniques must be chosen carefully, and post-sterilization validation is a crucial step in the creation of biomaterials.

Stability is also impacted by storage conditions, specifically humidity, temperature, and light exposure. UV-sensitive materials may experience photo-oxidation, while hydrolytic polymers, for example, are susceptible to pre-degradation under humid conditions. Barrier packing, stabilizers, and antioxidants can lessen these effects and guarantee that the material maintains its intended qualities until implantation. As a result, processing parameters which need strict control and standardization represent a crucial connection between material design and clinical performance.

3.6.4 *Surface Modification and Coating Strategies for Corrosion and Hydrolysis Control*

Surface modification is essential for improving biomaterials' functioning and durability, especially when it comes to reducing hydrolytic degradation and corrosion. Since biological interactions and the early phases of degradation are controlled by surface reactions, interface engineering provides a practical means of enhancing long-term performance.

The development or improvement of passive films is frequently used to provide corrosion protection for metallic biomaterials. On titanium and magnesium alloys, oxide layers are thickened and stabilized using methods like anodization, ion implantation, and plasma surface modification. In addition to providing corrosion protection, hydroxyapatite or bioactive glass coatings encourage osteointegration. By acting as physical barriers to ion exchange, polymer-based coatings like polylactic acid or polyurethane lessen electrochemical reactions in physiological fluids.

By lowering water permeability and enhancing chemical stability, surface modification for polymeric materials seeks to regulate hydrolysis. Surface grafting, fluorination, and plasma treatment are among techniques that can change hydrophobicity and surface energy. When controlled breakdown is needed, hydrophilic changes can improve cell adherence and biocompatibility, while hydrophobic coatings slow hydrolytic chain scission by reducing water penetration. Modern innovations like self-healing and stimuli-responsive coatings enable materials to fix surface flaws or adjust to changes in the environment, including oxidative stress or pH.

Coating can stop phase dissolution or interfacial deterioration in ceramic and composite systems. For example, silane coupling agents increase stability and decrease microcracking in polymer-ceramic composites by improving filler-matrix adhesion. All things considered, surface engineering offers a flexible and scalable way to manage deterioration without changing the bulk composition of the material, increasing its biological safety and functional longevity.

3.6.5 Integration of Biocompatibility, Mechanical Demands and Environmental Exposure in Design Optimization

Biocompatibility, mechanical performance, and environmental resistance must all be incorporated into a coherent design framework for biomaterials to be designed successfully. A system-level approach to material design is necessary since these elements are interrelated and maximizing one frequently affects the others.

Degradation byproducts and surface contacts are prevented from causing harmful immunological or toxicological reactions by biocompatibility. It is necessary to choose material formulations that produce degradation products that are pH-neutral, metabolizable, and non-toxic. Additionally, the surface chemistry should minimize inflammation and bacterial colonization while promoting advantageous protein adsorption and cellular adhesion.

The application determines the mechanical requirements; for example, soft-tissue scaffolds need to be flexible and compliant, while load-bearing implants need to be extremely strong and fatigue resistant. Until the tissue regains enough strength, the degradation profile needs to be adjusted to preserve mechanical integrity. Predicting long-term stability and failure behavior requires the use of mechanical testing under physiological load simulations and finite element modeling (FEM).

Degradation pathways are greatly impacted by environmental exposure, which includes temperature, pH, enzymatic activity, and oxidative conditions. Different biochemical milieus are experienced by materials placed in soft connective tissues, vascular tissue, or bone. Therefore, site-specific degrading processes must be taken into consideration when optimizing designs. Predicting material behavior across many biological settings is made possible by sophisticated techniques including multi-scale modeling, accelerated aging studies, and in situ monitoring.

Adaptive and intelligent systems that dynamically modify stability and degradation in response to biological feedback are the key to the future of biomaterial design. By combining additive manufacturing, molecular simulation, and computational design, material properties may be precisely tailored at various scales. Functional, safe, and predictable therapeutic outcomes are ultimately ensured by modern biomaterial design, which is based on the integration of biocompatibility, mechanical performance, and environmental adaptation [24].

3.7 Applications and Case Studies

The performance of biomaterials in physiological and therapeutic settings is just as important to their practical success as their chemical makeup and structural soundness. From scaffolds that direct tissue regeneration to drug carriers that release medicines at exact rates, controlled degradation and stability are essential to the operation of many biomedical applications. To guarantee consistent results, each application needs a different balance of mechanical stability, biocompatibility, and degradation kinetics. To demonstrate how degradation concepts are used in the design and optimization of biomaterials for a variety of medical applications, this examines important applications and illustrative case studies.

3.7.1 Tissue Engineering Scaffolds—Controlled Degradation Enabling Cell Infiltration and Matrix Deposition

Biodegradable scaffolds, which momentarily replace extracellular matrices and offer structural support while encouraging cell adhesion, proliferation, and differentiation, are crucial to tissue engineering. Such scaffolds must be able to break down in tandem with tissue regeneration in order to provide gradual load transfer and the development of room for the deposition of new matrix.

Because of their adjustable rates of breakdown, polymers including poly(lactic acid) (PLA), poly(glycolic acid) (PGA), and their copolymers (PLGA) are used extensively. These polymers remain biocompatible because the hydrolysis of their ester linkages produces lactic and glycolic acid, which can be metabolized by regular cellular processes. Timelines for scaffold deterioration in bone tissue engineering usually correspond with osteogenesis and last a few weeks to months, allowing for vascular infiltration and mineralization prior to total resorption.

While breakdown produces calcium and phosphate ions that promote bone rebuilding, recent research on nanocomposite scaffolds combining PLGA with bioactive ceramics like hydroxyapatite (HA) has shown enhanced mechanical strength and osteoconductivity. Additionally, the construction of porous structures with regulated pore interconnectivity has been made possible by 3D printing and electrospinning methods, which improve cell motility and nutrient transport. These developments highlight how crucial it is to combine biological and structural design with degradation control in order to achieve functional tissue regeneration.

3.7.2 Orthopedic Implants, Biodegradable Screws, Pins, and Plates (e.g., Magnesium Alloys)

Biomaterials with regulated biodegradability and mechanical toughness are essential for orthopedic applications. Metallic implants, including titanium and stainless steel, have historically offered structural support but needed to be surgically removed because of their long-term persistence. Orthopedic implant design has been transformed by the development of biodegradable metals, especially magnesium (Mg) alloys, which allow for in vivo breakdown and resorption after a brief period of mechanical support.

The mechanical characteristics of magnesium-based screws, pins, and fixation plates are similar to those of natural bone (elastic modulus = 45 GPa). As they progressively corrode in physiological settings, biocompatible Mg2+ ions are released, which can promote osteogenesis. Controlling the rate of corrosion is crucial, though, since severe deterioration can result in the early loss of mechanical integrity and the development of hydrogen gas. Stabilizing corrosion rates has been achieved by alloying magnesium with calcium, zinc, or rare earth metals (Y, Nd), as well as by applying surface coatings (such as fluoride, calcium phosphate, or polymer layers).

The use of MAGNEZIX® screws and other clinical case studies show excellent fracture repair with complete bone healing and implant resorption over a period of 12 to 18 months, hence avoiding the necessity for follow-up procedures. These findings highlight the interdependence between clinical outcomes, deterioration control, and material design. There is potential for next-generation resorbable orthopedic devices with ongoing alloy composition and coating strategy optimization.

3.7.3 Drug Delivery Systems—Polymers with Tunable Degradation for Sustained Release

The exact control of drug release kinetics in drug delivery is made possible by the controlled breakdown of polymeric carriers. Through hydrolysis or enzymatic cleavage, biodegradable polymers ensure the drug's continuous release while also shielding it from premature destruction [25]. For degradable drug delivery systems, the most popular matrices are polyanhydrides, polycaprolactone (PCL), and PLGA. The polymer molecular weight, copolymer ratio, and crystallinity can all be changed to alter the degradation rate and, consequently, the release profile. For example, increasing glycolic acid content promotes PLGA decomposition, producing quick release, while increased lactic acid content or crystallinity produces extended release patterns.

This idea is best shown by microsphere and nanoparticle systems, such as PLGA-based formulations for hormone delivery or cancer treatment. As an example of how degradation-controlled design can be translated into therapeutic efficacy, Lupron Depot® (leuprolide acetate), a PLGA microsphere formulation, offers sustained drug release over several months for the treatment of prostate cancer in clinical practice.

Stimuli-responsive degradable systems where degradation and release are triggered by environmental factors including pH, temperature, or enzyme activity are the subject of recent research. By enabling geographical and temporal precision, these technologies improve treatment targeting and lessen systemic toxicity. Polymer degradation is therefore an active design aspect for intelligent drug delivery platforms rather than just a passive process.

3.7.4 Wound Healing and Regenerative Dressings—Hydrogel Degradation Matching Tissue Repair Rate

Hydrogels are widely utilized in wound care because of their high water content, biocompatibility, and capacity to replicate natural extracellular matrix. They are made up of networks of crosslinked hydrophilic polymers. Controlled breakdown rate is a key component of hydrogel performance; it must align with tissue restoration to preserve a moist environment while permitting gradual replacement by new tissue.

Hydrogels made of natural polymers, such collagen, gelatin, chitosan, or alginate, break down via hydrolytic and enzymatic processes. Degradation rates can be adjusted to correspond with stages of wound healing by changing the crosslink density, chemical makeup, or addition of labile linkages. For example, β-glycerophosphate-containing chitosan hydrogels break down over a few days to weeks, which corresponds with the granulation and epithelialization processes in chronic wound care.

Bioactive substances, such as growth factors, antimicrobials, or stem cells, are included into advanced smart hydrogel dressings and released concurrently with hydrogel disintegration. Adaptive healing dynamics are ensured by case studies of PEG-based hydrogels functionalized with matrix metalloproteinase (MMP)-sensitive peptides, which exhibit selective breakdown in response to enzyme production during tissue remodeling. The shift from passive wound coverings to biointeractive regenerative dressings is best illustrated by this combination of biological responsiveness and degradation control.

3.7.5 Cardiovascular Devices—Resorbable Stents and Coatings

Bioresorbable vascular scaffolds (BVS) and resorbable coatings have been developed in cardiovascular medicine in response to the requirement for short-term mechanical support with few long-term consequences. Resorbable metal stents restore natural vascular mobility by gradually degrading following vessel healing, in contrast to permanent metal stents that may cause persistent inflammation or restenosis.

With controlled hydrolysis over two to three years, poly(L-lactic acid) (PLLA) has been the most prominent polymer in this field. Despite initial issues with mechanical durability and partial resorption, the Absorb™ Bioresorbable Vascular Scaffold marked a significant advancement in clinical translation. Degradation of uniformity and radial strength have been increased by ongoing optimization, which has been achieved through polymer molecular alignment, crystallinity management, and better strut design.

Resorbable stents based on magnesium, like BIOTRONIK's Magmaris, provide a metallic substitute with advantageous endothelialization profiles and quicker disintegration (9–12 months). To prevent quick corrosion and maintain structural stability while the vessel heals, surface passivation and fluoride coatings are used. Comparative clinical studies highlight the therapeutic value of controlled degradation in cardiovascular treatments by demonstrating that these next-generation stents considerably lower the risk of late thrombosis when compared to their permanent equivalents.

3.7.6 Comparative Analysis of Degradation Outcomes in Preclinical and Clinical Settings

Although laboratory-based (preclinical) degradation studies offer fundamental knowledge, it is nevertheless very difficult to translate these findings into clinical performance. Because biological environments are complex and include factors including enzyme activity, mechanical stress, local pH, and immunological response, degradation kinetics seen in vitro frequently deviate significantly from in vivo results.

For instance, PLGA scaffolds may hydrolyze uniformly in buffered solutions but degrade differently in vivo because of macrophage infiltration and localized acidic microenvironments. Similarly, protein adsorption and inflammatory cell interactions may cause magnesium implants that exhibit controlled corrosion in saline-based conditions to corrode in an unpredictable manner in vivo. Thus, to close this gap, multiscale modeling and accelerated aging tests are being employed more and more to mimic physiological stressors that affect degradation pathways.

The variation in patient outcomes associated with degrading behavior is emphasized by comparative clinical data. While certain vascular stents show slower-than-expected polymer resorption, magnesium screws show complete resorption within 18 months with good bone regeneration in orthopedic trials. These variations highlight the significance of site-specific degradation models and customized material choices.

Comprehensive degradation profiling, including in vitro testing, animal studies, and long-term human follow-up, is currently required by regulatory frameworks to correlate degradation pathways with clinical performance to guarantee predictability and safety. A potent approach for directing the design of next-generation biomaterials is the combination of AI-driven prediction modeling and real-time imaging of degradation in vivo.

Controlled deterioration is both a design tool and a functional requirement across biomaterial systems, as demonstrated by the various applications and case studies that are provided. Clinical success for tissue scaffolds and vascular devices depends on striking the correct balance between mechanical performance, biological responsiveness, and degradation rate [26]. A new era of biomaterials, where deterioration is not a constraint but rather an engineered road toward regeneration, healing, and therapeutic precision, is promised by ongoing research into intelligent, adaptive materials that can interact with biological environments in real-time.

3.8 Recent Advances and Innovations

The need for materials that not only satisfy mechanical and biocompatibility standards but also dynamically interact with their biological environment has fueled the rapid evolution of the biomaterials industry. Recent developments have produced smart, adaptive, and sustainable materials that can react to physiological stimuli, providing precise control over stability and degradation. Traditional biomaterials were intended to be either inert or uniformly degradable. The next generation of intelligent biomaterials for environmental and medicinal applications is made possible by advancements in computational modeling, additive manufacturing, and nanotechnology. With an emphasis on how they reinterpret degradation management and long-term performance, this section examines these new paradigms in biomaterial design.

3.8.1 Smart and Responsive Biomaterials—Stimuli-Triggered Degradation (pH, Temperature, Enzymes)

By selectively reacting to environmental cues like pH, temperature, enzymatic concentration, or redox status, smart biomaterials mark a revolutionary transition from passive degradation to stimuli-responsive degradation. By limiting off-target effects and increasing treatment precision, these materials are designed to break down only under biological or pathological circumstances.

Because localized pH fluctuations can cause deterioration, pH-sensitive biomaterials are especially useful in wound healing, infection control, and tumor therapy. For instance, in acidic microenvironments, polymers with acid-labile links, like acetals or hydrazones, break down, allowing for regulated medication release at tumor locations. Like this, poly(β-amino esters) hydrolyze more quickly in acidic conditions, allowing for targeted administration in inflammatory and cancerous tissues.

Utilizing polymers that experience phase transitions at physiological temperatures, such as poly(N-isopropylacrylamide) (PNIPAM), temperature-responsive systems enable regulated swelling and breakdown for injectable hydrogels or on-demand therapeutic release. Conversely, enzyme-responsive materials use peptide or polysaccharide bonds that are broken down by enzymes like lysozymes or matrix metalloproteinases (MMPs), which are elevated during inflammation or tissue remodeling. By facilitating site-specific degradation, these technologies match the breakdown of materials with biological processes.

One prominent example is MMP-sensitive PEG hydrogels, which enable cell-mediated matrix remodeling in regenerative therapies by breaking down when exposed to enzymes released by invasive cells. When taken as a whole, these smart materials demonstrate how biochemical feedback mechanisms can be included in biomaterial design to provide patient-specific impairment control that is adaptive.

3.8.2 Nanostructured Materials—Enhanced Control of Degradation through Nanocomposites and Coatings

The development of nanostructured biomaterials has made it possible to manipulate material behavior at the molecular and nanoscale levels, which has completely changed the way degradation is controlled. By adding nanoparticles, nanofibers, or nanolayers to biomaterials, it is possible to drastically alter their mechanical integrity, diffusion rates, and surface reactivity, which can be used to customize stability profiles and degradation kinetics.

Polymer matrices supplemented with nanoclays, graphene oxide, or hydroxyapatite nanoparticles are examples of nanocomposite biomaterials that provide enhanced mechanical strength and more consistent degradation. By acting as physical barriers and delaying the entry of ions and water, the nanoscale fillers lower the rates of oxidative or hydrolytic breakdown. PLGA-hydroxyapatite nanocomposites have demonstrated improved osteoconductivity and a more progressive degradation pattern in tissue engineering, which corresponds with the timeliness of bone regeneration [27].

Additionally, nanostructured surface coatings offer exact control over hydrolysis and corrosion. For example, titanium implants coated with arrays of TiO_2 nanotubes have self-passivating qualities that support cellular attachment and minimize ion leaching and controlled deterioration. Diffusion barriers produced by nanostructured fluoride or calcium-phosphate coatings in biodegradable metals, such as magnesium, control corrosion rates without sacrificing bioactivity.

The use of core-shell nanoparticles and nanocarriers for drug administration is another significant advancement, in which the release profile of the encapsulating agent is controlled by the breakdown of the outer shell. These nanosystems adjustable degradation enables spatiotemporal control in intricate biological settings. As a result, nanostructuring offers a flexible method for maximizing the fine balance between functioning and degradation, which promotes improved biological integration and a longer material lifespan.

3.8.3 Additive Manufacturing—3D and 4D Printing for Spatially Controlled Degradation

A potent method for creating biomaterials with spatially controlled degrading qualities is additive manufacturing (AM), which includes 3D and 4D printing. AM makes it possible to create specialized geometries, graded compositions, and hierarchical structures by exact layer-by-layer deposition. These structures can be configured to break down at certain rates in various areas of a single construct.

Because 3D printing makes it possible to combine materials with different degradation profiles into a single scaffold, it has already revolutionized tissue engineering and implant design. To promote vascular infiltration, a bone scaffold might, for example, include a slower-degrading polymer in load-bearing areas and a faster-degrading component in porous zones. Degradation rates can be adjusted to correspond with site-specific tissue regeneration timescales by modifying characteristics including porosity, infill density, and crosslinking patterns.

The development of 4D printing adds a dynamic element to deterioration management by introducing materials that alter their shape or qualities over time in response to environmental stimuli like heat, moisture, or pH. Hydrogels and shape-memory polymers are two examples that break down in response to mechanical stress or hydration, allowing for time-programmed changes in vivo.

Recent studies have shown that 4D-printed biodegradable scaffolds and stents can self-expand or disintegrate in response to body temperature, providing patient-specific flexibility and minimally invasive deployment. These developments lessen the surgical risks connected to non-biodegradable implants while also improving functional integration. The integration of spatial degradation into biological systems will continue to be redefined by additive manufacturing as multimaterial printing and computational design technologies advance.

3.8.4 Computational Modeling—AI-Driven Prediction of Long-Term Stability and In Vivo Degradation

Given the diversity of vivo settings, predicting long-term deterioration and stability has long been one of the biggest concerns in biomaterials science. Artificial intelligence (AI) and computational modeling have recently advanced to the point where they offer strong tools for simulating deterioration behavior and improving material design prior to clinical application.

Crack development, mass loss, and the diffusion of degradation byproducts are examples of mechanical qualities that are altered by degradation and are increasingly being modeled using finite element analysis (FEA) and molecular dynamics (MD) simulations. These models, which incorporate experimental data, can forecast the behavior of materials under physiological pressures, directing design improvements for enhanced performance.

By examining enormous databases of material compositions, structural characteristics, and degradation trends, artificial intelligence (AI) and machine learning (ML) expand these capabilities even further. Under a variety of circumstances, ML algorithms can spot trends and forecast failure mechanisms, half-lives, or rates of degradation. For instance, using chemical characteristics like bond energy and hydrophilicity, neural networks trained on polymer degradation data can predict hydrolysis rates. Artificial intelligence (AI)-driven corrosion prediction models model passive film disintegration and electrochemical behavior in metallic biomaterials at different ion concentrations and pH levels. In a similar vein, machine learning algorithms help optimize filler-matrix ratios for biodegradable composites in order to attain the required stability.

These computational tools enable real-time monitoring and adaptive design modifications when combined with digital twin frameworks, which are virtual representations of biomaterial systems that change in tandem with their physical counterparts. Because it allows for the virtual testing of long-term deterioration scenarios, the incorporation of computational prediction into biomaterial development speeds up innovation, lowers experimental costs, and improves safety.

3.8.5 Green and Sustainable Biomaterials—Eco-Friendly Degradation Pathways and Recyclability

Research on biomaterials has become more concerned with environmentally benign degradation processes and circular design concepts as the importance of sustainability on a global scale increase. Green biomaterials integrate biomedical innovation with sustainable development goals by minimizing environmental effect during synthesis, use, and post-disposal degradation.

Biodegradable substitutes for petroleum-based products are provided by biopolymers made from renewable resources, such as polylactic acid (PLA), polyhydroxyalkanoates (PHAs), and cellulose derivatives. Through microbial or hydrolytic processes, their breakdown products which are non-toxic and environmentally benign break down into biomass, carbon dioxide, and water. These substances are increasingly being used in bioresorbable packaging, wound dressings, and temporary implants.

Green design prioritizes safe synthesis methods that minimize the use of hazardous solvents, catalysts, and crosslinkers, in addition to renewable sourcing. Advances in solvent-free additive manufacturing and enzyme-mediated polymerization improve material purity and sustainability.

Furthermore, a new paradigm in the design of circular biomaterials is emerging recyclable biomaterials, or those that can undergo controlled depolymerization and reprocessing.

Environmental biotechnology and sustainable degradation are related. Biomaterials are utilized in eco-remediation and biofiltration processes, which break down pollutants and recover nutrients. This makes degradation of science more widely applicable outside of the biological field and establishes biomaterials as important players in international sustainability initiatives.

The intersection of materials science, biotechnology, computational modeling, and environmental engineering is reflected in the latest developments and breakthroughs in biomaterial stability and degradation. These developments signal a shift toward intelligent, predictive, and sustainable biomaterials, from nanostructured and additively made structures with spatially controlled degradation to intelligent responsive systems that adjust to physiological inputs. Green chemistry makes sure that innovation happens in a responsible manner, and AI-driven modeling currently fills the gap between laboratory forecasts and clinical performance [28]. When combined, these technologies are changing the paradigm of degradation from one of difficulty to one of design opportunity, opening the door for biomaterials that are ecologically friendly, patient-centered, and adaptable in future biomedical applications.

3.9 Challenges and Limitations

Despite being essential to biomedical innovation, the stability and degradation of biomaterials continue to present numerous obstacles that prevent their predictable and secure clinical translation. It is challenging to regulate, forecast, and assess how biomaterials behave in the human body due to a number of internal and external elements, even with notable advancements in materials science, computer modeling, and manufacturing technology as shown in Fig. 3.2. The distinction between in vitro and in vivo degradation, the trade-off between mechanical integrity and

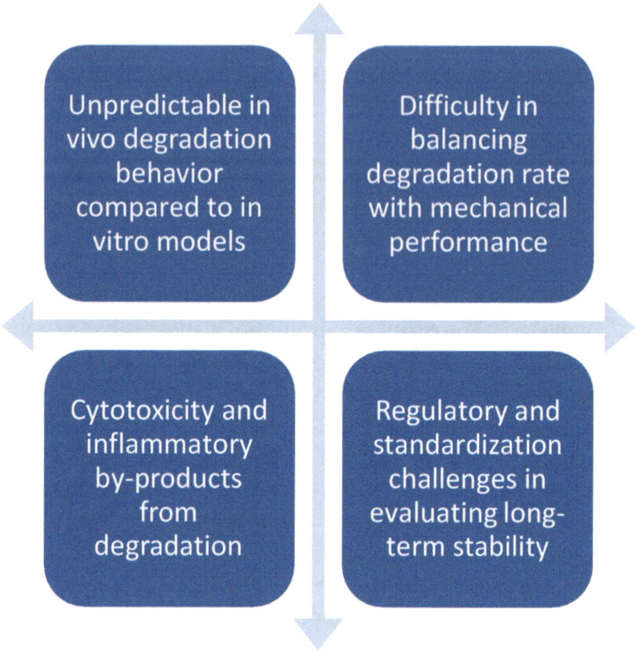

Fig. 3.2 Challenges and limitations associated with biomaterial degradation and stability, highlighting key issues such as unpredictable in vivo behavior, mechanical–degradation trade-offs, cytotoxicity of degradation by-products, regulatory and standardization gaps, and the lack of real-time in vivo monitoring tools

degradation kinetics, the toxicity of degradation byproducts, the lack of real-time monitoring tools, and regulatory and standards gaps are some of the main problems. Each of these difficulties emphasizes how urgently stronger design-to-clinic connections and a deeper multidisciplinary knowledge are needed.

3.9.1 Unpredictable in Vivo Degradation Behavior Compared to in Vitro Models

The discrepancy between in vitro degradation studies and real in vivo performance is one of the most enduring constraints in biomaterial development. Though they are essential for preliminary screening and optimization, laboratory-based models are unable to adequately represent the physiological complexity of living systems. The dynamic metabolic, mechanical, and immunological milieu of human tissues are rarely replicated in vitro under settings of controlled temperature, static pH, and homogeneous fluid exposure.

Biomaterials are subjected to varying pH gradients, enzymatic activity, mechanical stressors, and immunological responses in vivo, which differ depending on the tissue type and patient circumstances. For example, local acidity and inflammatory cell enzymatic secretions might cause a biodegradable polymer that breaks down reliably in phosphate-buffered saline to break down unpredictable in a wound site. Similarly, due to local galvanic effects, proteins, and chloride ions that are not present in simplified laboratory testing, metallic implants, like magnesium alloys, exhibit faster corrosion in vivo.

Additionally, it is difficult to represent the stochastic unpredictability introduced by the physiological environment, which includes variations in hydration, vascularization, and local cell density. Clinical translation is eventually made more difficult by this unpredictability, which causes variations in mechanical performance, by-product release, and degradation rate. Degradation research is still severely limited by the unreliability of in vitro-to-in vivo correlation (IVIVC), necessitating the creation of sophisticated, biomimetic testing setups that more accurately capture physiological complexity.

3.9.2 Difficulty in Balancing Degradation Rate with Mechanical Performance

Finding the ideal balance between mechanical performance and deterioration kinetics is another significant difficulty. Before safely decomposing, biomaterials, especially those utilized in load-bearing applications like vascular scaffolds and orthopedic implants must retain their structural integrity long enough to promote mechanical function or tissue healing.

Degradation, on the other hand, weakens materials by causing microcracks, crystalline structure disruption, and molecular weight reduction. While increasing strength usually slows degradation, accelerating degradation for fast resorption frequently compromises mechanical strength. High crystalline poly(L-lactic acid) (PLLA), for example, has excellent mechanical qualities but degrades slowly and remains long after tissue regeneration is finished. On the other hand, PLGA and other amorphous copolymers break down quickly but may lose their strength too soon, which could result in implant collapse or insufficient tissue integration.

The trade-off for metallic biomaterials is comparable. Despite being technically compatible with bone and biodegradable, magnesium alloys break down too quickly in vivo, creating hydrogen gas pockets and jeopardizing structural stability. Although surface coatings can reduce corrosion, they can increase complexity and the possibility of delamination.

Patient-specific factors that affect degradation behavior, such as age, loading circumstances, and metabolic rate, make the problem much more difficult. Therefore, exact control over composition, microstructure, and porosity is necessary to design materials that display controlled degradation while maintaining strength. This area still requires advanced material engineering and predictive modeling.

3.9.3 *Cytotoxicity and Inflammatory By-products from Degradation*

Although material resorption and remodeling are made possible by degradation, the breakdown of products themselves may pose new biological hazards. Degradation byproduct-induced cytotoxicity and inflammation pose serious clinical problems. Degradation of polymeric biomaterials frequently produces acidic byproducts like lactic and glycolic acid (from PLA and PGA), which can cause cellular stress and reduce the local pH. When these acids build up in small tissue areas, it can lead to fibrosis, inflammation, and slow recovery. Similarly, reactive carbonyl compounds and free radicals are produced during the oxidative breakdown of polyurethanes and polyethylene, which aids in the activation of macrophages and the development of chronic inflammation.

Ions that are known to be cytotoxic or allergic, including nickel, chromium, or cobalt, are released when corrosion occurs in metallic implants. Nanoscale debris released by even biocompatible materials, such as titanium, can cause oxidative stress and immunological activation [29]. Despite being bioresorbable, magnesium breakdown produces hydrogen gas and hydroxides, which may irritate tissue and cause local pH imbalances. Degradation products also can change systemic physiology. Wear debris nanoparticles have the potential to spread to distant organs, where they could cause immunogenicity or oxidative stress. The necessity for materials that not only decompose reliably but also produce non-toxic, bio-assimilable compounds is highlighted by the poorly known interaction between degradation chemistry and biological response.

Toxicological evaluation of degradation by-products is further complicated by the difficulty of long-term in vivo tracking. Consequently, cytotoxicity testing protocols remain conservative, often delaying approval and clinical translation of novel materials.

3.9.4 *Regulatory and Standardization Challenges in Evaluating Long-Term Stability*

Another significant obstacle is the biomaterials regulatory environment. Standardized techniques for assessing degradation, stability, and biocompatibility are still scarce and unevenly implemented across jurisdictions, despite the increasing diversity of biodegradable and smart materials.

Existing international standards, including ASTM recommendations for polymer degradation and ISO 10993 for biological evaluation, offer broad frameworks but frequently overlook the special properties of emerging materials like hybrid composites, nanostructured coatings, and 4D biomaterials. Complex degradation routes in these new systems make it impossible to assess using traditional chemical or mechanical techniques.

Long-term stability evaluation also presents ethical and practical difficulties. Accelerated aging tests may not accurately mimic normal degradation pathways, and real-time in vivo investigations can take years and a lot of resources. Establishing trustworthy degradation benchmarks and safety profiles before clinical implementation is challenging due to this regulatory gap. The absence of coordination amongst regulatory bodies is another drawback. The European Medicines Agency (EMA), the U.S. Food and Drug Administration (FDA), and other agencies have different acceptance criteria and testing procedures, which causes confusion for producers and delays product approval. Furthermore, because degradation science is constantly changing, regulatory frameworks frequently lag technological advancement, leaving new materials without obvious assessment routes, such bioresorbable electronics or adaptable hydrogels.

The challenge, therefore, lies in developing adaptable, data-driven regulatory systems that integrate mechanistic modeling, in vitro–in vivo correlations, and standardized predictive simulations to evaluate long-term biomaterial stability with greater precision and efficiency.

3.9.5 Limited Real-Time Monitoring Tools for Degradation Tracking In Vivo

The lack of trustworthy, real-time monitoring instruments that can evaluate biomaterial deterioration in vivo is another barrier impeding the development of degradation research. The majority of evaluation techniques now in use focus on post-explant analysis, which only offers endpoint data and is unable to capture the dynamic, time-varying progression of degradation processes. The sensitivity of conventional imaging techniques like CT, MRI, and X-ray scans to chemical or microstructural alterations during deterioration is restricted. Although more specificity is offered by more recent methods like Raman spectroscopy, optical coherence tomography (OCT), and positron emission tomography (PET), their clinical use is still limited by factors including cost, resolution limitations, and signal interference from nearby tissues.

Although they are currently mostly at the experimental stage, emerging techniques such as embedded biosensors, fluorescent tagging, and smart materials that may self-report degradation via colorimetric or electrical signals show promise. Creating high-resolution, biocompatible, and non-invasive instruments that can track degradation dynamics continually, identify early failure, and link structural alterations to physiological reactions is the difficult part. In addition to improving knowledge of degradation mechanisms, real-time tracking would allow for tailored biomaterial performance, enabling physicians to modify treatment regimens in response to patient reactions. Degradation monitoring is still mostly indirect and retrospective until such technologies are developed, which restricts feedback-driven optimization in clinical practice.

The difficulties and constraints in studying biomaterial degradation highlight how difficult it is to create materials that will interact with the human body in a predictable and safe manner. The translation of biomaterials from laboratory to clinic is hampered by several factors, including cytotoxic byproducts, unpredictable in vivo behavior, the mechanical–chemical trade-off, unclear regulations, and insufficient monitoring systems.

An integrative approach is needed to overcome these obstacles, combining improved imaging, computational modeling, biomimetic testing systems, and adaptive regulatory frameworks. For deterioration to become a manageable, quantifiable, and advantageous process, interdisciplinary cooperation between materials scientists, physicians, toxicologists, and regulatory specialists will be essential to future advancement. The entire potential of biomaterials as dynamic, safe, and regenerative elements of contemporary medicine can only be realized with such coordinated efforts [30].

3.10 Future Directions

Advanced computation, bioinspired design, and sustainable engineering are the nexus of biomaterial degradation and stability research's future. Understanding and managing degradation processes will be even more important as biomedical technologies advance toward more intelligent, individualized, and ecologically conscious systems. To ensure that biomaterials can safely and successfully interact with dynamic biological settings, emerging directions place a strong emphasis on predictive modeling, adaptive materials, and worldwide standardization. Important topics influencing the future wave of biomaterials research and application are examined in the next subsections.

3.10.1 Integration of AI and Machine Learning for Degradation Prediction and Optimization

A revolutionary approach for anticipating degrading behavior, improving material qualities, and spurring innovation is the incorporation of artificial intelligence (AI) and machine learning (ML) into biomaterial science. Long-term, expensive, and time-consuming in vitro and in vivo investigations are a major component of traditional degradation studies. By simulating degradation mechanisms with previously unheard-of accuracy, AI-driven modeling may lessen the need for empirical testing.

Large-scale datasets of material compositions, structural characteristics, and environmental factors can be analyzed by machine learning algorithms to forecast the creation of byproducts, mechanical stability, and degradation kinetics. For instance, using bond energies, hydrophilicity, and molecular structure, neural network models have been created to predict the rates at which polymers will hydrolyze. Similarly, under varying physiological conditions, AI-assisted corrosion modeling may forecast passive film degradation and electrochemical reactions in metallic biomaterials.

Additionally, through iterative design feedback loops, reinforcement learning techniques are being used to optimize material formulations. In these loops, algorithms automatically determine the best parameters for striking a balance between mechanical performance and deterioration rate. Real-time monitoring and predictive maintenance of medical equipment are made possible by the idea of the "digital twin," a virtual representation of a biomaterial system that develops concurrently with its physical counterpart.

AI will not only be able to forecast deterioration behavior as datasets grow and computational models advance, but it will also make it possible for inverse material design, in which the system determines material compositions that meet desired degradation characteristics after defining them first. The creation of biomaterials will be transformed by this paradigm, producing more dependable, patient-specific, and legally compliant goods.

3.10.2 Development of Bioinspired and Adaptive Degradation Systems

In an effort to emulate how natural tissues react dynamically to external stimuli, bioinspired and adaptive design principles are increasingly influencing the next generation of biomaterials. Enzymatic extracellular matrix breakdown and mechanical stress-guided bone remodeling are examples of controlled degradation and renewal found in biological systems. Converting these processes into artificial materials offers a model for context-sensitive and self-regulating deterioration.

Utilizing enzymatically cleavable sequences or hierarchical structures that break down in response to biological stimuli, bioinspired materials incorporate molecular motifs or architectures taken from natural polymers such as collagen, chitin, and elastin [31]. Materials with MMP-sensitive peptide connections, for example, enable cells to reshape scaffolds during the healing process, guaranteeing synchronous tissue development and material resorption.

By incorporating feedback mechanisms, emerging adaptive degradation systems go one step farther and react instantly to mechanical or biological cues. Examples of this direction include metallic coatings that self-heal when microcracks emerge or smart hydrogels that change their consistency in response to strain. Furthermore, materials can reversibly disintegrate and re-form under physiological conditions thanks to dynamic covalent chemistry and self-assembling nanostructures, which promote robustness and longevity. Achieving homeostatic biomaterials systems that can independently maintain equilibrium between degradation and regeneration is the ultimate goal of these designs. In regenerative medicine, where materials must adjust to shifting tissue environments while retaining functional stability, such advancements will be essential.

3.10.3 Advancements in Multi-Scale Modeling for Lifetime Prediction

Accurately forecasting the long-term lifespan of biomaterials under physiological settings is still difficult, despite tremendous experimental advancements. Multi-scale modeling, which combines atomic, molecular, and macroscopic investigations to fully reflect the complexity of material behavior across time, is the way of the future for degradation research.

Bond breakage mechanisms and water transport during hydrolysis are clarified at the molecular level by simulations employing molecular dynamics (MD) and quantum mechanics (QM). At the macroscale, system-level models forecast how implants will function under load-bearing and biological stress, whereas at the mesoscale, finite element analysis (FEA) connects local degradation patterns to mechanical weakness. Accurate and therapeutically applicable lifetime prediction models will be made possible by combining these scales into a single computational framework.

Real-time data from spectroscopic and imaging techniques can be used to calibrate simulations thanks to recent advancements in hybrid experimental–computational models. For instance, FEA predictions of mass loss and porosity evolution can be verified by time-lapse micro-CT imaging of deteriorating scaffolds. By combining these strategies with AI-driven analytics, predictive accuracy will be improved and patient-specific material performance estimates will be possible. Multi-scale modeling will eventually be a commonplace part of biomaterial design, assisting regulatory approval procedures by offering quantifiable proof of durability and safety. The reliability of next-generation biodegradable devices will be improved and development times shortened by this combination.

3.10.4 Expansion of Biodegradable Metallic Systems for Orthopedic and Cardiovascular Use

For orthopedic and cardiovascular applications in particular, the creation of biodegradable metallic biomaterials is one of the most promising areas of biomaterial innovation. Metals having the ability to safely decompose within the body, such magnesium (Mg), iron (Fe), and zinc (Zn), provide mechanical qualities that are significantly superior to those of polymers.

In orthopaedic fixation systems, magnesium-based alloys have already shown promise by offering initial mechanical strength followed by progressive resorption that promotes bone repair. By using surface modification, rare-earth alloying, and nanostructuring, the next generation of magnesium alloys is being developed with corrosion rates that are carefully controlled. Zinc alloys are also becoming more popular for cardiovascular implants because they have slower corrosion kinetics and less hydrogen evolution than magnesium, which makes them appropriate for bioresorbable vascular scaffolds [32].

By enabling precisely calibrated porosity and degradation gradients, developments in additive manufacturing (AM) are speeding up the personalization of metallic implants. For instance, gradient pore architectures in 3D-printed magnesium scaffolds can be used to control mechanical stress distribution and ion release, coordinating tissue remodeling and breakdown.

Multi-metallic composites and hybrid coatings, which combine metals with polymers or ceramics to balance strength and degradation control, will be the focus of future research. Biodegradable metals will become essential components for regenerative and minimally invasive medical devices as biocompatible corrosion inhibitors and bioactive coatings advance concurrently, improving safety and performance even further.

3.10.5 Regulatory Harmonization and Sustainability-Driven Design Frameworks

Maintaining sustainability and regulatory harmonization is crucial as biomaterial technologies develop. Different testing methods and degradation mechanisms have led to disparities in safety evaluations between jurisdictions. Global harmonization of metrics, standards, and assessment frameworks that appropriately represent in vivo performance is essential for future advancement.

Guidelines for biodegradation testing are being expanded by organizations like ISO and ASTM International to include biocompatibility evaluations, accelerated aging models, and in situ corrosion evaluation. But the quick development of smart and hybrid materials necessitates new standards that include AI-assisted design verification and computational validation. Harmonization will increase reproducibility in both industry and research and speed up clinical translation.

Integrating sustainability-driven design frameworks is equally important. The move to green biomaterials, which are non-toxic, biodegradable, and derived from renewable resources, is consistent with the circular economy's tenets and lessens the environmental impact of products across their whole existence. Biomedical materials are being subjected to adaptations of life cycle assessment (LCA) approaches, which cover extraction, processing, use, degradation, and environmental fate. “Eco-biocompatibility,” which strikes a balance between environmental responsibility and biological safety, will be embraced by future design philosophies. This strategy reduces the long-term waste accumulation from medical equipment by promoting the development of biomaterials that break down into innocuous or recyclable byproducts.

Convergence of artificial intelligence and materials science, of biological inspiration and engineering accuracy, and of innovation and sustainability define the future of biomaterial degradation research. Intelligent materials customized for each patient will be made possible by predictive modeling and machine learning, and bioinspired adaptive systems will close the gap between artificial and live materials. With the help of internationally standardized and environmentally conscientious regulatory frameworks, multi-scale simulations and biodegradable metals will increase material lifetimes and expand therapeutic uses. Collectively, these directions will transform degradation from a limiting factor into a strategic design element driving the creation of smart, sustainable, and patient-centered biomaterials that embody the next evolution of medical technology [33, 34].

3.11 Conclusion

3.11.1 Summary of Key Insights on Degradation–Stability Interplay

One of the most dynamic and multidisciplinary areas of biomedical engineering is the research of biomaterial stability and degradation. The complex interactions between degradation kinetics, chemical composition, mechanical integrity, and biological response have been gradually revealed by scientific research over the past few decades. The realization that stability and degradation are complementing factors that need to be balanced for safe and effective biomaterial performance rather than being mutually exclusive occurrences is fundamental to this concept. While stability controls a biomaterial’s ability to retain structural and functional integrity under mechanical, chemical, and biological stress, degradation controls a biomaterial’s lifespan within the physiological environment. The optimal biomaterial, therefore, is not one that simply resists degradation indefinitely, but one that degrades predictably and synchronously with tissue regeneration or therapeutic intent.

Degradation pathways hydrolysis, oxidation, corrosion, and enzymatic breakdown determine how materials interact with the biological environment in metallic, polymeric, and ceramic systems. For example, titanium’s stable oxide layer guarantees long-term mechanical performance in permanent implants, whereas regulated hydrolysis of polyesters allows bioresorbable scaffolds to vanish after completing their regenerative function. Therefore, depending on its intended biological purpose, the degradation–stability relationship determines a biomaterial’s clinical identity, whether it be transitory, semi-permanent, or permanent.

Furthermore, this interaction controls both biocompatibility and functional performance. The necessity of controlling chemistry degradation at the molecular level is highlighted by the way degradation by-products affect local pH, cellular viability, and immunological response. The fundamental scientific and engineering problem is still striking a balance between stability and degradation, which calls for accuracy in fabrication, design, and predictive modeling.

3.11.2 Reinforcement of Degradation Control as a Cornerstone of Biomaterial Safety and Performance

The foundation of biomaterial safety and performance is now understood to be the ability to regulate degradational terms of rate, mechanism, and by-product composition. Degradation control dictates how a material behaves throughout its lifecycle, from implantation to full integration or removal, regardless of the objective resorption, durability, or biofunctionality.

Precise degradation control in bioresorbable systems, like PLA or implants made of magnesium, guarantees that structural integrity is maintained during tissue healing and only lost when the new tissue is able to withstand physiological demands. Degradation control, on the other hand, reduces wear and corrosion in permanent implants and stops the discharge of harmful ions or particles. Strategies like surface engineering (coatings, passivation layers), environmental stability (antioxidants, buffering agents), and molecular design (copolymerization, crosslinking) are used to achieve this control.

Furthermore, maintaining consistent performance under a range of physiological circumstances depends on degradation control. Materials must be designed with adaptive stability properties because localized inflammation, infection, and mechanical loading can change the way things degrade.

Degradation management is crucial from the standpoint of clinical safety to avoid negative reactions like fibrosis, persistent inflammation, or mechanical failure. It connects laboratory performance with practical results and serves as the foundation for regulatory evaluation and quality assurance. Thus, one of the key areas of biomaterials science is the development of materials with programmable degradation profiles that react to pH values, enzyme activity, or mechanical stress.

3.11.3 Importance of Interdisciplinary Integration Chemistry, Biology, and Engineering in Stability Design

The search for improved stability and controlled deterioration is intrinsically multidisciplinary, combining knowledge from engineering, biology, and chemistry. Every field offers a distinct viewpoint that is crucial for converting materials from conceptual design to practical use.

From a chemical perspective, the basis for forecasting degradation routes is an understanding of molecule structure, bond energy, and reactivity under physiological settings. Materials with specific chemical stability and regulated breakdown mechanisms can be designed thanks to methods in surface modification, electrochemistry, and polymer chemistry.

Another crucial component is biology, which sheds light on the interactions between materials and immune cells, enzymes, and tissue microenvironments. Degradation behavior is directly influenced by cellular reactions like oxidative stress, enzymatic secretion, and macrophage activation. By incorporating biological knowledge, materials are guaranteed to be both mechanically compatible and biologically intelligent, allowing them to interact with natural healing processes without causing negative reactions.

Degradation–stability relationships can be simulated, optimized, and validated from an engineering standpoint using computer modeling, materials processing, and mechanical testing. For example, additive manufacturing enables fine-grained control over design and porosity, affecting mechanical strength, diffusion, and degradation kinetics all at once. The process from prototype to patient can be sped up by using machine learning methods and finite element modeling to forecast deterioration behavior under intricate physiological settings.

Innovation in contemporary biomaterials is fueled by the collaboration of these fields. Material characteristics are determined by chemistry, its behavior in vivo by biology, and its long-term dependability by engineering. By combining these fields, the scientific triangle of stability design is created, guaranteeing that materials are both biologically sensitive and structurally robust.

3.11.4 Outlook on the Evolving Paradigm Toward Adaptive, Predictive, and Regenerative Biomaterial Systems

Research on biomaterial stability and degradation is changing significantly in the future, moving from empirical observation to paradigms that are predictive, adaptive, and regenerative. This change is a result of developments in systems biology, nanotechnology, artificial intelligence (AI), and computational modeling, all of which are working together to create a new class of materials that can react to their surroundings in a clever way. In response to physiological stimuli, adaptive biomaterials are being developed that can dynamically modify their rate of disintegration. Hydrogels that are sensitive to pH or enzymes, for instance, can degrade more quickly in inflammatory tissues while staying stable in other circumstances. In a similar vein, self-healing oxide coatings on bioresorbable metallic implants can modify corrosion behavior to preserve peak mechanical performance during the healing process.

Predictive modeling is yet another significant development. Long-term behavior may now be predicted with surprising precision using machine learning algorithms that have been trained on large datasets of material properties and degradation profiles. These solutions decrease the time and expense involved in clinical validation while also improving safety and dependability. Personalized biomaterials, whose stability and degradation are adapted to each patient's unique healing pace and physiological circumstances, are made possible by integration with patient-specific data. The ultimate objective is the development of regenerative biomaterial systems, which are materials that actively aid in the healing process by releasing bioactive chemicals, directing cell proliferation, and remodeling into natural tissue, in addition to safely degrading. These systems represent the fusion of regenerative medicine with degradation control, progressing from passive biocompatibility to biofunctionality and restoration.

This evolving paradigm redefines stability not as resistance to change but as a controlled transformation aligned with biological adaptation. The future of biomaterials thus lies in their capacity to be both transient and transformative to degrade with purpose, stability, and intelligence.

The scientific basis for safe, efficient, and regenerative medical devices is the degradation and stability of biomaterials. The future requires dedication to sustainability and patient-centered design, as well as ongoing interdisciplinary integration and cutting-edge modeling and monitoring technology. Biomaterials have the potential to develop from static implants into dynamic, self-regulating systems that adjust to human physiology and encourage internal healing as research advances. This view sees the mastery of degradation control as a deep manifestation of biomaterials research at the nexus of chemistry, biology, and technology, rather than merely a technical accomplishment.

References

1. Gałko, G., Sajdak, M.: Trends for the thermal degradation of polymeric materials: analysis of available techniques, issues, and opportunities. Appl. Sci. **12**(18), 9138 (2022)
2. Veskova, J., Sbordone, F., Frisch, H.: Trends in polymer degradation across all scales. Macromol. Chem. Phys. **223**(13), 2100472 (2022)
3. Ma, B., Martín, C., Kurapati, R., Bianco, A.: Degradation-by-design: how chemical functionalization enhances the biodegradability and safety of 2D materials. Chem. Soc. Rev. **49**(17), 6224–6247 (2020)
4. Remya, R.R., Julius, A., Suman, T.Y., Mohanavel, V., Karthick, A., Pazhanimuthu, C., Samrot, A.V., Muhibbullah, M.: Role of nanoparticles in biodegradation and their importance in environmental and biomedical applications. J. Nanomater. **1**, 6090846 (2022)
5. Al-Zyoud, W., Haddadin, D., Hasan, S.A., Jaradat, H., Kanoun, O.: Biocompatibility testing for implants: a novel tool for selection and characterization. Materials. **16**(21), 6881 (2023)
6. Ebrahimi, M.: Standardization and regulation of biomaterials. In: Handbook of Biomaterials Biocompatibility, pp. 251–265. Woodhead Publishing (2020)
7. Prasad, A., Chakraborty, G.a., Kumar, A.: Bio-based environmentally benign polymeric resorbable materials for orthopedic fixation applications. In: Adv. Mater. Biomed. Appl., pp. 251–266. CRC Press (2022)
8. Raut, H.K., Das, R., Liu, Z., Liu, X., Ramakrishna, S.: Biocompatibility of biomaterials for tissue regeneration or replacement. Biotechnol. J. **15**(12), 2000160 (2020)

9. Seehaam, A., Pullichola, A.H.: Transformative advances in the durability and stimuli-responsiveness of intrinsic and extrinsic self-healing polymer coatings: a comprehensive review. Polym. Adv. Technol. **37**(2), e70535 (2026). https://doi.org/10.1002/pat.70535
10. Sobhana, K.S., Kizhakudan, S.J., George, G., Sukumaran, S., Sharma, S.R., Edison, S.J., Muktha, M., Bindu, J., Chakraborty, K., Jayasankar, J., Shinoj, P.: XVI Agricultural Science Congress 2023: Transformation of agri-food systems for achieving sustainable development goals. XVI Agricultural Science Congress 2023 2023
11. Liu, X., Chen, Y., Mao, A.S., Xuan, C., Wang, Z., Gao, H., An, G., Zhu, Y., Shi, X., Mao, C.: Molecular recognition-directed site-specific release of stem cell differentiation inducers for enhanced joint repair. Biomaterials. **232**, 119644 (2020)
12. Maddock, R.M., Pollard, G.J., Moreau, N.G., Perry, J.J.a., Race, P.R.: Enzyme-catalysed polymer cross-linking: biocatalytic tools for chemical biology, materials science and beyond. Biopolymers. **111**(9), e23390 (2020)
13. Hassna, E., Huang, Y., Yan, T.: Biodegradable metals for cardiovascular and orthopaedic implants: a comparative review of magnesium, iron and zinc. Met. Adv. **39**, 68–82 (2026). https://doi.org/10.1016/j.metadv.2025.12.001
14. Park, H.J., Hong, H., Thangam, R., Song, M.G., Kim, J.E., Jo, E.H., Jang, Y.J., Choi, W.H., Lee, M.Y., Kang, H., Lee, K.B.: Static and dynamic biomaterial engineering for cell modulation. Nano. **12**(8), 1377 (2022)
15. Shi, H., Wang, C., Ma, Z.: Stimuli-responsive biomaterials for cardiac tissue engineering and dynamic mechanobiology. APL Bioeng. **5**(1), 011506 (2021)
16. Akhtar, N., Syakir Ishak, M.I., Bhawani, S.A., Umar, K.: Various natural and anthropogenic factors responsible for water quality degradation: a review. Water. **13**(19), 2660 (2021)
17. Visan, A.I., Popescu-Pelin, G., Socol, G.: Degradation behavior of polymers used as coating materials for drug deliveryA basic review. Polymers. **13**(8), 1272 (2021)
18. Hu, F., Lu, Y., Tai, Z., Zhu, Q., He, H., Chen, Z., Wu, W.: Internal water-induced acceleration, chemical pathways, and contributing factors in the degradation of poly(lactic-co-glycolic acid) (PLGA) microparticles and devices. ACS Biomater. Sci. Eng. **11**(7), 3932–3948 (2025). https://doi.org/10.1021/acsbiomaterials.5c00419
19. Lim, J.I., Park, H., Kim, Y., Oh, S.: Study on enzymatic degradation of polycaprolactone-based composite scaffolds for tissue engineering applications. ACS Appl. Bio Mater. **8**(10), 9058–9071 (2025). https://doi.org/10.1021/acsabm.5c01203
20. Morgan, F.L., Moroni, L., Baker, M.B.: Dynamic bioinks to advance bioprinting. Adv. Healthc. Mater. **9**(15), 1901798 (2020)
21. Suwardi, A., Wang, F., Xue, K., Han, M.Y., Teo, P., Wang, P., Wang, S., Liu, Y., Ye, E., Li, Z.a., Loh, X.J.: Machine learning-driven biomaterials evolution. Adv. Mater. **34**(1), 2102703 (2022)
22. Rynkus, B., Scano, A., Puxeddu, S., Angius, F., Ennas, G., Szewczenko, J.: Biodegradable magnesium alloys for short-term orthopedic implants: properties, surface modification and biological response. J. Mater. Res. Technol. **40**, 488–503 (2026). https://doi.org/10.1016/j.jmrt.2025.12.038
23. Dai, X., Chen, Y.: Computational biomaterials: computational simulations for biomedicine. Adv. Mater. **35**(7), 2204798 (2023)
24. Xue, K., Wang, F., Suwardi, A., Han, M.Y., Teo, P., Wang, P., Wang, S., Ye, E., Li, Z., Loh, X.J.: Biomaterials by design: harnessing data for future development. Mater. Today Bio. **12**, 100165 (2021)
25. Tsung, T.H., Tsai, Y.C., Lee, H.P., Chen, Y.H., Lu, D.W.: Biodegradable polymer-based drug-delivery systems for ocular diseases. Int. J. Mol. Sci. **24**(16), 12976 (2023)
26. Zia, A.W., Liu, R., Wu, X.: Structural design and mechanical performance of composite vascular grafts. Bio-Des. Manuf. **5**(4), 757–785 (2022)
27. Ielo, I., Calabrese, G., De Luca, G., Conoci, S.: Recent advances in hydroxyapatite-based biocomposites for bone tissue regeneration in orthopedics. Int. J. Mol. Sci. **23**(17), 9721 (2022)
28. Alowais, S.A., Alghamdi, S.S., Alsuhebany, N., Alqahtani, T., Alshaya, A.I., Almohareb, S.N., Aldairem, A., Alrashed, M., Bin Saleh, K., Badreldin, H.A., Al Yami, M.S.: Revolutionizing

healthcare: the role of artificial intelligence in clinical practice. BMC Med. Educ. **23**(1), 689 (2023)
29. Messous, R., Henriques, B., Bousbaa, H., Silva, F.S., Teughels, W., Souza, J.C.: Cytotoxic effects of submicron-and nano-scale titanium debris released from dental implants: An integrative review. Clin. Oral Investig. **25**(4), 1627–1640 (2021)
30. Jovic, T.H., Combellack, E.J., Jessop, Z.M., Whitaker, I.S.: 3D bioprinting and the future of surgery. Front. Surg. **7**, 609836 (2020)
31. Ganewatta, M.S., Wang, Z., Tang, C.: Chemical syntheses of bioinspired and biomimetic polymers toward biobased materials. Nat. Rev. Chem. **5**(11), 753–772 (2021)
32. Prasadh, S., Raguraman, S., Wong, R., Gupta, M.: Current status and outlook of temporary implants (magnesium/zinc) in cardiovascular applications. Meta. **12**(6), 999 (2022)
33. Bibri, S.E.: A novel model for data-driven smart sustainable cities of the future: the institutional transformations required for balancing and advancing the three goals of sustainability. Energy Inform. **4**(1), 4 (2021)
34. Dixit, K.K., Dharme, A., Singh, D.P., Kalra, R., Bhavani, B., Asha, V., Abdulsada, Z.R.: Sustainability by design: innovative ways of revolutionizing production practices for a better tomorrow. In: E3S Web of Conferences, vol. 453, p. 01026. EDP Sciences (2023)

Chapter 4
Surface Properties and Modification Techniques

Abstract The way biomaterials interact with biological surroundings is largely determined by their surface characteristics, which also affect biocompatibility, corrosion resistance, protein adsorption, cell adhesion, and overall clinical performance. The surface, which serves as the interface between the substance and the tissue, controls the first biological reaction, determining whether integration, encapsulation, or rejection takes place. As a result, one of the main pillars of biomaterial engineering is the accurate control and manipulation of surface properties. This study looks at the basic ideas that control surface characteristics as well as cutting-edge modification methods intended to maximize the performance of biomaterials. At the molecular and cellular levels, surface characteristics such as topography, chemistry, charge, wettability, and energy influence biological interactions. Technological developments in surface modification have made it possible to customize these parameters without sacrificing the material's bulk characteristics. Physical techniques including laser texturing, ion implantation, and plasma treatment alter surface energy and morphology to improve protein compatibility and cell affinity. Covalent grafting, salinization, and self-assembled monolayers are examples of chemical modification techniques that enable precise functionalization with bioactive compounds that stimulate biological responses. Biomimetic interfaces that promote cell differentiation and tissue regeneration are made possible by biological modification techniques including the immobilization of peptides, growth factors, or extracellular matrix (ECM) components. Stimuli-responsive and nanostructured surfaces that can dynamically adapt to physiological inputs like pH, temperature, or enzyme activity are the subject of recent advances. Complex tissue interfaces can now have gradient patterns thanks to the increased spatial control over surface topologies made possible by additive manufacturing and nanocoating technology. New green surface modification techniques that make use of biopolymers and environmentally friendly procedures complement sustainability objectives in the creation of biomaterials. All things considered, the combination of surface science, nanotechnology, and bioengineering offers a way to develop next-generation biomaterials with improved durability, adaptive biological performance, and tun-

M. Adeoba, T. Pandelani, *Application of Biomaterials in Biomedical Engineering*, Series in BioEngineering,
https://doi.org/10.1007/978-3-032-34477-9_4

able interfacial functionality all of which are essential for developing implantable technology, smart therapeutic systems, and regenerative medicine.

4.1 Introduction

The primary factor influencing biocompatibility, functioning, and long-term clinical success is a biomaterial's surface, which serves as the crucial interface between synthetic and biological systems. The surface controls both the initial and continuing biological reactions after implantation, in contrast to bulk qualities, which control structural strength, elasticity, and durability. The way proteins adsorption, cells attach, and tissues integrate is determined by several factors, including surface chemistry, topography, charge, roughness, wettability, and surface energy [1, 2]. A material's biological destiny can be significantly changed by even minor changes in these properties. For instance, although a hydrophobic or contaminated surface may cause fibrotic encapsulation or immunological rejection, a hydrophilic surface often encourages advantageous protein adsorption and cell spreading.

Surface properties are especially important because biomolecules interact with a material's outermost atomic layers at the nanoscale, which is where biological recognition starts. For example, a titanium implant with a modified oxide layer can increase osteoblast activity, and polymer surface coatings can decrease bacterial adhesion. Likewise, surface phenomena are the primary determinant of hydrolytic resistance in polymers and corrosion resistance in metallic implants [3, 4]. To improve implants' long-term performance, durability, and safety as well as their initial biocompatibility, surface qualities must be optimized. A fundamental idea in biomedical design is the ability to precisely control and engineer surfaces as the field of biomaterials moves toward multifunctional, adaptable systems.

4.1.1 Role of Surface–Tissue Interactions in Determining Biocompatibility, Adhesion, and Osseointegration

The clinical behavior of a biomaterial is determined by the interaction between its surface and the biological environment around it. The surface of a biomaterial is instantly covered with a coating of blood or interstitial fluid proteins, ions, and water molecules after implantation. Subsequent cell attachment, differentiation, and tissue integration are controlled by this first layer of protein adsorption [5, 6]. The physicochemical properties of the surface determine the makeup and shape of adsorbed proteins, including albumin, vitronectin, and fibronectin. Integrin-mediated cell attachment is supported by a favorable protein layer, which creates a stable interface between the implant and tissue. On the other hand, foreign body reactions or inflammatory cascades may result from non-physiological protein adsorption.

Osteointegration, or the direct structural and functional bond between living bone and the implant surface, is a critical success factor in bone-contacting implants, such as titanium and magnesium alloys. It has been demonstrated that surface roughness, chemical makeup, and oxide layer thickness greatly increase osteoblastic activity and bone apposition. To increase the mechanical interlocking and biochemical affinity between the implant and tissue, methods like sandblasting, acid etching, anodization, and plasma spraying have been used. Like this, improved surface contacts can reduce thrombosis, inflammation, and infection in soft tissue applications including wound dressings and cardiovascular stents.

Therefore, regulating surface–tissue interactions involve more than just averting negative reactions; it also involves guiding biological outcomes, such as immune behavior modulation, cell differentiation guidance, and angiogenesis promotion. To promote healing and regeneration, this paradigm has changed the design of biomaterial surfaces from passive biocompatibility to bioactivity, where surfaces actively interact with the biological environment.

4.1.2 Relationship Between Surface Chemistry, Topography, and Biological Response

Communication between biomaterials and biological systems is largely dependent on the interaction between surface chemistry and topography. The kinds of chemical bonds, functional groups, and elements that can interact with biomolecules are determined by surface chemistry. Protein adsorption in conformations that reveal cell-binding domains is often encouraged by hydrophilic and functionalized surfaces, which facilitates cellular adherence and proliferation [7]. For instance, carboxyl and hydroxyl groups raise polymer's surface energy, which improves wettability and protein-cell interactions.

Surface topography, on the other hand, influences how cells physically interact with the material. This ranges from micro-scale roughness to nano-scale texture. While nanoscale shapes can imitate the natural extracellular matrix (ECM), improving cell attachment and differentiation, microscale features can affect mechanical anchoring and cellular orientation. According to studies, osteoblasts grown on titanium surfaces with nanostructures show improved mineralization and bone-formation-related gene expression. Additionally, it is crucial that chemistry and topography work together harmoniously since a surface that is chemically inert but topographically tailored may produce a more positive reaction than one that is smooth yet bioactive.

In addition to these traditional factors, surface charge and wettability also affect how proteins and cells interact. It is necessary to achieve equilibrium through hybrid or dynamic surface treatments because positively charged surfaces frequently improve initial protein adsorption but may also encourage undesired bacterial adherence. Wettability indirectly shapes immunological and healing responses by influencing the thickness and orientation of protein layers. These interconnected elements are viewed as a multifaceted interface system in contemporary biomaterial design, necessitating integrated control to produce the intended biological effects [8, 9].

4.1.3 Scope of the Chapter Covering Surface Science Principles, Modification Strategies, and Emerging Innovations

This chapter offers a thorough examination of surface characteristics and modification methods in relation to biomaterials. It starts by summarizing the basic ideas of surface science and explaining how properties at the atomic level affect biological performance at the macroscopic level. These guidelines cover the physicochemical characteristics that control the interface dynamics between biomaterials and biological systems, including surface energy, charge distribution, and roughness [10, 11]. The talk will focus on how these characteristics can be measured, described, and altered to maximize biological reactions.

The chapter next looks at surface alteration techniques, which are divided into three primary groups: chemical, biological, and physical methods. We'll talk about physical methods like ion implantation, laser texturing and plasma treatment because they can change energy and shape without compromising the bulk integrity of the material. Fine-tuning of chemical functions and wettability is made possible by chemical alterations, such as polymer grafting, silane coupling, and self-assembled monolayers [12, 13]. By immobilizing peptides, growth factors, or extracellular matrix constituents, biological surface engineering produces biomimetic surfaces that actively direct tissue regeneration.

The new developments in the field are next examined in this chapter, including smart and stimuli-responsive surfaces that may dynamically adapt to physiological inputs (temperature, pH, or enzyme activity). The spatially controlled modulation of biological activity across complicated geometries is made possible by advancements in nanostructured and gradient surfaces, which are made possible by additive manufacturing and nanocoating techniques. Green surface modification techniques, which use environmentally friendly materials and procedures, are also becoming more popular and are bringing biomaterial development into line with international sustainability objectives.

The chapter also discusses cutting-edge analytical methods for characterizing and measuring surface properties at the micro- and nanoscales, such as contact angle measurements, X-ray photoelectron spectroscopy (XPS), and atomic force microscopy (AFM). The logical design of next-generation materials is guided by these technologies, which allow connections between structural characteristics and biological performance. From basic interactions to sophisticated engineering techniques, this chapter offers a comprehensive view of how surface science supports the success of biomaterials. It emphasizes the critical role that surface modification plays in moving biomaterials toward adaptable, intelligent, and regenerative systems by tying molecular-scale knowledge to macro-scale design. The knowledge acquired will help create a coherent framework for maximizing surface-driven biological functionality in contemporary biomedical materials, which will guide further sections on mechanisms, processing methods and applications [14, 15].

4.2 Key Concepts and Definitions

A key component of biomaterials science is the investigation of surface characteristics and modification methods since interactions between biomaterials and their biological environments mostly take place at the interface. According to Rahmati et al. [16] and Vaiani et al. [17], surface qualities control a material's biocompatibility, bioactivity, and integration with surrounding tissues, whereas bulk properties influence its mechanical and structural performance. It is crucial to comprehend the basic terminology and ideas pertaining to surface chemistry, energy, shape, and functionalization to strategically design biomaterials that elicit desired biological reactions. The fundamental ideas of surface science in biomaterials are covered in detail here, covering surface characteristics, biointerfaces, modification methods, and characterisation criteria.

4.2.1 Definition of Surface Properties: Chemistry, Energy, Wettability, Charge, and Roughness

The physicochemical features that specify a biomaterial's interfacial behavior with biological fluids, proteins, and cells are referred to as its surface properties. These characteristics include roughness, energy, wettability, charge, and surface chemistry determine the material's molecular interactions with its surroundings. The elemental makeup, functional groups, and chemical bonds at a material's outermost atomic layers are all described by surface chemistry. It determines the surface's stability, reactivity, and capacity to facilitate biomolecules' covalent attachment or molecular adsorption. For instance, inert coatings like polyethylene glycol (PEG) inhibit biofouling by blocking protein attachment, whereas hydroxyl or carboxyl groups encourage hydrophilicity and protein adsorption.

The thermodynamic potential of a surface to interact with its environment is measured by surface energy. It symbolizes the disparity between the intermolecular forces that atoms near the surface and those in the bulk experience. Metals and ceramics are examples of high-energy surfaces that are generally more reactive and encourage robust adhesive interactions with biological components [4, 18]. Fluoropolymers and other low-energy surfaces, on the other hand, are more hydrophobic and do not adsorb. Wettability, which describes how liquids spread across a solid surface, is the macroscopic expression of surface energy. The contact angle that forms between a liquid droplet and the surface is typically used to measure it; hydrophilic surfaces have low contact angles (<90°), whereas hydrophobic surfaces have high contact angles (>90°). Protein structure, cell adhesion, and biofilm development are all impacted by wettability.

Ionizable functional groups, adsorbed ions, or surface dipolar orientation are the sources of surface charge. It influences protein adsorption and cell adhesion by altering electrostatic interactions with charged biomolecules. This charge is measured in aquatic environments by the zeta potential, which also acts as a gauge of biological reactivity and colloidal stability. Lastly, topographical abnormalities detected at the micro or nanoscale are referred to as surface roughness. Roughness affects tissue integration, migration, and cell attachment in addition to changing the effective surface area. On titanium implants, a higher roughness can promote osteoblast activity, but if left unchecked, it can also promote bacterial colonization. These five characteristics chemistry, energy, wettability, charge and roughness collectively determine the biological performance of biomaterial surfaces and establish their physicochemical identity.

4.2.2 *Concepts of Biointerface, Bioactivity, and Surface Functionalization*

The dynamic barrier layer that separates the surface of a biomaterial from the biological milieu, which is made up of proteins, cells, and extracellular matrix (ECM) constituents, is known as the biointerface. The first biocompatibility events are identified within this nanometric zone. Protein adsorption takes place seconds after implantation and determines immune recognition, cell adhesion, and differentiation later. Thus, regulating chemistry and topography of the interface is essential for guiding biological reactions.

The ability of a substance to produce biological effects, such adhering to tissue, triggering cell differentiation, or accelerating healing, is known as bioactivity. For instance, calcium phosphate coatings and bioactive glasses release ions that promote osteogenesis, but bioinert materials such as alumina function as stable structural supports despite not interacting chemically. Surface modification is frequently used to engineer bioactivity by adding growth factors, peptides, or chemical cues that control cell behavior.

The intentional modification of surface chemistry to add desired functional groups or bioactive compounds without changing bulk characteristics is known as surface functionalization. Covalent grafting, adsorption, or layer-by-layer deposition of biomolecules such peptides, polysaccharides, or antifouling polymers are examples of functionalization techniques. For example, heparin functionalization gives vascular grafts anticoagulant qualities, whereas immobilizing RGD (arginine–glycine–aspartic acid) peptides improves integrin-mediated cell adhesion [19]. Thus, functionalization offers a way to convert inert materials into surfaces that interact with biology at the molecular level.

4.2.3 *Distinction Between Bulk and Surface Modifications*

The difference between bulk and surface modification is a key idea in biomaterials engineering. The degree to which material qualities are changed and the fundamental reason for modification vary between these two approaches. To obtain desired mechanical, thermal, or degrading properties, bulk modification entails changing the material's total volume or internal composition. This includes operations that alter the material's inherent qualities, such as copolymerization, blending, or alloying. For instance, PLGA, a copolymer with adjustable breakdown rates and flexibility, is created when glycolic acid is added to polylactic acid. Likewise, titanium's mechanical strength and fatigue resistance are enhanced by alloying it with aluminum or vanadium.

Surface modification, on the other hand, only modifies the outermost atomic or molecular layers; the bulk structure remains unaltered. This method is particularly useful when the surface needs improved biological compatibility, but the bulk material already offers sufficient mechanical support. Methods including thin-film deposition, ion implantation, and plasma treatment can enhance wettability, introduce chemical functions, or encourage protein interactions [20]. For instance, titanium surfaces coated with hydroxyapatite improve bone integration without sacrificing the mechanical integrity of the substrate, whereas polyethylene surfaces can be plasma oxidized to increase hydrophilicity and encourage cell adherence. The difference is in the scope and purpose: surface modification maximizes biological reaction at the interface, whereas bulk modification customizes material performance from within. For synergistic functionality, these methodologies are frequently integrated into effective biomaterial design.

4.2.4 *Measurement Parameters: Contact Angle, Zeta Potential, Surface Free Energy, and Roughness Average (Ra)*

Quantitative measurement parameters that offer objective, repeatable insight into interfacial behavior are necessary for characterizing surface attributes. The main indicator of wettability is the contact angle. It offers details on hydrophilicity, surface cleanliness, and energy state using dynamic or sessile drop techniques. After treatment, such as plasma activation or coating deposition, changes in the contact angle show changed surface chemistry or morphology. The effective surface charge in a liquid medium is measured by the zeta potential. The stability of colloidal dispersions and the possibility of electrostatic interactions with proteins and cells are both reflected in electrophoretic mobility measurements. Although they may cause unintended immunological reactions, surfaces with extremely positive or negative zeta potential frequently show improved protein adsorption.

The thermodynamic propensity of a surface to create interfacial bonds is represented by surface free energy (SFE). Contact angle measurements of liquids with various polarity can be combined to determine it. Low-SFE surfaces are usually non-fouling, but high-SFE surfaces show strong adhesive behavior and quick protein adsorption. The arithmetic mean of height deviations from the mean line, which is commonly determined by profilometry or atomic force microscopy (AFM), is the roughness average (Ra), which quantifies surface topography [21]. Ra values offer a consistent way to quantify micro- and nanoscale abnormalities, which are related to biological attachment and mechanical anchoring. The quantitative basis for assessing and contrasting biomaterial surfaces across investigations is formed by these metrics taken together: contact angle, zeta potential, SFE, and Ra.

4.2.5 Terminology in Surface Engineering Plasma Treatment, Grafting, Coating, Texturing

The various techniques used to alter and improve material interfaces for biological applications are collectively referred to as surface engineering. The most popular methods are defined by a few essential terms: Plasma treatment introduces polar functional groups like hydroxyl or carboxyl groups to the surface by using ionized gas to activate or clean it. As a prelude to additional coating or grafting, it improves hydrophilicity, adhesion, and chemical reactivity. Grafting is the process of covalently adhering biomolecules or polymers to the surface to accomplish desired chemical functionality. While "grafting-to" procedures connect premade polymers, "grafting-from" approaches create polymer chains straight from surface initiators. Heparin-grafting for anticoagulant coatings and PEG-grafting for antifouling surfaces are two examples. The process of applying a thin layer of a different substance to the surface of a substrate is called coating. Methods for producing bioactive, protective, or lubricating layers include dip-coating, sputtering, sol-gel deposition, and layer-by-layer assembly. Titanium implants with hydroxyapatite coatings are well-known examples of osseointegration enhancement. Through micro- or nanostructuring, texturing alters the physical topography, affecting cell adherence and orientation. Biological integration is improved by methods like laser ablation, etching, and additive manufacturing, which create patterns that resemble the extracellular matrix seen in nature.

Each method provides distinct advantages depending on the target property whether chemical, mechanical, or biological. The selection of technique depends on the biomaterial type, intended clinical application, and desired functional outcome.

Designing biomaterials requires an understanding of surface characteristics and how to modify them. The initial interactions between a biomaterial and the body are governed by surface chemistry, energy, wettability, charge, and roughness, which determine tissue integration, cell adhesion, and protein adsorption. Scientists can precisely modify these features to obtain optimal biological results through controlled surface engineering, which includes grafting, coating, texturing, and plasma treatment [22, 23]. The development of biomaterials that are both structurally sound and intelligently interact with the human body is made possible by surface science, which is still acting as a link between material engineering and biological functionality.

4.3 Historical Background

The investigation of corrosion and passivation events in early metallic implants is a fundamental aspect of the historical evolution of surface modification in biomaterials. Because of their mechanical strength and seeming inertness, metals like gold, silver, and stainless steel were utilized in dental and surgical procedures as early as the late nineteenth and early twentieth centuries. Clinicians quickly realized, however, that direct metal-to-physiological fluid contact frequently resulted in electrochemical corrosion, releasing ions that triggered cytotoxicity, mechanical failure, or inflammatory reactions. The scientific community's interest in comprehending and managing surface-environment interactions began with this awareness.

The discovery of surface passivation, especially in alloys containing chromium, was one of the first significant developments. Significant corrosion resistance in physiological settings was offered by the thin, adhering oxide layer that spontaneously formed on stainless steel, mostly composed of chromium oxide. By highlighting the fact that surface chemistry, not only bulk composition, determines biocompatibility and lifespan, this passivation mechanism established the groundwork for contemporary surface engineering. Biomedical implantology was later transformed by the mid-twentieth century advent of titanium and related alloys. Titanium has been widely used in dental implants, orthopedic prostheses, and cardiovascular devices due to its extraordinary corrosion resistance and biocompatibility, which are attributed to its unique ability to produce a durable, self-healing oxide coating (TiO_2) [24, 25].

Standards for implant corrosion testing were established by the 1950s and 1960s because of methodical studies into the electrochemical behavior of metallic surfaces in bodily fluid simulations. Researchers like Venable, Brown, and Branemark showed that ion release kinetics, oxidation behavior, and surface stability were critical factors in the long-term success of metallic implants. The knowledge that surfaces phenomena controlled both chemical stability and biological integration was solidified during this time and this idea still influences the design of biomaterials today.

4.3.1 Development of Surface Polishing and Anodization for Dental and Orthopedic Materials

As metallic biomaterials became more popular, focus shifted to surface modification and finishing methods that improved tissue compatibility, decreased corrosion, and improved appearance. Anodization, electropolishing, and mechanical polishing were introduced as important surface treatments in the 1960s and 1970s. By increasing smoothness, mechanical polishing decreased surface flaws that could harbor bacteria or function as sites for corrosion. In dental applications, titanium and polished cobalt-chromium alloys showed reduced plaque accumulation and improved lifespan. By employing regulated electrochemical dissolution, electropolishing produced surfaces that were cleaner, more consistent, and had less micro-roughness and residual stress. This technique worked especially well for cardiovascular stents and stainless steel orthopedic wires, where surface imperfections could cause thrombosis or fatigue.

When anodization was initially used on titanium in the 1970s, it was a significant advancement. Titanium surfaces could develop a porous and adherent oxide layer by introducing an electrical current into an electrolyte. Along with improving corrosion resistance, this layer made it possible to regulate surface charge, thickness, and porosity all of which are essential for osseointegration and cell adhesion. Because anodized titanium implants showed better bone anchoring than untreated surfaces, they were widely used in orthopedic and dental prosthesis [26, 27]. To further promote osteoconductivity, the development of anodization processes also made it possible to incorporate bioactive ions (such as calcium, phosphorus, or fluoride) into the oxide layer.

By the end of the twentieth century, surface finishing had evolved from purely mechanical smoothing toward chemical and electrochemical modification, setting the stage for functional biomaterial surfaces that could actively influence biological outcomes rather than merely resist corrosion.

4.3.2 Introduction of Plasma Spraying and Chemical Vapor Deposition (CVD) in the Late Twentieth Century

The introduction of chemical vapor deposition (CVD) and plasma spraying technologies in the late twentieth century brought about a paradigm change in surface modification by making it possible to apply coatings with precise composition, thickness, and microstructure. The main goals of these techniques' development were to improve bioactivity, corrosion protection, and wear resistance of metallic and ceramic biomaterials.

Deposition of hydroxyapatite (HA) coatings on metallic implants, particularly titanium and its alloys, was made possible by plasma spraying, which was first used in the 1970s and improved upon in the 1980s. Because of its chemical resemblance to the mineral phase of bone, HA offered a bioactive surface that supported direct bone bonding and aided in osseointegration. In orthopaedic and dental implants, plasma-sprayed HA coatings dramatically sped up bone development and shortened healing periods. However, issues including phase instability and coating delamination prompted continued study into enhancing adhesion and crystallinity using post-treatment methods and adjusted plasma conditions [28, 29].

Diamond-like carbon (DLC) films, carbides, and nitrides (TiN, ZrN) are now among the coating options made feasible by chemical vapor deposition (CVD) and its variation, physical vapor deposition (PVD). These coatings were perfect for cardiovascular stents and joint replacements because of their exceptional hardness, reduced friction, and resilience to wear. Furthermore, precise control over layer thickness and homogeneity both essential for preserving dimensional tolerances in load-bearing implants was made possible by CVD and PVD procedures. The combination of vapor and plasma deposition methods marked a shift from passive protective coatings to biofunctional surfaces that may enhance both biological performance and mechanical durability at the same time [30, 31]. The increasing multidisciplinary cooperation among materials science, surface chemistry, and biomedical engineering was reflected in these developments.

4.3.3 Emergence of Biomimetic and Nanostructured Coatings in the Twenty-First Century

A new wave of biologically inspired surface technologies, known as biomimetic and nanostructured coatings, emerged at the turn of the twenty-first century. These coatings are intended to mimic the dynamic functionality and hierarchical organization of natural tissues. By emphasizing the chemical and structural mimicry of the extracellular matrix (ECM), biomimetic techniques made it possible for surfaces to interact directly with cells by means of biochemical signals [32, 33].

Methods including electrophoretic deposition, layer-by-layer (LbL) assembly, and sol–gel processing were created to create thin, bioactive films enhanced with peptides, collagen, or calcium phosphates. These coatings provided customizable degradation rates, enhanced adhesion, and regulated composition. Concurrently, developments in nanotechnology made it possible to create nanostructured surfaces that closely resemble the chemistry and nanoscale roughness of genuine bones. It has been demonstrated that titanium and polymer surfaces with nanorod, nanotube, or nanopore patterns improve protein adsorption and promote osteogenic differentiation. Silica, graphene, or silver nanoparticles gave multifunctionality to nanocomposite coatings by fusing mechanical reinforcement, antibacterial, or bioactivity.

Static coatings gave way to biointeractive interfaces that might guide cellular pathways and promote tissue regeneration because of this biomimetic and nanoscale revolution [11]. The next frontier, dynamic, adaptable, and responsive biomaterial surfaces was made possible by the fusion of surface science and nanotechnology.

4.3.4 Transition from Passive Surfaces to Functionalized and Responsive Interfaces

The shift from passive, corrosion-resistant surfaces to functionalized, stimuli-responsive interfaces that intelligently interact with the biological environment is reflected in the most recent stage of surface modification's historical progression. The modern objective is to actively control biological processes including inflammation, angiogenesis, and tissue remodeling in addition to preventing negative effects.

Surface functionalization is the process of creating surfaces that stimulate biological responses by affixing bioactive chemicals, such as polysaccharides, growth factors, or peptides (RGD sequences). Self-assembled monolayers (SAMs), click chemistry, and covalent grafting have emerged as crucial methods for obtaining regulated biological activity. Similarly, stimuli-responsive coatings, sometimes referred to as "smart" surfaces, can change their characteristics in reaction to mechanical stress, pH, temperature, or enzyme activity. These technologies extend the usefulness of implants beyond structural support by enabling self-healing, anti-fouling behavior, or on-demand drug delivery. Furthermore, spatially resolved surface design with micron and submicron precision is now possible thanks to the convergence of computational modeling, microfabrication, and additive manufacturing. This versatility is extended to dynamic tissue environments through 4D printing, where materials alter shape or function over time.

Surface modification in biomaterials has historically followed a path from corrosion control to bioactivity and, eventually, adaptivity. Every period improved on earlier knowledge; for example, mechanical polishing followed electrochemical passivation, which in turn gave rise to sophisticated coatings, biomimetic design, and responsive interfaces. Surface modification is currently a multidisciplinary field where materials science, nanotechnology, and regenerative biology come together to produce biomaterials that actively aid in healing and regeneration in addition to being long-lasting inside the body [34, 35].

4.4 Material Types and Properties

The performance and biocompatibility of a biomaterial are intimately linked to its surface characteristics, which dictate interactions with biological systems [36]. Each material class consists of polymers, metals, ceramics, and composites possess

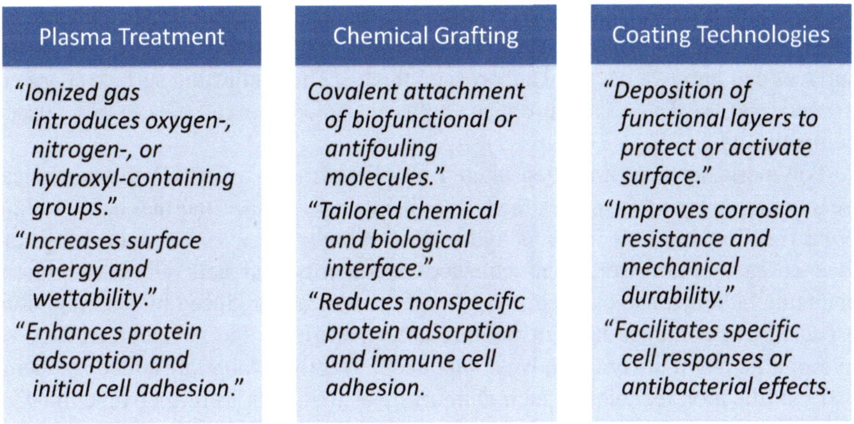

Fig. 4.1 Summary of key surface modification techniques used to alter biomaterial topography, chemistry, and functionality to enhance biological performance

unique surface attributes influencing properties such as hydrophobicity, charge, topography, and energy. These, in turn, govern protein adsorption, cell adhesion, and tissue integration. Accordingly, the choice of surface modification technique must be tailored to the material's intrinsic chemistry, mechanical behavior, and clinical application as shown in Fig. 4.1. This provides a detailed examination of the major biomaterial categories and their surface-related properties, exploring how specific modification methods enhance biological performance and functionality.

4.4.1 Polymeric Biomaterials

From scaffolds and sutures to medication delivery systems and prosthetic coverings, polymeric biomaterials are extensively used in biomedical applications. Their surface characteristics control biological performance and compatibility, especially hydrophobicity, charge distribution, and protein adsorption behavior. Low wettability and inadequate protein adsorption control are caused by the surface hydrophobicity of polymers like polyethylene (PE), polypropylene (PP), and polytetrafluoroethylene (PTFE). Bacterial colonization, undesired immunological reactions, or nonspecific protein fouling may arise from this. On the other hand, more hydrophilic polymers, including poly(ethylene glycol) (PEG) or poly(vinyl alcohol) (PVA), are frequently utilized for implantable device stealth coatings since they do not adhere to proteins. The type of protein adsorption is determined by the balance between hydrophilicity and hydrophobicity; moderate hydrophilicity frequently encourages advantageous cell adhesion, but severe hydrophobicity or hydrophilicity may impede stable connections [37].

The distribution of surface charges also has a big impact on how cells respond. Positively charged serum proteins like fibronectin, which facilitate cell adhesion, are drawn to negatively charged surfaces, such as those with carboxyl or phosphate groups. In addition to promoting fibroblast growth, positively charged amine-rich surfaces can improve bacterial adherence [38, 39]. Thus, adjusting surface charge is a tactic to strike a compromise between infection resistance and tissue compatibility.

Polymeric surfaces are often altered by plasma, ultraviolet (UV), or chemical treatments to get around the drawbacks of intrinsic surface inertness. By adding polar functional groups (such as hydroxyl, carbonyl, or carboxyl) and raising surface energy, plasma treatment enhances wettability and cell adhesion without changing bulk mechanical characteristics. Free radicals produced by UV radiation, especially in conjunction with photoinitiators, facilitate the covalent grafting of hydrophilic polymers or bioactive compounds. Reactive groups are added by chemical modification techniques such aminolysis or oxidation to further functionalize peptides, medications, or biomimetic coatings.

4.4.2 *Metallic Biomaterials*

The great strength, fatigue resistance, and structural stability of metallic biomaterials, such as titanium (Ti), stainless steel, cobalt-chromium (Co–Cr) alloys, and magnesium (Mg) alloys, make them valuable. Their surface characteristics are essential for biocompatibility and corrosion resistance, especially the production of oxide layers and electrochemical stability.

Most metallic biomaterials spontaneously develop oxide layers on their surfaces, which serve as passive defenses against ion release and corrosion. For example, titanium naturally creates a persistent TiO_2 layer that shields against oxidative deterioration and encourages osseointegration. In a similar vein, the passive CrO_3 film keeps stainless steel resistant to corrosion. These oxide films could, however, deteriorate under physiological circumstances because of pH changes, mechanical wear, or chloride ion attack, which could cause ion leaching and possible inflammatory responses.

Several surface modification methods, such as anodization, ion implantation, and laser texturing, are used to improve biological performance and durability; By thickening the oxide layer through an electrochemical process called anodization, corrosion resistance is increased and controlled surface nanotopography development is made possible [40]. Bone-implant integration and osteoblast adhesion are improved by anodized titanium with nanoporous or nanotubular features. To change the composition of the metal surface and produce a hard, wear-resistant surface, ion implantation entails blasting it with energetic ions (such as oxygen or nitrogen). For instance, adding nitrogen to stainless steel increases its hardness and decreases the release of metal ions. High-intensity laser pulses are used in laser texturing to reshape and ablate surface topography at the micro- and nanoscale. This promotes protein adsorption and wettability in addition to mechanical interlocking with tissues. A systematic evaluation of biomedical implant surface coating routes comparing plasma spraying, pulsed laser deposition, atomic layer deposition, and plasma-enhanced CVD for hydroxyapatite, protective hard coatings, and antibacterial layers demonstrates that nanostructured and multifunctional coatings consistently accelerate osteogenic responses, with ALD-deposited ultrathin conformal films offering superior corrosion resistance on complex implant geometries without impairing cell viability [41].

These techniques collectively ensure that metallic biomaterials combine mechanical robustness with biofunctional performance, making them indispensable for orthopedic, dental, and cardiovascular implants.

4.4.3 Ceramic Biomaterials

Ceramic biomaterials with outstanding biocompatibility, hardness, and wear resistance include hydroxyapatite (HA), zirconia (ZrO_2), alumina (AlO_3), and bioactive glasses. Their ability to interact with biological tissues is largely dependent on their porosity, surface energy, and bioactive ion release properties. Both biological integration and mechanical integrity are determined by porosity. Protein adsorption is facilitated by microporous structures (less than 10 μm), but bone ingrowth and vascularization are made possible by macroporous networks (greater than 100 μm). Therefore, it is essential to regulate pore size and interconnectivity to balance biological and mechanical performance.

Strong ionic and covalent bonds in ceramics tend to have a high surface energy, which encourages protein adsorption and cellular adhesion. Additionally, when exposed to physiological fluids, this high energy promotes the production of a bioactive layer, especially in bioactive glasses that release ions like Ca^{2+}, Si^{2+}, and PO_4^{3-} that promote the formation of apatite and osteoblast differentiation. Both biochemical cues for tissue regeneration and the mediating of local pH changes that promote bone mineralization are functions of bioactive ion release. The kinetics of dissolution must be carefully controlled, though, as excessive ion release may result in localized irritation or cytotoxicity.

Ceramics are frequently modified using coating techniques like sol–gel processing and biomimetic deposition to improve their biological performance and integration; sol–gel coatings allow for the creation of thin, homogeneous sheets with regulated porosity and content. For instance, titanium coated with HA produced from sol-gel enhances osteoconductivity and chemical adherence to bone. By submerging materials in simulated bodily fluid (SBF), biomimetic deposition mimics physiological mineralization processes and produces apatite layers that resemble bone [42]. This method works especially well for producing bioactive surfaces on polymer or ceramic substrates that would otherwise be inert. Because they combine chemical stability, surface reactivity, and bioactivity, ceramic biomaterials are therefore excellent options for coating and hard-tissue healing applications.

4.4.4 Composites and Hybrid Materials

Composite and hybrid biomaterials integrate two or more distinct material phases, often metals, ceramics, and polymers, to achieve synergistic combinations of mechanical strength, toughness, and biological functioning. Important factors influencing performance include component interfacial bonding and multi-material surface compatibility.

Stress transfer between phases and mechanical integrity are guaranteed by interfacial bonding. Under physiological loads, weak interfaces may delaminate or fail. To improve interphase adhesion, techniques such gradient interfaces, silane coupling agents, and plasma activation are used. Strong interfacial chemical connections, for example, are necessary for the transfer of mechanical stresses while preserving bioactivity in hydroxyapatite-reinforced polymer composites [43].

One of the biggest problems with hybrid systems is surface compatibility across many materials. For instance, surface adjustments are necessary for polymer–ceramic composites to reduce the discrepancy between surface energy and thermal expansion coefficients. Surface customization, such as chemical grafting or plasma etching, encourages improved stability and adhesion between disparate phases. Additionally, composites provide synergistic optimization: metallic inclusions add conductivity or strength, polymers offer flexibility and degradability, and ceramics give stiffness and bioactivity. Bioresorbable composites like PLA/β-TCP, which combine ceramic osteoconductivity and polymeric flexibility, and Ti–HA composites, which combine biointegration and mechanical robustness, are prime examples of this kind of synergy. Composites offer a framework for creating multifunctional biomaterials with dynamic mechanical and biological responses by utilizing interfacial engineering.

4.4.5 Correlation Between Material Type and Preferred Surface Modification Method

The inherent chemistry and structure of the biomaterial have a significant influence on the choice of surface modification techniques. Due to their chemical inertness and sensitivity to heat, polymers are best changed by wet chemical functionalization, UV activation, or low-energy plasma treatment to add reactive groups without causing bulk damage. Techniques including anodization, ion implantation, and laser texturing which produce stable oxide layers and customized topographies are necessary for metals to improve corrosion resistance and biocompatibility [30, 44]. Sol-gel and biomimetic coatings improve bioactivity while maintaining the underlying stability and robustness of ceramics. To balance the physicochemical characteristics of disparate phases and guarantee cohesive performance, composites require gradient surface engineering and interfacial coupling.

Rational surface design that satisfies mechanical and biological constraints is made possible by an understanding of the relationship between material type and modification technique. The development of adaptive biomaterial surfaces engineered not just for compatibility but also for active participation in tissue healing and regeneration is made possible by the integration of hybrid and nanostructured modification approaches as the field progresses.

Modern biomaterials research is based on surface qualities specific to a certain material. Every material class requires a different modification technique, from the hydrophobic-to-hydrophilic conversions of polymers to the oxide-passivation of metals and the ion-releasing bioactivity of ceramics. These ideas are combined in composites, which use interfacial engineering to achieve multifunctional synergy. The ability to customize biomaterials for clinical outcomes is ultimately supported by the relationship between material type and surface modification technique, bringing in a new era of intelligent, adaptable, and biologically responsive materials for next-generation medical applications [45].

4.5 Mechanisms and Processes

One of the most important methods for adjusting biological reactions in biomaterials without compromising the material's bulk mechanical or chemical integrity is surface modification. By improving characteristics including biocompatibility, corrosion resistance, wear resistance, and bioactivity, these modification approaches let implants and scaffolds function at their best in intricate physiological settings as shown in Fig. 4.2. Each of the physical, chemical, biological, and physicochemical mechanisms that underline these activities modulate surface shape, energy, charge, and reactivity. Furthermore, surface modification is now an active method of controlling cellular behavior rather than a passive enhancing strategy because of the development of nanotechnology and biofunctionalization.

4.5.1 Physical Modification Techniques

To change a biomaterial's surface morphology, texture, or topography without altering its overall chemical makeup, physical surface modification uses mechanical or energetic techniques. Mechanical polishing, sandblasting, laser ablation, plasma treatment, and thermal spraying are examples of common methods. By utilizing abrasives to remove surface defects, mechanical polishing creates a smoother finish and less roughness, which can serve as a breeding ground for bacteria or corrosion. Electropolishing and mechanical finishing are frequently used in metallic implants to provide atomically clean surfaces that reduce fatigue failure and ion leaching. On the other hand, regulated roughness improves mechanical interlocking and osteoblastic adhesion in some applications, such as bone-contacting implants. A

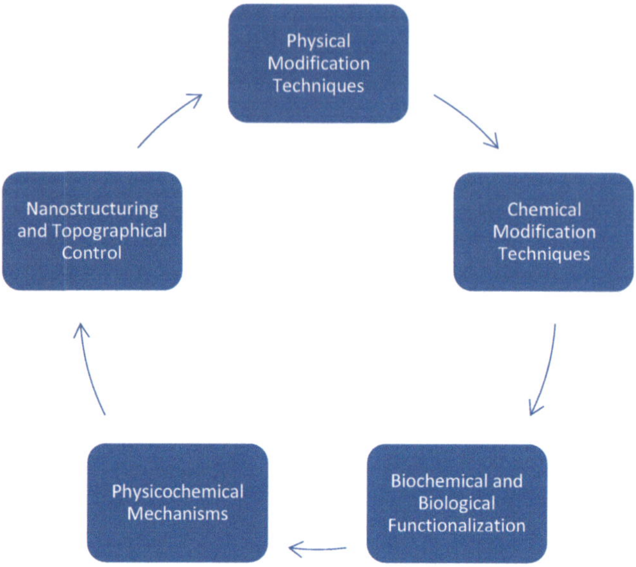

Fig. 4.2 Illustration of major surface modification techniques used to alter biomaterial topography, chemistry, and biofunctionality

comprehensive review of advanced surface modification techniques for titanium implants covering ion doping, hydroxyapatite coatings, nanostructured surfaces, and graphene-based modifications quantifies their osteogenic and antibacterial outcomes, demonstrating that zinc-doped coatings increase osteoblast proliferation by 25% and copper-doped coatings achieve >99% antibacterial efficacy against *S. aureus*, establishing a performance benchmark for multifunctional surface design [46].

Sandblasting, or grit blasting, modifies surface roughness by bombarding the material with high-velocity abrasive particles (e.g., alumina or silica). The resulting micro-roughened surface increases surface area and improves the anchorage of coatings or bone tissue. Sandblasting is particularly valuable for dental and orthopedic titanium implants, where it promotes osseointegration by providing mechanical cues that guide bone cell attachment. Laser ablation represents a more advanced physical modification technique that employs focused laser pulses to precisely sculpt surface features at micro- and nanoscales [47]. By adjusting parameters such as wavelength, pulse duration, and intensity, laser ablation can create ordered patterns, microgrooves, or hierarchical textures that influence protein adsorption and cellular orientation. The process is clean, reproducible, and suitable for diverse materials including metals, ceramics, and polymers.

By employing molten materials or high-energy gases, thermal spraying and plasma treatment broaden the scope of physical alterations. By introducing polar groups or reactive sites, ionized gases (oxygen, nitrogen, or argon plasma) can clean, activate, or functionalize surfaces. This process is known as plasma treatment. It improves cell adhesion and protein binding by raising surface energy and hydrophilicity. On the other hand, molten or semi-molten particles are deposited onto a substrate via thermal spraying, which includes plasma and flame spraying, to create coatings like titanium oxide or hydroxyapatite. These coatings produce stable surfaces for tissue integration by improving bioactivity and corrosion resistance.

4.5.2 Chemical Modification Techniques

By introducing or changing functional groups through controlled reactions, chemical modification techniques change the surface chemistry of biomaterials. In order to improve surface reactivity, wettability, and compatibility with biological molecules, these procedures are essential. Surface grafting, oxidation, silanization, wet chemical etching, and covalent bonding are the primary methods. By selectively dissolving surface layers with acids or bases, wet chemical etching creates micro- and nano-textures that raise surface energy and roughness [48]. For example, titanium surfaces that have been acid-etched encourage the growth of new bones by promoting osteoblast proliferation and protein adsorption. A unified thermodynamic framework for protein adsorption and cell adhesion on metallic biomaterial surfaces distinguishing the roles of effective surface charge density and surface deformation energy provides a quantitative basis for classifying surface modification strategies into direct charge control, direct deformation energy control, or coupled control, enabling more predictable design of biointerfaces for cell-selective adhesion [49]. Additionally, the procedure can eliminate impurities or passive oxide coatings, improving adherence for later coatings.

Stable oxide layers are frequently formed on metals by thermal, anodic, or chemical oxidation processes. For instance, anodic oxidation of titanium produces porous TiO_2 layers that offer nanotopographical cues for cell guiding in addition to corrosion protection. Similar to this, carbon-based materials undergo chemical oxidation to produce carboxyl or hydroxyl groups, which enhance hydrophilicity and offer reactive sites for the attachment of biomolecules. One important chemical modification method that is mostly applied to glass, silica, and polymeric materials is silanization [50]. It entails attaching silane coupling agents with reactive end groups (like epoxy or amine) that can create covalent connections with organic molecules as well as inorganic substrates. In hybrid biomaterials, this technique is crucial for tying together bioactive ingredients, improving coating adherence, and managing surface chemistry.

By directly introducing polymer chains or functional molecules onto a substrate, surface grafting and covalent bonding processes produce surfaces with specific chemical and biological characteristics [51]. The "grafting-to" and "grafting-from" methods enable the regulated development of polymer brushes that alter charge density, protein adsorption, and hydrophobicity. Functional groups like carboxyl, amine, or hydroxyl can be covalently bonded to form persistent anchoring sites for additional biofunctionalization. This allows surfaces to either selectively attach cells and biomolecules or resist nonspecific fouling. Researchers bridge the gap between inert substrates and physiologically active interfaces by achieving long-term stability and usefulness in biomaterials through these chemical changes.

4.5.3 Biochemical and Biological Functionalization

As biomaterials have developed, biochemical and biological functionalization where surface modification directly incorporates biological components to achieve biomimicry and bioactivity has grown in significance. The immobilization of peptides, proteins, and growth factors, as well as techniques like layer-by-layer assembly (LbL) and self-assembled monolayers (SAMs), are key components of this approach. The immobilization of bioactive molecules provides specific biochemical cues that guide cellular adhesion, proliferation, and differentiation. Short peptide sequences such as RGD (arginine-glycine-aspartic acid) are commonly attached to surfaces to mimic extracellular matrix (ECM) attachment sites sensed by integrins. Similarly, at implant sites, immobilized growth factors (such bone morphogenetic proteins or vascular endothelial growth factor) stimulate angiogenesis and osteogenesis. Depending on the required release kinetics and stability, immobilization can be accomplished by covalent bonding, physical adsorption, or entrapment inside polymeric matrices [52].

Electrostatic or hydrogen-bonding interactions are used to deposit oppositely charged polymers, proteins, or nanoparticles in alternating layers during layer-by-layer (LbL) assembly. The functionality, composition, and thickness of the film can all be precisely controlled with this technique. LbL coatings can incorporate bioactive substances, antimicrobial agents, or nanoparticles to produce multifunctional surfaces with controlled release and dynamic reactivity. Self-assembled monolayers (SAMs), often composed of silanes or alkanethiols, provide molecular-level order on metal or oxide surfaces. SAMs offer controlled surface chemistry through certain terminal groups that affect wettability, charge, and biological affinity. Their uniformity and chemical tunability make them ideal substrates for studying cell-surface interactions and creating model biointerfaces. Smart biomaterials for cardiovascular, bone, and skin tissue engineering including shape-memory polymers, stimuli-responsive hydrogels, and multifunctional nanocomposites demonstrate dynamic on-demand modification of physicochemical properties in response to pH, temperature, light, and magnetic fields, enabling active guidance of cell behaviour toward osteogenesis, wound healing, and myocardial repair beyond passive surface compatibility [53].

Together, these biofunctionalization strategies transform inert materials into bioactive interfaces that communicate with the biological environment, facilitating integration and promoting regenerative outcomes.

4.5.4 Physicochemical Mechanisms

The success of surface modification depends on the basic physicochemical mechanisms that govern the interactions between atoms, ions, and molecules. Diffusion and adsorption kinetics, together with surface energy modulation and charge redistribution, are two important phenomena that significantly influence the final surface state. Surface energy modulation is the technique of altering a surface's thermodynamic potential to either attract or repel molecules. Processes like chemical grafting and plasma treatment, which enhance wettability and promote protein adsorption, raise surface energy. Conversely, hydrophobic coatings or low-energy fluorinated layers reduce surface energy to create anti-fouling qualities.

Charge redistribution is the process by which modification adds or rearranges surface charges by adsorption, reduction, or oxidation of charged species. Surface charge affects cell adhesion, protein orientation, and ion adsorption. For example, positively charged surfaces must be fine-tuned because they can attract negatively charged proteins or cell membranes and increase bacterial adherence. Diffusion and adsorption kinetics regulate the rate and consistency of modifying activities. Reactive species must diffuse to the surface and adsorb before a reaction occurs in plasma or wet chemical treatments. A few factors that influence these kinetics are temperature, concentration, and surface shape. Reproducibility and long-term stability are ensured by controlling coating thickness, functional group density, and bioactivity through an understanding of these dynamics [54].

4.5.5 Nanostructuring and Topographical Control

The development of topographical control and nanostructuring has revolutionized surface modification and brought material science and cell biology together. Since cells perceive and respond to features at the micro- and nanoscale, controlling these parameters enables the guidance of biological activities such as adhesion, proliferation, and differentiation. Lithography techniques like as photolithography, electron-beam lithography, and nanoimprint lithography enable the precise patterning of micro- and nanoscale features that mimic real tissue structures. Electrospinning is another versatile technique that produces fibrous scaffolds with a wide surface area and tunable porosity that closely resemble the extracellular matrix. Electrospun fibers functionalized with bioactive compounds or nanoparticles serve as scaffolds to control cell alignment and promote tissue regeneration.

The incorporation of nanoparticles into surfaces or coatings enables the simultaneous enhancement of mechanical, antibacterial, and biological properties. To enhance multifunctionality, graphene, hydroxyapatite, and silver nanoparticles are commonly used. Nanocomposite coatings can modify degradation rates and improve surface roughness to optimize cell–material interactions. Cell alignment and differentiation are particularly impacted by topographical signals at the nanoscale

[55]. For example, elongated microgrooves promote fibroblast orientation, while nanorough titanium enhances osteogenic differentiation of stem cells. These effects stem from mechanotransduction pathways, where cytoskeletal tension and focal adhesion organization are modulated by the physical geometry of the surface.

In essence, by making it possible to create surfaces that both support and direct biological behavior, nanostructuring closes the gap between materials engineering and regenerative biology. Surface modification techniques and methods include physical and chemical alterations as well as intricate biofunctional and nanostructured strategies. Together, they allow for the exact control of surface chemistry, energy, and topography, all of which influence the way biomaterials interact with biological systems. By combining several strategies that are guided by physicochemical principles and biological insights, inert materials have been transformed into dynamic and flexible interfaces. As the area develops, new technologies like self-assembly, additive manufacturing, and smart coatings will keep enhancing surface engineering's potential and propel the creation of biomaterials that actively contribute to long-term clinical success, healing, and regeneration [56, 57].

4.6 Design Considerations

Designing biomaterial surfaces is an essential part of biomedical engineering, as the material's interaction with the biological environment largely determines its clinical efficacy. Although a biomaterial's bulk properties provide mechanical stability and load-bearing ability, its surface dictates how it interacts with fluids, proteins, and cells, influencing its bioactivity, biocompatibility, and long-term performance. Effective surface design requires a comprehensive approach that adheres to clinical and regulatory standards while balancing chemical, physical, mechanical, and biological components as shown in Table 4.1 [58]. This looks at the key design

Table 4.1 Surface property comparisons before and after modification

Material type/ technique	Surface property (before modification)	Surface property (after modification)	Modification method(s)	Key functional outcome/biomedical relevance
Metallic biomaterials (Ti, stainless steel, Mg alloys)	• Rough, heterogeneous oxide layer • Susceptible to corrosion in physiological media • Moderate protein adsorption, variable wettability	• Uniform and stable oxide/ passive film • Reduced corrosion and ion release • Enhanced hydrophilicity and protein adhesion	• Anodization (TiO_2 nanotube formation) • Plasma spraying or ion implantation • Electrochemical polishing/ passivation	Improved osseointegration, corrosion resistance, and cell adhesion for orthopedic and dental implants

(continued)

Table 4.1 (continued)

Material type/ technique	Surface property (before modification)	Surface property (after modification)	Modification method(s)	Key functional outcome/biomedical relevance
Ceramic biomaterials (Al_2O_3, ZrO_2, HA, bioglass)	• Chemically stable but inert surface • Low protein adsorption and poor cell attachment • Brittle and microcracked structure	• Bioactive or functionalized surface (e.g., silanized, HA-coated) • Improved surface energy and wettability • Increased bioaffinity and bone bonding	• Plasma coating with bioactive layers • Surface silanization or acid etching • Sol–gel or laser texturing	Enhanced cell adhesion, bone–material interface strength, and bioactivity for bone regeneration
Polymeric biomaterials (PLA, PEG, PCL, collagen)	• Hydrophobic, low surface energy • Poor cell adhesion and protein binding • Chemically inert, smooth morphology	• Increased hydrophilicity and surface charge • Functional groups (–COOH, $-NH_2$, –OH) introduced • Improved roughness and biofunctional molecule attachment	• Plasma treatment (oxygen, nitrogen plasma) • UV/ozone exposure • Grafting or coating with peptides/ polysaccharides	Enhanced biocompatibility, selective cell adhesion, and controlled degradation for tissue scaffolds
Composite biomaterials (polymer–ceramic, metal–ceramic)	• Interfacial mismatch between phases • Irregular topography and poor wettability • Localized corrosion or debonding risk	• Chemically bonded or graded interface • Controlled roughness for mechanical interlocking • Enhanced hydrophilicity and stress transfer	• Sol–gel infiltration • Laser patterning • Bioactive coating (e.g., HA or collagen layer)	Increased interfacial stability, improved mechanical strength, and biointegration for hybrid implants
Carbon-based biomaterials (graphene, carbon nanotubes, diamond-like carbon)	• Chemically inert, hydrophobic • Smooth and nonreactive surface • Limited protein adsorption	• Functionalized with oxygen/ nitrogen groups • Enhanced electrical conductivity and wettability • Controlled nanoscale roughness	• Chemical vapor deposition (CVD) • Plasma functionalization • Electrochemical oxidation	Bioelectronic compatibility; promotes neural and cardiac cell adhesion and minimizes fouling

(continued)

Table 4.1 (continued)

Material type/ technique	Surface property (before modification)	Surface property (after modification)	Modification method(s)	Key functional outcome/biomedical relevance
General comparison	• Native surfaces often inert, hydrophobic, or corrosion-prone • Limited biomolecular interactions	• Tailored surface chemistry, charge, and topography • Tunable hydrophilicity, corrosion resistance, and bioactivity		Surface modification transforms passive biomaterials into biointeractive systems, enabling improved tissue integration and functional performance

elements for biomaterial surface engineering, emphasizing how tactical changes can optimize adhesion, stability, biological response, and regulatory compliance.

4.6.1 Tailoring Surface Chemistry for Specific Cellular Interactions

A key idea in surface design is tailoring chemistry to produce particular biological interactions. Endothelial cells, fibroblasts, and osteoblasts are among the cell types that respond differentially to chemical signals on the biomaterial's surface. By influencing downstream signaling cascades, protein adsorption, and integrin-mediated adhesion, surface chemistry ultimately controls cell proliferation, differentiation, and tissue integration. For instance, surfaces containing functional groups of phosphate, calcium, or hydroxyl promote osteoblast adhesion and bone formation by facilitating apatite nucleation and mimicking the mineral makeup of bone. The hydroxyapatite coatings on titanium implants, which offer topographical and chemical cues to encourage osteointegration, are a well-known example.

However, endothelial cell adhesion to vascular grafts is enhanced by surfaces that include arginine–glycine–aspartic acid (RGD) peptides, heparin, or sulfated polysaccharides. These functional groups maintain a hemocompatible interface, reduce thrombogenicity, and encourage endothelialization. Advanced surface functionalization techniques that offer precise control over surface chemistry include chemical derivatization, UV-induced immobilization, and plasma-assisted grafting. The spatial arrangement and density of functional groups can be changed to create cell-selective surfaces that optimize desired tissue responses and reduce unwanted adhesion, including bacterial colonization or fibroblast expansion. In the end, sensible chemical customization makes it possible to create surfaces that actively direct biological processes, converting inert substrates into biointeractive scaffolds for regenerative medicine and tissue engineering [59].

4.6.2 Optimizing Roughness and Wettability to Enhance Adhesion or Reduce Fouling

Two essential physical factors that affect microbial colonization, protein adsorption, and cell attachment are surface roughness and wettability. To get the intended functional results, these attributes must be properly balanced. Micro- and nanoscale surface roughness can enhance cellular adherence by increasing the effective contact area and providing mechanical anchorage sites. For example, titanium implants with micro-roughened surfaces (~1–5 μm) promote osteoblast growth and bone matrix synthesis, while nanoscale topographies can change protein adsorption and integrin clustering [60, 61]. However, excessive roughness may encourage bacterial adherence or biofilm formation, depending on the clinical scenario, necessitating optimal design.

Surface energy has a high correlation with wettability, which is a measure of how fluids interact with the biomaterial. Hydrophilic surfaces (low contact angle) generally encourage uniform protein adsorption and beneficial cell attachment, whereas hydrophobic surfaces inhibit bacterial colonization and protein fouling. Vascular implants with moderate hydrophilic surfaces, for instance, balance the requirements of biocompatibility and anti-thrombogenicity by promoting endothelialization and decreasing platelet aggregation. By combining roughness and wettability optimization, surfaces can reduce nonspecific adsorption and microbial colonization in some applications (like indwelling catheters or cardiovascular grafts) while selectively improving cellular adherence where it is needed (like in osteoconductive scaffolds).

4.6.3 Compatibility Between Surface Treatments and Bulk Material Integrity

Surface modifications must preserve the mechanical and structural integrity of the bulk material. Aggressive treatments including laser ablation, deep chemical functionalization, and high-energy plasma etching may inadvertently weaken the substrate, create microcracks, or alter fatigue behavior, especially in metals and polymers used in load-bearing applications. For example, extensive acid etching on stainless steel might increase surface roughness for bone implantation; however, excessive etching may reduce the tensile strength of the material. However, when physiological pressures are applied, UV-induced crosslinking of polymers may improve surface functionalization while reducing elasticity and ductility, potentially leading to brittle fracture. To ensure that modifications are consistent, superficial, and compliant with the mechanical requirements of the implant, surface engineering must be carefully calibrated.

Computational modeling, finite element analysis, and microstructural evaluation are increasingly employed to predict the impact of surface treatments on bulk behavior. This integrative approach allows designers to balance surface functionality with mechanical reliability, ensuring long-term implant performance.

4.6.4 Balancing Stability, Durability, and Functionality of Surface Coatings

Adding bioactivity, antimicrobial, or anti-fouling properties is effectively accomplished through surface coatings. Designers must carefully combine stability, durability, and biological functionality to provide outcomes that are clinically beneficial. Durability is essential for implants that will be used for a long time or load. Coatings such as hydroxyapatite on titanium and diamond-like carbon on stainless steel must withstand micro-motion, cyclic loading, and mechanical wear without delamination. Coatings must not degrade or dissolve in physiological fluids, particularly under challenging circumstances with varying pH, ionic strength, or oxidative stress [62]. This is equally critical as chemical stability.

Biological characteristics such as peptide presentation, controlled ion release, and antibacterial activity should still be present in coatings. For instance, calcium phosphate coatings must dissolve gradually to release calcium and phosphate ions for bone mineralization, whereas polymeric antifouling layers should be non-toxic but resistant to protein adsorption. To reach this balance, it is often necessary to use surface nanostructuring, gradient coatings, or multilayer architectures that optimize mechanical robustness and biological interaction.

4.6.5 Regulatory and Biocompatibility Implications of Surface-Modified Implants

Surface-modified implants may alter clinical performance and biocompatibility, hence they are closely regulated. Evidence that surface therapies do not result in cytotoxicity, inflammation, or unanticipated systemic effects is required by the FDA, EMA, and other regulatory bodies. When evaluating biocompatibility, in vitro cytotoxicity tests, hemocompatibility tests, and in vivo implantation studies are frequently employed. Coating or surface functionalizations must be stable, non-toxic, and have predictable interactions with cells and proteins. Surface modification methods need to be hygienic, reproducible, and well-characterized because even little chemical alterations, such as undesired oxidation products or residual grafting chemicals, can trigger immunological or foreign body reactions.

In order to ensure that the functionalized surface is safe and effective for the duration of its shelf life and clinical use, regulatory compliance also requires documentation of production methods, quality control measures, and sterilizing procedures. To connect surface engineering tactics with both performance goals and safety criteria, designers must incorporate regulatory considerations early in the development process [63].

4.6.6 Long-Term Stability and Sterilization Resilience of Surface Modifications

A key aspect of surface design is ensuring that changes endure over the intended life of the implant and can withstand sterilization procedures without losing their efficacy. Chemical, mechanical, and biological resilience are all components of long-term stability. In vivo, surfaces need to be impervious to oxidation, hydrolytic breakdown, and mechanical wear. For instance, polymeric coatings on metal implants may hydrolyze, while bioactive ceramic layers may crack or dissolve in physiological settings. Controlled crosslinking, surface densification, or covalent functionalization can enhance long-term stability while maintaining the necessary bioactivity and mechanical integrity.

Sterilization resistance is also crucial. Common sterilization techniques that alter mechanical, wettability, or surface chemistry include autoclaving, ethylene oxide (EtO), gamma irradiation, and electron-beam irradiation. For example, gamma irradiation may cause chain scission in polymer coatings, altering protein adsorption and reducing hydrophilicity. As a result, designers must either select surface treatments that complement sterilization methods or employ protective strategies such post-sterilization functionalization, stabilizing compounds, or sacrificial layers. The possibility of losing bioactivity, delamination, or implant failure if long-term stability or sterilization resilience are not achieved emphasizes the importance of thorough testing procedures that assess surface performance under physiological and clinical preparation conditions [64, 65].

Incorporating these design considerations requires a thorough, multidisciplinary approach. The optimization of surface chemistry, roughness, and wettability must be balanced against mechanical integrity, coating longevity, and regulatory compliance. Advanced computational modeling combined with experimental characterization (e.g., contact angle measurement, zeta potential, and surface roughness analysis) supports predictive design and informed modification technique selection. Furthermore, iterative testing, which encompasses in vitro, ex vivo, and in vivo evaluations, ensures that surface-engineered biomaterials function in a manner that is safe, practical, and advantageous from a clinical standpoint.

Effective biomaterial surface design is a complex and multidimensional process that requires careful consideration of topography, chemistry, durability, mechanical compatibility, and regulatory constraints. Surface modification for specific cellular interactions, wettability and roughness adjustment, and compatibility with bulk materials are necessary for predictable biological outcomes. When coating stability, durability, and functionality are balanced while maintaining biocompatibility and regulatory compliance, implants work consistently over long periods of time. By combining these ideas, designers can create next-generation biomaterials that are both structurally sound and biologically intelligent, capable of interacting with tissues in a controlled and beneficial manner for therapy [66]. The creation of scaffolds and implants that promote regenerative medicine, enhance patient outcomes, and establish new benchmarks for biomaterial performance is supported by this comprehensive design concept.

4.7 Applications and Case Studies

The functionalization and modification of biomaterial surfaces has changed the performance of medical devices and the outcomes of therapy, directly affecting biocompatibility, tissue integration, and clinical efficacy. Because surface engineering allows for controlled interactions with biological systems, materials perform better in orthopedic, dental, cardiovascular, and drug delivery applications. Furthermore, nanostructuring, biofunctionalization, and physicochemical modification have led to a surge in the use of biomaterials in tissue engineering, wound healing, and the development of biosensors [67]. By looking at various applications, this shows how crucial surface modification is to achieving clinical success.

4.7.1 Orthopedic and Dental Implants

For dental and orthopedic implants to be mechanically stable and successful over the long term, strong osseointegration is required. Surface engineering techniques like acid etching, sandblasting, roughening, and coating with bioactive chemicals have been significantly responsible for this advancement [68]. For instance, titanium and its alloys are widely employed in orthopedic and dental applications due to its exceptional mechanical properties and corrosion resistance. On flat titanium surfaces, however, osteoblastic adhesion is only partially feasible.

Studies have demonstrated that micro and nanoscale surface roughening significantly enhances osteoblast growth and multiplication. While sandblasting and acid-etching titanium surfaces enhance surface area and mechanical interlocking with bone, anodization produces nanoporous oxide layers that improve hydrophilicity and protein adsorption. Often applied via sol-gel or plasma spraying methods, calcium phosphate and hydroxyapatite (HA) coatings provide osteoconductive surfaces that speed up bone integration and deposition. Clinical studies indicate improved bone–implant contact, faster healing times, and higher implant survival rates when compared to untreated controls. Advanced biomimetic coating enhances osteoinductive potential and guide tissue remodeling and localized bone creation by including peptides or growth factors such as BMP-2. These strategies demonstrate how biological, chemical, and topographical elements work together to optimize implant performance. A translational review of innovations in implant osseointegration demonstrates that the field is shifting from static 2D surface modifications toward functional 3D nanofiber constructs and biomimetic scaffolds replicating ECM architecture with nanostructured surfaces and bioactive coatings consistently accelerating early-stage osteogenesis, while long-term clinical validation of their durability and infection resistance remains an outstanding priority [69].

4.7.2 Cardiovascular Devices

The interactions between blood and materials present special difficulties for cardiovascular implants, such as heart valves, grafts, and stents. Device failure is frequently caused by thrombosis, inflammation, and endothelial dysfunction brought on by unmodified surfaces [70]. Strategies for surface modification seek to limit immunological responses, encourage endothelialization, and lessen platelet adhesion. While preserving material compatibility, anti-thrombogenic coatings, such as immobilized heparin or nitric oxide-releasing layers, stop clots from forming. Heparin-coated stents, for instance, lessen thrombus development and platelet activation in the early phases of implantation. On the other hand, endothelialization-promoting surfaces use RGD peptides or ECM proteins to promote quick endothelial cell coverage and produce a non-thrombogenic interface. Vascular healing is improved by nanostructured and micropatterned surfaces, which also affect cell alignment and function.

In preclinical and clinical trials, surface-engineered cardiovascular devices have shown notable benefits, such as decreased rates of restenosis, accelerated endothelial healing, and less need on systemic anticoagulant medication [71]. These findings highlight how crucial it is to adjust surface chemistry, topography, and biofunctionalization to satisfy the particular physiological needs of the cardiovascular system.

4.7.3 Drug Delivery Systems

In drug delivery, surface modification is essential, especially for focused therapy, controlled release, and increased bioavailability. Functionalization of hydrogels, liposomes, and nanoparticles is used to enhance cellular absorption, circulation time, and selective binding to target tissues. PEGylation and ligand conjugation are two examples of functionalized nanoparticle surfaces that decrease immunogenic clearance and allow for targeted distribution to cell types. For instance, cancer cells can be selectively bound by nanoparticles coated with peptides or antibodies, limiting systemic toxicity while permitting high medication concentrations at the problematic site. Like this, drug release kinetics can be adjusted by hydrogels with adjustable surface chemistry in response to environmental cues like pH, temperature, or enzymatic activity. Therapeutic time and dosage may be precisely controlled thanks to these responsive surfaces.

Combination therapies are also made easier by surface modification in drug delivery. Materials can simultaneously carry medications, encourage cell adhesion, and alter immune responses by including multifunctional coatings [72]. The effectiveness of these strategies in preclinical models is demonstrated by recent case studies, which show better tissue targeting, decreased off-target effects, and improved pharmacokinetics.

4.7.4 Wound Healing and Tissue Engineering

Surface characteristics have a direct impact on angiogenesis, microbial control, cell adhesion, and proliferation in wound healing and tissue engineering. Hydrophilic materials promote nutrition transfer and cell penetration, whereas antimicrobial coatings lower the danger of infection. To promote healing, functional groups, growth factors, or silver nanoparticles are commonly incorporated into hydrogels, electrospun scaffolds, and bioactive dressings [73]. For example, dressing functionalized with silver nanoparticles have strong antibacterial properties without sacrificing cell viability. In a similar vein, scaffolds coated with collagen or extracellular matrix promote fibroblast adhesion and extracellular matrix deposition, speeding up tissue regeneration. Additionally, cellular orientation is guided by surface nanostructures and micropatterns, which facilitate the creation of ordered tissues.

Comparing wounds treated with surface-engineered materials to those treated with conventional bandages, clinical case studies show decreased infection rates, decreased scarring, and quicker epithelialization. These illustrations show how integrating biological, chemical, and topographical changes can maximize the results of tissue restoration.

4.7.5 Biosensors and Diagnostic Platforms

Surface engineering is equally critical in biosensors and diagnostic devices, where molecular-level control over surface chemistry and topography directly influences sensitivity, specificity, and signal stability [74]. Target analyte selective detection is made possible by immobilizing recognition elements such as enzymes, antibodies, or aptamers onto functionalized surfaces. Signal responses are enhanced by nanostructured surfaces, such as graphene sheets, carbon nanotubes, and gold nanoparticles, which improve surface area and electron transfer efficiency. For instance, compared to electrodes that have not been altered, electrochemical glucose sensors with electrodes treated with gold nanoparticles exhibit increased sensitivity and quicker reaction times. In a similar manner, surface patterning is used in microfluidic devices to regulate fluid flow and cell adhesion, enhancing analytical accuracy.

In order to reduce non-specific adsorption, guarantee reproducibility, and facilitate incorporation into point-of-care diagnostic systems, surface changes in biosensors are essential. Case studies illustrate the revolutionary potential of surface science in clinical diagnostics by proving that precisely designed surfaces may identify biomarkers at picomolar concentrations.

4.7.6 Comparative Evaluation of Clinical Outcomes Based on Surface Engineering Strategies

The substantial influence of surface modification on therapeutic results is highlighted by the combined data from orthopedic, dental, cardiovascular, drug delivery, wound healing, and biosensor applications. Engineered surfaces regularly perform better than untreated or traditionally processed materials, according to comparative research [75]. For instance, endothelialized stents with bioactive coatings lower restenosis rates in comparison to bare-metal stents, whereas sandblasted and HA-coated dental implants show higher osseointegration rates than smooth titanium implants. Antimicrobial and hydrophilic surfaces accelerate epithelialization and decrease infection during wound healing, which results in shorter hospital stays and better patient outcomes. Functionalized surfaces in drug delivery devices minimize systemic side effects while achieving more consistent release profiles and increased therapeutic efficacy. Likewise, biosensors featuring nanostructured surfaces have improved analytical capabilities, which are essential for early disease monitoring and diagnosis.

These parallels demonstrate that surface engineering is a key factor in determining clinical efficacy rather than just a supporting component of material design. By combining topographical, chemical, and biological cues, multifunctional, patient-specific biomaterials that can dynamically interact with the physiological environment can be created [76]. Additionally, continued advancements in stimuli-responsive coatings, additive manufacturing, and nanotechnology hold promise for enhancing results, increasing therapeutic applications, and lowering problems in a variety of biomedical fields.

Engineering techniques and surface modification are essential to the development of contemporary biomaterials. These methods allow for the precise regulation of biological responses, tissue integration, and device performance through the manipulation of topography, chemistry, and biofunctionalization. The adaptability and influence of surface engineering on therapeutic results are demonstrated by applications in tissue engineering, wound healing, medication delivery, cardiovascular devices, orthopedic and dental implants, and biosensors. Optimized surfaces improve long-term performance, safety, and efficacy, according to comparative case studies. The development of next-generation biomaterials that are not only robust and biocompatible but also intelligent and regenerative will be fueled by the integration of nanostructures, bioactive coatings, and responsive interfaces as the field develops. These materials will be able to precisely address complex clinical challenges with never-before-seen precision [68].

4.8 Recent Advances and Innovations

Over the past 10 years, nanotechnology, biomimetic design, smart materials, additive manufacturing, and computational modeling have all significantly changed the field of biomaterial surface engineering. In order to achieve improved bioactivity, decreased fouling, and adaptive functionality, the interface between the biomaterial and the biological environment is carefully tailored in modern implants and scaffolds, which no longer rely only on bulk material qualities [77]. This demonstrates how state-of-the-art methods are changing the field of biomaterial design by highlighting recent developments and breakthroughs in surface science.

4.8.1 Nanotechnology-Driven Surface Engineering

Surface engineering has been transformed by nanotechnology, which allows for control over surface topography, composition, and functioning at the atomic and molecular level. Atomic layer deposition (ALD) and nanocomposite coatings are two well-known techniques that have shown great promise in improving implant performance. A vapor-phase process called atomic layer deposition (ALD) creates atomic-level precision deposits of ultra-thin, conformal layers. Without changing the bulk properties, ALD enables consistent coating of intricate geometries, such as microstructured implants and porous scaffolds. Titanium dioxide (TiO_2) or alumina ALD coatings, for example, enhance corrosion resistance and offer adjustable surface roughness to encourage osteoblast adherence on titanium implants. Additionally, ALD makes it easier to functionalize bioactive compounds or antibacterial agents, giving cells precise spatial control over chemical cues that trigger a response.

Nanoparticles like graphene, carbon nanotubes, hydroxyapatite, or silver are incorporated into a polymeric or ceramic matrix to create nanocomposite coatings. The mechanical, chemical, and biological benefits of several materials are combined in these coatings. For instance, silver-doped nanocomposites offer persistent antibacterial activity, while hydroxyapatite–graphene nanocomposites on titanium surfaces improve osteoconductivity and mechanical resilience. These coatings create a nanoscale topography that resembles the natural extracellular matrix (ECM) architecture, which facilitates tissue integration, integrin clustering, and protein adsorption [78, 79]. When combined, surface engineering powered by nanotechnology allows for precise biointerface design, bridging the gap between the functionality of cells and the performance of bulk materials.

4.8.2 Bioinspired and Biomimetic Approaches

Inspired by nature, bioinspired and biomimetic surfaces achieve exceptional control over adhesion, wettability, and self-cleaning by replicating functional patterns found in plants and animals [80]. By using evolutionary concepts, these techniques produce surfaces that actively control biological interactions. Superhydrophobicity, in which hierarchical patterns at the micro and nanoscale provide self-cleaning surfaces, is best illustrated by the lotus leaf effect. By applying these phenomena to medical implants, long-term sterility and biocompatibility are improved by lowering protein fouling and bacterial colonization. Surfaces inspired by geckos also resemble fibrillar structures, which promote reversible adhesion without the need for chemical bonding. This idea has been used in biomedical settings to provide regulated mechanical engagement with soft tissues using tissue scaffolds, wearable biosensors, and microneedle arrays.

Additional biomimetic techniques include electrospinning, soft molding, and lithography to replicate extracellular matrix topographies. These surfaces improve regenerative outcomes in orthopedic, cardiovascular, and brain implants by directing cell alignment, proliferation, and differentiation by imitating the natural fibrous architecture of tissues [81]. Bioinspired surfaces show that biological behavior can be determined by functional topography rather than just chemical composition. By combining mechanical signals, surface chemistry, and hierarchical structures, materials can actively interact with cells to replicate the conditions seen in real tissues.

4.8.3 Smart and Responsive Surfaces

The creation of intelligent, stimuli-responsive coatings that dynamically modify their characteristics in response to environmental inputs is a significant advancement in surface engineering. These coatings improve therapeutic performance and safety by providing spatially and temporally regulated functionality. pH-sensitive surfaces use the local acidity to cause exposure to bioactive molecules, drug release, or degradation. To minimize systemic effects, tumor-targeted implants or antimicrobial coatings, for instance, release medicines preferentially in acidic microenvironments. Poly(*N*-isopropylacrylamide) (PNIPAM) hydrogels are examples of temperature-sensitive surfaces that experience reversible swelling or contraction close to physiological temperatures, regulating drug release, surface wettability, and cell adhesion. Enzyme-responsive coatings offer feedback-regulated material performance by selectively degrading when enzymes released during inflammation or tissue remodeling are present.

Implants can interact dynamically with tissues thanks to these responsive surfaces, which can gradually adjust to variations in temperature, enzyme activity, or pH. By bringing material behavior into line with biological processes, the capacity to modify surface attributes in situ marks a substantial advancement above static surface engineering [22].

4.8.4 4D Surface Modification

Traditional surface engineering is expanded by the idea of 4D surface modification, which adds time as a functional dimension [75]. Because 4D surfaces are made to change dynamically in physiological settings, they can function adaptively in response to mechanical, chemical, or biological stimuli. For instance, 4D hydrogel coatings could gradually change stiffness or topography, directing tissue regeneration or stem cell differentiation. After implantation, shape-memory polymers with 4D capabilities can alter their shape, allowing for less invasive delivery and subsequent expansion for the best possible tissue contact. Surfaces that dynamically modify their hydrophilicity or ligand presentation in response to flow shear stress enhance endothelialization and reduce thrombosis in vascular grafts.

4D surface modifications merge material science, biomechanics, and bioengineering, creating implants capable of temporal adaptation, an essential requirement for long-term integration in dynamic biological environments.

4.8.5 Additive Manufacturing Integration

Surface engineering has changed because of additive manufacturing (AM), which includes 3D and newer 4D printing methods. AM allows for layer-by-layer control over chemistry, porosity, and topography. At the micro- and nanoscale resolution, AM enables the creation of intricate structures with integrated surface characteristics. For example, in a single manufacturing process, 3D-printed titanium scaffolds can integrate bioactive coatings, porosity gradients, and controlled roughness. Time-evolving surfaces, in which printed materials react to stimuli after implantation by changing their shape, stiffness, or wettability to correspond with the process of tissue healing, are made possible by 4D printing. Customized, patient-specific implants are made possible by AM integration, in which surface characteristics are carefully adjusted to meet biological objectives and anatomical specifications. Furthermore, AM can be used with post-processing methods like surface grafting or laser ablation to create multifunctional surfaces that integrate mechanical support, bioactivity, and anti-fouling qualities in a harmonious way [82].

4.8.6 Computational and AI-Guided Design

The intricacy of contemporary surface engineering has made the prediction and optimization of material–biological interactions possible using computational modeling and artificial intelligence (AI) [83]. Cost, time, and the enormous combinatorial space of surface chemistry, topographies, and coatings are the constraints of traditional experimental methods. Finite element analysis, molecular dynamics, and Monte Carlo simulations are used in predictive modeling to predict mechanical response, cell adhesion, and protein adsorption. These models lessen the need for intensive in vitro and in vivo testing by enabling virtual testing of surface alterations under physiological circumstances.

This is furthered by AI-guided design, which analyzes vast databases of surface characteristics, material compositions, and biological effects using machine learning algorithms. AI can recommend the best surface alterations for tissue types, patient situations, or clinical applications by finding correlations and forecasting patterns. AI models have been utilized, for instance, to enhance polymer coatings for controlled drug delivery or forecast osteoblast adherence on titanium nanotopographies. Rational surface design is accelerated by the combination of computational tools and experimental validation, shifting the discipline away from empirical methods and toward predictive, data-driven engineering of biomaterial interfaces.

The design of biomaterials has changed from static, one-size-fits-all methods to dynamic, multifunctional, and adaptive interfaces due to recent developments in surface properties and modification techniques. Atomic-scale control and nanocomposite coatings are made possible by nanotechnology, and bioinspired surfaces mimic natural functions to direct cell behavior and lessen fouling. For long-term integration, 4D surface modification adds temporal evolution, while smart and responsive surfaces offer environmental adaptation. Precision layer-by-layer patterning made possible by additive printing supports patient-specific tailoring, and predictive design made possible by computational modeling with AI lessens the load of experiments and improves safety [84].

Together, these developments completely reinterpret the function of the biomaterial surface, transforming it from a passive interface to an intelligent, active player in tissue regeneration, healing, and medicinal delivery. The next generation of biomaterials promises surfaces that are precisely tailored, dynamically adaptive and optimized for clinical performance, ushering in a new era of functional and regenerative medicine. This is due to ongoing research that integrates nanotechnology, biomimicry, responsive systems, and data-driven design.

4.9 Challenges and Limitations

Surface modification of biomaterials has emerged as a critical strategy for enhancing biocompatibility, bioactivity, and clinical performance. Techniques ranging from physical roughening and chemical functionalization to nanostructuring and biofunctional coating have significantly expanded the functionality of implants, scaffolds, drug delivery systems, and diagnostic devices. Despite these advances, multiple challenges and limitations continue to constrain the widespread implementation and clinical translation of surface-engineered biomaterials. These issues encompass technical, biological, regulatory, and economic aspects, reflecting the complex interplay between material science and physiological environments.

4.9.1 Lack of Universal Characterization Standards for Modified Surfaces

The lack of defined methods for describing changed surfaces is one of the main issues facing the subject. Surface features like roughness, chemistry, energy, and topography necessitate specific methods, in contrast to bulk materials, whose qualities may be measured using tried-and-true mechanical, thermal, and chemical tests [85]. Although techniques such as scanning electron microscopy (SEM), atomic force microscopy (AFM), X-ray photoelectron spectroscopy (XPS), and contact angle measurements offer comprehensive information, the outcomes can differ based on sample preparation, analytical procedures, and instrument calibration.

It is challenging to establish unambiguous relationships between surface alterations and biological consequences due to the absence of universal standards, which also makes inter-study comparisons and reproducibility more challenging. Although regulatory organizations like ISO and ASTM have produced certain rules regarding coating thickness, corrosion, and biocompatibility, full standards addressing multi-functional and nanostructured surfaces are still lacking. This gap slows clinical translation and provider acceptability by limiting the capacity to thoroughly assess and validate surface alterations.

4.9.2 Difficulty in Maintaining Coating Adhesion and Mechanical Durability Under Physiological Stress

Surface modifications and coatings must withstand chemical exposure, cyclic loading, and mechanical stress in the human body. Adhesion failure, cracking, or delamination are problems that many modern coatings, especially hydroxyapatite or polymeric layers put to orthopedic and dental implants, face over time. The integrity of the implant may be jeopardized if physiological stressors, including as tensile, compressive, and shear forces, cause microfractures at the coating–substrate interface. Although initially strong, thermal or plasma-deposited coatings may also show lingering stresses from the deposition process, which would shorten their mechanical endurance over time. Stents and grafts in cardiovascular applications are exposed to pulsatile pressure, dynamic blood flow, and endothelial shear stress, all of which can worsen coating deterioration [86]. One of the significant engineering challenges is maintaining uniform adhesion and mechanical stability under various implant geometries and stress scenarios.

4.9.3 Degradation or Delamination of Bioactive Layers over Time

Many surface alterations, such as the addition of growth factors, peptides, or nanocomposite layers that improve cellular responses, are made to be bioactive or resorbable. Despite their initial effectiveness, these bioactive layers are frequently prone to delamination or disintegration in physiological settings. Surface coatings may be broken down more quickly than anticipated by hydrolytic, enzymatic, or oxidative processes, which could reduce their effectiveness and expose the underlying substrate to corrosion or immunological recognition [87].

For instance, hydroxyapatite coatings sprayed with plasma may partially disintegrate in bodily fluids, changing the topography of the surface and the patterns of protein adsorption. Likewise, polymer brushes or peptide-functionalized layers may lose their functionality due to hydrolysis or conformational changes. Variability in patient physiology, local pH, enzymatic activity, and mechanical loading make it difficult to predict and regulate the lifetime of bioactive layers. Long-term reliability and clinical results are complicated by this unpredictability [88].

4.9.4 Potential Cytotoxicity or Immune Response from Residual Chemicals or Nanoparticles

Chemicals, solvents, or nanoparticles that may stay on the material after production are commonly used in surface modification procedures. Unreacted monomers, crosslinkers, or residual reagents might cause cytotoxicity or unfavorable immunological responses. For example, solvent residues, silanization agents, and precursors of plasma polymerization can all have an impact on cell survival if they are not sufficiently eliminated. Coatings containing nanoparticles like graphene, titanium dioxide, or silver may produce reactive oxygen species, cause inflammation, or build up in tissues, all of which could compromise biocompatibility [89].

Surface chemistry and topography further complicate immune responses by activating complement pathways, dendritic cells, or macrophages. Unintentional immune cell activation can lead to fibrous encapsulation, implant rejection, or persistent inflammation, even when surface biofunctionalization seeks to enhance cellular interactions. Therefore, thorough in vitro and in vivo toxicological evaluation is crucial nevertheless, present models prediction ability is constrained, especially for complex or multifunctional surfaces.

4.9.5 Cost, Scalability, and Reproducibility Issues in Advanced Surface Modification Techniques

Numerous advanced surface modification methods are resource-intensive and technically complex, including plasma spraying, atomic layer deposition, nanolithography, and 3D/4D printing of functionalized surfaces. These procedures raise production costs because they call for specialist knowledge, regulated settings, and high-precision equipment. There are additional difficulties in scaling these techniques from lab prototypes to commercial manufacture. At industrial sizes, it is challenging to achieve reproducible bioactivity, maintain homogeneity across batches, and guarantee consistent coating thickness. Clinical performance may be impacted by discrepancies resulting from variations in raw materials, process parameters, or environmental circumstances [90]. The broad use of sophisticated surface-modified biomaterials is hampered by these manufacturing and financial constraints, especially in healthcare environments with limited resources.

4.9.6 Balancing Multifunctionality with Simplicity and Manufacturability

Multifunctional surfaces are frequently the goal of contemporary surface engineering, combining characteristics like mechanical reinforcement, bioactivity, antibacterial activity, and stimuli-responsiveness. Although multifunctionality improves performance, it also makes design, manufacturing, and regulatory approval more difficult. The possibility of process mistakes, instability, or unexpected interactions between surface components increases when complex surfaces necessitate several deposition processes, careful control of nanostructures, and integration of bioactive molecules. Additionally, excessively complicated surfaces could be hard to replicate, sterilize, or inspect, which would make quality control and regulatory compliance challenging. In certain instances, less complex surface alterations with moderate functionality could produce more dependable clinical results than extremely complex designs that are susceptible to manufacturing and environmental fluctuations [91].

When designing biomaterials, the trade-off between manufacturability and multifunctionality must be carefully considered. Maintaining enough bioactivity while maximizing cost, scalability, and clinical safety continues to be a crucial balancing act. This difficulty emphasizes how crucial iterative testing, predictive modeling, and logical design frameworks are to producing surfaces that are useful and efficient for actual medical applications.

Although surface modification has advanced significantly, there are still major obstacles that prevent synthetic biomaterials from reaching their full potential. While coating adhesion, mechanical durability, and bioactive layer stability are susceptible to physiological stressors and degradation processes, the absence of common characterization standards makes comparison and reproducibility across investigations more difficult. Clinical translation is made more difficult by the possibility of cytotoxicity or immunological activation from leftover compounds or nanoparticles. Furthermore, there are practical and financial obstacles due to the cost, scalability, and reproducibility of sophisticated surface modification methods. Lastly, to guarantee dependable clinical performance, the pursuit of multifunctionality must be weighed against simplicity, manufacturability, and regulatory viability. In addition to established procedures, stringent testing, and scalable production techniques, addressing these issues calls for an integrated strategy that incorporates materials science, surface chemistry, nanotechnology, and biological evaluation. Overcoming these limitations is essential for advancing surface-engineered biomaterials from experimental innovation to widely adopted clinical solutions, ultimately improving patient outcomes across orthopedic, cardiovascular, wound healing, drug delivery, and diagnostic applications [22, 92].

4.10 Future Directions

Advanced materials science, computer modeling, nanotechnology, and bioengineering are all coming together to drive the development of biomaterial surface engineering. The future of surface science places an emphasis on dynamic, multifunctional, and adaptable surfaces that can react to the complex physiological environment, whereas past surface alterations concentrated on static advances in mechanical performance or biocompatibility. This section examines new developments that have the potential to revolutionize the functionality, appearance, and therapeutic efficacy of biomaterial surfaces.

4.10.1 Integration of Artificial Intelligence for Predictive Surface Design and Optimization

Rapid prototyping, optimization, and predictive design are made possible by artificial intelligence (AI) and machine learning, which have the potential to completely transform biomaterial surface engineering. Iterative cycles of fabrication, characterisation, and in vitro or in vivo testing are necessary for traditional experimental approaches to surface modification, which are time-consuming and resource intensive. Large datasets of surface chemical, topography, mechanical characteristics, and biological effects can be analyzed by AI algorithms to find patterns that would otherwise be hard to spot [93].

For instance, using chemical functionalization and nanoscale surface properties, machine learning models can forecast the likelihood of bacterial colonization, protein adsorption profiles, or cell adhesion behavior. AI can also help with multi-objective optimization, which involves juggling conflicting requirements like mechanical stability, hydrophilicity, and antibacterial activity. Researchers can design surfaces more logically rather than experimentally thanks to these predictive capabilities, which speeds up development and improves implant safety and effectiveness. Moreover, virtual screening of surface alterations before physical production is made possible by integration with computational models, which lowers expenses and experimental iterations.

4.10.2 Development of Self-Healing and Regenerative Surface Coatings

Surface engineering is taking a revolutionary turn with the development of regenerative and self-healing coatings. When mechanical damage, chemical deterioration, or biological wear occurs, these coatings are made to automatically regain their structure or bioactivity. In order to successfully repair microcracks, delamination, or erosion, self-healing surfaces can be designed utilizing microcapsules or polymer networks that release restorative chemicals upon injury [94, 95]. Regenerative coatings in bone and tissue engineering can actively stimulate tissue regeneration while preserving structural integrity by releasing growth hormones, ions, or bioactive compounds in response to inflammatory or cellular cues. For example, a titanium implant coated with a calcium phosphate-polymer composite may be able to maintain osteoconductivity throughout time by self-renewing its bioactive layer in situ.

The development of these adaptive surfaces has the potential to extend implant lifespan, reduce revision surgeries, and enhance tissue integration, representing a paradigm shift from static coatings toward dynamic, self-regulating interfaces.

4.10.3 Sustainable and Green Surface Modification Technologies

The development of ecologically friendly surface modification techniques is being driven by the growing importance of sustainability in biomaterials engineering. Conventional techniques include metal ion deposition, chemical grafting, and plasma treatments can use dangerous chemicals, a lot of energy, or a lot of waste. Future directions will focus on green chemistry concepts such solvent-free deposition methods, enzymatic catalysis, and aqueous-based functionalization. For instance, sol-gel coatings made under ambient settings with biodegradable precursors or biomimetic mineralization techniques preserve bioactivity while minimizing their negative effects on the environment. Furthermore, reducing energy-intensive high-temperature treatments, recycling leftover precursors, and using sustainable polymeric coatings all help to make manufacturing more environmentally friendly without sacrificing efficiency [96].

Such sustainable approaches are particularly relevant for large-scale production of implants and medical devices, aligning surface engineering practices with global environmental and regulatory goals.

4.10.4 Multi-functional Coatings Combining Antimicrobial, Anti-inflammatory, and Regenerative Properties

Multifunctional coatings that can handle several clinical issues at once are the direction of the next generation of surface modifications. The complex requirements of dynamic physiological settings are frequently not met by conventional single-function coatings, such as silver for antibacterial activity or hydroxyapatite for osteoconduction [97, 98]. New multifunctional coatings combine regeneration elements, antimicrobials, and anti-inflammatory medications into one interface. For instance, composite coating may include osteogenic peptides to promote bone regeneration, regulated release of anti-inflammatory cytokines to reduce tissue reaction, and silver nanoparticles to limit infection. These functions can be controlled spatially and temporally by layered, gradient, or nanostructured designs, guaranteeing that therapeutic effects are administered at the right timings and concentrations.

Such multifunctional approaches are particularly important for high-risk implants including orthopedic, cardiovascular, and dental devices, where infection, inflammation, and tissue integration must be concurrently managed.

4.10.5 Interdisciplinary Convergence of Materials Science, Nanotechnology, and Bioengineering

Surface engineering's future depends on the multidisciplinary fusion of bioengineering, nanotechnology, and materials science. Bioengineering offers insights into cellular function and tissue integration, while advances in nanoscale fabrication allow for exact control of surface chemistry and topography. The study of materials science advances our understanding of chemical stability, mechanical characteristics, and degradation dynamics. The logical design of interfaces that replicate the intricacy of natural tissues is made easier by this convergence [99]. For example, extracellular matrix patterns can be replicated by nanostructured surfaces, and growth factors can be delivered by bioengineered coatings in response to mechanical loading. By developing patient-specific, adaptable surfaces, such integrated techniques promote personalized therapy and enhance therapeutic results.

Interdisciplinary collaboration also supports the translation of laboratory innovations into scalable, regulatory-compliant medical devices, bridging the gap between research and clinical application.

4.10.6 Real-Time Monitoring and Adaptive Feedback Systems for Surface Performance In Vivo

The use of adaptive feedback systems and real-time monitoring to evaluate and control surface performance in vivo represents another frontier in surface engineering. Conventional assessment techniques, including ex vivo analysis or periodic imaging, offer little understanding of dynamic biological interactions. Biosensors, embedded electronics, or sensitive coatings that may identify local variations in pH, enzyme activity, or mechanical stress are examples of emerging technology. These systems can react to physiological cues by releasing bioactive chemicals, changing wettability, or triggering self-healing mechanisms in real-time when paired with AI-driven control algorithms.

For example, a vascular stent with a smart coating could detect early inflammation or thrombus formation and release anti-inflammatory or anticoagulant agents on demand, preventing complications before they become clinically significant. Such adaptive surfaces represent a move toward closed-loop, intelligent biomaterials, capable of maintaining optimal performance throughout the implant's lifecycle.

Advanced materials, nanotechnology, bioengineering, and computational intelligence are all integrated into dynamic, adaptable, and multifunctional interfaces that define the future of biomaterial surface engineering. While self-healing and regenerative coatings increase implant longevity and functional performance, AI-guided predictive modeling allows for logical design and optimization [100]. Multifunctional coatings tackle the intricate relationship between infection, inflammation, and tissue regeneration, while sustainable, green modification technologies lessen their negative effects on the environment. The development of patient-specific, adaptable surfaces that closely resemble natural tissue interfaces is made possible by interdisciplinary convergence, which speeds up innovation. Finally, adaptive feedback and real-time monitoring systems offer previously unheard-of control over in vivo surface performance, creating new possibilities for smart, responsive implants. Collectively, these future directions signal a paradigm shift in biomaterial design toward interfaces that are not only structurally robust but actively therapeutic, adaptive, and aligned with the dynamic needs of the human body.

4.11 Conclusion

It is becoming more widely acknowledged that a biomaterial's surface, which serves as the main contact between artificial materials and the biological environment, is a key factor in determining its clinical effectiveness. The performance of biomaterials is influenced more by their surface features than by their bulk qualities in a variety of biomedical applications, including tissue engineering scaffolds, drug delivery systems, cardiovascular devices, and orthopedic and dental implants. Protein adsorption, cell adhesion, tissue integration, and immunological response are all influenced by surface chemistry, topography, charge, wettability, and energy. The biological reaction can be significantly changed by even little changes in these parameters, highlighting the significance of exact surface engineering and control to produce reliable and secure results.

4.11.1 Summary of the Central Role of Surface Properties in Biomaterial Function and Success

For all biological processes surrounding an implant or device, surface characteristics serve as the first point of contact. They control the development of protein layers, which in turn control the attachment, growth, and differentiation of cells. For example, hydrophilic polymer coatings improve fibroblast attachment and vascularization, while roughened titanium surfaces promote osteoblast adhesion and osseointegration. Surface charge and nanoscale patterning in cardiovascular devices affect endothelialization and platelet adhesion, lowering the risk of thrombosis. In order to accomplish regulated release and targeted absorption, drug delivery systems depend on functionalized surfaces, proving that surface engineering is essential to biomaterial function rather than an afterthought.

Surface characteristics play a variety of roles, including supporting dynamic interactions with the physiological environment, facilitating bioactive signaling, and offering mechanical and chemical stability. Biomaterials that are not carefully designed may fail to integrate, delaminate, or trigger immunological responses, highlighting the need for surface-focused approaches to achieve clinical success.

4.11.2 Reinforcement of Modification Techniques as Tools for Enhancing Biological Integration and Longevity

Techniques for surface modification, including physical, chemical, and biochemical methods, are crucial instruments for improving the biomaterials' durability and biological function. Physical methods that modify surface roughness and energy to encourage cellular adherence or prevent microbial colonization include mechanical polishing, sandblasting, laser ablation, and plasma therapy. Functional groups that affect wettability, protein adsorption, and bioactivity can be included through chemical changes such as oxidation, silanization, and polymer grafting. Biomimetic cues that direct cellular behavior and tissue regeneration are provided by biochemical techniques including growth factor inclusion, peptide immobilization, and self-assembled monolayers (SAMs).

Combining these methods frequently results in multifunctional surfaces that include controlled deterioration, bioactivity, and mechanical resilience. Properly developed surfaces enhance osseointegration, endothelialization, and therapeutic efficacy while lowering problems like infection, thrombosis, or inflammatory response, as shown by case studies spanning orthopedic implants, cardiovascular devices, and drug delivery systems. Therefore, surface modification serves as a proactive mediator of biological integration and long-term gadget longevity, going beyond simple protection or passive functionality.

4.11.3 Emphasis on the Synergy Between Chemistry, Physics, and Biology in Surface Design

The multidisciplinary integration of chemical, physical, and biological factors is essential for the design of successful biomaterial surfaces. Surface topography and nanostructuring offer mechanical signals that affect cellular alignment and differentiation, while surface chemistry dictates the kinds of interactions that can occur with proteins, ions, and cells. Roughness, hardness, and elasticity are examples of physical characteristics that affect tissue adhesion and mechanical stability. The selection and functionalization of surface characteristics are simultaneously guided by biological factors, including extracellular matrix mimicry, cell type specificity, and immunogenicity.

These areas are not taken into consideration separately in the design of contemporary biomaterial surfaces, which are increasingly being created as holistic interfaces. For instance, to improve osseointegration, a nanopatterned titanium implant may incorporate adsorbed osteogenic peptides (biological modification), micro-grooved topography (physical modification), and anodization (chemical modification). This integration emphasizes that multifaceted knowledge is necessary for successful surface engineering, balancing mechanical, chemical, and biological performance for predictable and efficient results.

4.11.4 Outlook on the Evolution Toward Intelligent, Adaptive, and Bioresponsive Surfaces

As we look to the future, surface modification is changing from passive, static designs to bioresponsive, intelligent, and adaptive surfaces that can interact dynamically with their surroundings. Surfaces that may alter their characteristics in response to temperature, enzyme activity, pH, or mechanical stress are made possible by developments in nanotechnology, additive manufacturing, and stimuli-responsive materials. These "smart" surfaces could self-heal minor damage, release medications as needed and change cellular behavior in real time.

Predictive surface design is made possible by the combination of computer modeling, machine learning, and high-throughput screening, which maximizes mechanical performance, bioactivity, and degradation before implantation. Additionally, the creation of green and sustainable surface modification techniques places a strong emphasis on recyclable materials, biocompatible coatings, and eco-friendly manufacturing, bringing the field into line with larger ecological and healthcare objectives. Surfaces that are both biocompatible and functionally instructive that is, able to direct tissue regeneration, stop infection, and adjust to the physiological conditions of individual patients will be more necessary for future biomedical applications. A new generation of intelligent, multipurpose, and regenerative biomaterials that combine chemistry, physics, biology, and computational science could revolutionize therapeutic outcomes in a variety of clinical specialties.

The engineering of surface characteristics is still essential to the development of biomaterials. In orthopedic, dental, cardiovascular, drug delivery, and tissue engineering applications, they determine biological interactions, promote mechanical stability, and affect long-term clinical outcomes. For improving biocompatibility, integration, and lifespan, modification techniques from physical and chemical to biochemical and nanostructured approaches are crucial instruments. To enhance cellular responses and functional performance, surface design necessitates a synergistic approach that integrates chemical, physical, and biological understanding. In the future, the creation of intelligent, bioresponsive, and adaptive surfaces presents previously unheard-of possibilities for next-generation biomaterials that may dynamically interact with the biological environment to support tailored therapy, healing, and regeneration. By bridging fundamental science with translational innovation, surface engineering will continue to define the forefront of biomedical materials research and application.

References

1. Chambers, L., Roach, P., Shirtcliffe, N.: Recent innovations in surface topography. Surf. Innov. **10**(6), 341–372 (2022)
2. Mitra, S.P.: Protein adsorption on biomaterial surfaces: subsequent conformational and biological consequences: a review. J. Surf. Sci. Technol. **36**(1), 7–38 (2020)
3. Nagay, B.E., Cordeiro, J.M., Barao, V.A.: Insight into corrosion of dental implants: from biochemical mechanisms to designing corrosion-resistant materials. Curr. Oral Health Rep. **9**(2), 7–21 (2022)
4. Thakur, A., Kumar, A., Kaya, S., Marzouki, R., Zhang, F., Guo, L.: Recent advancements in surface modification, characterization and functionalization for enhancing the biocompatibility and corrosion resistance of biomedical implants. Coatings. **12**(10), 1459 (2022)

5. Cintra, C.V., Sepúlveda, R.V., Valente, F.L., Reis, E.C.C., Borges, A.P.B.: Cellular interactions with implanted surfaces in the living organism and osseointegration of implants. Revista Saúde e Meio Ambiente. **12**(1), 102–120 (2021)
6. Zhu, G., Wang, G., Li, J.J.: Advances in implant surface modifications to improve osseointegration. Mater. Adv. **2**(21), 6901–6927 (2021)
7. Maynard, S.A., Winter, C.W., Cunnane, E.M., Stevens, M.M.: Advancing cell-instructive biomaterials through increased understanding of cell receptor spacing and material surface functionalization. Regen. Eng. Transl. Med. **7**(4), 533–547 (2021)
8. Guimarães, C.F., Marques, A.P., Reis, R.L.: Pushing the natural frontier: progress on the integration of biomaterial cues toward combinatorial biofabrication and tissue engineering. Adv. Mater. **34**(33), 2105645 (2022)
9. Mirzaali, M.J., Moosabeiki, V., Rajaai, S.M., Zhou, J., Zadpoor, A.A.: Additive manufacturing of biomaterials—design principles and their implementation. Materials. **15**(15), 5457 (2022)
10. Barberi, J., Spriano, S.: Titanium and protein adsorption: an overview of mechanisms and effects of surface features. Materials. **14**(7), 1590 (2021)
11. Lee, C.Y., Hu, S.M., Christy, J., Chou, F.Y., Ramli, T.C., Chen, H.Y.: Biointerface coatings with structural and biochemical properties modifications of biomaterials. Adv. Mater. Interfaces. **10**(10), 2202286 (2023)
12. Chen, H., Zhang, W., Li, M., He, G., Guo, X.: Interface engineering in organic field-effect transistors: principles, applications, and perspectives. Chem. Rev. **120**(5), 2879–2949 (2020)
13. Purohit, P., Bhatt, A., Mittal, R.K., Abdellattif, M.H., Farghaly, T.A.: Polymer grafting and its chemical reactions. Front. Bioeng. Biotechnol. **10**, 1044927 (2023)
14. Bowick, M.J., Fakhri, N., Marchetti, M.C., Ramaswamy, S.: Symmetry, thermodynamics, and topology in active matter. Phys. Rev. X. **12**(1), 010501 (2022)
15. Martinsen, O.G., Heiskanen, A.: Bioimpedance and Bioelectricity Basics. Elsevier (2023)
16. Rahmati, M., Silva, E.A., Reseland, J.E., Heyward, C.A., Haugen, H.J.: Biological responses to physicochemical properties of biomaterial surface. Chem. Soc. Rev. **49**(15), 5178–5224 (2020)
17. Vaiani, L., Boccaccio, A., Uva, A.E., Palumbo, G., Piccininni, A., Guglielmi, P., Cantore, S., Santacroce, L., Charitos, I.A., Ballini, A.: Ceramic materials for biomedical applications: an overview on properties and fabrication processes. J. Funct. Biomater. **14**(3), 146 (2023)
18. Arun, K.L., Udhayakumar, M., Radhika, N.: A comprehensive review on various ceramic nanomaterial coatings over metallic substrates: applications, challenges and future trends. J. Bio- and Tribo-Corros. **9**(1), 11 (2023)
19. Wolfe, J.T., Shradhanjali, A., Tefft, B.J.: Strategies for improving endothelial cell adhesion to blood-contacting medical devices. Tissue Eng. Part B Rev. **28**(5), 1067–1092 (2022)
20. Kligman, S., Ren, Z., Chung, C.H., Perillo, M.A., Chang, Y.C., Koo, H., Zheng, Z., Li, C.: The impact of dental implant surface modifications on osseointegration and biofilm formation. J. Clin. Med. **10**(8), 1641 (2021)
21. Chrostowski, R., Mangolini, F.: On the nature and propagation of errors in roughness parameters obtained from spectral analysis of atomic force microscopy topographic images. J. Vac. Sci. Technol. A. **40**(5), 053204 (2022)
22. Sultana, A., Zare, M., Luo, H., Ramakrishna, S.: Surface engineering strategies to enhance the in situ performance of medical devices including atomic scale engineering. Int. J. Mol. Sci. **22**(21), 11788 (2021)
23. Zhianmanesh, M., Gilmour, A., Bilek, M.M., Akhavan, B.: Plasma surface functionalization: a comprehensive review of advances in the quest for bioinstructive materials and interfaces. Appl. Phys. Rev. **10**(2), 021301 (2023)
24. Hanawa, T.: Biocompatibility of titanium from the viewpoint of its surface. Sci. Technol. Adv. Mater. **23**(1), 457–472 (2022)
25. Marin, E., Lanzutti, A.: Biomedical applications of titanium alloys: a comprehensive review. Materials. **17**(1), 114 (2023)

26. Alipal, J., Lee, T.C., Koshy, P., Abdullah, H.Z., Idris, M.I.: Evolution of anodised titanium for implant applications. Heliyon. **7**(7), e07408 (2021)
27. Gulati, K., Zhang, Y., Di, P., Liu, Y., Ivanovski, S.: Research to clinics: clinical translation considerations for anodized nano-engineered titanium implants. ACS Biomater. Sci. Eng. **8**(10), 4077–4091 (2021)
28. Levchenko, I., Xu, S., Baranov, O., Bazaka, O., Ivanova, E.P., Bazaka, K.: Plasma and polymers: recent progress and trends. Molecules. **26**(13), 4091 (2021)
29. Winnicki, M., Łatka, L., Jasiorski, M., Baszczuk, A.: Mechanical properties of TiO2 coatings deposited by low pressure cold spraying. Surf. Coat. Technol. **405**, 126516 (2021)
30. Badiceanu, M., Anghel, S., Mihailescu, N., Visan, A.I., Mihailescu, C.N., Mihailescu, I.N.: Coatings functionalization via laser versus other deposition techniques for medical applications: a comparative review. Coatings. **12**(1), 71 (2022)
31. Roh, S., Jang, Y., Yoo, J., Seong, H.: Surface modification strategies for biomedical applications: enhancing cell–biomaterial interfaces and biochip performances. Biochip J. **17**(2), 174–191 (2023)
32. Anouz, R., Groth, T.: Biomimetic surface modifications of biomaterials using a layer-by-layer technique (2021)
33. Urciuolo, F., Imparato, G., Netti, P.A.: In vitro strategies for mimicking dynamic cell–ECM reciprocity in 3D culture models. Front. Bioeng. Biotechnol. **11**, 1197075 (2023)
34. Khalilov, R.: A comprehensive review of advanced nano-biomaterials in regenerative medicine and drug delivery. Adv. Biol. Earth Sci. **8**(1), 5–18 (2023)
35. Li, Z., Wang, Y., Liu, J., Rawding, P., Bu, J., Hong, S., Hu, Q.: Chemically and biologically engineered bacteria-based delivery systems for emerging diagnosis and advanced therapy. Adv. Mater. **33**(38), 2102580 (2021)
36. Liu, Z., Wan, X., Wang, Z.L., Li, L.: Electroactive biomaterials and systems for cell fate determination and tissue regeneration: design and applications. Adv. Mater. **33**(32), 2007429 (2021)
37. Chen, X., Chen, J., Huang, N.: The structure, formation, and effect of plasma protein layer on the blood contact materials: a review. Biosurf. Biotribol. **8**(1), 1–14 (2022)
38. Martocq, L., Douglas, T.E.: Amine-rich coatings to potentially promote cell adhesion, proliferation and differentiation, and reduce microbial colonization: strategies for generation and characterization. Coatings. **11**(8), 983 (2021)
39. Özgüzar, H.F., Evren, E., Meydan, A.E., Kabay, G., Göçmen, J.S., Buyukserin, F., Erogul, O.: Plasma-assisted surface modification and heparin immobilization: dual-functionalized blood-contacting biomaterials with improved hemocompatibility and antibacterial features. Adv. Mater. Interfaces. **10**(6), 2202009 (2023)
40. Herath, I., Davies, J., Will, G., Tran, P.A., Velic, A., Sarvghad, M., Islam, M., Paritala, P.K., Jaggessar, A., Schuetz, M., Chatterjee, K.: Anodization of medical grade stainless steel for improved corrosion resistance and nanostructure formation targeting biomedical applications. Electrochim. Acta. **416**, 140274 (2022)
41. Zaheer, M.U., Razzaq, M.H., Coy, E., Aycan, M.F., Mishra, Y.K.: Engineered surfaces for biomedical implants: advances in coatings, materials, and techniques. Prog. Biomed. Eng. **8**(2), 022006 (2026)
42. Hong, M.H., Lee, J.H., Jung, H.S., Shin, H., Shin, H.: Biomineralization of bone tissue: calcium phosphate-based inorganics in collagen fibrillar organic matrices. Biomater. Res. **26**(1), 42 (2022)
43. Radulescu, D.E., Neacsu, I.A., Grumezescu, A.M., Andronescu, E.: Novel trends into the development of natural hydroxyapatite-based polymeric composites for bone tissue engineering. Polymers. **14**(5), 899 (2022)
44. Omarov, S., Nauryz, N., Talamona, D., Perveen, A.: Surface modification techniques for metallic biomedical alloys: a concise review. Metals. **13**(1), 82 (2022)
45. Thanigaivel, S., Priya, A.K., Balakrishnan, D., Dutta, K., Rajendran, S., Soto-Moscoso, M.: Insight on recent development in metallic biomaterials: strategies involving synthesis, types

and surface modification for advanced therapeutic and biomedical applications. Biochem. Eng. J. **187**, 108522 (2022)

46. Zhang, H., Wu, Z., Wang, Z., Yan, X., Duan, X., Sun, H.: Advanced surface modification techniques for titanium implants: a review of osteogenic and antibacterial strategies. Front. Bioeng. Biotechnol. **13**, 1549439 (2025). https://doi.org/10.3389/fbioe.2025.1549439
47. Babu, B., Dhamotharan, S., Jayaram, R., Saravanamuthukumar, P.: A summary of recent breakthroughs in micro- and nano-machining technologies. Periodico. **91**(4), 749–765 (2022)
48. Pratap, T., Patra, K.: Micro–nano surface texturing, characterization, and their impact on biointerfaces. In: Advanced Machining and Finishing, pp. 577–610. Elsevier (2021)
49. Migita, S., Sato, M.: Protein adsorption and cell adhesion on metallic biomaterial surfaces. Adhesives. **1**(4), 15 (2025)
50. Aziz, T., Ullah, A., Fan, H., Jamil, M.I., Khan, F.U., Ullah, R., Iqbal, M., Ali, A., Ullah, B.: Recent progress in silane coupling agent with its emerging applications. J. Polym. Environ. **29**(11), 3427–3443 (2021)
51. Hu, X., Wang, T., Li, F., Mao, X.: Surface modifications of biomaterials in different applied fields. RSC Adv. **13**(30), 20495–20511 (2023)
52. Imam, H.T., Marr, P.C., Marr, A.C.: Enzyme entrapment, biocatalyst immobilization without covalent attachment. Green Chem. **23**(14), 4980–5005 (2021)
53. Mirza, E.H., Almubarak, A.A., Majeed, S., Al-Obaidi, J.R., Mohammed, A.A.: Smart biomaterials for cardiovascular, bone, and skin tissue engineering: mechanisms, applications, and future prospects. J. Biol. Eng. **20**, 7 (2026). https://doi.org/10.1186/s13036-025-00607-8
54. Zeng, Q., Huang, Z.: Challenges and opportunities of implantable neural interfaces: from material, electrochemical and biological perspectives. Adv. Funct. Mater. **33**(32), 2301223 (2023)
55. Xiao, L., Sun, Y., Liao, L., Su, X.: Response of mesenchymal stem cells to surface topography of scaffolds and the underlying mechanisms. J. Mater. Chem. B. **11**(12), 2550–2567 (2023)
56. Dubey, A., Vahabi, H., Kumaravel, V.: Antimicrobial and biodegradable 3D printed scaffolds for orthopedic infections. ACS Biomater. Sci. Eng. **9**(7), 4020–4044 (2023)
57. Rodrigo-Navarro, A., Sankaran, S., Dalby, M.J., Del Campo, A., Salmeron-Sanchez, M.: Engineered living biomaterials. Nat. Rev. Mater. **6**(12), 1175–1190 (2021)
58. Jin, Z., He, C., Fu, J., Han, Q., He, Y.: Balancing the customization and standardization: exploration and layout surrounding the regulation of the growing field of 3D-printed medical devices in China. Bio-Des. Manuf. **5**(3), 580–606 (2022)
59. Ying, Y.L., Hu, Z.L., Zhang, S., Qing, Y., Fragasso, A., Maglia, G., Meller, A., Bayley, H., Dekker, C., Long, Y.T.: Nanopore-based technologies beyond DNA sequencing. Nat. Nanotechnol. **17**(11), 1136–1146 (2022)
60. Guo, T., Ivanovski, S., Gulati, K.: From micro to nano: surface modification for enhanced bioactivity of titanium dental implants. In: Surface Modification of Titanium Dental Implants, pp. 117–151. Springer International Publishing (2023)
61. Stich, T., Alagboso, F., Křenek, T., Kovářík, T., Alt, V., Docheva, D.: Implant-bone-interface: reviewing the impact of titanium surface modifications on osteogenic processes in vitro and in vivo. Bioeng. Transl. Med. **7**(1), e10239 (2022)
62. Visan, A.I., Popescu-Pelin, G., Socol, G.: Degradation behavior of polymers used as coating materials for drug delivery: a basic review. Polymers. **13**(8), 1272 (2021)
63. Jiao, R., Commuri, S., Panchal, J., Milisavljevic-Syed, J., Allen, J.K., Mistree, F., Schaefer, D.: Design engineering in the age of industry 4.0. J. Mech. Des. **143**(7), 070801 (2021)
64. Auditee, M.M.: Design and fabrication of biocompatible copper based shape memory alloy by spark plasma sintering (2022)
65. Djisalov, M., Knežić, T., Podunavac, I., Živojević, K., Radonic, V., Knežević, N.Ž., Bobrinetskiy, I., Gadjanski, I.: Cultivating multidisciplinarity: manufacturing and sensing challenges in cultured meat production. Biology. **10**(3), 204 (2021)
66. Tang, T.C., An, B., Huang, Y., Vasikaran, S., Wang, Y., Jiang, X., Lu, T.K., Zhong, C.: Materials design by synthetic biology. Nat. Rev. Mater. **6**(4), 332–350 (2021)

67. Harish, V., Tewari, D., Gaur, M., Yadav, A.B., Swaroop, S., Bechelany, M., Barhoum, A.: Review on nanoparticles and nanostructured materials: bioimaging, biosensing, drug delivery, tissue engineering, antimicrobial, and agro-food applications. Nanomaterials. **12**(3), 457 (2022)
68. Nilawar, S., Uddin, M., Chatterjee, K.: Surface engineering of biodegradable implants: emerging trends in bioactive ceramic coatings and mechanical treatments. Mater. Adv. **2**(24), 7820–7841 (2021)
69. Ahn, J., Kim, M., Park, S., Lee, H., Choi, J.: Innovations in implant osseointegration: biomaterials, surface engineering, and translational strategies. J. Biomed. Mater. Res. A. **114**, e70081 (2026). https://doi.org/10.1002/jbm.a.70081
70. Manivasagam, V.K., Sabino, R.M., Kantam, P., Popat, K.C.: Surface modification strategies to improve titanium hemocompatibility: a comprehensive review. Mater. Adv. **2**(18), 5824–5842 (2021)
71. Raikar, A.S., Priya, S., Bhilegaonkar, S.P., Somnache, S.N., Kalaskar, D.M.: Surface engineering of bioactive coatings for improved stent hemocompatibility: a comprehensive review. Materials. **16**(21), 6940 (2023)
72. He, M., Yang, B., Huo, F., Xie, L., Yang, M., Tian, W.: A novel coating with universal adhesion and inflammation-responsive drug release functions to manipulate the osteoimmunomodulation of implants. J. Mater. Chem. B. **9**(26), 5272–5283 (2021)
73. Alven, S., Buyana, B., Feketshane, Z., Aderibigbe, B.A.: Electrospun nanofibers/nanofibrous scaffolds loaded with silver nanoparticles as effective antibacterial wound dressing materials. Pharmaceutics. **13**(7), 964 (2021)
74. Frutiger, A., Tanno, A., Hwu, S., Tiefenauer, R.F., Voros, J., Nakatsuka, N.: Nonspecific binding fundamental concepts and consequences for biosensing applications. Chem. Rev. **121**(13), 8095–8160 (2021)
75. Ramezani, M., Mohd Ripin, Z., Pasang, T., Jiang, C.P.: Surface engineering of metals: techniques, characterizations and applications. Metals. **13**(7), 1299 (2023)
76. Serna, J.A., Rueda-Gensini, L., Céspedes-Valenzuela, D.N., Cifuentes, J., Cruz, J.C., Muñoz-Camargo, C.: Recent advances on stimuli-responsive hydrogels based on tissue-derived ECMs and their components: towards improving functionality for tissue engineering and controlled drug delivery. Polymers. **13**(19), 3263 (2021)
77. Reddy, M.S.B., Ponnamma, D., Choudhary, R., Sadasivuni, K.K.: A comparative review of natural and synthetic biopolymer composite scaffolds. Polymers. **13**(7), 1105 (2021)
78. Ligorio, C., Mata, A.: Synthetic extracellular matrices with function-encoding peptides. Nat. Rev. Bioeng. **1**(7), 518–536 (2023)
79. Xie, W., Wei, X., Kang, H., Jiang, H., Chu, Z., Lin, Y., Hou, Y., Wei, Q.: Static and dynamic: evolving biomaterial mechanical properties to control cellular mechanotransduction. Adv. Sci. **10**(9), 2204594 (2023)
80. Deo, D., Singh, S.P., Mohanty, S., Guhathakurata, S., Pal, D., Mallik, S.: Biomimicking of phyto-based super-hydrophobic surfaces towards prospective applications: a review. J. Mater. Sci. **57**(19), 8569–8596 (2022)
81. Carotenuto, F., Politi, S., Ul Haq, A., De Matteis, F., Tamburri, E., Terranova, M.L., Teodori, L., Pasquo, A., Di Nardo, P.: From soft to hard biomimetic materials: tuning micro/nano-architecture of scaffolds for tissue regeneration. Micromachines. **13**(5), 780 (2022)
82. Syrlybayev, D., Seisekulova, A., Talamona, D., Perveen, A.: The post-processing of additive manufactured polymeric and metallic parts. J. Manuf. Mater. Proc. **6**(5), 116 (2022)
83. Vinoth, A., Datta, S.: Computational intelligence based design of biomaterials. Comput. Methods Mater. Sci. **22**(4), 229–262 (2022)
84. Bax, M., Thorpe, J., Romanov, V.: The future of personalized cardiovascular medicine demands 3D and 4D printing, stem cells, and artificial intelligence. Front. Sens. **4**, 1294721 (2023)
85. Drobota, M., Ursache, S., Aflori, M.: Surface functionalities of polymers for biomaterial applications. Polymers. **14**(12), 2307 (2022)

86. Zia, A.W., Liu, R., Wu, X.: Structural design and mechanical performance of composite vascular grafts. Bio-Des. Manuf. **5**(4), 757–785 (2022)
87. Aljibori, H.S., Alamiery, A., Kadhum, A.A.H.: Advances in corrosion protection coatings: a comprehensive review. Int. J. Corros. Scale Inhib. **12**(4), 1476–1520 (2023)
88. Yogev, D., Goldberg, T., Arami, A., Tejman-Yarden, S., Winkler, T.E., Maoz, B.M.: Current state of the art and future directions for implantable sensors in medical technology: clinical needs and engineering challenges. APL Bioeng. **7**(3), 031506 (2023)
89. Yadav, S., Singh Raman, A.P., Meena, H., Goswami, A.G., Bhawna, Kumar, V., Jain, P., Kumar, G., Sagar, M., Rana, D.K., Bahadur, I.: An update on graphene oxide: applications and toxicity. ACS Omega. **7**(40), 35387–35445 (2022)
90. Wixmerten, A., Miot, S., Bittorf, P., Wolf, F., Feliciano, S., Hackenberg, S., Häusner, S., Krenger, W., Haug, M., Martin, I., Pullig, O.: Good manufacturing practice–compliant change of raw material in the manufacturing process of a clinically used advanced therapy medicinal product—a comparability study. Cytotherapy. **25**(5), 548–558 (2023)
91. Leung, C.M., De Haan, P., Ronaldson-Bouchard, K., Kim, G.A., Ko, J., Rho, H.S., Chen, Z., Habibovic, P., Jeon, N.L., Takayama, S., Shuler, M.L.: A guide to the organ-on-a-chip. Nat. Rev. Methods Primers. **2**(1), 33 (2022)
92. Jang, S., Jeong, J.G., Oh, T.I., Lee, E.: Biomaterials for cell-surface engineering and their efficacy. J. Funct. Biomater. **12**(3), 41 (2021)
93. Rickert, C.A., Hayta, E.N., Selle, D.M., Kouroudis, I., Harth, M., Gagliardi, A., Lieleg, O.: Machine learning approach to analyze the surface properties of biological materials. ACS Biomater. Sci. Eng. **7**(9), 4614–4625 (2021)
94. Cioffi, M.O.H., Bomfim, A.S., Ambrogi, V., Advani, S.G.: A review on self-healing polymers and polymer composites for structural applications. Polym. Compos. **43**(11), 7643–7668 (2022)
95. He, S., Gao, Y., Gong, X., Wu, C., Cen, H.: Advance of design and application in self-healing anticorrosive coating: a review. J. Coat. Technol. Res. **20**(3), 819–841 (2023)
96. Petersen, H.A., Myren, T.H., O'Sullivan, S.J., Luca, O.R.: Electrochemical methods for materials recycling. Mater. Adv. **2**(4), 1113–1138 (2021)
97. Gildersleeve, E.J., Vaßen, R.: Thermally sprayed functional coatings and multilayers: a selection of historical applications and potential pathways for future innovation. J. Therm. Spray Technol. **32**(4), 778–817 (2023)
98. Mahafdeh, R.M., Moore, J.V., Wylie, M.P., McCoy, C.P.: Antibacterial assessment of TMPyP-incorporated p (HEMA-co-MMA). In: Northern Ireland Biomedical Engineering Society: Annual Symposium 2023 (2023)
99. Fang, Y., Yang, X., Lin, Y., Shi, J., Prominski, A., Clayton, C., Ostroff, E., Tian, B.: Dissecting biological and synthetic soft–hard interfaces for tissue-like systems. Chem. Rev. **122**(5), 5233–5276 (2021)
100. Stevens, R., Taylor, V., Nichols, J., Maccabe, A.B., Yelick, K., Brown, D.: AI for Science: report on the Department of Energy (DOE) Town Halls on Artificial Intelligence (AI) for Science (No. ANL-20/17). Argonne National Lab. (ANL), Argonne (2020)

Chapter 5
Biomaterials in Tissue Engineering and Wound Healing

Abstract Biomaterials are essential for tissue engineering and wound healing because they support cell proliferation, differentiation, and tissue regeneration structurally and biochemically. These materials, which can be synthetic, natural, or hybrid, are designed to function similarly to the extracellular matrix (ECM) and aid in the repair of injured tissues by means of regulated interactions with biological processes. In tissue engineering, biomaterials act as scaffolds that offer a three-dimensional space that promotes neovascularization, cellular adhesion, and proliferation. The creation of biomimetic scaffolds with adjustable mechanical characteristics and breakdown rates that correspond with the dynamics of tissue remodeling has been made possible by developments in biodegradable polymers, hydrogels, and nanocomposites. Biomaterials serve as active dressings in wound healing, promoting cellular recruitment, hemostasis, and moisture balance in addition to shielding the site from infection. By delivering growth factors, antimicrobial agents, and stem cells straight to the wound site, innovations including hydrogel matrices, bioactive coatings, and electrospun nanofibers have improved healing results. Additionally, by combining additive printing with nanotechnology, tailored biomaterial systems with precise architecture and biofunctionalization can be fabricated, enhancing tissue integration and lowering immunological rejection. Complete vascularization, immunomodulation, and long-term functional integration of synthetic tissues remain difficult to achieve despite tremendous advancements. Smart and sensitive biomaterials that can sense and adjust to the physiological environment are the focus of future research. All things considered, biomaterials have revolutionized regenerative medicine by linking the fields of biology and materials science and providing potential treatment options for intricate wounds and tissue defects that traditional methods are unable to effectively treat.

M. Adeoba, T. Pandelani, *Application of Biomaterials in Biomedical Engineering*, Series in BioEngineering,
https://doi.org/10.1007/978-3-032-34477-9_5

5.1 Introduction

One of the most revolutionary areas of biomedical science is regenerative medicine, which combines biology, materials science, and engineering to repair, replace, or regenerate damaged tissues and organs. Biomaterials are used as both structural frameworks and functional mediators of biological processes, making them essential to this interdisciplinary field. Biomaterials give cells the physical support and metabolic environment they need to connect, proliferate, differentiate, and eventually form tissues in tissue engineering and wound healing. From passive implants to dynamic, bioresponsive systems that actively engage with the host environment and direct the body's natural regeneration potential, biomaterial design has advanced [1, 2]. The function of biomaterials in regulating immune responses, promoting angiogenesis, and aiding integration with native tissues has grown more crucial as regenerative therapies move from research to clinical use.

5.1.1 Overview of the Role of Biomaterials in Regenerative Medicine

As synthetic matrices that mimic the composition and functionality of the natural extracellular matrix (ECM), biomaterials serve as the cornerstone of regenerative medicine. Their main responsibility is to establish a milieu that supports tissue regeneration and cell survival. Regenerative biomaterials are intended to take part in biological signaling and remodeling, in contrast to conventional prosthetic or inert implants. The gradual transmission of mechanical load to the regenerating tissue is made possible by materials including hydrogels, composites, ceramics, and biodegradable polymers that are designed to break down in tandem with tissue creation [3, 4].

Furthermore, biomaterials can operate as transporters for bioactive substances that affect cellular activity, including nucleic acids, cytokines, and growth factors. The ability to administer regulated biochemical signals has transformed treatment approaches for the regeneration of bone, cartilage, skin, heart, and nerves. Collagen-based scaffolds, for instance, encourage angiogenesis and fibroblast migration during wound healing, whereas calcium phosphate ceramics improve osteogenesis during bone regeneration. By using surface modification techniques, biomaterials can be given properties that increase targeted cell adhesion, lower the risk of infection, and improve biocompatibility. Therefore, biomaterials are both active players in coordinating tissue regeneration and inert structural supports.

5.1.2 Importance of Tissue Engineering and Wound Healing for Restoring Function and Aesthetics

Restoring tissue integrity, function, and appearance following damage or illness is the goal of both tissue engineering and wound healing, two complementary but separate subfields of regenerative medicine. The main goal of tissue engineering is to create biological replacements that can sustain or replace damaged tissues. Three elements are necessary for this process: scaffolding materials, signaling chemicals, and cells. The crucial third component is made up of biomaterials, which offer both mechanical stability and a microenvironment that promotes cell proliferation. Applications range from cardiac patches and nerve conduits to bone and cartilage regeneration, all of which need for exact control over material characteristics like porosity, stiffness, and rate of deterioration [5, 6].

In contrast, wound healing entails a complicated series of biological processes, including remodeling, inflammation, proliferation, and hemostasis. Burns, diabetic ulcers, and chronic wounds continue to present significant clinical problems because of their compromised tissue regeneration and infection risks. By acting as bioactive wound dressings that can absorb exudate, maintain a moist healing environment, and administer pro-regenerative or antibacterial agents, biomaterials have helped to overcome these difficulties [7, 8]. For instance, hydrogel-based dressings encourage cellular migration and provide hydration, simulating the natural extracellular matrix. Meanwhile, electrospun nanofibrous mats improve tissue granulation and oxygen exchange.

These technologies seek to enhance aesthetic results in addition to functional restoration, which is becoming a more significant factor in reconstructive and cosmetic medicine. Biomaterial-based treatments promote tissue remodeling that closely mimics the original architecture and scarless healing, which aids in both physical and mental rehabilitation.

5.1.3 Integration of Biomaterials with Biological Cues to Promote Repair and Regeneration

The capacity of next-generation biomaterials to actively direct cellular responses through integration with biological cues is one of its distinguishing characteristics. Providing mechanical, chemical, and topographical cues, the extracellular matrix (ECM) in real tissues is a dynamic regulator of cell behavior rather than just a passive scaffold. One of the main challenges in the creation of biomaterials is to mimic this complexity. Bioactive ligands, such as RGD peptides, which facilitate certain cell adhesion through integrin binding, can be functionalized into biomaterials by molecular engineering [9, 10]. Similar to this, growth factors that promote angiogenesis or differentiation at the site of damage, such as transforming growth factor-beta (TGF-β) or vascular endothelial growth factor (VEGF), can be added to scaffolds for regulated release.

Furthermore, mechanobiology has demonstrated that cells react to the substrate's stiffness, elasticity, and nanotopography. For example, harder settings foster osteogenesis, whereas softer matrices promote neural development. As a result, biomechanical tunability is now incorporated into biomaterial design to match the native environment of the target tissue. The accuracy with which such biological cues can be integrated has been further improved by recent developments in additive manufacturing and nanotechnology. The diverse structure of actual tissues can be replicated by spatially arranging cells and signaling molecules using methods like 3D bioprinting.

Regenerative potential has also been increased by the combination of biomaterials and cell-based therapies, such as stem cells and genetically modified cells. Biomaterial scaffolds improve the survival and integration of transplanted cells by giving them the support and localization they need [11, 12]. When combined, these tactics highlight the transition from inert implants to physiologically active structures that may coordinate intricate healing processes.

5.1.4 Scope of the Chapter

This chapter offers a thorough examination of biomaterials in wound healing and tissue engineering, highlighting the multidisciplinary ideas that propel advancements in regenerative medicine. The selection of materials is covered first, along with the characteristics, benefits, and drawbacks of natural, synthetic, and composite biomaterials. The effects of several factors on cell behavior and tissue outcomes will be examined, including biocompatibility, mechanical strength, degradation rate, and surface chemistry [13, 14].

The chapter next looks at design strategies, including surface modification techniques that improve bioactivity and immunological tolerance and scaffold production methods like electrospinning, freeze-drying, and 3D bioprinting. To clarify how materials promote tissue regeneration at the molecular and cellular levels, the mechanisms of action such as growth factor release, immunomodulation, and angiogenesis produced by biomaterials will be covered. Lastly, the focus will shift to translational applications, emphasizing clinical case studies and regulatory factors in the commercialization of biomaterial-based treatments [15]. Examples from the fields of orthopedics, cardiovascular disease, dermatology, and neural tissue regeneration are included, along with information on how additive manufacturing can be used to create implants that are customized for each patient.

This chapter highlights the revolutionary potential of biomaterials as regenerative healing catalysts by linking the fields of materials science, biology, and clinical translation. Biomaterials have the potential to revolutionize therapeutic paradigms for repairing the functionality and appearance of injured tissues through ongoing innovation in material design and integration with biological systems.

5.2 Key Concepts and Definitions

The goal of the multidisciplinary area of tissue engineering, which sits at the intersection of biology, materials science, and engineering, is to preserve, improve, or restore tissue function [16]. The field's effectiveness hinges on a thorough comprehension of its fundamental ideas, such as how biological systems and constructed structures interact, how wounds naturally heal, and the characteristics of materials made to interact with live tissue. The three components of biomaterials-based tissue engineering, the stages of wound healing, material classifications, scaffold and hydrogel design, and important biological performance measures are all covered in detail in this article.

5.2.1 Definition of Tissue Engineering and Its Triad: Cells, Scaffolds, and Signaling Molecules

Tissue engineering is the process of restoring, maintaining, or enhancing biological tissues or organs by combining cells, engineering techniques, biochemical and physicochemical elements. The three interconnected components of tissue engineering cells, scaffolds, and signaling molecules are the foundation of this subject. The main functional units in charge of tissue development and repair are cells. Depending on the intended use, these could be autologous (derived from the patient), allogeneic (derived from the donor), or stem cells (embryonic, mesenchymal, or induced pluripotent) [17, 18]. Mesenchymal stem cells (MSCs), for example, are frequently employed because of their immunomodulatory and multipotent characteristics.

The three-dimensional (3D) structural framework that facilitates cell adhesion, proliferation, and differentiation is supplied by scaffolds. Scaffolds should ideally have a microarchitecture that allows for waste elimination and nutrition diffusion, as well as be mechanically stable, biocompatible, and biodegradable. Natural polymers like collagen and chitosan as well as synthetic ones like polylactic acid and polyethylene glycol are among the materials employed.

Growth factors and cytokines are examples of signaling molecules that coordinate the cellular activity required for tissue growth and remodeling. These include transforming growth factor-beta (TGF-β) for the synthesis of extracellular matrix (ECM), bone morphogenetic proteins (BMPs) for osteogenesis, and vascular endothelial growth factor (VEGF) for angiogenesis. By simulating native tissue microenvironments, the scaffold's-controlled release of these bioactive chemicals improves the effectiveness of regeneration. By directing cellular activity within engineered constructions toward effective tissue regeneration, this triad works in concert to mimic the natural processes of tissue development.

5.2.2 Wound Healing Phases: Hemostasis, Inflammation, Proliferation, and Remodeling

Hemostasis, inflammation, proliferation, and remodeling (also known as maturation) are the four overlapping and tightly controlled stages that make up the biological process of wound healing. Designing biomaterials that actively promote or speed tissue restoration requires an understanding of these stages.

Vasoconstriction and platelet aggregation create a fibrin clot that closes the wound and serves as a temporary matrix for cell migration during the hemostasis phase, the body's initial reaction to injury. Growth factors including TGF-β and platelet-derived growth factors (PDGF) are released by platelets and start the subsequent healing processes. During the inflammatory phase, immune cells such as neutrophils and macrophages infiltrate the body, removing debris and pathogens while releasing cytokines that control angiogenesis and the recruitment of fibroblasts. However, excessive or protracted inflammation might hinder regeneration and result in fibrosis. Granulation tissue development, fibroblast proliferation, and angiogenesis are the hallmarks of the proliferation phase. Endothelial cells and keratinocytes, respectively, aid in the development of new vessels and epithelialization. Through the controlled release of bioactive substances, biomaterials intended for this phase frequently encourage cell proliferation and neovascularization. The remodeling (maturation) phase increases tensile strength by modifying the newly generated extracellular matrix (ECM) and replacing type III collagen with type I collagen [19, 20]. The tissue gradually regains its structural and functional integrity as vascular networks develop. To facilitate a smooth transition from synthetic to biological structure, biodegradable scaffolds are optimally engineered to break down at rates that correspond with tissue maturity.

Each phase provides cues for biomaterial design such as surface chemistry, degradation profile, and mechanical properties that must align with the body's temporal healing response.

5.2.3 Bioactive vs. Bioinert Materials and Their Impact on Tissue Regeneration

Based on how they interact with biological tissues, biomaterials can be roughly divided into two categories: bioactive and bioinert. In order to encourage tissue integration and regeneration, bioactive materials are made to trigger particular biological reactions at the interface. Calcium phosphate ceramics and bioactive glasses are two examples; they can create chemical connections with bone tissue and release ions that promote osteogenesis [21]. This group also includes polymers functionalized with growth factors or peptides (such RGD sequences), which actively promote cell adhesion and signaling.

Bioinert materials, on the other hand, aim to reduce contact with surrounding tissue, which lowers fibrous encapsulation and immune response. Examples include titanium and alumina, which are frequently utilized in dental and orthopedic implants due to their chemical stability and mechanical strength. Their inertness, though, may restrict tissue integration. Therefore, methods of surface modification, including chemical grafting or plasma treatment, are frequently used to improve bioactivity while preserving bulk mechanical qualities. A paradigm changes toward functional biomaterials that actively direct biological processes necessary for healing and regeneration in addition to provide mechanical support is represented by the switch from bioinert to bioactive biomaterials.

5.2.4 Definition of Scaffold, Hydrogel, and Extracellular Matrix (ECM) Mimics

A scaffold is a three-dimensional porous structure that offers a transient physical setting for cell migration, adhesion, and differentiation. Its structure and function are like those of the extracellular matrix (ECM), enabling cells to create their own matrix and gradually modify the structure. Pore size, interconnectivity, degradation rate, and mechanical strength are important design factors that affect tissue formation and cell behavior. The design of effective biomaterial scaffolds increasingly draws on detailed knowledge of extracellular matrix (ECM) biology, as the structural and functional relationships within native ECM including its composition, mechanical properties, and remodeling dynamics provide critical blueprints for engineering biomimetic constructs that support wound repair and tissue integration [22].

Large volumes of water can be absorbed by hydrogels, which are networks of hydrophilic polymers that retain their structural integrity. Cells and medicinal compounds are perfectly encapsulated by them because of their soft, tissue-like mechanical characteristics. Hydrogels can be produced synthetically using polymers like polyethylene glycol (PEG) or naturally from sources including hyaluronic acid, gelatin, and alginate [23]. Applications for hydrogels include soft tissue engineering, wound dressings, and medication administration due to their adjustable physicochemical characteristics.

Biomaterials intended to mimic the biochemical and biomechanical properties of native extracellular matrix (ECM) are known as ECM mimics. These structures frequently include synthetic analogues that mimic the structure of natural ECM components like collagen, laminin, and fibronectin. Another strategy that maintains the original microarchitecture and biochemical signals while promoting natural tissue regeneration is the use of decellularized extracellular matrix (ECM) produced from donor tissues. The design of biomaterials for tissue engineering is based on scaffolds, hydrogels, and ECM mimics, all of which have unique benefits for simulating the complexity of natural tissue environments [24].

5.2.5 *Metrics for Evaluation: Cell Adhesion, Proliferation, Differentiation, and Vascularization*

Evaluating the performance of biomaterials and tissue-engineered constructs relies on specific biological and functional metrics that reflect their capacity to support and integrate with host tissue.

Cell adhesion measures how well cells adhere to the surface of the biomaterial, which is an essential first stage in the creation of future tissue. Microscopy or adhesion assays can be used to quantify adhesion, which is influenced by surface chemical, topography, and stiffness. The rate of cellular growth over time, or cell proliferation, is a measure of the scaffold environment's nutritional sufficiency and biocompatibility. Proliferation rates are frequently assessed using methods like MTT or DNA quantification assays. The ability of progenitor or stem cells within the construct to develop into the intended tissue-specific lineages such as osteogenic, chondrogenic, or myogenic is determined by cell differentiation. Gene expression analysis and lineage-specific marker immunostaining are frequently used to validate this.

One of the most important markers of long-term construct viability is vascularization, or the development of new blood vessels. Especially in dense tissue structures, adequate vascular networks provide the transport of nutrients and oxygen as well as the elimination of waste [25]. Using co-culture systems with endothelial cells or adding angiogenic agents can both encourage vascularization. When taken as a whole, these measurements offer a multifaceted evaluation of a biomaterial's capacity for regeneration. Transforming laboratory constructs into clinically successful tissue-engineered medicines is made possible by optimizing them through iterative design and testing.

In order to construct functional tissues, the fundamental ideas of tissue engineering rely on the combination of cells, scaffolds, and signaling molecules. Knowing the stages of wound healing gives biomaterial designers a biological context and knowing the differences between bioactive and bioinert materials helps them choose the right materials. The significance of structural and metabolic simulation of native tissues is highlighted by the definitions of scaffolds, hydrogels, and ECM mimics. Lastly, strong assessment measures, such as vascularization and cell adhesion, guarantee that engineered constructions can successfully restore form and function, propelling the field of regenerative medicine closer to clinical reality [26, 27].

5.3 Material Types and Properties

For tissue engineering and wound healing applications to be successful, the right biomaterials must be chosen. Different physicochemical and biological properties of natural polymers, synthetic polymers, ceramics, and composites affect tissue integration, cellular behavior, and overall therapeutic results. The ideal biomaterial should guarantee immunocompatibility and regulatory compliance while striking a balance between mechanical integrity, biodegradability, and bioactivity as shown in Table 5.1. The main categories of biomaterials, their distinguishing characteristics, and their applications in regenerative medicine are covered in the sections that follow.

5.3.1 Natural Polymers

Naturally occurring polymers have biochemical patterns that promote cell adhesion, proliferation, and differentiation since they are derived from biological sources. Their bioactivity and biocompatibility make them perfect for scaffolds that are meant to resemble the extracellular matrix (ECM). Common examples are alginate, chitosan, collagen, and gelatin; each has special structural and functional characteristics.

The most prevalent protein in the extracellular matrix (ECM), collagen is essential for both cellular signaling and structural integrity. Collagen-based scaffolds encourage angiogenesis, tissue remodeling, and fibroblast adhesion. They are also very biocompatible. To increase stability, however, crosslinking or mixing with synthetic polymers is frequently required due to their mechanical fragility and quick deterioration. Derived from denatured collagen, gelatin is frequently utilized in hydrogel formulations because it preserves comparable cell-binding domains. Controlled gelation and drug delivery are made possible by its thermoresponsive nature and simplicity of chemical modification, especially in injectable scaffolds and wound dressings.

The polysaccharide chitosan, which is produced by deacetylating chitin, is well-known for its inherent antibacterial and hemostatic qualities. Cell adhesion and the retention of bioactive molecules are facilitated by its positive charge, which permits electrostatic interaction with negatively charged cell membranes and growth factors [28]. The non-toxic byproducts of lysozyme's breakdown of chitosan promote tissue regeneration even more. Brown seaweed alginate crosslinks with divalent cations like calcium to generate ionic hydrogels. Alginate can be functionalized with peptides or mixed with extracellular matrix proteins to improve cell adhesion and bioactivity, despite its intrinsic bioinertness.

Tissue remodeling is significantly impacted by these natural polymers' breakdown characteristics. Collagenases and proteases break down collagen and gelatin enzymatically at a rate that corresponds to the development of new tissue. The degree of deacetylation or crosslink density can alter the pace of hydrolytic and

Table 5.1 Biomaterials used in different types of tissue

Tissue type	Common biomaterials	Examples	Key functions	Design considerations
Bone and orthopedic tissue	Metals, ceramics, composites, bioresorbable polymers	Titanium alloys (Ti-6Al-4V), hydroxyapatite, poly(L-lactic acid) (PLLA)	Structural support, osteoconduction, load-bearing capability	High compressive strength, osteointegration, controlled degradation, radiopacity
Cartilage tissue	Hydrogels, collagen-based matrices, PEG derivatives	Agarose, hyaluronic acid, polyethylene glycol diacrylate (PEGDA)	Shock absorption, chondrocyte proliferation, ECM mimicry	Elasticity, nutrient diffusion, viscoelastic properties, biocompatibility
Cardiovascular tissue	Elastomers, bioresorbable polymers, metallic stents	Poly(glycerol sebacate) (PGS), polylactic-*co*-glycolic acid (PLGA), nitinol	Elastic recoil, blood compatibility, endothelialization	Hemocompatibility, fatigue resistance, controlled degradation, mechanical compliance
Skin and wound healing	Natural polymers, hydrogels, nanofibrous mats	Collagen, chitosan, gelatin, PCL nanofibers	Cell migration, wound closure, antibacterial activity	Moisture retention, oxygen permeability, antimicrobial surface modification
Neural tissue	Conductive polymers, hydrogels, biodegradable scaffolds	Polypyrrole (PPy), poly(3,4-ethylenedioxythiophene) (PEDOT), alginate	Electrical conductivity, neural regeneration, axonal growth	Softness, conductivity, minimal inflammation, neurocompatibility
Muscle tissue	Elastomeric polymers, ECM-based scaffolds, peptide hydrogels	Polyurethane, collagen-gel scaffolds, fibrin gels	Mechanical contractility, myoblast alignment, signal transduction	Elastic modulus matching, electrical stimulation capability, bioactivity
Dental and craniofacial tissue	Ceramics, composites, biodegradable polymers	Calcium phosphate cements, zirconia, PLA composites	Hard tissue regeneration, implant stability	High hardness, biocompatibility, aesthetic integration, minimal wear
Liver and pancreatic tissue	Natural polymers, synthetic hydrogels, decellularized matrices	Alginate, GelMA, PEG hydrogels	Hepatocyte viability, vascular integration, metabolic function	Porosity, oxygen transport, bioactivity, tunable stiffness
Vascular and endothelial tissue	Biodegradable elastomers, ECM mimics, synthetic grafts	PGS, Polycaprolactone (PCL), collagen-elastin composites	Compliance, endothelial cell growth, anti-thrombogenic surface	Mechanical compliance, hemocompatibility, porosity for tissue ingrowth

Tissue type	Common biomaterials	Examples	Key functions	Design considerations
Corneal and ocular tissue	Transparent hydrogels, collagen mimics, PEG derivatives	Collagen type I, PEGDA, methacrylated gelatin (GelMA)	Optical clarity, epithelial cell support, minimal inflammation	Transparency, refractive index matching, oxygen diffusion

enzymatic breakdown of chitosan and alginate. In order to minimize mechanical failure and prevent premature scaffold collapse, controlled degradation guarantees a gradual transfer of stress to regenerated tissue. Therefore, natural polymers offer physiologically informative settings; yet, for wider therapeutic utility, hybridization is required due to their mechanical constraints and unpredictability.

5.3.2 Synthetic Polymers

Compared to their natural equivalents, synthetic polymers have the advantages of controlled composition, predictable degradation, tunable mechanics, and superior processing versatility. Synthetic biomaterials such as polyethylene glycol (PEG), polylactic acid (PLA), polyglycolic acid (PGA), and polycaprolactone (PCL) are frequently utilized. Aliphatic polyesters like PLA and PGA break down by hydrolyzing ester linkages producing lactic and glycolic acids, which are then broken down by natural processes. By varying the PLA:PGA ratio, their copolymer, PLGA, allows for exact manipulation of the breakdown rate [29]. While PLA degrades more slowly and offers longer mechanical support, especially in bone and cartilage applications, PGA degrades more quickly, making it ideal for short-term scaffolding in soft tissue regeneration.

Another aliphatic polyester, PCL, has a high mechanical flexibility and a low rate of degradation, which makes it appropriate for load-bearing tissues and long-term implants [30, 31]. Its semi-crystalline structure makes it possible to 3D print into intricate geometries and electrospin into nanofibers, which makes it useful for dermal scaffolds, vascular grafts, and nerve conduits. In contrast, PEG is a non-biodegradable, hydrophilic polymer that is frequently employed to make surface coatings and hydrogels. PEG improves biocompatibility and decreases immunogenicity due to its resistance to protein adsorption. Scientists have created responsive scaffolds that can supply growth factors or medications in situ by functionalizing PEG with bioactive peptides or degradable linkers.

By adjusting molecular weight, crystallinity, and copolymer composition, synthetic polymers' mechanical characteristics and rate of breakdown can be accurately controlled. Design freedom is further increased by processing methods including solvent casting, electrospinning, and additive manufacturing. However, localized irritation may be caused by the acidic degradation byproducts of polyesters, necessitating careful regulation of degradation rates and the use of basic ceramics or buffering agents. Synthetic polymers are nonetheless essential despite these drawbacks because of their scalability, repeatability, and ability to be tailored to specific clinical needs [32].

5.3.3 Ceramic Biomaterials

Ceramic biomaterials are inorganic, non-metallic materials that are especially useful for bone and dental applications because of their high compressive strength, bioactivity, and osteoconductivity. Calcium phosphates, including hydroxyapatite (HA) and tricalcium phosphate (TCP), and bioactive glasses are the two most common types.

Chemically comparable to the mineral phase of bone, hydroxyapatite ($Ca_{10}(PO_4)_6(OH)_2$) offers the perfect surface for osteoblast mineralization and adhesion. With modest resorption rates that promote long-term bone integration, it is bioactive but comparatively stable. On the other hand, β-tricalcium phosphate (β-TCP) breaks down more quickly, releasing phosphate and calcium ions that promote osteogenic development. These complementary qualities are combined in HA and TCP composites to balance resorbability and structural support.

In physiological fluids, bioactive glasses, which are mostly made of SiO_2, CaO, NaO_2, and P_2O_5, undergo surface reactions that result in the formation of a hydroxycarbonate apatite (HCA) layer, which strengthens the interaction with bone. In addition to altering cellular activity, the release of ionic dissolution products triggers signaling pathways linked to osteogenesis and angiogenesis. Additionally, porous foams, granules, or fibers can be created from bioactive glasses, allowing them to be used in both load-bearing and non-load-bearing applications. Under tensile stress, ceramic biomaterials become brittle due to their low toughness and exceptional bioactivity. To get around this, ceramics are frequently mixed with fibers or polymers to create composite structures that increase mechanical robustness while preserving bioactivity [33, 34].

5.3.4 Composite and Hybrid Materials

The goal of developing composite and hybrid biomaterials is to combine the biological usefulness of natural polymers or ceramics with the mechanical durability of synthetic materials. The hierarchical structure of native tissues, where organic and inorganic components live harmoniously, is modeled by these materials. PCL/HA and PLGA/TCP are examples of polymer-ceramic composites that combine the flexibility and processability of polymers with the osteoconductivity of ceramics. These scaffolds encourage mineral deposition and tissue regeneration by offering increased mechanical strength and bioactivity. Similarly, cell-friendly biochemical signals are combined with adjustable degradation and flexibility in natural-synthetic polymer hybrids, such as collagen-PEG or chitosan-PCL.

Using nanoparticles, nanotubes, or nanofibers to improve mechanical, electrical, or biological performance, nanocomposites are an advanced subclass. For instance, silver or zinc oxide nanoparticles provide antibacterial action, lowering the risk of infection during wound healing, whereas nanohydroxyapatite-reinforced polymers increase stiffness and encourage osteogenic differentiation. In applications involving nerve regeneration, carbon-based nanostructures like graphene and carbon nanotubes can also promote neuronal development and enhance electrical conductivity. Nanocomposites have established themselves as the next generation of scaffolds in regenerative medicine due to their capacity to affect cell signaling pathways via surface topography and ion release [13, 35].

5.3.5 Key Properties of Biomaterials

The clinical appropriateness of biomaterials is determined by several important physicochemical and biological characteristics that affect their effectiveness in tissue engineering. Cell migration, vascularization, and nutrient diffusion all depend on porosity and pore interconnectivity. Depending on the tissue type, the ideal pore diameters range from 100 to 300 μm for bone and 20 to 60 μm for skin. These can be customized by fabrication techniques like 3D printing or freeze-drying. Mechanical Strength: To avoid deformation or stress shielding, materials must fit the target tissue's mechanical profile. Ceramics and hard polymers are used in orthopedic settings, whereas elastomers are best suited for soft tissues.

Degradation rate and tissue regeneration should be in sync to guarantee steady replacement without sacrificing support. The equilibrium between structural integrity and resorption is preserved by controlled degradation achieved by crosslinking, copolymerization, or crystallinity modification. The ability to stimulate biological processes, including protein adsorption, cell adhesion, and differentiation, is known as bioactivity. Bioactivity is greatly influenced by surface topography and chemistry, as well as by the presence of ions, growth factors, or peptides. Long-term integration depends on immunocompatibility and reducing inflammatory and foreign body reactions. Techniques include hydrophilic coatings, surface passivation, and the controlled release of anti-inflammatory drugs [36].

From naturally occurring polymers to designed nanocomposites, the variety of biomaterial types allows for customized solutions for a range of regenerative problems. Ceramics give osteoconductivity, synthetic polymers offer tunable mechanics, and natural polymers offer intrinsic bioactivity [37, 38]. Composites combine these advantages to mimic the complexity of native tissues. Through the optimization of critical characteristics including porosity, degradation, bioactivity, and immunocompatibility, scientists are working to create biomaterials that actively guide biological healing processes in addition to restoring structure and function.

5.4 Mechanisms and Processes

The intricate interactions of biological, chemical, and physical processes that regulate cellular activity and tissue creation are essential to tissue engineering and regenerative medicine. Designing biomaterials that actively promote tissue regeneration through regulated biological interactions and maintain structural integrity requires an understanding of these mechanisms. The key mechanisms and procedures that support successful tissue engineering are covered in this section. These include matrix remodeling, angiogenesis, cell–material interactions, immunological regulation, and biochemical signaling. Each of these procedures works in concert to produce integrated, functional tissue constructs that can replace or repair damaged biological structures.

5.4.1 Cell–Material Interactions

Effective cell–material interactions, which control how cells identify, adhere to, and react to the material surface, are the first step towards the success of any tissue-engineered product. The first and most important phase is cell adhesion, which is mostly mediated by integrin receptors that attach to motifs (such the RGD sequence) found in extracellular matrix (ECM) proteins found in nature or coatings made of artificial biomaterials. Cells are anchored to the scaffold by this contact, which also starts intracellular signaling cascades and affects later behaviors including spreading, proliferation, and differentiation.

Cell proliferation after attachment makes ensuring that there are enough cells on the scaffold to create new tissue [39]. Material characteristics including stiffness, surface energy, and nutrient permeability affect proliferation. For instance, firmer substrates are better for osteogenic lineage commitment, whereas softer hydrogels can encourage the growth of fibroblasts and chondrocytes. Both biochemical and biophysical cues from the scaffold direct cell differentiation, the process by which progenitor or stem cells develop into certain cell types. Lineage-specific differentiation is influenced by topographical characteristics, matrix elasticity, and mechanical stiffness. As an example, mesenchymal stem cells (MSCs) tend to differentiate into neural cells on softer matrices (in the kilopascal range) and osteoblasts on stiff substrates (in the gigapascal range).

At the material interface, surface topography and chemistry are crucial in regulating biological responses. Cell adhesion and signaling are directly impacted by the kind and density of adsorbed proteins, which are determined by surface chemistry. Compared to hydrophobic surfaces, hydrophilic surfaces frequently encourage more consistent protein adsorption and improved cell spreading. By simulating natural ECM interactions, functionalization with bioactive ligands or peptides improves cell recognition and attachment.

Through mechanotransduction, surface topography including characteristics at the nano and microscales influences gene expression and cytoskeletal architecture. By strengthening cell–matrix interactions and encouraging the establishment of focal adhesions, nanostructured surfaces can improve osteogenic differentiation. Thanks to developments in microfabrication and additive manufacturing, topographical cues may now be precisely controlled, allowing the creation of biomaterials that influence biological outcomes. The delicate balance between biochemical and biomechanical cues is essential for successful cell material interactions, highlighting the necessity of scaffold designs that combine biofunctionality with the best possible physical architecture [40].

5.4.2 Matrix Remodeling and ECM Deposition

The dynamic interaction of extracellular matrix (ECM) formation and scaffold breakdown is necessary for tissue regeneration. ECM proteins including collagen, fibronectin, and elastin are secreted by cells during their proliferation and differentiation, gradually replacing the transient scaffold structure. The smooth transition of the designed tissue from a synthetic to a biological state is guaranteed by this procedure, which is called matrix remodeling. For best results, scaffold breakdown must be timed to coincide with tissue formation. The scaffold might not give the growing tissue enough mechanical support if it breaks down too quickly. On the other hand, delayed breakdown can impede tissue maturation by obstructing cell migration and extracellular matrix deposition. To preserve structural integrity and permit biological remodeling, scaffold degradation should ideally happen at a rate that corresponds with the development of new tissue.

Depending on the kind of material, either hydrolytic or enzymatic methods may be used to cause the breakdown process. Natural polymers like collagen and chitosan are broken down by proteases and lysozymes, whereas synthetic polylactic acid (PLA) break down mostly by the hydrolysis of ester linkages. Bioactive degradation products released by the scaffold's breakdown may have further effects on tissue growth and cell behavior. Additionally, scaffold remodeling is influenced by the mechanical forces produced by cells during ECM deposition. Fibers are rearranged by cell-mediated traction forces, which affect tissue anisotropy, porosity, and alignment [41]. The logical design of scaffolds that change with developing tissues is made possible by an understanding of these interconnected biochemical and biomechanical processes.

5.4.3 Angiogenesis and Vascularization

A key component of successful tissue regeneration is angiogenesis, which is the process by which new blood vessels are formed from pre-existing vasculature. Necrosis and poor integration with host tissue result from created tissues experiencing nutrition and oxygen deficiencies due to inadequate vascularization. Endothelial cell activation, basement membrane breakdown, migration toward angiogenic stimuli, proliferation, tube formation, and pericyte stabilization are all coordinated phases in the angiogenic process [42, 43]. By using both structural and biological cues, biomaterials can be designed to encourage these processes.

Scaffold porosity and interconnectivity are critical structural features that facilitate vessel ingrowth and fluid transport. Highly porous scaffolds with interconnected pores larger than 100 μm are generally favorable for microvascular formation. Additionally, the inclusion of angiogenic growth factors such as vascular endothelial growth factor (VEGF) and fibroblast growth factor-2 (FGF-2) enhances endothelial cell recruitment and vessel sprouting.

Important structural elements that promote fluid flow and vessel ingrowth are scaffold porosity and interconnectivity. For microvascular development, highly porous scaffolds with interconnected pores bigger than 100 μm are typically advantageous. Furthermore, endothelial cell recruitment and vessel sprouting are improved by the addition of angiogenic growth factors, such as fibroblast growth factor-2 (FGF-2) and vascular endothelial growth factor (VEGF). Pre-vascularized scaffolds, in which endothelial cells are co-cultured with supportive cells like smooth muscle or pericytes prior to implantation, and bioprinting, which enables accurate spatial patterning of vascular networks, are examples of emerging vascularization techniques. Controlled oxygen supply, accomplished with oxygen-releasing materials, is another promising strategy to promote cell viability in the initial post-implantation phases.

5.4.4 Immune Modulation in Wound Healing

In tissue regeneration, the immune system can either promote healing or result in long-term inflammation and fibrosis. In order to improve tissue repair without triggering unfavorable immune responses, immune regulation is therefore a crucial technique for successful tissue engineering. Biomaterials cause an initial inflammatory response after implantation, which is typified by the influx of macrophages and neutrophils. Macrophages can change from pro-inflammatory (M1) to anti-inflammatory (M2) phenotypes, demonstrating their extraordinary adaptability. While the M2 phenotype fosters tissue remodeling and regeneration, the M1 phenotype encourages debris removal and infection defense.

Macrophage polarization is influenced by biomaterial characteristics such as stiffness, degradation products, and surface chemistry [44]. For example, surfaces that are hydrophilic and negatively charged tend to encourage M2 polarization, which supports regeneration results. The inflammatory response can be further fine-tuned by including immunomodulatory molecules into scaffolds, such as transforming growth factor-beta (TGF-β) or interleukin-10 (IL-10). To use the immune response as a beneficial element of healing rather than a barrier, recent strategies entail creating immuno-informed biomaterials that intelligently interact with immune cells. The use of immune-integrative designs that capitalize on the body's inherent defense and healing systems is a paradigm change from conventional "immune-evasive" materials.

5.4.5 *Biochemical Signaling*

The precise coordination of biochemical signals that control cellular functions like migration, proliferation, and differentiation is essential for effective tissue engineering. Growth factors, cytokines, and other bioactive substances can be included into scaffolds to create a microenvironment that stimulates regeneration signaling cascades and resembles the original extracellular matrix. Growth factors that are essential for angiogenesis, osteogenesis, and chondrogenesis include VEGF, basic fibroblast growth factor (bFGF), and bone morphogenetic proteins (BMPs). To ensure prolonged and localized release, these compounds can be integrated into scaffolds by physical entrapment, covalent bonding, or encapsulation within micro- or nanoparticles [45].

Cell recruitment and immunological responses are further regulated by cytokines and chemokines. For instance, stromal cell-derived factor-1 (SDF-1) enhances regeneration by encouraging stem cell homing to damaged areas. These signals can be spatially and temporally regulated by controlled delivery systems, avoiding quick deterioration or undesirable systemic consequences. Because of their increased stability and tunability, small molecules and peptides are being employed more to simulate natural signaling pathways in addition to protein-based stimuli. Mechanochemical signaling, in which mechanical inputs (such as shear stress or strain) are transformed into biochemical signals that direct cell function, is another area of emerging research. The future of biomaterial design lies in the combination of biochemical, mechanical, and electrical signaling modalities, which allows for intricate control over tissue morphogenesis and functional repair.

Tissue engineering is controlled by a complex web of interrelated mechanisms and processes, including vascularization, scaffold remodeling, cellular adhesion, immunological regulation, and signaling dynamics. Designing biomaterials that actively direct biological processes toward functional regeneration in addition to provide mechanical support is made possible by a comprehensive understanding of these mechanisms [46]. Dynamic and responsive biomaterials systems that can adjust to biological feedback and coordinate regeneration through regulated biochemical, mechanical, and immunological interactions are becoming increasingly important as research progresses. These developments bode well for the next wave of tissue-engineered treatments that are clinically successful and work in harmony with the body's own healing processes.

5.5 Design Considerations

The effective use of biomaterials in tissue engineering and wound healing requires rigorous design considerations that incorporate structural, mechanical, biochemical, and translational variables in addition to material selection. To provide both biological cues for tissue regeneration and physical support, an effective scaffold design must replicate important elements of the natural extracellular matrix (ECM) as shown in

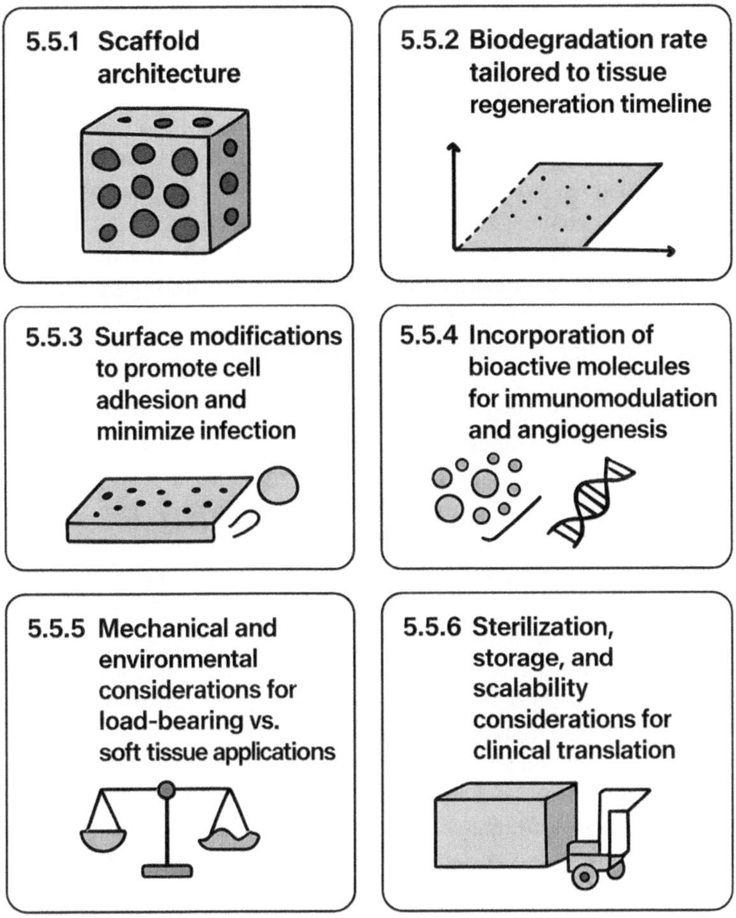

Fig. 5.1 Schematic representation of scaffold designs for tissue engineering, illustrating variations in pore size, porosity, interconnectivity, and architectural features that influence cell infiltration, nutrient diffusion, mechanical performance, and overall regenerative outcomes

Fig. 5.1. Cellular reactions and long-term results are determined by the interaction of architecture, degradation, surface functionality, and mechanical behavior. Clinical translation also depends on practical factors including sterilization, storage stability, and large-scale manufacturing [47]. The main design guidelines that direct the creation of biomaterial scaffolds for regenerative medicine are described in this section.

5.5.1 Scaffold Architecture: Porosity, Interconnectivity, and Mechanical Properties

A key factor in determining the biological performance of biomaterials is scaffold architecture. The scaffold must combine porosity, connectedness, and the right amount of mechanical strength to replicate the hierarchical structure of native tissues. The volume percentage of empty areas in a scaffold is called porosity, and it has a direct impact on waste elimination, cell infiltration, and nutrient diffusion. Although it promotes vascularization and tissue ingrowth, high porosity (usually 70–90%) may jeopardize mechanical stability. As a result, maintaining both strength and functionality requires the ideal balance. Additionally, the pore size needs to be customized for the target tissue. Smaller pores (20–80 μm) are appropriate for soft tissues like skin or cartilage, while larger pores (100–300 μm) are best for bone regeneration because they allow osteoblast migration and capillary development.

The scaffold's effective transport of oxygen, nutrients, and signaling chemicals is ensured by the interconnectivity of its pores. Uneven tissue growth and necrotic areas might result from poorly connected designs. By precisely controlling the geometry and distribution of pores, methods like electrospinning, freeze-drying, and 3D bioprinting make it possible to create gradient structures that closely resemble the variability of actual tissue [48, 49].

For mechanical mismatches and stress shielding to be avoided, mechanical characteristics must match those of the host tissue. Soft tissue scaffolds should have low modulus values (<1 MPa) and great elasticity, while bone scaffolds need compressive strengths between 2 and 20 MPa. Finite element analysis (FEA) and computational modeling are being used more to optimize designs prior to manufacturing and forecast mechanical performance. Incorporating mechanical signals into scaffold architecture promotes cell differentiation via mechanotransduction pathways in addition to ensuring structural stability.

5.5.2 Biodegradation Rate Tailored to Tissue Regeneration Timeline

The biodegradation rate is a crucial design parameter in the development of biomaterials, and it needs to be in sync with the rate at which new tissue is formed. A scaffold should ideally break down gradually as the regenerated tissue takes on structural and load-bearing roles. Mechanical support is removed too soon if deterioration happens too quickly; if it happens too slowly, leftover material may prevent tissue reorganization or cause chronic inflammation. Depending on the material's chemical makeup, degradation can take place by oxidative, enzymatic, or hydrolytic processes. Crystallinity, molecular weight, and copolymer ratio all affect the rates at which synthetic polymers like poly(lactic acid) (PLA), polycaprolactone (PCL), and polyglycolic acid (PGA) hydrolyze. Proteases or lysozymes break down natural polymers like collagen, chitosan, and gelatin enzymatically, producing physiologically acceptable byproducts that further encourage cell division.

By adjusting the crosslinking density, polymer blends, or composite compositions, degradation rates can be fine-tuned. For example, adding calcium phosphate ceramics to polymer scaffolds can improve osteoconductivity and slow down deterioration. Degradation kinetics are also influenced by environmental factors including pH, temperature, and local enzymatic activity, which calls for material design that may be adjusted to physiological fluctuation [50, 51]. In the end, the scaffold serves as a temporary template rather than a permanent implant thanks to the timing of tissue regeneration and degradation, enabling natural tissue restoration without sacrificing mechanical integrity or biocompatibility.

5.5.3 Surface Modifications to Promote Cell Adhesion and Minimize Infection

One of the most effective methods for maximizing cell–material interactions is surface modification of the scaffold, which serves as the main contact between the biomaterial and the biological environment. Because native synthetic polymers frequently lack bioactive sites for cell attachment, they are modified chemically or physically to enhance their antibacterial, protein-adsorption, and cell-adhesion capabilities. Physical modification methods that change surface energy and roughness, like laser ablation, plasma treatment, and ultraviolet (UV) irradiation, improve wettability and encourage integrin-mediated cell attachment. Bioactive ligands like fibronectin, collagen fragments, or RGD peptides can be immobilized chemically to simulate ECM signaling [52]. For tissue regeneration to be successful, these functionalized surfaces promote cell adhesion, proliferation, and differentiation.

Antimicrobial coatings are used concurrently to stop infections, which is one of the biggest problems with implanted biomaterials. Quaternary ammonium compounds, zinc oxide, and silver nanoparticles are commonly used to break down bacterial membranes while preserving cytocompatibility. New approaches employ bacteriophage-based systems and coatings that release nitric oxide to provide long-lasting antibacterial activity without encouraging drug resistance. Hence, surface modification has two functions: it facilitates favorable cellular contacts and reduces unfavorable immunological or microbial reactions, both of which are necessary for long-term scaffold integration and healing.

5.5.4 *Incorporation of Bioactive Molecules for Immunomodulation and Angiogenesis*

Beyond optimizing their structure and mechanics, biomaterials can be created as bioactive platforms that send signaling molecules to guide tissue regeneration. Complex biological processes like immunomodulation and angiogenesis depend on the precise integration and release of growth factors, cytokines, and genetic elements [53]. An overabundance of inflammation during wound healing can prevent regeneration. In order to change the polarization of macrophages from a pro-inflammatory (M1) to a pro-regenerative (M2) phenotype, biomaterials are being designed to release immunomodulatory drugs or anti-inflammatory cytokines (like IL-10). Likewise, the incorporation of VEGF (vascular endothelial growth factor), FGF (fibroblast growth factor), or PDGF (platelet-derived growth factor) into scaffolds guarantees sufficient vascularization for waste evacuation and nutrient delivery in newly formed tissues by promoting angiogenesis.

Different techniques, such gradient deposition, covalent anchoring, or encapsulation in microspheres, enable temporal and geographic control of molecular release. Particularly, hydrogels work well as continuous release carriers, and 3D bioprinting makes it possible to precisely locate growth factors inside scaffold structures. Furthermore, high surface area and adjustable release profiles are provided by nanomaterials such as polymeric nanocarriers and mesoporous silica nanoparticles, which improve therapeutic efficacy. By incorporating bioactive molecules, scaffolds become bio-instructive systems that may actively direct the development of circulatory networks and immunological balance, two processes necessary for stable and effective tissue regeneration.

5.5.5 *Mechanical and Environmental Considerations for Load Bearing vs. Soft Tissue Applications*

The design of biomaterials is subject to unique mechanical and environmental restrictions depending on the kind of tissue. In order to endure repeated loads, load-bearing tissues like bone, cartilage, and tendons need scaffolds with high stiffness, compressive strength, and fatigue resistance. On the other hand, materials with elasticity, flexibility, and compliance are necessary for soft tissues, such as skin, muscle, and nerves, to permit dynamic movement and deformation without failure. Materials like titanium-coated composites and hydroxyapatite-reinforced polymers offer osteoconductivity and mechanical durability in bone engineering. For these purposes, scaffold topologies need to include anisotropic features that mimic the patterns of trabecular bone. On the other hand, in order to mimic native viscoelastic behavior, soft tissue scaffolds frequently use elastomeric polymers (such as collagen–elastin blends, poly(glycerol sebacate), or polyurethane).

Environmental elements like electrical conductivity, oxygen permeability, and moisture retention are also crucial. For instance, skin scaffolds need to preserve their barrier and moisture properties, but cardiac or brain scaffolds require electrical conductivity to facilitate signal transmission. The seamless integration of biomaterials with their surrounding tissues, which supports both functional and physiological demands, is ensured by achieving mechanical–biological harmony [26].

5.5.6 Sterilization, Storage, and Scalability Considerations for Clinical Translation

Clinical translation requires biomaterials to fulfill practical and regulatory requirements in addition to laboratory performance. Scalability, storage stability, and sterilization all affect how safely and effectively a scaffold may be used in medical environments. To avoid infection and immunological problems, sterilization is necessary. However, traditional techniques like ethylene oxide exposure, autoclaving, and gamma irradiation can change the structure of the material and break down delicate bioactive ingredients [54]. As a result, scaffold integrity must be maintained in the sterilizing procedure selection. For example, to preserve their mechanical and biological qualities, hydrogels and polymeric scaffolds frequently need low-temperature techniques such supercritical CO_2 sterilization or UV treatment.

Biomaterials' shelf life and functionality are impacted by storage stability. For hydrogels and porous scaffolds, lyophilization (freeze-drying) is frequently utilized to extend storage life without sacrificing bioactivity. Controlling temperature and humidity is essential, especially for formulations that contain cells, growth hormones or proteins. Reproducibility and scalability continue to be significant obstacles in the development of biomaterials for clinical use. Complex designs can be consistently produced at an industrial scale thanks to advanced fabrication methods like automated electrospinning and 3D bioprinting. Patient safety and quality assurance are guaranteed by adherence to regulatory requirements and Good Manufacturing Practice (GMP).

Ultimately, the clinical viability of biomaterial-based scaffolds depends on the ability to balance biological functionality with manufacturing practicality achieving consistent, sterile, and cost-effective products suitable for large-scale deployment in regenerative medicine.

A comprehensive grasp of the interactions between structure, degradation, surface functioning, and biological signaling is necessary for designing biomaterials for tissue engineering and wound healing. Mechanical and cellular performance is determined by scaffold architecture; cellular communication and immune control are fueled by surface changes and bioactive integration; degradation kinetics must coincide with regeneration timescales. Furthermore, long-term stability, scalability, and sterilization must all be carefully considered for translation to be successful [55]. Biomaterials can be designed as dynamic, responsive systems that precisely and effectively coordinate tissue regeneration rather than just as inert supports by including these complex design factors.

5.6 Applications and Case Studies

From theoretical models to real-world clinical uses that tackle a variety of medical issues, tissue engineering has progressed. Regenerative techniques for skin, bone, cartilage, and cardiovascular tissues have been completely transformed by the creation of biomaterial scaffolds, hydrogels, and bioactive constructions [56]. Every tissue system has unique mechanical and biological needs, necessitating unique scaffold designs and material characteristics as shown in Fig. 5.2. Key applications and illustrative case studies from the main tissue engineering areas are reviewed in this section, with an emphasis on material selection, fabrication techniques, and comparative preclinical and clinical results that show the effectiveness of scaffolds.

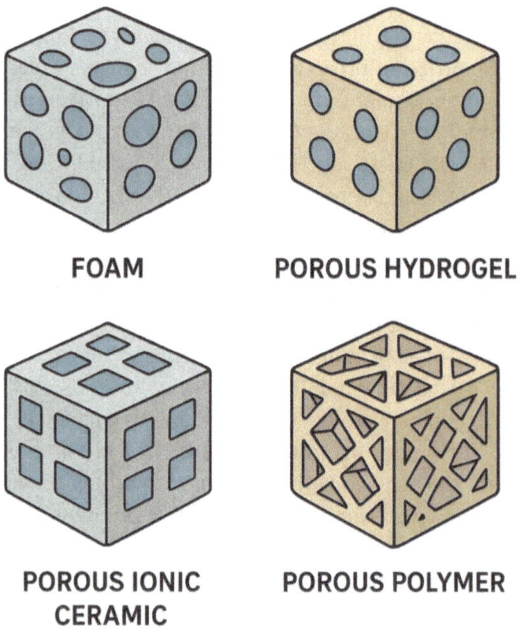

Fig. 5.2 Examples of 3D scaffold architecture used in tissue engineering applications, demonstrating variations in pore structure, material composition, and fabrication methods that influence mechanical performance, cell infiltration, nutrient transport, and overall regenerative outcomes

5.6.1 Skin and Wound Healing: Hydrogel Dressings and Bioengineered Skin Substitutes

Restoring the protective layer and functional integrity of injured skin after burns, chronic wounds, or trauma is the main goal of skin tissue engineering. Biomaterial-based therapies, such hydrogel dressings and bioengineered skin substitutes, have emerged as game-changing options since conventional wound management is frequently constrained by infection, scarring, and delayed healing. Hydrogel dressings, which are made of networks of hydrophilic polymers like chitosan, alginate, or polyethylene glycol (PEG), keep the wound wet, which promotes re-epithelialization and lessens discomfort. They operate as carriers for the delivery of growth factors or antimicrobial agents (e.g., VEGF and epidermal growth factor), absorb exudates, and offer oxygen permeability. For instance, in diabetic wound models, hydrogels based on chitosan and loaded with silver nanoparticles show both antibacterial and pro-healing properties.

Bioengineered skin substitutes replicate the structure of the natural dermis and epidermis by combining cells and scaffolds. Commercial products that have shown clinical efficacy in treating chronic ulcers include Integra® Dermal Regeneration Template, which is a bilayer of collagen–glycosaminoglycan with a silicone epidermal layer, and Apligraf®, which is made of bovine collagen and human fibroblasts/keratinocytes. Compared to traditional grafts, preclinical research in pig and mouse wound models demonstrates decreased fibrosis and increased vascularization. These alternatives represent a significant advancement in regenerative dermatology since they reduce healing timeframes and enhance cosmetic results in clinical settings.

5.6.2 Bone Tissue Engineering: Bioceramic Scaffolds and 3D-Printed Implants

Bone regeneration represents one of the most studied areas in tissue engineering due to the high incidence of fractures, osteoporosis, and tumor-related defects. Bioceramic scaffolds and 3D-printed implants have proven particularly effective in supporting osteogenesis through structural and biochemical mimicry of native bone.

Highly biocompatible and osteoconductive, bioceramic scaffolds are composed of materials including hydroxyapatite (HA), β-tricalcium phosphate (β-TCP), and bioactive glass. Their innate resemblance to the mineral phase of bone encourages mineral deposition, cell adhesion, and proliferation. Composite scaffolds further improve mechanical flexibility and degradation control by combining biodegradable polymers (such polycaprolactone or polylactic acid) with ceramics [57]. Comparing HA-collagen scaffolds implanted in rabbit femoral defects to polymer-only controls in preclinical trials, the former showed noticeably greater bone mineral density and vascularization.

A technological advancement in creating patient-specific designs is represented by 3D-printed bone implants. Porosity, architecture, and mechanical qualities can all be precisely controlled with additive manufacturing. For example, in large-animal models, scaffolds made of titanium and polyetheretherketone (PEEK) that were 3D printed showed excellent osseointegration and mechanical stability. When compared to autologous grafts, clinical trials of bespoke 3D-printed mandibular and craniofacial implants have demonstrated superior biocompatibility, long-term function, and lower donor site morbidity. Together, these findings demonstrate that combining bioceramics and 3D printing produces scaffolds that establish new benchmarks for orthopedic restoration by integrating with host bone physiologically and offering mechanical strength.

5.6.3 Cartilage and Joint Repair: Injectable Hydrogels, Polymeric Scaffolds, and ECM-Mimetic Constructs

The problem of mending avascular, aneural, and non-regenerative articular cartilage is addressed via cartilage tissue engineering. Novel biomaterial systems, such as polymeric scaffolds, injectable hydrogels, and ECM-mimetic structures, present encouraging substitutes for traditional surgical procedures such autologous chondrocyte implantation or microfracture. Injectable hydrogels made of PEG derivatives, hyaluronic acid (HA), or gelatin methacrylate (GelMA) can be applied minimally invasively and harden in place to fit the forms of defects. They promote mechanical robustness, matrix formation, and chondrocyte encapsulation. In comparison to untreated controls, studies employing HA-chondroitin sulfate hydrogels have demonstrated improved glycosaminoglycan (GAG) deposition and chondrogenic development in rabbit joint defect models [58].

Polymeric scaffolds, such polylactic-*co*-glycolic acid (PLGA) and polycaprolactone (PCL), allow for waste movement and nutrition diffusion while offering structural support. Hyaline cartilage regeneration and matrix production are improved by the addition of growth factors such as transforming growth factor-beta (TGF-β3). The biochemical environment of native cartilage is replicated by ECM-mimetic constructs, which can be made from decellularized cartilage or created with collagen type II and proteoglycans. At the defect–tissue interface, these scaffolds promote mechanical integration and chondrocyte-specific gene expression [59]. In early cases of osteoarthritis, clinical studies of cell-seeded extracellular matrix scaffolds have shown enhanced joint function and long-term durability.

Overall, cartilage engineering strategies exemplify how materials design, biochemical signaling, and minimally invasive delivery converge to address one of the most complex challenges in regenerative orthopedics.

5.6.4 *Cardiovascular Regeneration: Vascular Grafts and Endothelialized Scaffolds*

The goal of cardiovascular tissue engineering is to replace or repair damaged heart tissue and blood vessels using endothelialized scaffolds and vascular grafts that blend in perfectly with the host's circulatory system. Vascular grafts need to be biocompatible, thrombosis-resistant, and mechanically strong. Small-diameter grafts have been made using synthetic polymers such poly(ε-caprolactone) (PCL), poly(glycolic acid) (PGA), and polyurethane; nonetheless, thrombosis and intimal hyperplasia still present difficulties. Hybrid structures that combine synthetic backbones with natural materials like collagen or elastin have been created to get around these restrictions. In canine and porcine models, for instance, electrospun PCL–collagen grafts seeded with endothelial progenitor cells have demonstrated decreased thrombosis and increased patency.

By imitating the inner lining of natural vessels, endothelialized scaffolds decrease platelet adhesion and increase the production of nitric oxide. Hemocompatibility is improved by methods such surface modification with heparin or peptide sequences (like REDV, which is unique to endothelial cell binding). Clinical-grade grafts with little immunological rejection and long-term patency, like Humacyte's human acellular vascular (HAV), have demonstrated encouraging results in phase II trials for dialysis access. Novel strategies that promote oxygen transport and myocardial regeneration after myocardial infarction include hydrogel-based microvascular networks and bioprinted cardiac patches [60]. With these developments, passive vascular conduits give way to dynamic, cell-responsive structures that may integrate and repair themselves.

5.6.5 *Comparative Studies of Preclinical and Clinical Outcomes Demonstrating Scaffold Efficacy*

Translating laboratory discoveries into practical treatments requires comparing preclinical and clinical research. From tiny rodents to massive animals, preclinical models shed light on host response, mechanical performance, degradation, and biocompatibility. Other difficulties, such as size, immunological heterogeneity, and integration with local tissues, are also revealed by clinical translation. For example, preclinical research on collagen-based skin substitutes showed low scarring and quick epithelialization, which are results that are mostly repeated in clinical settings for burns and chronic ulcers. Similar to human maxillofacial and orthopaedic repairs, animal models of HA-TCP bone scaffolds showed nearly total defect closure, which was highly linked with increased bone density.

On the other hand, there are occasionally differences; cartilage scaffolds that work well for tiny animals could break down too soon or not provide enough mechanical strength for people. These variations highlight how crucial it is to scale research and improve vascularization and degradation kinetics for bigger, more metabolically demanding tissues. Overall, the ability of biomaterial scaffolds to support functional regeneration with lower donor morbidity and better patient outcomes is continuously confirmed by clinical validation. The development of regenerative biomaterial design still depends on ongoing improvement via iterative feedback between preclinical research and clinical experience.

From 3D-printed bone implants to hydrogel-based wound dressings, the various uses of tissue-engineered scaffolds demonstrate the adaptability and revolutionary potential of biomaterials in contemporary medicine [61, 62]. The requirements for mechanical integrity, controlled degradation, biocompatibility, and biological responsiveness are universal across tissues. Critical feedback loops for improving scaffold designs and guaranteeing translational success are provided by comparative preclinical and clinical investigations. Tissue engineering holds promises for more individualized, useful, and sustainable regenerative treatments in the future as materials science, stem cell biology, and digital manufacturing come together.

5.7 Recent Advances and Innovations

The advent of sophisticated biomaterial technologies and production techniques has significantly changed the fields of tissue engineering and wound healing. Current developments in biomaterials seek to mimic the intricacy, responsiveness, and adaptability of biological tissues, whereas traditional biomaterials were mainly created to offer structural support. Modern biomaterials allow for exact control over architecture, cellular relationships, and biochemical signaling by combining ideas from nanotechnology, additive manufacturing, smart materials, and customized medicine. By improving clinical results, biocompatibility, and functioning, these innovations are revolutionizing regenerative medicine.

5.7.1 3D and 4D Bioprinting: Spatial Control over Scaffold Architecture and Cell Distribution

By enabling previously unheard-of spatial precision in the deposition of biomaterials, cells, and bioactive compounds, three-dimensional (3D) bioprinting has completely transformed the scaffold production process. 3D bioprinting uses computer-aided design (CAD) to create layer-by-layer designs that closely resemble the structural variability of real tissues, in contrast to conventional scaffold production techniques. Pore size, geometry, and interconnectedness can be fine-tuned with this method, which is essential for vascularization and nutrient diffusion. Recent advances in biomaterial engineering and 3D bioprinting have accelerated the development of highly customized, tissue-mimicking constructs for wound healing and skin tissue restoration, enabling precise spatial control over scaffold architecture, cellular composition, and bioactive molecule distribution [63].

The use of "bioinks," which are usually hydrogels containing cells and signaling molecules, is permitted by several bioprinting modalities, including as inkjet, extrusion, and laser-assisted printing. Because of their biocompatibility and adjustable rheological characteristics, hydrogels like collagen, alginate, and gelatin methacrylate (GelMA) are frequently utilized. Co-culture systems, in which various cell types are deposited in spatially defined patterns to replicate tissue interfaces like skin, cartilage, or vasculature, are made possible by 3D bioprinting [64].

Four-dimensional (4D) bioprinting adds the idea of time as a dynamic design parameter to 3D bioprinting. When exposed to external stimuli like pH, temperature, or magnetic fields, 4D-printed structures can alter their shape, stiffness, or functionality. Stimuli-responsive hydrogels and shape-memory polymers are examples of smart materials that enable scaffolds to adjust to the physiological environment after implantation. For instance, a cartilage scaffold may stiffen in reaction to mechanical loading, or a 4D-printed vascular graft may expand on its own when hydrated. Instead of acting as passive templates, this dynamic flexibility is a step toward biomaterials that actively contribute to the regeneration process.

5.7.2 *Smart Biomaterials: Stimuli-Responsive Hydrogels for Controlled Drug Release and Dynamic Remodeling*

A novel class of responsive systems that can recognize environmental inputs and modify their behavior in response is represented by smart biomaterials. Stimuli-responsive hydrogels stand out among them because of their ability to modify tissue, change shape, and release drugs under regulated conditions. Reversible physicochemical changes occur in these hydrogels in response to light, electric fields, enzymes, temperature, and pH [65]. Emerging intelligent biomaterials are being engineered not only to promote tissue regeneration but also to actively reprogram the wound immune microenvironment, enabling precise delivery of therapeutic agents that minimize scar formation and improve aesthetic and functional outcomes in wound healing [66].

Injectable delivery methods that solidify in situ to conform to wound geometries are made possible by thermoresponsive hydrogels, such as poly(*N*-isopropylacrylamide) (PNIPAAm), which exhibit sol–gel transitions around physiological temperature. Because changes in wound pH can cause the release of growth factors or antimicrobial agents at the infection site, pH-responsive hydrogels are especially useful for managing chronic wounds. When tissue remodeling takes place, enzyme-responsive systems use matrix metalloproteinases (MMPs) or other enzymatic cues to start scaffold disintegration or release encapsulated compounds [67].

Smart hydrogels can be used as dynamic ECM mimics in addition to drug delivery, promoting cell migration and remodeling through gradual changes in stiffness or crosslinking density. Additionally, hybrid systems that contain conductive polymers or nanoparticles can react to electrical or magnetic stimuli, creating opportunities for the regeneration of heart and brain tissue. Smart biomaterials facilitate real-time responsiveness to biological signals by combining sensing and actuation capabilities, opening the door for "intelligent" regenerative scaffolds.

5.7.3 *Nanotechnology Integration: Nanofibers, Nanoparticles, and Nanocomposites Enhancing Bioactivity and Antimicrobial Properties*

Metal-organic framework (MOF) based biomaterials have emerged as a promising class of wound care materials, offering exceptional advantages including high porosity, tunable structural properties, and intrinsic multifunctionality that enable controlled drug delivery, stimuli-responsive behavior, and potent antibacterial, immunomodulatory, angiogenic, and neurogenic effects at the wound site [68]. The ability to manipulate surface characteristics and structures at the nanoscale scale made possible by nanotechnology has greatly increased the functional potential of biomaterials. Materials' nanoscale arrangement is very similar to that of the natural extracellular matrix (ECM), offering biological cues that affect cell adhesion, proliferation, and differentiation. For example, electrospun nanofibers with fiber diameters between 50 and 500 nm form extremely flexible and porous matrices. By simulating collagen fibrils, these fibers can guide cell development through contact and allow for the prolonged release of medicinal compounds by encapsulation or surface adsorption. Nanofibrous scaffolds have been shown to improve wound healing effectiveness by speeding up angiogenesis and epithelialization.

Growth factors, genes, and antimicrobial agents can be delivered precisely via nanoparticles, such as liposomes, polymeric nanocarriers, and metallic nanoparticles (such as silver, gold, and zinc oxide). Systemic toxicity is decreased by their large surface area-to-volume ratio, which is for effective loading and regulated release [69]. For instance, wound dressings containing silver nanoparticles offer broad-spectrum antibacterial action that inhibits the formation of biofilms and the recurrence of infections. Nanocomposites improve mechanical and biological performance by combining nanoscale fillers with polymeric or ceramic matrix. While carbon-based nanomaterials (graphene, carbon nanotubes) improve electrical conductivity for brain and cardiac applications, the addition of nanohydroxyapatite increases osteoconductivity and mechanical strength. To further support functional tissue regeneration, nanocomposite scaffolds can also use mechanical and electrical cues to activate cell signaling pathways.

Through nanotechnology integration, biomaterials achieve superior bioactivity, antimicrobial defense, and regenerative efficiency key characteristics for next-generation wound and tissue therapies.

5.7.4 Growth Factor Delivery Systems: Controlled Spatiotemporal Release for Accelerated Healing

During tissue repair, growth hormones play a crucial role in controlling angiogenesis, differentiation, and cell proliferation. However, systemic side effects, short half-lives, and quick disintegration frequently restrict their direct use. Controlled growth factor delivery methods have been created to address these obstacles by achieving spatiotemporal manipulation of release kinetics within biomaterial scaffolds. VEGF, PDGF, TGF-β, and BMP-2 can be delivered locally and sustainably using hydrogels, microspheres, and nanoparticle carriers. These proteins are shielded from enzymatic breakdown by encapsulation in biodegradable matrices, which also permits regulated diffusion in response to environmental or degradation stimuli [70, 71]. Dual-delivery systems, for instance, can coordinate the regeneration of bone and vascular tissue by releasing angiogenic factors and osteogenic cues in a sequential manner.

Spatial patterning of growth factors within scaffolds is made possible by advanced fabrication techniques, including 3D printing and layer-by-layer assembly, which replicate the natural gradients present in tissue formation. Additionally, "on-demand" delivery during crucial healing phases is made possible by smart release mechanisms that react to pH or enzyme activity. These systems optimize treatment efficacy while reducing inflammation or fibrosis by precisely regulating dosage and timing. Clinical success has resulted from these advancements, especially in the areas of soft tissue regeneration, bone defect repair, and diabetic wound healing, where coordinated molecular signaling is essential for functional recovery.

5.7.5 Personalized Medicine Approaches: Patient-Specific Scaffolds and Regenerative Constructs

Regenerative healthcare is undergoing a paradigm shift because of the combination of customized treatment and biomaterials technology. To recreate unique anatomical features and physiological conditions, patient-specific scaffolds are currently being created using medical imaging data, computational modeling, and 3D printing technologies rather than one-size-fits-all approaches.

Researchers may create implants that are perfectly matched to patient geometry by combining 3D bioprinting with CT or MRI images. Examples of these implants include skin substitutes that fit to the shapes of wounds or craniofacial bone transplants. These unique constructions increase integration, shorten operating times, and produce better functional and cosmetic results.

Additionally, autologous cell sourcing using a patient's own stem or progenitor cells improves regeneration and reduces immunological rejection. The development of living tissues tailored to particular restorative requirements is made possible by customized bioinks that contain growth hormones and patient-derived cells. Based on biological information unique to each patient, artificial intelligence (AI) and machine learning are being employed more and more to forecast material performance and improve scaffold settings. Precision therapies, where biomaterial formulations can be tailored to the patient's metabolic profile, wound microenvironment, or genetic predispositions, is another area where this individualized approach goes beyond structural modification [72, 73]. Consequently, individualized biomaterials are improving long-term functional recovery, safety, and efficacy while bringing in a new era of precision tissue engineering.

The breadth and accuracy of regenerative medicine have been increased by recent developments in biomaterial science, including 3D/4D bioprinting, smart hydrogels, nanotechnology integration, targeted growth factor delivery, and customized scaffold design [74]. Beyond static implants, these advancements allow for dynamic, patient-responsive devices that achieve active healing participation. A future where biomaterials are patient-specific, intelligent, and adaptive capable of recreating intricate tissue functions with previously unheard-of fidelity and efficiency is promised by the convergence of material engineering, biotechnology, and digital design.

5.8 Challenges and Limitations

Transforming laboratory discoveries into functional and therapeutically feasible treatments is still a problem, despite the impressive advancements in tissue engineering and biomaterials research. Technical obstacles, regulatory impediments, and biological complexity limit the field and affect patient outcomes and scaffold effectiveness. Effective tissue regeneration requires precise synchronization of vascularization, immunological response, material degradation, and mechanical integrity, all of which are challenging to maximize at the same time. The main obstacles to advancement in biomaterials-based tissue engineering are discussed in this section. These include problems with vascularization, immunological modulation, degradation kinetics, mechanical trade-offs, regulatory translation, and scalability. Smart biomaterials have evolved beyond passive structural supports into dynamic therapeutic platforms capable of integrating antimicrobial, immunomodulatory, and angiogenic functions within a single wound dressing system, addressing the multifactorial challenges of chronic wound management through intelligent, stimuli-responsive design.

5.8.1 *Matching Scaffold Degradation with Tissue Regeneration Kinetics*

Synchronizing the dynamics of scaffold degradation and tissue regeneration is a basic difficulty in scaffold design. A biomaterial scaffold should ideally break down at a pace that corresponds with the growth of new tissue, offering structural and mechanical support until the regenerated tissue is able to support itself. Achieving this dynamic balance is extremely difficult, though, as a number of variables, such as material composition, porosity, local enzymatic activity, and mechanical loads, affect tissue growth and breakdown [75, 76].

A scaffold may lose structural integrity before enough tissue has grown if it breaks down too quickly, which could result in mechanical failure or insufficient healing. On the other hand, sluggish breakdown can prevent nutrients from diffusing, delay the development of extracellular matrix (ECM), and impede cell invasion. For instance, in some applications, poly(lactic acid) (PLA) and polycaprolactone (PCL) break down excessively slowly, leaving behind leftover particles that could cause inflammation. However, without crosslinking or chemical modification, natural polymers like collagen or gelatin sometimes break down too quickly.

Designing intelligent or stimuli-responsive biomaterials whose degradation may be controlled by environmental cues like pH, enzyme concentration, or mechanical stress is one emerging strategy to solve this difficulty. Despite these developments, patient-specific differences in metabolism, vascularization, and immunological activity make it challenging to estimate breakdown kinetics in vivo. As a result, optimizing deterioration profiles remains a crucial obstacle to reliable clinical results.

5.8.2 *Controlling Immune Response and Inflammation In Vivo*

Implanting biomaterials invariably sets off an immunological reaction that may promote tissue repair or result in long-term inflammation and fibrosis. One of the most enduring problems in tissue engineering is still managing this reaction. Proteins quickly adsorb onto the scaffold surface during implantation, creating a temporary matrix that affects immunological pathways and macrophage activation. A fibrous capsule is frequently formed because of the foreign body response (FBR), which isolates the scaffold from the surrounding tissue and hinders integration [77]. Modulating macrophage polarization, encouraging the pro-regenerative M2 phenotype while reducing the pro-inflammatory M1 phenotype is the key to overcoming this.

Individual immune responses, however, differ greatly based on tissue type, genetics, and coexisting diseases like infection or diabetes. Furthermore, degradation products from PLA and other polymers can cause local pH to drop, which exacerbates irritation. Although methods like adding immunomodulatory nanoparticles or surface functionalization with anti-inflammatory molecules (such TGF-β or IL-10) show promise, total immunological control is still difficult. Immune tolerance and pathogen defense must be balanced, which is a difficult and unsolved balance. In order to guide immune responses rather than just try to suppress them, future biomaterials must incorporate immune-instructive design concepts.

5.8.3 Vascularization Limitations in Large Tissue Constructs

In engineering of big, metabolically active tissues like bone, muscle, or the heart, vascularization continues to be a significant bottleneck. Cells inside scaffolds depend on the diffusion of nutrients and oxygen, which is restricted to 100–200 μm from a capillary. Necrosis and insufficient tissue development happen when there is insufficient vascular integration. Large tissue constructs need active vascularization techniques, whereas thin, compact constructs can rely on passive diffusion. Although they have shown better results in animal models, pre-vascularization, co-culturing with endothelial cells, and the administration of angiogenic growth factors (e.g., VEGF, FGF-2) frequently fall short of producing stable, perfused networks in vivo. Furthermore, the inability of designed capillaries to successfully anastomose with the host vasculature sometimes results in temporary or non-functional arteries.

Vascular patterning can be precisely controlled thanks to recent developments in 3D bioprinting and microfluidic technology, however these methods have limits in terms of scalability and reproducibility. Complexity is further increased by the fact that local immunological and mechanical factors have an impact on vascular integration [78]. Since it supports the survivability of all thick tissue constructs, achieving quick and functional vascularization continues to be one of the defining frontiers of tissue engineering.

5.8.4 Mechanical Strength vs. Biocompatibility Trade-Offs

A recurring design conundrum is striking a balance between biocompatibility and mechanical strength. Scaffolds must encourage cell adhesion, proliferation, and remodeling while simultaneously offering enough mechanical support to endure physiological stressors. However, highly biocompatible natural polymers typically lack mechanical robustness, whereas mechanically strong materials, including metals and some ceramics, are frequently bioinert and rigid. For example, titanium alloys have limited degradability and weak bioactivity, yet they have an excellent load-bearing capacity for orthopedic applications. On the other hand, scaffolds based on collagen and gelatin promote cell attachment and the deposition of extracellular matrix (ECM), but they are weak mechanically and quickly degrade. Although PCL-collagen blends and other hybrid composites that include natural and synthetic materials try to close this gap, it is still difficult to maximize their interfacial bonding and degrading uniformity [79].

Furthermore, stress shielding or micromotion at the interface due to mechanical incompatibilities between the native tissue and the implant might result in inflammation or implant failure. Although scaffold architecture may now be more precisely controlled to customize stiffness and elasticity thanks to additive manufacturing, real biomimetic mechanical performance that dynamically adjusts to tissue remodeling is still a goal.

5.8.5 *Regulatory Hurdles and Clinical Translation Challenges*

Translational and regulatory constraints obstruct the path from laboratory discovery to clinical application. Because biomaterial-based therapies frequently incorporate cells, scaffolds, and bioactive chemicals, they are categorized as combination goods that are subject to several regulatory frameworks (e.g., FDA, EMA). As a result, they occupy a complex regulatory space. Extensive in vitro and in vivo testing for biocompatibility, toxicity, and long-term performance is necessary for preclinical validation, and this can be costly and time-consuming. Widespread adoption may be delayed even after approval because of variations in long-term safety data and patient outcomes. International commercialization is further complicated by variations in regional regulatory constraints and ethical considerations.

The inability to replicate biological variability in preclinical models and the absence of uniform testing procedures further impede clinical translation. Transparency, traceability, and ethical sourcing of biological materials are being emphasized by regulatory authorities more and more, which makes the development pipeline more complicated [80]. Accelerating safe and efficient clinical adoption requires the establishment of standardized international protocols for biomaterials evaluation.

5.8.6 *Scalability and Reproducibility of Complex Biomaterial Scaffolds*

Achieving the scalability and reproducibility of complex biomaterial scaffolds is another significant obstacle in the research. Although laboratory-scale fabrication techniques like electrospinning, freeze-drying, and bioprinting yield outstanding small-scale structures, they are challenging to scale up for mass production without sacrificing functionality or accuracy. Pore structure, rate of degradation, and mechanical strength can all be strongly impacted by batch-to-batch variations in raw materials, processing parameters, and crosslinking chemistry [4]. Additionally, preserving sterility, viability, and regulatory compliance during large-scale manufacturing becomes more difficult when living cells or bioactive chemicals are added.

Automated biomanufacturing and Good Manufacturing Practice (GMP)-compliant bioprinting technologies are emerging options, but they remain pricey and technically demanding. Furthermore, problems with reproducibility can arise in preclinical research; differences within labs can obfuscate important comparisons and impede advancement. For next-generation biomaterial scaffolds to be widely used in clinical settings, these scaling and standardization issues must be resolved.

Tissue engineering presents several difficulties and constraints, from basic material–biological interactions to extensive production and regulatory monitoring. Managing immunological reactions, attaining vascularization in big structures, coordinating scaffold degradation with tissue growth, and striking a balance between mechanical performance and biocompatibility are all unresolved scientific and engineering issues. Clinical adoption is further delayed outside of the lab by manufacturing and translational obstacles. It will take integrative, multidisciplinary approaches that incorporate systems biology, bioengineering, materials science, and regulatory innovation to overcome these challenges. To close the gap between experimental promise and therapeutic reality, the ultimate goal is to develop dynamic, adaptable biomaterials that not only satisfy biological demands but also achieve consistency, safety, and scalability in clinical use [81, 82].

5.9 Future Directions

Biomaterials used in tissue engineering and wound healing are heading toward intelligent, flexible, and sustainable systems that can precisely coordinate intricate biological processes. In order to develop next-generation materials that actively interact with the host environment and promote tissue growth, emerging research combines artificial intelligence (AI), computational modeling, immunomodulation, and biofabrication [83]. As the area develops, the focus is moving from static scaffolds to patient-specific, multifunctional, and responsive platforms intended for customized regeneration results.

5.9.1 Integration of AI and Computational Modeling for Scaffold Design Optimization

A paradigm change toward data-driven and predictive tissue engineering is signaled using AI and computational modeling into the creation of biomaterials. Empirical testing, which can be time- and resource-intensive, is a major component of traditional scaffold design. However, before scaffolds are made, mechanical, biological, and mass transport behaviors can be simulated using computer models such as finite element analysis (FEA), computational fluid dynamics (CFD), and agent-based modeling.

Large datasets can be analyzed using AI-driven design techniques, such as machine learning and generative design tools, to optimize scaffold properties including stiffness, diffusion paths, pore geometry, and degradation rate. AI makes it possible to quickly identify design combinations that optimize mechanical integrity, nutrient delivery, and cell viability by establishing a correlation between material qualities and biological performance. For example, based on topological properties, deep learning frameworks have been used to forecast tissue ingrowth and cell migration within 3D-printed objects. Furthermore, in silico testing of scaffold performance under physiological conditions is made possible by digital twins, which are virtual replicas of patient-specific tissues. This reduces experimental errors and speeds up clinical translation. By creating precisely constructed scaffolds that meet mechanical and biological requirements, this computational integration is anticipated to transform regenerative medicine and drastically shorten the time between concept and clinical implementation [84].

5.9.2 Development of Multifunctional, Smart Biomaterials for Dynamic Tissue Repair

Biomaterials of the future will develop into multipurpose intelligent systems that can perceive, react, and adjust to their physiological surroundings. Instead of acting as passive templates, these materials actively contribute to tissue restoration by combining biochemical, mechanical, and electrical responsiveness. For instance, stimuli-responsive hydrogels can react to particular environmental cues like pH, temperature, or enzyme activity by releasing growth nutrients or medications. Biosensing components that identify inflammation or infection and automatically initiate therapeutic reactions might be incorporated into the next generation of these materials. Additionally, electroactive tissue regeneration, particularly for brain and heart repair, can be facilitated by combining conductive polymers and piezoelectric materials [85].

Incorporating antibacterial, antioxidant, and angiogenic qualities into a single material system is another example of multifunctionality that speeds up healing and minimizes problems. It is possible to create hybrid composites that imitate the multi-scale structure of real tissues by combining nanoparticles, bioactive ceramics, and polymers to provide hierarchical activity. By enabling real-time adaptation in intricate physiological contexts, these dynamic, intelligent biomaterials will close the gap between artificial materials and live systems.

5.9.3 Immunomodulatory Scaffolds for Personalized Regenerative Therapy

The emphasis has turned to immunomodulatory biomaterials intended to actively direct host immune responses as a result of a better knowledge of the immune system's function in tissue regeneration [86]. These scaffolds seek to coordinate immune signals to encourage positive tissue integration and remodeling rather than inhibit immunity. In order to control macrophage polarization and promote a transition from the pro-inflammatory (M1) to the pro-regenerative (M2) phenotype, future immunomodulatory scaffolds will be developed. Surface-immobilized peptides, extracellular vesicles, or cytokine-mimetic compounds can be used to guide the activation and recruitment of immune cells. Materials functionalized with transforming growth factor-beta (TGF-β) or interleukin-4 (IL-4) have demonstrated potential in fostering regenerative immunological settings.

Patient-specific immune profile will probably be used in personalized immunomodulation to enable scaffold compositions that are customized to each patient's immunological status. By combining bioinformatics and AI-driven analytics, immunotherapeutic approaches may be further improved, guaranteeing maximum biocompatibility and a lower risk of fibrosis or chronic inflammation. With the help of these developments, biomaterials will become active immune mediators that support integration and tolerance in customized regenerative medicine.

5.9.4 Advanced Vascularization Strategies for Large Tissue Constructs

Vascularization of large metabolically demanding structures continues to be one of the most persistent issues in tissue engineering. The development of pre-vascularized networks that can quickly anastomose with host vasculature after implantation will be the focus of future strategies. Vascularized scaffolds with spatially ordered capillary channels are being created by combining techniques including angiogenic factor gradients, endothelial cell bioprinting, and microfluidic patterning. Furthermore, angiogenic nanoparticles and oxygen-releasing materials are being created to support cells throughout the crucial pre-vascularization phase.

Vascular organoids, which are tiny, self-assembling networks of vessels made from stem cells, are a breakthrough in the in vitro construction of perfusable tissues. By combining computational fluid dynamics with these biological techniques, nutrient flow and shear stress may be optimized, guaranteeing physiological function [87]. One of the main obstacles in regenerative medicine will be addressed when these vascularization technologies advance and make it possible to create therapeutically relevant tissues including the liver, myocardium, and skeletal muscle.

5.9.5 *Sustainable and Biodegradable Biomaterials for Eco-Friendly Regenerative Medicine*

Sustainability has become a crucial factor in the creation of biomaterials. Synthetic polymer manufacturing and disposal frequently use non-renewable resources and produce waste for the environment. Future developments will likely focus on environmentally benign, biodegradable biomaterials made from renewable resources such marine biopolymers, bacterial cellulose, and plant polysaccharides. Green chemistry techniques are being used to reduce the amount of energy, solvents, and hazardous byproducts produced during synthesis. Furthermore, biodegradable composites can be designed to break down into innocuous metabolites, obviating the necessity for surgical excision. Sustainable biomaterials ensure that regenerative medicine develops without compromising the environment by encouraging environmental stewardship and adhering to the circular bioeconomy's tenets.

These materials are particularly relevant for low-resource settings, where cost-effective, sustainable solutions can democratize access to advanced wound and tissue therapies.

5.9.6 *Synergy Between Biomaterials, Stem Cells, and Gene Therapy Approaches*

One of the most exciting areas of regenerative medicine is the intersection of gene therapy, stem cell biology, and biomaterials. These days, biomaterial scaffolds improve stem cell survival, differentiation, and integration by acting as microenvironmental regulators and delivery systems. Cell behavior can be controlled both spatially and biochemically by encasing stem cells or genetically modified cells in biomaterial matrices. Additionally, scaffolds can be designed to transport viral vectors, CRISPR-Cas9 systems, or nucleic acids, facilitating endogenous repair pathways and enabling localized gene regulation [88].

Precision regenerative medicine is made possible by this synergistic triangle, in which gene therapy provides molecular control, stem cells offer regenerative potential, and biomaterials provide structure. For instance, vascular endothelial growth factor (VEGF) plasmids delivered by gene-activated scaffolds can promote tissue remodeling and angiogenesis at the same time. Real-time feedback methods via biosensors will probably be incorporated into future systems, enabling adaptive control of gene expression in situ. Integration, intelligence, and sustainability determine the future paths of biomaterials research. A new era of regenerative medicine is being ushered in by AI-driven design, intelligent multifunctional systems, immunomodulatory scaffolds, sophisticated vascularization techniques, and environmentally friendly materials. The sector is ready to move from passive tissue replacement to active, customized, and sustained tissue regeneration by combining biomaterials with stem cell and gene therapy technologies [89]. This will change clinical outcomes as well as the paradigms of healthcare around the world.

5.10 Conclusion

5.10.1 Summary of Biomaterials' Role in Tissue Engineering and Wound Healing

Since they offer the structural and biochemical foundation required to preserve, enhance, or restore tissue function, biomaterials have become the mainstay of contemporary tissue engineering and wound healing. Regenerative medicine has evolved from a theoretical area to a therapeutically significant subject thanks to their development from inert synthetic polymers to bioactive and cleverly constructed scaffolds. Biomaterials like hydrogels, bioengineered skin substitutes, and nanocomposites have shown promise in wound healing by delivering therapeutic compounds that speed tissue repair, promoting cell migration, and maintaining moist conditions. Biomaterial scaffolds serve as transient extracellular matrix (ECM) analogs in more general tissue engineering applications, promoting angiogenesis and ECM deposition while promoting cell adhesion, proliferation, and differentiation.

Their ability to integrate biological, chemical, and physical stimuli that replicates the dynamic milieu of native tissues is what makes them successful. For instance, bone, cartilage, and vascular tissues have been rebuilt using polymeric matrices and bio-ceramic scaffolds with progressively more biomimetic structures. Furthermore, the development of biofabrication and additive manufacturing technology has made it possible to precisely tailor pore size, mechanical strength, and degradation kinetics, matching scaffold features to the unique functional requirements of various tissues. Altogether, biomaterials have changed the paradigm of tissue repair and regeneration by evolving from passive fillers to active players in the healing process that can perceive, react, and adjust to biological cues.

5.10.2 Emphasis on Design Strategies Integrating Biocompatibility, Degradation, and Bioactivity

The comprehensive integration of biocompatibility, degradation behavior, and bioactivity three interdependent factors that together determine scaffold performance are key to the future of biomaterials. Materials that are biocompatible are guaranteed to provide the right biological reactions without producing harmful or toxic side effects. However, to retain mechanical support and room for the development of new tissue during the healing process, degradation needs to be carefully regulated to correspond with the kinetics of tissue regeneration. A further dimension is added by bioactivity, which makes it possible for scaffolds to behave as biofunctional systems that can provide growth factors, regulate immunological responses, and direct cell destiny decisions in addition to passive frameworks.

The structural and chemical complexity of the natural extracellular matrix (ECM) acts as a blueprint for design tactics that are increasingly informed by biomimetic and bioinspired principles. To improve protein adsorption and integrin-mediated cell attachment, methods like surface functionalization, peptide grafting, and nanoscale topographical patterning have been used. Stimuli-responsive materials, on the other hand, provide dynamic control over degradation and release patterns by changing their characteristics in response to mechanical stress, enzyme activity, or pH.

Furthermore, scaffold design is being redefined by the combination of artificial intelligence (AI) and computer modeling, which enables predictive simulations of mechanical performance, cell-material interactions, and degradation kinetics. By reducing trial-and-error testing, these data-driven methods speed up the creation of customized biomaterials with ideal performance profiles for certain tissue types and patient groups. The combination of these design approaches signifies a change from static biomaterials to systems that are adaptable and functionally synergistic, able to coordinate the many biological mechanisms that underlie tissue regeneration.

5.10.3 Recognition of Recent Innovations and Interdisciplinary Approaches Driving Regenerative Medicine

Interdisciplinary cooperation across materials science, bioengineering, molecular biology, and clinical medicine provides the foundation for the quick advancement in regenerative medicine. Recent developments demonstrate how these cooperative efforts can have a transformational effect. By producing patient-specific scaffolds with microscale accuracy, 3D bioprinting and biofabrication technologies have made it easier to arrange cells, biomolecules, and other materials spatially to create architecturally intricate tissue structures. Nanotechnology breakthroughs have created multipurpose scaffolds that combine real-time biosensing, tailored medication delivery, and mechanical reinforcement.

Furthermore, the therapeutic landscape is growing thanks to intelligent and responsive biomaterials that may change their characteristics in reaction to external stimuli. These include immunomodulatory scaffolds that guide host immune responses toward pro-regenerative pathways, electrically conductive hydrogels for brain and cardiac regeneration, and shape-memory polymers for dynamic tissue interfaces. The distinction between natural and synthetic materials is further blurred using bioprintable hydrogels, nanofibrous composites, and decellularized matrices in hybrid systems, which result in scaffolds that are mechanically durable, biocompatible, and physiologically instructive.

The transfer of bench side innovation to bedside use is also being propelled by interdisciplinary research. To overcome manufacturing, scalability, and regulatory obstacles, academic labs, physicians, and industry must form collaborative networks. Successful clinical uses such vascular conduits, osteogenic implants, and bioengineered skin grafts have resulted from these collaborations. A new era in regenerative healthcare is being ushered in by the ongoing feedback between basic science and clinical practice, which is promoting the creation of next-generation biomaterials that can both replace damaged tissues and stimulate endogenous repair mechanisms.

5.10.4 Outlook on the Evolution Toward Adaptive, Patient-Specific, and Multifunctional Biomaterials for Clinical Translation

The direction of biomaterials research indicates that multifunctional, patient-specific, and adaptable systems for customized regenerative medicine will be developed in the future. Advanced biomaterial design combined with precision medicine concepts will allow scaffolds to be tailored to the biological, genetic, and biomechanical characteristics of individual patients. Individualized treatment plans that reduce immunological rejection and maximize functional results will be possible because to technologies like 3D bioprinting using patient-derived cells and computer modeling of tissue–material interactions.

Multifunctionality at several scales combining mechanical reinforcement, immunomodulation, drug administration, and biosensing in a single construct is probably going to be a feature of the future generation of biomaterials. For example, bioactive coatings may release signaling molecules in response to biological signals, and scaffolds embedded with nanosensors may offer real-time input on tissue repair. Additionally, sustainability and environmentally sensitive design will become more popular, supporting renewable and biodegradable materials that reduce environmental effect while upholding high clinical performance standards.

The development of intelligent biomaterials that not only blend in perfectly with the host environment but also change dynamically with it is ultimately what will determine the future of tissue engineering. These materials will help regenerative medicine progress from restorative therapies to truly regenerative solutions by bridging the gap between artificial structures and living systems. Biomaterials will continue to provide the essential foundation for the clinical realization of the goal of customized, flexible, and sustainable tissue regeneration as interdisciplinary cooperation deepens and computational and manufacturing technologies advance.

References

1. Kantaros, A., Ganetsos, T.: From static to dynamic: smart materials pioneering additive manufacturing in regenerative medicine. Int. J. Mol. Sci. **24**(21), 15748 (2023)
2. Wei, H., Cui, J., Lin, K., Xie, J., Wang, X.: Recent advances in smart stimuli-responsive biomaterials for bone therapeutics and regeneration. Bone Res. **10**(1), 17 (2022)
3. Koch, S.M., Goldhahn, C., Müller, F.J., Yan, W., Pilz-Allen, C., Bidan, C.M., Ciabattoni, B., Stricker, L., Fratzl, P., Keplinger, T., Burgert, I.: Anisotropic wood-hydrogel composites: extending mechanical properties of wood towards soft materials' applications. Mater. Today Bio. **22**, 100772 (2023)
4. Li, J., Fleetwood, J., Hawley, W.B., Kays, W.: From materials to cell: state-of-the-art and prospective technologies for lithium-ion battery electrode processing. Chem. Rev. **122**(1), 903–956 (2021)
5. Shokrollahi, P., Omidi, Y., Cubeddu, L.X., Omidian, H.: Conductive polymers for cardiac tissue engineering and regeneration. J. Biomed. Mater. Res. B Appl. Biomater. **111**(11), 1979–1995 (2023)
6. Zhang, Y., Mu, W., Zhang, Y., He, X., Wang, Y., Ma, H., Zhu, T., Li, A., Hou, Q., Yang, W., Ding, Y.: Recent advances in cardiac patches: materials, preparations, and properties. ACS Biomater. Sci. Eng. **8**(9), 3659–3675 (2022)
7. Su, L., Jia, Y., Fu, L., Guo, K., Xie, S.: The emerging progress on wound dressings and their application in clinic wound management. Heliyon. **9**(12), e22520 (2023)
8. Tiwari, R., Pathak, K.: Local drug delivery strategies towards wound healing. Pharmaceutics. **15**(2), 634 (2023)
9. Kumar, V.B., Tiwari, O.S., Finkelstein-Zuta, G., Rencus-Lazar, S., Gazit, E.: Design of functional RGD peptide-based biomaterials for tissue engineering. Pharmaceutics. **15**(2), 345 (2023)
10. Ludwig, B.S., Kessler, H., Kossatz, S., Reuning, U.: RGD-binding integrins revisited: how recently discovered functions and novel synthetic ligands (re-)shape an ever-evolving field. Cancer. **13**(7), 1711 (2021)
11. Lv, B., Zhang, X., Yuan, J., Chen, Y., Ding, H., Cao, X., Huang, A.: Biomaterial-supported MSC transplantation enhances cell–cell communication for spinal cord injury. Stem Cell Res. Ther. **12**(1), 36 (2021)
12. Wong, J.K.U., Mehta, A., Vũ, T.T., Yeo, G.C.: Cellular modifications and biomaterial design to improve mesenchymal stem cell transplantation. Biomater. Sci. **11**(14), 4752–4773 (2023)
13. Daneshmandi, L., Barajaa, M., Tahmasbi Rad, A., Sydlik, S.A., Laurencin, C.T.: Graphene-based biomaterials for bone regenerative engineering: a comprehensive review of the field and considerations regarding biocompatibility and biodegradation. Adv. Healthc. Mater. **10**(1), 2001414 (2021)
14. Kim, H.S., Kumbar, S.G., Nukavarapu, S.P.: Biomaterial-directed cell behavior for tissue engineering. Curr. Opin. Biomed. Eng. **17**, 100260 (2021)
15. Todros, S., Todesco, M., Bagno, A.: Biomaterials and their biomedical applications: from replacement to regeneration. Processes. **9**(11), 1949 (2021)
16. Ashammakhi, N., GhavamiNejad, A., Tutar, R., Fricker, A., Roy, I., Chatzistavrou, X., Hoque Apu, E., Nguyen, K.L., Ahsan, T., Pountos, I., Caterson, E.J.: Highlights on advancing frontiers in tissue engineering. Tissue Eng. Part B Rev. **28**(3), 633–664 (2022)
17. Dashnau, J.L., Xue, Q., Nelson, M., Law, E., Cao, L., Hei, D.: A risk-based approach for cell line development, manufacturing and characterization of genetically engineered, induced pluripotent stem cell–derived allogeneic cell therapies. Cytotherapy. **25**(1), 1–13 (2023)
18. Marinkovic, M., Tran, O.N., Wang, H., Abdul-Azees, P., Dean, D.D., Chen, X.D., Yeh, C.K.: Autologous mesenchymal stem cells offer a new paradigm for salivary gland regeneration. Int. J. Oral Sci. **15**(1), 18 (2023)

19. Amirrah, I.N., Lokanathan, Y., Zulkiflee, I., Wee, M.M.R., Motta, A., Fauzi, M.B.: A comprehensive review on collagen type I development of biomaterials for tissue engineering: from biosynthesis to bioscaffold. Biomedicine. **10**(9), 2307 (2022)
20. Dzobo, K., Dandara, C.: The extracellular matrix: its composition, function, remodeling, and role in tumorigenesis. Biomimetics. **8**(2), 146 (2023)
21. Xu, C., Sun, Y., Jansen, J., Li, M., Wei, L., Wu, Y., Liu, Y.: Calcium phosphate ceramics and synergistic bioactive agents for osteogenesis in implant dentistry. Tissue Eng. Part C Methods. **29**(5), 197–215 (2023)
22. Abolhasani, S., Ahmadi, Y., Rostami, Y., Baravar, E., Fattahi, D.: Biomaterials in tissue repair and regeneration: key insights from extracellular matrix biology. Front. Med. Technol. **7**, 1565810 (2025). https://doi.org/10.3389/fmedt.2025.1565810
23. Serafin, A., Culebras, M., Collins, M.N.: Synthesis and evaluation of alginate, gelatin, and hyaluronic acid hybrid hydrogels for tissue engineering applications. Int. J. Biol. Macromol. **233**, 123438 (2023)
24. Nitti, P., Narayanan, A., Pellegrino, R., Villani, S., Madaghiele, M., Demitri, C.: Cell-tissue interaction: the biomimetic approach to design tissue engineered biomaterials. Bioengineering. **10**(10), 1122 (2023)
25. Paul, O., Tao, J.Q., Guo, X., Chatterjee, S.: The vascular system: components, signaling, and regulation. In: Endothelial Signaling in Vascular Dysfunction and Disease, pp. 3–13. Elsevier (2021)
26. Choi, J., Lee, E.J., Jang, W.B., Kwon, S.M.: Development of biocompatible 3D-printed artificial blood vessels through multidimensional approaches. J. Funct. Biomater. **14**(10), 497 (2023)
27. Mohammadi, A.T., Ghanbarzadeh, E., Darestani, N.G., Nouri, M., Rasoulzadehzali, M., Moghadamnia, M., Nazarizadeh, S., Nahavandi, R., Jahedi, M.: Advancements in Medical Science and the Pharmaceutical Industry: Artificial Intelligence in Medicine, Regenerative Medicine and Stem Cells, New Developments in Pharmaceuticals (Nano Drugs). Nobel Sciences (2023)
28. Samrot, A.V., Abubakar Mohamed, A., Faradjeva, E., Si Jie, L., Hooi Sze, C., Arif, A., Chuan Sean, T., Norbert Michael, E., Yeok Mun, C., Xiao Qi, N., Ling Mok, P.: Mechanisms and impact of biofilms and targeting of biofilms using bioactive compounds—a review. Medicina. **57**(8), 839 (2021)
29. Yoon, S.K., Chung, D.J.: In vivo degradation studies of PGA-PLA block copolymer and their histochemical analysis for spinal-fixing application. Polymers. **14**(16), 3322 (2022)
30. Archer, E., Torretti, M., Madbouly, S.: Biodegradable polycaprolactone (PCL) based polymer and composites. Phys. Sci. Rev. **8**(11), 4391–4414 (2023)
31. Naseem, R., Tzivelekis, C., German, M.J., Gentile, P., Ferreira, A.M., Dalgarno, K.: Strategies for enhancing polyester-based materials for bone fixation applications. Molecules. **26**(4), 992 (2021)
32. Arefin, A.M., Khatri, N.R., Kulkarni, N., Egan, P.F.: Polymer 3D printing review: materials, process, and design strategies for medical applications. Polymers. **13**(9), 1499 (2021)
33. Abbas, Z., Dapporto, M., Tampieri, A., Sprio, S.: Toughening of bioceramic composites for bone regeneration. J. Compos. Sci. **5**(10), 259 (2021)
34. Vaiani, L., Boccaccio, A., Uva, A.E., Palumbo, G., Piccininni, A., Guglielmi, P., Cantore, S., Santacroce, L., Charitos, I.A., Ballini, A.: Ceramic materials for biomedical applications: an overview on properties and fabrication processes. J. Funct. Biomater. **14**(3), 146 (2023)
35. Karmakar, R., Dey, S., Alam, A., Khandelwal, M., Pati, F., Rengan, A.K.: Attributes of nanomaterials and nanotopographies for improved bone tissue engineering and regeneration. ACS Appl. Bio Mater. **6**(10), 4020–4041 (2023)
36. Lebaudy, E., Fournel, S., Lavalle, P., Vrana, N.E., Gribova, V.: Recent advances in antiinflammatory material design. Adv. Healthc. Mater. **10**(1), 2001373 (2021)

37. Kumari, S., Katiyar, S., Darshna, Anand, A., Singh, D., Singh, B.N., Mallick, S.P., Mishra, A., Srivastava, P.: Design strategies for composite matrix and multifunctional polymeric scaffolds with enhanced bioactivity for bone tissue engineering. Front. Chem. **10**, 1051678 (2022)
38. Ruffini, A., Sandri, M., Dapporto, M., Campodoni, E., Tampieri, A., Sprio, S.: Nature-inspired unconventional approaches to develop 3D bioceramic scaffolds with enhanced regenerative ability. Biomedicine. **9**(8), 916 (2021)
39. Valdoz, J.C., Johnson, B.C., Jacobs, D.J., Franks, N.A., Dodson, E.L., Sanders, C., Cribbs, C.G., Van Ry, P.M.: The ECM: to scaffold, or not to scaffold, that is the question. Int. J. Mol. Sci. **22**(23), 12690 (2021)
40. Guimarães, C.F., Marques, A.P., Reis, R.L.: Pushing the natural frontier: progress on the integration of biomaterial cues toward combinatorial biofabrication and tissue engineering. Adv. Mater. **34**(33), 2105645 (2022)
41. Dolgin, J., Hanumantharao, S.N., Farias, S., Simon Jr., C.G., Rao, S.: Mechanical properties and morphological alterations in fiber-based scaffolds affecting tissue engineering outcomes. Fibers. **11**(5), 39 (2023)
42. Ivanov, A.N., Chabbarov, Y.R.: Mechanisms of physiological angiogenesis. J. Evol. Biochem. Physiol. **59**(3), 914–929 (2023)
43. Mukwaya, A., Jensen, L., Lagali, N.: Relapse of pathological angiogenesis: functional role of the basement membrane and potential treatment strategies. Exp. Mol. Med. **53**(2), 189–201 (2021)
44. Mao, J., Chen, L., Cai, Z., Qian, S., Liu, Z., Zhao, B., Zhang, Y., Sun, X., Cui, W.: Advanced biomaterials for regulating polarization of macrophages in wound healing. Adv. Funct. Mater. **32**(12), 2111003 (2022)
45. Sharma, S., Sudhakara, P., Singh, J., Ilyas, R.A., Asyraf, M.R.M., Razman, M.R.: Critical review of biodegradable and bioactive polymer composites for bone tissue engineering and drug delivery applications. Polymers. **13**(16), 2623 (2021)
46. Zohorsky, K., Mequanint, K.: Designing biomaterials to modulate notch signaling in tissue engineering and regenerative medicine. Tissue Eng. Part B Rev. **27**(5), 383–410 (2021)
47. Jere, D., Sediq, A.S., Huwyler, J., Vollrath, I., Kardorff, M., Mahler, H.C.: Challenges for cell-based medicinal products from a pharmaceutical product perspective. J. Pharm. Sci. **110**(5), 1900–1908 (2021)
48. John, J.V., McCarthy, A., Wang, H., Luo, Z., Li, H., Wang, Z., Cheng, F., Zhang, Y.S., Xie, J.: Freeze-casting with 3D-printed templates creates anisotropic microchannels and patterned macrochannels within biomimetic nanofiber aerogels for rapid cellular infiltration. Adv. Healthc. Mater. **10**(12), 2100238 (2021)
49. Joukhdar, H., Seifert, A., Jüngst, T., Groll, J., Lord, M.S., Rnjak-Kovacina, J.: Ice templating soft matter: fundamental principles and fabrication approaches to tailor pore structure and morphology and their biomedical applications. Adv. Mater. **33**(34), 2100091 (2021)
50. Kabir, M.F., Ju, L.K.: On optimization of enzymatic processes: temperature effects on activity and long-term deactivation kinetics. Process Biochem. **130**, 734–746 (2023)
51. Pardeshi, S., Damiri, F., Zehravi, M., Joshi, R., Kapare, H., Prajapati, M.K., Munot, N., Berrada, M., Giram, P.S., Rojekar, S., Ali, F.: Functional thermoresponsive hydrogel molecule to material design for biomedical applications. Polymers. **14**(15), 3126 (2022)
52. Joyce, K., Fabra, G.T., Bozkurt, Y., Pandit, A.: Bioactive potential of natural biomaterials: identification, retention and assessment of biological properties. Signal Transduct. Target. Ther. **6**(1), 122 (2021)
53. Akbarian, M., Bertassoni, L.E., Tayebi, L.: Biological aspects in controlling angiogenesis: current progress. Cell. Mol. Life Sci. **79**(7), 349 (2022)
54. Naikwadi, A.T., Sharma, B.K., Bhatt, K.D., Mahanwar, P.A.: Gamma radiation processed polymeric materials for high performance applications: a review. Front. Chem. **10**, 837111 (2022)
55. Wang, Z., Wang, X., Xu, W., Li, Y., Lai, R., Qiu, X., Chen, X., Chen, Z., Mi, B., Wu, M., Wang, J.: Translational challenges and prospective solutions in the implementation of biomimetic delivery systems. Pharmaceutics. **15**(11), 2623 (2023)

56. Farag, M.M.: Recent trends on biomaterials for tissue regeneration applications. J. Mater. Sci. **58**(2), 527–558 (2023)
57. Maadani, A.M., Salahinejad, E.: Performance comparison of PLA- and PLGA-coated porous bioceramic scaffolds: mechanical, biodegradability, bioactivity, delivery and biocompatibility assessments. J. Control. Release. **351**, 1–7 (2022)
58. Alessio, N., Stellavato, A., Aprile, D., Cimini, D., Vassallo, V., Di Bernardo, G., Galderisi, U., Schiraldi, C.: Timely supplementation of hydrogels containing sulfated or unsulfated chondroitin and hyaluronic acid affects mesenchymal stromal cells commitment toward chondrogenic differentiation. Front. Cell Dev. Biol. **9**, 641529 (2021)
59. Jia, Y., Le, H., Wang, X., Zhang, J., Liu, Y., Ding, J., Zheng, C., Chang, F.: Double-edged role of mechanical stimuli and underlying mechanisms in cartilage tissue engineering. Front. Bioeng. Biotechnol. **11**, 1271762 (2023)
60. Basara, G., Bahcecioglu, G., Ozcebe, S.G., Ellis, B.W., Ronan, G., Zorlutuna, P.: Myocardial infarction from a tissue engineering and regenerative medicine point of view: a comprehensive review on models and treatments. Biophys. Rev. **3**(3), 031305 (2022)
61. Shabbirahmed, A.M., Sekar, R., Gomez, L.A., Sekhar, M.R., Hiruthyaswamy, S.P., Basavegowda, N., Somu, P.: Recent developments of silk-based scaffolds for tissue engineering and regenerative medicine applications: a special focus on the advancement of 3D printing. Biomimetics. **8**(1), 16 (2023)
62. Vyas, J., Shah, I., Singh, S., Prajapati, B.G.: Biomaterials-based additive manufacturing for customized bioengineering in management of otolaryngology: a comprehensive review. Front. Bioeng. Biotechnol. **11**, 1234340 (2023)
63. Syed, M.B., Ahmed, T.A.E., Hincke, M.T.: The promise of 3D biomaterial bioprinting for wound-healing and skin tissue restoration. Life. **16**(5), 718 (2026). https://doi.org/10.3390/life16050718
64. Shahabipour, F., Tavafoghi, M., Aninwene, G.E., Bonakdar, S., Oskuee, R.K., Shokrgozar, M.A., Potyondy, T., Alambeigi, F., Ahadian, S.: Coaxial 3D bioprinting of tri-polymer scaffolds to improve the osteogenic and vasculogenic potential of cells in co-culture models. J. Biomed. Mater. Res. A. **110**(5), 1077–1089 (2022)
65. Andrade, F., Roca-Melendres, M.M., Durán-Lara, E.F., Rafael, D., Schwartz Jr., S.: Stimuli-responsive hydrogels for cancer treatment: the role of pH, light, ionic strength and magnetic field. Cancer. **13**(5), 1164 (2021)
66. Weng, T., Zhang, L., Liu, Y., Zhao, X., Yue, X.: Advances in tissue engineering and biomaterials for minimizing wound scarring: current status and future challenges. J. Funct. Biomater. **17**(1), 3 (2026). https://doi.org/10.3390/jfb17010003
67. Minehan, R.L., Del Borgo, M.P.: Controlled release of therapeutics from enzyme-responsive biomaterials. Front. Biomater. Sci. **1**, 916985 (2022)
68. Zhou, X., Feng, Z., Liu, P., Song, Y., Shakir, I., Sun, X., et al.: Mechanisms of MOF-based biomaterials in skin wound healing: antibacterial, immunomodulatory, angiogenic, and neurogenic effects. Adv. Healthc. Mater. **15**(11), e03944 (2026)
69. Abbasi, R., Shineh, G., Mobaraki, M., Doughty, S., Tayebi, L.: Structural parameters of nanoparticles affecting their toxicity for biomedical applications: a review. J. Nanopart. Res. **25**(3), 43 (2023)
70. Bretherton, R.C., Haack, A.J., Kopyeva, I., Rahman, F., Kern, J.D., Bugg, D., Theberge, A.B., Davis, J., DeForest, C.A.: User-controlled 4D biomaterial degradation with substrate-selective sortase transpeptidases for single-cell biology. Adv. Mater. **35**(19), 2209904 (2023)
71. Rizzo, F., Kehr, N.S.: Recent advances in injectable hydrogels for controlled and local drug delivery. Adv. Healthc. Mater. **10**(1), 2001341 (2021)
72. Alghamdi, M.A., Fallica, A.N., Virzì, N., Kesharwani, P., Pittalà, V., Greish, K.: The promise of nanotechnology in personalized medicine. J. Pers. Med. **12**(5), 673 (2022)
73. Serrano, D.R., Kara, A., Yuste, I., Luciano, F.C., Ongoren, B., Anaya, B.J., Molina, G., Diez, L., Ramirez, B.I., Ramirez, I.O., Sánchez-Guirales, S.A.: 3D printing technologies in personalized medicine, nanomedicines, and biopharmaceuticals. Pharmaceutics. **15**(2), 313 (2023)

74. Pourmasoumi, P., Moghaddam, A., Nemati Mahand, S., Heidari, F., Salehi Moghaddam, Z., Arjmand, M., Kühnert, I., Kruppke, B., Wiesmann, H.P., Khonakdar, H.A.: A review on the recent progress, opportunities, and challenges of 4D printing and bioprinting in regenerative medicine. J. Biomater. Sci. Polym. Ed. **34**(1), 108–146 (2023)
75. Ansari, M.A.A., Golebiowska, A.A., Dash, M., Kumar, P., Jain, P.K., Nukavarapu, S.P., Ramakrishna, S., Nanda, H.S.: Engineering biomaterials to 3D-print scaffolds for bone regeneration: practical and theoretical consideration. Biomater. Sci. **10**(11), 2789–2816 (2022)
76. Lou, J., Mooney, D.J.: Chemical strategies to engineer hydrogels for cell culture. Nat. Rev. Chem. **6**(10), 726–744 (2022)
77. Capuani, S., Malgir, G., Chua, C.Y.X., Grattoni, A.: Advanced strategies to thwart foreign body response to implantable devices. Bioeng. Transl. Med. **7**(3), e10300 (2022)
78. O'Connor, C., Brady, E., Zheng, Y., Moore, E., Stevens, K.R.: Engineering the multiscale complexity of vascular networks. Nat. Rev. Mater. **7**(9), 702–716 (2022)
79. Kazemzadeh, G., Jirofti, N., Kazemi Mehrjerdi, H., Rajabioun, M., Alamdaran, S.A., Mohebbi-Kalhori, D., Mirbagheri, M.S., Taheri, R.: A review on developments of in-vitro and in-vivo evaluation of hybrid PCL-based natural polymers nanofibers scaffolds for vascular tissue engineering. J. Ind. Text. **52**, 15280837221128314 (2022)
80. Trump, B., Cummings, C., Klasa, K., Galaitsi, S., Linkov, I.: Governing biotechnology to provide safety and security and address ethical, legal, and social implications. Front. Genet. **13**, 1052371 (2023)
81. Chekroud, A.M., Bondar, J., Delgadillo, J., Doherty, G., Wasil, A., Fokkema, M., Cohen, Z., Belgrave, D., DeRubeis, R., Iniesta, R., Dwyer, D.: The promise of machine learning in predicting treatment outcomes in psychiatry. World Psychiatry. **20**(2), 154–170 (2021)
82. Coppersmith, D.D., Dempsey, W., Kleiman, E.M., Bentley, K.H., Murphy, S.A., Nock, M.K.: Just-in-time adaptive interventions for suicide prevention: promise, challenges, and future directions. Psychiatry. **85**(4), 317–333 (2022)
83. Hayat, H., Nukala, A., Nyamira, A., Fan, J., Wang, P.: A concise review: the synergy between artificial intelligence and biomedical nanomaterials that empowers nanomedicine. Biomed. Mater. **16**(5), 052001 (2021)
84. Srivastava, S.: Integrating Computational Modeling and Biological Data for Predictive Analysis of Tissue Engineering Outcomes: A Review. SSRN 4951069 (2022)
85. Liu, Z., Wan, X., Wang, Z.L., Li, L.: Electroactive biomaterials and systems for cell fate determination and tissue regeneration: design and applications. Adv. Mater. **33**(32), 2007429 (2021)
86. Whitaker, R., Hernaez-Estrada, B., Hernandez, R.M., Santos-Vizcaino, E., Spiller, K.L.: Immunomodulatory biomaterials for tissue repair. Chem. Rev. **121**(18), 11305–11335 (2021)
87. Omar, A.M., Hassan, M.H., Daskalakis, E., Ates, G., Bright, C.J., Xu, Z., Powell, E.J., Mirihanage, W., Bartolo, P.J.: Geometry-based computational fluid dynamic model for predicting the biological behavior of bone tissue engineering scaffolds. J. Funct. Biomater. **13**(3), 104 (2022)
88. Iqbal, Z., Rehman, K., Xia, J., Shabbir, M., Zaman, M., Liang, Y., Duan, L.: Biomaterial-assisted targeted and controlled delivery of CRISPR/Cas9 for precise gene editing. Biomater. Sci. **11**(11), 3762–3783 (2023)
89. Ławkowska, K., Rosenbaum, C., Petrasz, P., Kluth, L., Koper, K., Drewa, T., Pokrywczynska, M., Adamowicz, J., Trauma and Reconstructive Urology Working Party of the European Association of Urology Young Academic Urologists: Tissue engineering in reconstructive urology—the current status and critical insights to set future directions—critical review. Front. Bioeng. Biotechnol. **10**, 1040987 (2023)

Chapter 6
Drug Delivery Systems and Biosensors

Abstract Biosensors and drug delivery systems are two quickly developing fields at the nexus of biomedical engineering, nanotechnology, and biomaterials research. Both aim to improve diagnostic sensitivity and treatment precision, tackling important issues in real-time health monitoring and personalized medicine. Polymers, liposomes, hydrogels, and nanoparticles are examples of engineered carriers that are used in drug delivery systems to administer therapeutic compounds in a sustained, targeted, and regulated way. These systems enhance drug bioavailability, reduce systemic toxicity, and allow localized treatment through processes like diffusion, degradation, and environmental responsiveness. In order to match therapy with changing physiological demands, recent advancements in stimulus-responsive and intelligent delivery systems enable on-demand release that is triggered by pH, temperature, enzyme activity, or external inputs like magnetic or light stimuli. The detection of biomarkers, pathogens, or metabolic analytes with high specificity and sensitivity is made possible by biosensors, which are analytical tools that transform biological recognition events into quantifiable signals. Contemporary biosensors combine transducers based on electrochemical, optical, or piezoelectric principles with biorecognition components (enzymes, antibodies, and nucleic acids). By boosting surface area, electron transfer efficiency, and biostability, the use of nanomaterials and biocompatible polymers has greatly improved sensor performance. Real-time early disease detection and ongoing health monitoring have been made possible by the combination of biosensors with wearable and implantable technology. Current developments place a strong emphasis on combining drug delivery and biosensing capabilities into cohesive "theranostic" platforms that can perform feedback-controlled drug release, targeted therapy, and diagnosis all at once. These hybrid systems use micro/nanofabrication and artificial intelligence (AI) to provide precision control, customization, and flexibility. The basic ideas, material design approaches, mechanisms, and translational applications of these systems are examined, highlighting their revolutionary potential in next-generation healthcare, where intelligent, responsive biomaterials combine diagnostics and therapy to produce genuinely customized, adaptable medical solutions.

M. Adeoba, T. Pandelani, *Application of Biomaterials in Biomedical Engineering*, Series in BioEngineering,
https://doi.org/10.1007/978-3-032-34477-9_6

6.1 Introduction

Biomaterials have transformed medicine by offering advanced platforms for the localized, regulated, and long-term administration of medicinal substances. Systemic toxicity and unsatisfactory efficacy might result from the limits of traditional drug delivery techniques, such as oral or systemic injection, which include quick clearance, poor bioavailability, and non-specific distribution [1, 2]. To address these issues, biomaterial-based drug delivery systems (DDS) modify the physicochemical characteristics of materials to control biodistribution and drug release kinetics. Therapeutic agents ranging from tiny molecules to proteins, nucleic acids, and even living cells can be encapsulated in these systems using polymers, liposomes, hydrogels, dendrimers, micelles, and inorganic nanoparticles. The development of intelligent and stimulus-responsive delivery systems that coordinate therapeutic release with the body's needs has been further advanced by biomaterials' capacity to react to physiological stimuli, such as pH, temperature, redox gradients, or enzyme activity. Biomaterial platforms are now crucial instruments for attaining spatiotemporal control of drug administration, which eventually improves therapeutic precision and patient outcomes [3]. This is achieved by precise engineering of degradation rates, porosity, and surface chemistry.

6.1.1 Role of Biosensors in Real-Time Monitoring of Physiological and Biochemical Parameters

Biosensors provide a continuous and quantitative evaluation of biological processes, which enhances the controlled medication administration made possible by biomaterials. A biosensor combines a transducer that transforms biological interactions into quantifiable electrical, optical, or mechanical signals with a biorecognition element (such as an enzyme, antibody, nucleic acid, or aptamer). With excellent specificity and sensitivity, these instruments can identify a broad range of analytes, such as glucose, lactate, hormones, cytokines, and disease biomarkers. For instance, electrochemical biosensors are frequently employed in metabolic tracking and glucose monitoring, but optical and piezoelectric biosensors have become popular for identifying cancer biomarkers and infectious pathogens. Biosensors have become smaller due to developments in microfabrication and nanotechnology, which has made it possible to include them into wearable, implantable, and point-of-care diagnostic devices. Biosensors are essential for early disease identification, medication optimization, and ongoing health monitoring, all of which are crucial elements in the shift to preventative and precision medicine by offering real-time, dynamic data on physiological and biochemical states [4]. Wearable biosensors are increasingly integrated into feedback-controlled drug delivery systems for diabetes and oncology [5].

6.1.2 Importance of Integrating Drug Delivery and Sensing Technologies for Personalized Medicine

The combination of biosensors with medication delivery devices is a revolutionary step toward tailored and flexible medicinal treatments. Conventional treatments follow set dosage schedules that don't take into consideration a patient's unique metabolism, disease course, or drug reaction. Closed-loop therapeutic platforms can be designed by combining feedback-controlled drug release devices with biosensors that can track biomarkers or therapeutic efficacy in real time. Recent AI-powered biosensors now enable adaptive dosing in real time, advancing closed-loop therapeutic platforms [6]. By automatically modifying medication dosage in response to physiological data, these systems reduce the risk of under- or over-treatment. In order to replicate pancreas regulation, glucose-responsive insulin delivery systems, for example, use biosensors to measure glucose levels and release insulin only when required. Biosensor-guided chemotherapy systems can accurately regulate drug release within malignant tissues by monitoring signals from the tumor microenvironment, such as pH or enzyme concentrations. In addition to improving treatment effectiveness, this mutually beneficial combination of sensing and administration also lowers side effects, encourages patient adherence, and permits ongoing therapeutic customization. Additionally, these systems are being enhanced by developments in artificial intelligence (AI) and machine learning (ML), which enable adaptive learning and predictive modeling from patient data to maximize therapy outcomes in real time [7, 8]. AI-enhanced biosensors can predict drug release profiles in oncology, optimizing chemotherapy outcomes [9].

6.1.3 Scope of the Chapter Covering Materials, Mechanisms, Applications, and Future Convergence Trends

The combination of biosensors with medication delivery devices is a revolutionary step toward tailored and flexible medicinal treatments. Conventional treatments follow set dosage schedules that don't take into consideration a patient's unique metabolism, disease course, or drug reaction. Closed-loop therapeutic platforms can be designed by combining feedback-controlled drug release devices with biosensors that can track biomarkers or therapeutic efficacy in real time. By automatically modifying medication dosage in response to physiological data, these systems reduce the risk of under- or over-treatment. To emulate pancreatic regulation, glucose-responsive insulin delivery systems utilize biosensors to monitor glucose levels and release insulin solely when necessary [10]. Biosensor-guided chemotherapy systems can accurately regulate drug release within malignant tissues by monitoring signals from the tumor microenvironment, such as pH or enzyme concentrations.

Applications in several biomedical domains, including cancer treatment, diabetes control, cardiovascular care, wound healing, and infectious disease detection, are examined in the following sections. Recent developments will be demonstrated through case studies that show how synthetic biomaterials have improved real-time physiological monitoring and tailored therapy. Current issues that obstruct large-scale clinical translation are also thoroughly evaluated in this chapter, including biocompatibility, long-term stability, signal drift, and regulatory concerns.

Emerging trends in convergence technologies are also highlighted, including theranostic systems, which combine therapeutic and diagnostic capabilities in a single device; bioelectronic medicine, which uses integrated sensors and actuators to modify physiological pathways; and 4D-printed biomaterials, which can adapt dynamically to environmental stimuli [11, 12]. These multidisciplinary developments represent the intelligent, responsive, and biologically integrated systems of the future for precision healthcare.

This chapter offers a thorough examination of biosensors and drug delivery systems as complementary technologies that shape the future of customized medicine. It highlights how the combination of delivery and sensing features can change therapeutic paradigms from reactive treatment models to adaptive, data-driven healthcare systems by linking the fields of material science, bioengineering, and clinical translation. These developments have the potential to transform the relationship between people and medical technology in the age of intelligent biomaterials, in addition to improving efficacy and safety.

6.2 Key Concepts and Definitions

A key concept in contemporary biomedical engineering is the combination of drug delivery systems (DDS) with biosensors, which provide sophisticated instruments for regulated therapeutic delivery and real-time physiological monitoring. For these systems to function effectively, precisely, and safely, molecular interactions and material–biological interfaces must be precisely manipulated. Designing next-generation devices that bridge diagnostics and therapies within the framework of customized and precision medicine requires an understanding of their basic definitions, guiding principles, classifications, and assessment metrics.

6.2.1 Definition of Drug Delivery Systems (DDS)

A drug delivery system (DDS) is a platform designed to deliver therapeutic compounds to body locations in a regulated way, maximizing therapeutic effectiveness and reducing side effects. Systemic exposure, variable plasma levels, and quick clearance are common outcomes of traditional drug delivery [13, 14]. DDSs, on the other hand, seek to regulate the drug release's pace, timing, and spatial distribution.

The term "controlled release" describes the gradual or time-programmed release of medications that are regulated by chemical activation, diffusion, or degradation processes. By employing ligands, antibodies, or nanoparticles that can identify disease indicators to guide medications to certain tissues, cells, or intracellular compartments, targeting improves therapeutic precision. By ensuring that the carrier material interacts favorably with biological systems, biocompatibility helps to prevent toxicity, inflammation, and immunological rejection. Microspheres, hydrogels, liposomes, polymeric nanoparticles, and implantable reservoirs are examples of DDS platforms that are made to preserve the best possible pharmacokinetics and pharmacodynamics. Achieving site-specific, temporally regulated therapy that adjusts to the physiology of the patient is the ultimate objective.

6.2.2 Definition of Biosensors: Biorecognition Element, Transducer, and Signal Processor

An analytical tool known as a biosensor uses biorecognition events to identify and measure biological or chemical components and transforms them into quantifiable signals. The biorecognition element, which oversees the analyte's selective binding, is one of its three main parts. Enzymes, antibodies, cells, nucleic acids, and artificial receptors are a few examples. The biorecognition event (such binding or an enzyme reaction) is transformed into a detectable physical signal via a transducer, usually an electrical, optical, or mechanical signal. Signal processors, which are frequently coupled with digital interfaces for real-time data display, amp up, filter, and transform signals into readable output [15].

Biosensors are integral to diagnostics, environmental monitoring, and drug delivery feedback systems, offering rapid, sensitive, and selective measurements. Their design is guided by specificity (selective recognition), sensitivity (signal strength at low analyte concentrations), and stability under physiological conditions.

6.2.3 Fundamental Principles: Diffusion, Degradation, and Molecular Recognition

Fundamental physicochemical and biological principles underpin the operation and performance of both DDS and biosensors. The passive passage of molecules (such as medications or analytes) across polymers or membranes along a concentration gradient is controlled by diffusion. It affects analyte delivery to the biorecognition interface in biosensors and regulates sustained release kinetics in DDS. The term "degradation" describes how hydrolysis, enzymatic activity, or oxidation breaks down carrier or sensing materials. While material degradation in biosensors can restrict stability or longevity, this process determines the release profile in biodegradable DDS. The selective binding between molecules that guarantee specificity, such as ligand-receptor interactions, enzyme-substrate interactions, or antigen-antibody interactions, is known as molecular recognition [16, 17]. This idea is essential to tailored medication delivery and biosensor selectivity.

These core mechanisms establish the functional basis for precision and reliability, enabling the synchronization of diagnostic feedback and therapeutic action an essential step toward closed-loop medical systems.

6.2.4 Classification of Drug Delivery Systems

Drug delivery Systems (DDSs) can be categorized according to their deployment tactics and release procedures, which represent different degrees of complexity and control; For a long time, sustained-release systems offer consistent and reliable medication delivery. Osmotic pumps, matrix tablets, and polymeric microspheres (like PLGA) are a few examples. They lessen the frequency of doses while maintaining therapeutic levels. In response to environmental signals, such as pH, temperature, enzyme concentration, or glucose levels, responsive-release systems also referred to as stimuli-responsive or smart systems modify drug release [18, 19]. These are essential for conditions like diabetes or cancer that call for dynamic dosing. Long-term drug delivery within the body is the goal of implantable systems. They can be reservoir-based devices that enable programmable or remotely controlled release, microchips, or biodegradable implants.

The transition from passive sustained-release platforms to intelligent, feedback-driven DDSs marks a significant evolution toward autonomous therapeutic regulation. Integration with biosensors enables real-time adaptive dosing, forming the basis of "theranostic" (therapy + diagnostic) systems. Nanoparticle-based theranostic systems combine biosensing and drug delivery in a single platform, enabling simultaneous diagnosis and therapy [20].

6.2.5 Types of Biosensors

Signal transduction mechanisms determine the sensitivity, speed, and application of biosensors and are used to classify them. Electrical signals produced by redox reactions or charge shifts at an electrode interface are measured by electrochemical biosensors. The most well-known example is glucose sensors, which depend on the catalysis of glucose oxidase. They provide wearable device compatibility, great sensitivity, and the possibility of downsizing. When analyte binding occurs, optical biosensors pick up on changes in light characteristics like absorbance, fluorescence, or surface plasmon resonance. They offer label-free, real-time detection, which is helpful for multiplexed experiments and ongoing monitoring. Crystal oscillation frequency alterations brought on by mass variations during analyte binding are exploited by piezoelectric biosensors. They can detect viruses or biomolecules at extremely low quantities because of their strong sensitivity to surface contacts. Rapid, low-sample-volume analysis is made possible by microfluidic biosensors, which combine fluidic channels and sensing components on a microchip. These "lab-on-a-chip" devices integrate drug delivery, processing, and sensing into small, portable packages. The applicability of biosensor platforms in clinical diagnostics, point-of-care monitoring, and intelligent drug delivery integration is improved by their diversity. In line with the objectives of precision health monitoring, the present trend places a strong emphasis on downsizing, wireless data transfer, and multi-analyte detection [21].

6.2.6 Metrics for Evaluation: Drug Release Kinetics, Sensitivity, Selectivity, and Response Time

Evaluating DDSs and biosensors requires quantifiable performance metrics that reflect their efficacy, reliability, and clinical relevance. Drug release kinetics, which are controlled by processes like swelling, degradation, and diffusion, explain how a drug is released over time. Consistent therapeutic concentrations are attained with ideal kinetics, which also prevent burst release and early tiredness. To forecast release behavior, mathematical models (such as Higuchi and Korsmeyer-Peppas) are frequently employed. Sensitivity quantifies a biosensor's capacity to pick up on minute variations in analyte concentration. Even in complicated biological contexts or at trace levels, high sensitivity guarantees precise identification. The ability of the sensor to differentiate the target analyte from chemicals that are structurally similar or interfere with it is measured by its selectivity. Surface engineering and extremely specialized recognition elements are used to accomplish this. Response time, which is important for both biosensors (signal production) and responsive DDSs, shows how soon the system produces a quantifiable or useful output after being exposed to a stimulus [22].

Other important parameters include stability, biocompatibility, and reproducibility, which ensure consistent operation in physiological conditions. Together, these metrics define the clinical feasibility and dependability of integrated diagnostic and treatment systems. Designing next-generation biomedical platforms requires a conceptual understanding of the fundamental ideas and terms underlying drug delivery systems and biosensors. The concepts of regulated, targeted, and biocompatible administration are embodied by DDSs, whereas biosensors, which use biorecognition and transduction, provide precise detection and real-time feedback. Because they both depend on diffusion, degradation, and molecular recognition, they create a common framework for theranostic convergence in which therapy and sensing act in concert. An era of intelligent, adaptive, and patient-centered healthcare technologies that combine monitoring, feedback, and precision-controlled treatment within a single responsive platform is being ushered in by the blurring of the lines between DDSs and biosensors due to advancements in materials science, microfabrication, and computational modeling [23, 24].

6.3 Material Types and Properties

The materials used to manufacture drug delivery systems (DDS) and biosensors have a fundamental impact on their performance as shown in Fig. 6.1. The choice of material determines the device's functional performance, including drug encapsulation, release kinetics, molecular recognition, and signal transduction, in addition to its biocompatibility and stability. A vast range of materials, from lipids and polymers to inorganic nanostructures and responsive hydrogels, have been developed during the past few decades to provide sensitive biochemical detection and accurate therapeutic delivery. An extensive review of these material classes, their inherent characteristics, and their contributions to the development of next-generation biomedical technologies are discussed. This chapter provides a comprehensive assessment of these material classes, their intrinsic properties, and their roles in advancing next-generation biomedical technology.

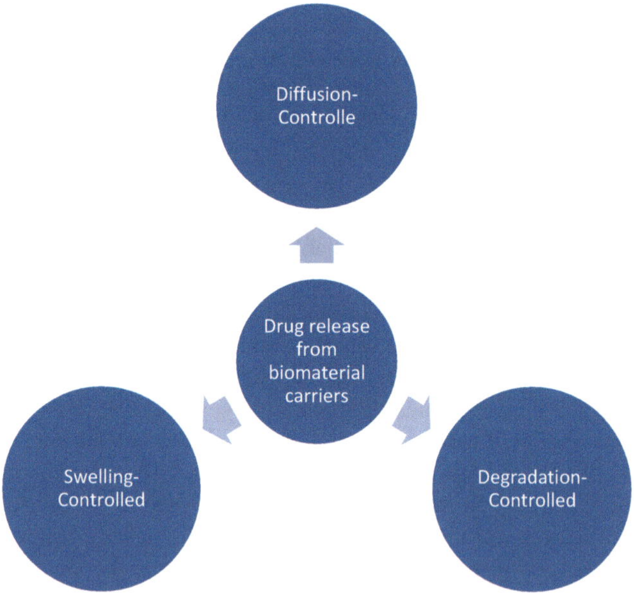

Fig. 6.1 Illustration of drug release from biomaterial carriers, showing how diffusion, degradation, and swelling mechanisms regulate therapeutic delivery in modern drug delivery systems

6.3.1 Polymeric Materials

Polymers represent the most versatile and widely utilized materials in both DDS and biosensors due to their tunable mechanical, chemical, and degradative properties [25]. They can be natural or synthetic, each offering distinct advantages for biomedical applications.

Natural polymers with intrinsic biocompatibility and bioactivity, such gelatin, chitosan, and alginate, come from biological sources. The polysaccharide alginate, which is derived from brown algae, is perfect for encapsulating proteins, cells, and hydrophilic medications because it forms ionically crosslinked hydrogels when calcium ions are present. The cationic functional groups of chitosan, which is produced by deacetylating chitin, improve mucoadhesion and allow for electrostatic interactions with negatively charged molecules, resulting in regulated release and increased bioavailability. Derived from collagen, gelatin promotes cell adhesion and proliferation, which makes it beneficial for biosensor scaffolds and tissue-regenerative DDS. Reproducibility and mechanical stability, however, may be impacted by batch-to-batch irregularities and variations in the natural polymer composition.

Poly(lactic-*co*-glycolic acid) (PLGA), polyethylene glycol (PEG), and polycaprolactone (PCL) are examples of synthetic polymers that provide better control over mechanical strength, degradation rate, and molecular weight. A biodegradable copolymer approved by the FDA, PLGA hydrolyzes to produce lactic and glycolic acids, allowing for consistent medication to release profiles over a period of weeks to months. Because of its hydrophilicity and "stealth" nature, PEG shortens the duration that nanocarriers circulate by reducing immunological recognition and protein adsorption. PCL is appropriate for long-term delivery systems and implantable biosensors due to its high flexibility and slower breakdown kinetics. Drug transport and degradation behavior are significantly influenced by the crosslinking density, polymer composition, and crystallinity [26]. While hydrophobic polymers offer prolonged delivery, hydrophilic polymers enable quicker medication release through improved water absorption. Hybrid polymeric systems can be designed to maximize drug loading capacity, release rate, and sensor sensitivity by combining natural and synthetic polymers or adding functional groups.

6.3.2 Lipid-Based Carriers

Lipid-based materials form another essential class of biomaterials for drug encapsulation and targeted delivery, owing to their ability to mimic biological membranes. The most prominent types include liposomes, solid lipid nanoparticles (SLNs), and micelles.

Drugs that are hydrophilic or hydrophobic can be encapsulated in liposomes, which are spherical vesicles made up of one or more phospholipid bilayers encircling an aqueous core [27, 28]. They are useful in gene therapy, cancer treatment, and vaccine delivery due to their biocompatibility, low toxicity, and ability to modify their surface. By decreasing opsonization and clearance by the reticuloendothelial system, the addition of polyethylene glycol (PEGylation) lengthens the duration of circulation.

The benefits of polymeric and liposome nanoparticles are combined in solid lipid nanoparticles, which provide labile chemical protection, controlled release, and physical stability. SLNs, which are made of physiological lipids, allow for the safe and long-term administration of drugs, especially hydrophobic ones. Micelles, on the other hand, are nanoscale carriers with a hydrophobic core and a hydrophilic shell that help solubilize poorly water-soluble medications. They are created when amphiphilic molecules self-assemble.

Lipid-based structures are used in biosensing to imitate cell membranes for receptor-mediated detection and stabilize biological recognition elements. Supported lipid bilayers, for example, are model biosensor interfaces that enhance biomolecule immobilization and selectivity. Lipid-based materials are essential to the development of therapeutic and diagnostic platforms because they provide a superior balance between biological compatibility and functional tunability [29, 30].

6.3.3 Inorganic and Hybrid Materials

The distinct physicochemical characteristics of inorganic materials, such quantum dots, gold and silver nanostructures, and silica nanoparticles, enhance organic systems. They are essential in sensing and controlled drug release technologies due to their electrical conductivity, optical tunability, and structural stability.

Because of their large surface areas and well-defined pore architecture, mesoporous silica nanoparticles (MSNs) allow for regulated diffusion-based release and effective drug loading. Stimuli-responsive gating, in which pH, temperature, or enzymatic activity can trigger drug release, is made possible by surface modification with functional groups or polymers. Because of their superior brightness and photostability over organic dyes, quantum dots (QDs), semiconductor nanocrystals with size-tunable fluorescence, are frequently used in biosensors for optical signal transduction and multiplexed detection.

The surface plasmon resonance (SPR) effects of metallic nanostructures, such as gold and silver nanoparticles, improve the sensitivity of optical and electrochemical sensors. In instance, gold nanoparticles offer biocompatible platforms for immobilizing enzymes and antibodies, whereas silver nanoparticles have antibacterial qualities that are advantageous for implanted biosensors and wound healing. For theranostic applications simultaneous therapy and diagnosis hybrid systems that combine inorganic cores with polymer or lipid coatings combine mechanical robustness, conductivity, and biological functioning to achieve synergistic performance [31, 32].

6.3.4 Hydrogels and Nanogels

Three-dimensional networks of hydrophilic polymers called hydrogels can absorb a lot of water without losing their structural integrity. They are excellent options for drug delivery and biosensing because of their biocompatibility, porosity, and resemblance to the natural extracellular matrix (ECM). Drugs, proteins, or cells can be encapsulated in hydrogels and released in a controlled way by diffusion or degradation-dependent mechanisms. Mechanical strength and release profiles can be adjusted thanks to the polymer composition and crosslinking density's tunability.

Hydrogels' tiny equivalents, nanogels, provide increased surface area and tissue penetration enabling quick reactions to external stimuli. They are especially well-suited for intracellular and targeted drug delivery, where exact control over payload release and degradation is crucial. Hydrogels serve as biocompatible surfaces in biosensors to immobilize enzymes, preserving the functional stability of biorecognition components while permitting analyte passage [33]. The development of self-regulated sensing systems is made possible by their sensitivity to temperature, pH, or ionic strength.

6.3.5 Smart and Responsive Materials

Systems that may dynamically interact with biological surroundings in response to internal or external inputs like pH, temperature, glucose content, magnetic fields, or enzymatic activity have been made possible by the development of smart materials. These materials enable adaptive biosensing and site-specific, on-demand medication release. For instance, polymers that are sensitive to pH, such poly (methacrylic acid), release medications in acidic conditions that are typical of tumor or inflammatory locations but stay stable at physiological pH. Temperature-triggered release or sensing modulation is made possible by thermoresponsive polymers, such poly(*N*-isopropylacrylamide) (PNIPAAm), which experience reversible phase shifts close to body temperature. By including glucose oxidase or phenylboronic acid moieties, glucose-responsive hydrogels enable self-regulated insulin administration in response to glucose concentration. 4D-printed hydrogels represent the next frontier in responsive biomaterials, offering dynamic adaptability in DDS and biosensors [34].

Smart materials in biosensors actively adjust to changing biological conditions, increasing sensitivity, stability, and selectivity. Additionally, they support antifouling and self-healing surfaces, which are essential for long-term implanted sensors. These adaptable systems serve as a link between active, intelligent biomedical interfaces and passive materials.

6.3.6 Correlation Between Material Structure and Function

The key to maximizing DDS and biosensor performance is the interaction between material structure and function. Fundamental behaviors including diffusion, degradation, adsorption, and electron transfer are governed by structural characteristics, including molecular weight, porosity, surface chemistry, and nanostructure geometry. For instance, increased porosity may jeopardize mechanical stability but improves medication diffusion and sensor analyte access. Analyte transport and biocompatibility are also enhanced by hydrophilic surfaces, while adhesion strength and electrical conductivity may be decreased.

By combining multi-component or hybrid architectures, these characteristics can be optimized simultaneously, striking a balance between functional performance, biocompatibility, and structural integrity [35]. The synthesis of next-generation DDS and biosensors with precisely tailored, adaptive functions will be directed by rational design driven by computer modeling and machine learning, which will progressively predict material behavior as research advances.

6.4 Mechanisms and Processes

The scientific basis for the efficacy, selectivity, and incorporation of drug delivery systems (DDS) and biosensors in contemporary biomedical technologies is found in the mechanisms and procedures that regulate these technologies. These systems depend on the exact regulation of transport, contact, and conversion processes at the interfaces between molecules and materials. While biosensors allow for the real-time detection of biochemical signals through identification and signal transduction, drug delivery systems seek to maximize therapeutic efficiency by regulating the spatial and temporal release of medications as shown in Table 6.1 [36, 37]. The development of theranostic platforms integrated systems that can perform targeted therapy, feedback, and diagnosis all at once is supported by the convergence of these mechanisms. The fundamental biological and physicochemical processes that govern the functionality and performance of drug delivery and biosensing devices are examined in this section.

6.4.1 Drug Release Mechanisms

The release of therapeutic agents from a carrier matrix is central to the design of DDS. Drug release mechanisms can be broadly classified into diffusion-controlled, degradation-controlled, and swelling-controlled processes, each determined by the physicochemical properties of the carrier and the environmental conditions.

Table 6.1 Drug delivery systems and their release profiles

	Mechanism/ process	Key features	Underlying principles	Applications/ examples
Drug release mechanisms	Diffusion-controlled release	Drug molecules diffuse through polymeric or lipid matrices	Fick's law governs release; dependent on concentration gradients and matrix porosity	Polymeric nanoparticles, liposomes, hydrogel depots
	Degradation-controlled release	Drug release coupled to matrix degradation rate	Hydrolytic or enzymatic cleavage of biodegradable polymers (e.g., PLGA, PCL)	Biodegradable implants and microspheres for sustained delivery
	Swelling-controlled release	Polymer swells upon fluid uptake, increasing mesh size for diffusion	Osmotic pressure and polymer relaxation kinetics control release rate	Hydrogels for peptide/protein release
	Burst vs. sustained release profiles	Rapid initial release (burst) vs. controlled, long-term release (sustained)	Controlled by surface adsorption, drug loading, and material microstructure	Vaccine depots, transdermal patches, ocular inserts
Targeting mechanisms	Passive targeting (EPR effect)	Accumulation in tumor tissue due to leaky vasculature and poor lymphatic drainage	Nanoparticle size (10–200 nm) and circulation time determine efficiency	Liposomal doxorubicin (Doxil®), polymeric micelles
	Active targeting (ligand–receptor binding)	Surface ligands (antibodies, peptides, aptamers) bind specific cell receptors	Enhances cell uptake and selectivity via receptor-mediated endocytosis	Folic acid–targeted nanoparticles, antibody–drug conjugates
	Magnetic targeting	Magnetically responsive carriers guided to target sites via external magnetic fields	Magnetite (Fe_3O_4) or iron oxide nanoparticles respond to applied fields	Magnetic hyperthermia, tumor-targeted delivery
	Ultrasonic targeting	Ultrasound waves enhance permeability or trigger release	Cavitation and acoustic pressure gradients modulate carrier structure	Ultrasound-triggered liposomes and microbubbles
	Photothermal targeting	Light-absorbing nanomaterials generate localized heat to trigger release	Near-infrared irradiation induces temperature-sensitive carrier disruption	Gold nanoshells for on-demand drug release

(continued)

Table 6.1 (continued)

	Mechanism/ process	Key features	Underlying principles	Applications/ examples
Biosensing mechanisms	Biorecognition	Specific molecular interaction with analyte (enzyme, antibody, aptamer)	Lock-and-key or conformational binding enhances detection specificity	Glucose sensors (GOx-based), immunosensors, aptamer sensors
	Signal transduction	Converts recognition event into measurable signal	Electrochemical (current/potential), optical (fluorescence/ plasmon), or piezoelectric (mass change)	Lab-on-chip biosensors, wearable glucose monitors
Signal amplification and data processing	Nanostructured electrodes	Increased surface area for higher signal-to-noise ratio and sensitivity	Use of nanowires, graphene, CNTs, or metallic nanoparticles	Electrochemical DNA sensors, neurotransmitter monitoring
	Microfluidic integration	Enables miniaturized, multiplexed analysis with small sample volumes	Controlled flow channels improve reaction kinetics and sensitivity	Point-of-care diagnostic chips
	Real-time monitoring	Continuous tracking via integrated electronic systems	Wireless data transfer using Bluetooth/NFC; flexible sensor substrates	Smart bandages, continuous glucose monitors, wearable diagnostics
System integration	Theranostic platforms	Combine therapy (drug delivery) and diagnostics (biosensing) in one device	Multifunctional nanostructures enable simultaneous treatment and feedback	Nanoparticle-based cancer theranostics, implantable biosensors
	Hybrid nonsystems	Integration of polymers, metals, and biomolecules for synergistic function	Cross-disciplinary design linking material science, bioengineering, and data analytics	Smart nanocomposites for precision medicine

When a medication moves along a concentration gradient across a polymeric matrix or membrane, it is said to exhibit diffusion-controlled release. The permeability, drug solubility, and matrix porosity of the polymer all affect the release rate. Diffusion is frequently the predominant process in systems such as lipid vesicles and implants made of non-biodegradable polymers [38]. Fick's law and the Higuchi model are frequently used to quantitatively explain this phenomenon.

Degradation-controlled release releases the medicine that is contained by breaking down the carrier material. Biodegradable polymers that break down by hydrolysis or enzymatic activity, like poly(lactic-*co*-glycolic acid) (PLGA) or polycaprolactone (PCL), enable regulated and predictable release profiles. Long-term implants benefit from this process since it removes the necessity for surgical removal when degradation aligns with therapeutic requirements. When hydrophilic polymers or hydrogels absorb water, they expand, allowing the medicine to diffuse via their swollen matrix. This phenomenon is known as swelling-controlled release. These systems are perfect for responsive delivery, in which the degree of swelling and, hence, the release kinetics are modulated by environmental cues such as temperature or pH. Burst release, as it relates to kinetics, is the quick initial release of surface-associated medications, which are sometimes unfavorable for reaching long-term therapeutic levels. Sustained release patterns, on the other hand, guarantee constant medication concentrations over long stretches of time, reducing adverse effects and enhancing patient compliance. A key component of DDS design is still striking a balance between these two modes, which is frequently accomplished via surface modification, multilayer coatings, or core-shell topologies that control diffusion pathways and degradation rates.

6.4.2 Targeting Mechanisms

Targeting mechanisms enable drugs to reach specific tissues, cells, or subcellular compartments, enhancing efficacy while minimizing systemic toxicity. Drug targeting can be categorized into passive and active mechanisms, complemented by physical targeting strategies such as magnetic, ultrasonic, and photothermal modulation.

The enhanced permeability and retention (EPR) effect, which is seen in tumors and inflammatory tissues with leaky vasculature and inadequate lymphatic drainage, is exploited by passive targeting. Because of their size (usually between 50 and 200 nm) and surface properties, nanoparticles, liposomes, and micelles preferentially concentrate at these locations, achieving localized drug concentration without the use of ligands. The process of functionalizing drug carriers with biorecognition ligands such as aptamers, peptides, or antibodies that attach to particular receptors that are overexpressed on target cells is known as active targeting [39]. For instance, RGD peptides improve endothelial cell identification by integrating with integrins, and folate-conjugated nanoparticles target cancer cells that exhibit high levels of folate receptor expression. This method improves treatment specificity by increasing cellular absorption and internalization.

Physical targeting techniques, such as magnetic targeting, which use superparamagnetic nanoparticles directed by external magnetic fields to direct drug accumulation at specific areas, are used in addition to biochemical targeting. Focused ultrasonic waves are used in ultrasonic targeting to increase tissue permeability and cause local medication to be released by cavitation. Drug release and hyperthermic therapy are made easier by photothermal targeting, which makes use of light-sensitive nanoparticles like gold nanorods that transform light energy into targeted heat.

Collectively, these mechanisms allow the spatiotemporal precision required for modern targeted therapies, supporting personalized treatment approaches in oncology, cardiology, and regenerative medicine.

6.4.3 Biosensing Mechanisms

Molecular recognition and signal transduction systems that convert biological events into measurable outputs control biosensing devices. Every biosensor consists of a transducer that transforms this biochemical event into a quantifiable physical signal and a biorecognition element that interacts uniquely with the analyte [40]. High affinity and specificity biomolecular interactions are essential to recognition mechanisms; Enzyme-based biosensors produce detectable products like hydrogen peroxide or electrons through catalytic processes (such as glucose oxidase accelerating glucose oxidation). High selectivity for biomarkers is provided by antibody-based biosensors, which take use of antigen–antibody interaction for immunoassays. Synthetic oligonucleotides that can fold into three-dimensional structures are used in aptamer-based biosensors to detect tiny chemicals or proteins with remarkable stability and specificity.

Through a variety of physical processes, transduction mechanisms transform recognition events into signals. Electrochemical transducers measure changes in current, voltage, or impedance brought on by redox reactions or charge shifts. When analyte binding occurs, optical transducers pick up changes in fluorescence, absorbance, or refractive index. Biomolecule binding correlates with mass-induced frequency shifts in quartz crystals, which are measured by piezoelectric transducers. The linkage between identification and transduction processes determines biosensing efficiency, and the total analytical performance is determined by the signal-to-noise ratio, detection limit, and response time. These properties have been significantly improved by developments in nanostructuring and surface modification, allowing for ultrasensitive, real-time biosensing for environmental and therapeutic applications.

6.4.4 Signal Amplification and Data Processing

Modern biosensors increasingly combine sophisticated data processing techniques and signal amplification to provide dependable and ultra-sensitive performance, especially in intricate biological contexts. The effective surface area and electron transfer rate of nanostructured electrodes, such as those made of graphene, gold nanoparticles, or carbon nanotubes, are significantly increased, improving electrochemical sensitivity. Analogously, optical biosensors with nanoplasmonic structures enhance the detection of trace analytes by amplifying local electromagnetic fields. With microfluidic integration, reaction kinetics, mixing, and fluid movement may all be precisely controlled in tiny channels. Multiplexed detection is made possible, repeatability is improved, and sample volume is decreased. Rapid, multi-analyte analysis at the point of care is made possible by microfluidics in conjunction with biosensors.

As sensors have become smaller, signal processing has also changed. Continuous, non-invasive monitoring is now possible with wearable and wireless systems that use Bluetooth or near-field communication (NFC) interfaces. Real-time signal processing using embedded microcontrollers uses algorithms for anomaly identification, calibration, and noise reduction. These devices offer ongoing feedback to help doctors make decisions, especially when it comes to treating long-term illnesses like diabetes or heart disease. Pattern identification, adaptive calibration, and early anomaly detection from complicated datasets are made possible by the incorporation of artificial intelligence (AI) into biosensor data processing, which further improves predictive capacity [41, 42]. A revolutionary step toward autonomous biosensing platforms that connect diagnosis and treatment is represented by the intersection of nanotechnology, microfluidics, and artificial intelligence.

6.4.5 System Integration

Theranostic systems hybrid platforms that can perform simultaneous diagnosis, feedback monitoring, and tailored treatment are the result of the integration of drug delivery with biosensing mechanisms. These systems are made to accomplish closed-loop therapeutic control, in which DDS components modify drug delivery in real time while biosensors identify physiological factors (such as glucose, pH, and cytokines). For instance, pH-sensitive hydrogels and enzymatic glucose sensors are combined in glucose-responsive insulin delivery systems to control insulin release in response to blood glucose levels. Similar to this, cancer theranostics employ nanoparticles that use biosensing to identify tumor markers and then activate signals to administer chemotherapeutics. These systems serve as an example of self-regulating medicine, in which the patient's physiological state is dynamically responded to by the treatment.

For such platforms to be realized, data analytics, biotechnology, and materials science must all be seamlessly integrated. Reliability of wireless connection, synchronization of sensing and release kinetics, and biocompatibility are major obstacles. However, these integrated systems are becoming more and more viable for clinical translation thanks to developments in bioresponsive polymers, flexible electronics, and nanofabrication. The workings of drug delivery systems and biosensors are the result of complex interactions between biological, physicochemical, and technical concepts. Targeting techniques improve site specificity, while controlling drug release mechanisms by diffusion, degradation, or swelling allow for precise therapeutic delivery. Using nanostructures and real-time data analytics, biosensing converts biological information into quantifiable signals through molecular recognition and transduction mechanisms. The future of individualized healthcare is marked by the incorporation of these elements into theranostic systems, which offer ongoing monitoring and therapy that is adaptive to the needs of each patient [43, 44]. An era of intelligent, responsive, and self-regulating biomedical systems that transform the field of diagnosis and treatment will be ushered in as nanotechnology, artificial intelligence, and materials engineering continue to advance, blurring the lines between sensing and therapy [45, 46].

6.5 Design Considerations

It takes a multidisciplinary approach that incorporates concepts from materials science, bioengineering, chemistry, and clinical medicine to design efficient drug delivery systems (DDS) and biosensors. The degree to which design parameters are in line with biological and functional needs has a significant impact on the devices' performance, safety, and translational success. To guarantee biocompatibility, stability, and responsiveness while satisfying regulatory requirements for clinical usage, every element from material selection to device architecture must be optimized. The main design factors that influence the creation of sophisticated DDS and biosensors are covered in this article, with special attention paid to material selection, drug release kinetics, surface chemistry, system miniaturization, power management, and safety.

6.5.1 Material Selection for Biocompatibility, Stability, and Responsiveness

The foundation of any DDS or biosensor design is the choice of material. When interacting with biological systems, the selected substance must be biocompatible, meaning it must not cause harmful immunological, inflammatory, or toxicological reactions. Responsiveness, which enables adaptive behavior to external stimuli, and chemical and structural stability, which preserve functionality over the device's operating lifespan, are equally significant.

For drug delivery methods, biodegradable polymers such as PLGA, PCL, and chitosan are favored due to their predictable breakdown kinetics and minimal toxicity. Since too slow degradation might lead to fibrotic encapsulation or drug retention and too quick degradation can cause a burst release, it is crucial to carefully balance the rate of degradation with the desired duration of drug release. On the other side, biosensors usually need non-biodegradable but biocompatible materials like silicon, gold, graphene, or PEG-modified surfaces to guarantee long-term durability without compromising sensor function [47, 48].

Both DDS and biosensors must be responsive, especially in smart systems. Adaptive sensing or controlled release can be achieved by materials that respond to pH, temperature, enzymes, or electromagnetic fields. For example, temperature-sensitive polymers allow thermally induced insulin delivery, and pH-sensitive hydrogels can release medications selectively in acidic tumor settings. Thus, to ensure prolonged performance in dynamic biological settings, material selection must strike a balance between mechanical integrity, functional responsiveness, and physiological compatibility.

6.5.2 Control of Drug Loading Efficiency and Release Rate

Key design elements affecting therapeutic results are the drug loading efficiency (DLE) and release rate. Achieving optimal DLE guarantees structural stability and maximal carrier capacity use. The therapeutic agent's temporal and spatial availability is determined by the release rate, which also affects toxicity, patient compliance, and efficacy. Drug loading and diffusion are controlled by material characteristics such hydrophobicity, crystallinity, molecular weight, and porosity. Hydrophobic polymer matrices allow for the prolonged diffusion-based release of lipophilic medicines, whereas porous materials such as mesoporous silica nanoparticles offer a high loading capacity due to their large surface areas [49, 50]. Furthermore, the drug and carrier material can interact electrostatically, hydrogen-bondingly, and covalently to improve encapsulation efficiency and modify release profiles.

In general, drug release mechanisms can be classified as stimuli-responsive, diffusion-controlled, or degradation-controlled. Drugs move through polymer matrices or pores in diffusion-controlled systems at varying rates that depend on the permeability and crosslinking density of the polymer. In degradation-controlled systems, the medication is released through enzymatic cleavage or hydrolysis of the carrier. On the other hand, stimuli-responsive systems use environmental cues, including changes in pH, redox conditions, or light exposure, to start release exactly where it is needed. Combining processes in a hybrid model to achieve the proper release kinetics frequently guarantees an initial loading dose followed by sustained therapeutic levels. The goal of tailored and adaptable drug delivery systems is being advanced by computational modeling and machine learning-based optimization, which now helps forecast release patterns and customize designs to meet patient-specific demands.

6.5.3 Surface Functionalization for Biosensor Specificity and Antifouling Properties

The way a biosensor or DDS interacts with the biological environment is directly influenced by its surface chemistry. Surface functionalization controls cellular uptake and biodistribution in DDS and selectivity, sensitivity, and stability in biosensors. Functionalization for biosensors is the process of immobilizing biorecognition components, including aptamers, enzymes, or antibodies, onto the transducer surface while maintaining their biological activity [51, 52]. These molecules can have their orientation and density regulated by methods including click chemistry, covalent coupling, and self-assembled monolayers (SAMs). The objective is to minimize nonspecific binding while achieving high affinity and specificity toward target analytes. For instance, thiol-based SAMs functionalized on gold surfaces offer a stable interface for immobilizing biomolecules, improving the accuracy of signals in optical and electrochemical biosensors.

In order to avoid protein adsorption or biofilm formation, which might impair sensor performance, antifouling qualities are equally important. Hydration layers produced by hydrophilic coatings, especially those based on zwitterionic or polyethylene glycol (PEG) polymers, thwart nonspecific adsorption. By keeping surfaces clean and functional even in the face of complicated physiological circumstances, nanostructured coatings, including graphene oxide or titanium dioxide nanofilms, can further increase signal-to-noise ratios. Surface functionalization makes targeted delivery easier in medication delivery systems. In certain tissues, ligands like folic acid, peptides, or antibodies can be affixed to the surface of nanoparticles to facilitate receptor-mediated endocytosis. Targeting and antifouling properties can also be combined in multifunctional coatings to increase accuracy and systemic circulation time. Therefore, surface engineering ensures selective, stable, and biocompatible performance by serving as a link between material science and biological functions.

6.5.4 Miniaturization and Integration with Microelectronic Components

The field of DDS and biosensors has seen radical change because of the need for integrated and compact systems. The development of small devices with high-resolution sensing, controlled release, and wireless communication all within microscale dimensions appropriate for wearing or implantation has been made possible by developments in microfabrication, nanolithography, and microelectromechanical systems (MEMS). Multiplexed sensing of numerous analytes at once is made possible by miniaturization, which also improves spatial precision and lessens invasiveness. Lab-on-a-chip systems, micro-and nanoneedles, and micropumps allow for localized, on-demand dosage in drug administration that is regulated by embedded electronics or external stimuli [53]. High sensitivity and quick signal transduction are provided in biosensing through integration with field-effect transistors (FETs), nanowire electrodes, or photonic components.

Real-time data collection, processing, and wireless connection are made easier by integration with microelectronic components, which is essential for ongoing monitoring in personalized treatment. This trend is demonstrated by wearable glucose sensors, heart monitors, and implantable electrochemical biosensors, where data accuracy and patient comfort are improved by miniaturization. Miniaturized systems, however, need to strike a balance between mechanical durability, biocompatibility, and power efficiency, necessitating careful selection of flexible substrates, encapsulating materials, and interconnects.

6.5.5 Energy Efficiency and Data Transmission in Implantable Biosensors

Energy economy and dependable data transmission are key design considerations for implantable biosensors since they must function independently for prolonged periods of time. Power management must maintain the continuous operation of sensing, signal processing, and communication components while reducing heat generation and preventing tissue damage. Miniaturized batteries, wireless power transfer (inductive coupling), or energy harvesting from physiological processes like body heat or motion are some of the energy sources for implantable devices. Sustainable, biocompatible energy solutions have been proved by recent developments in biofuel cells that use glucose and oxygen from bodily fluids.

Efficient data transport is crucial for establishing a real-time connection between the implant and external monitoring devices. Technologies that offer different tradeoffs in terms of battery consumption, data rate, and penetration depth include Bluetooth Low Energy (BLE), near-field communication (NFC), and ultrasound-based telemetry. Adaptive frequency modulation and safe data encryption are used to protect privacy and stop signal interference. New wireless and self-powered biosensors combine data transmission and energy harvesting components into biocompatible platforms, allowing for long-term use without the need for outside maintenance. These developments move biosensing closer to continuous, remote health management and smooth clinical integration.

6.5.6 Safety, Sterilization, and Regulatory Considerations for Clinical Translation

Safety, sterilization, and regulatory compliance are critical to the transition of DDS and biosensors from lab prototypes to clinical applications. To guarantee patient safety, every material and design decision must go through a thorough assessment for immunogenicity, mechanical stability, and toxicity [54]. Because conventional techniques like autoclaving, gamma irradiation, or ethylene oxide treatment may destroy delicate polymers, enzymes, or surface coatings, sterilization poses a unique problem. To preserve structural and functional integrity, there is a growing utilization of sterilization-compatible materials and alternate methods, including low-temperature plasma sterilization and supercritical CO_2.

Frameworks like the U.S. FDA, EMA, and ISO standards categorize these technologies according to risk categories from a regulatory standpoint, determining the degree of preclinical and clinical testing necessary. It is necessary to meet requirements including data integrity (FDA 21 CFR Part 11), electrical safety (IEC 60601), and biocompatibility (ISO 10993). Approval requires thorough documentation that addresses design validation, material traceability, sterilization validation, and performance reproducibility. Furthermore, in the era of networked biosensing, ethical issues pertaining to patient permission, data privacy, and long-term surveillance are becoming more and more significant. To guarantee public trust and adoption, a successful clinical translation necessitates not just technological proficiency but also a thorough comprehension of regulatory science, risk management, and ethical compliance.

A systems-level approach is necessary for designing biosensors and next-generation drug delivery systems, combining biological interactions, device architecture, and material properties. Accurate and secure therapeutic performance is ensured by paying close attention to surface functionality, drug release control, responsiveness, and biocompatibility. The development of completely autonomous, adaptive biomedical devices is being accelerated at the same time by developments in data communication, power management, and downsizing. The path toward therapeutically transferable, patient-specific, and intelligent healthcare technology becomes more accessible by coordinating scientific innovation with ethical and regulatory frameworks [55, 56].

6.6 Applications and Case Studies

Modern biomedical practice has been revolutionized by the combination of drug delivery systems (DDS) and biosensors, which allow for targeted, intelligent, and regulated therapeutic interventions across a range of disorders. In order to improve therapeutic precision, reduce side effects, and enable ongoing physiological monitoring, these technologies combine materials science, nanotechnology, and bioengineering. Their use in neurology and oncology demonstrates how real-time feedback, molecular recognition, and regulated release can be combined to create tailored and adaptable treatment. The primary application areas and real-world case studies that highlight how sensing and delivery mechanisms have come together to have a clinical impact are examined in this section.

6.6.1 Cancer Therapy

Cancer therapy remains one of the most advanced fields for the application of DDS and biosensor technologies. The challenge in oncology is to deliver high doses of chemotherapeutic agents specifically to tumor cells while sparing healthy tissue.

Targeted nanoparticles have become key tools in overcoming this challenge through both passive and active targeting mechanisms.

The enhanced permeability and retention (EPR) effect, in which nanoparticles gather inside tumor tissue because of leaky vasculature, is used in passive targeting. Micelles, liposomes (like Doxil®), and polymeric nanoparticles make use of these phenomena to lower systemic toxicity and raise local medication concentration. By adorning nanoparticles with ligands or antibodies that identify tumor-specific markers, active targeting expands on this idea. For example, folate-conjugated liposomes enhance intracellular absorption by binding to folate receptors that are overexpressed in breast and ovarian malignancies. Stimuli-responsive DDS, including temperature-activated, redox-responsive, and pH-sensitive systems, allow for controlled drug release throughout the tumor microenvironment in addition to targeting. For instance, when exposed to alternating magnetic fields or near-infrared light, gold nanoshells or magnetic nanoparticles can release medications, combining photothermal therapy and chemotherapy in a way that works well together.

Current theranostic technologies allow for the simultaneous identification and therapy of tumor markers by combining medication delivery with biosensing capabilities [57]. For example, nanocomposites containing quantum dots can release anticancer medications in reaction to changes in reactive oxygen species levels, enabling dynamic feedback during treatment. These multipurpose nanocarriers are a significant advancement in self-regulating cancer treatments.

6.6.2 Diabetes Management

The management of diabetes is a prime example of how biosensing and responsive medication delivery can be combined to achieve closed-loop therapeutic control. Glucose variations brought on by conventional insulin therapy can have long-term health consequences. Thus, the creation of glucose-responsive DDS has emerged as a key component of intelligent diabetes treatment. Polymeric matrices known as glucose-responsive hydrogels expand or contract in response to changes in blood glucose levels, adjusting insulin release appropriately. Glucose oxidase (GOx), which catalyzes glucose oxidation to produce gluconic acid, is commonly included in these systems. This lowers pH and causes insulin to be released from pH-sensitive hydrogels. As an alternative, hydrogels functionalized with phenylboronic acid bind glucose molecules reversibly, offering a biocompatible, adjustable sensing method.

These hydrogels and implantable glucose sensors offer ongoing observation and feedback, serving as the basis for artificial pancreas systems. Continuous glucose monitors (CGMs) such as Dexcom® and Medtronic Guardian® that relate to insulin pumps that automatically modify dosage in response to biosensor readings are examples of commercial advancements. These integrated systems have shown stable glucose control and fewer hypoglycemia episodes in clinical trials, indicating a move toward patient-specific, self-management of diabetes. For the management of chronic diseases, increased comfort and accessibility are anticipated with the further development of wearable and minimally invasive glucose-responsive systems [58].

6.6.3 Cardiovascular Diseases

Since cardiovascular diseases (CVDs) continue to be the world's leading cause of death, prevention, treatment, and monitoring require cutting-edge DDS and biosensor technology. This field is dominated by two main applications: biosensors for cardiac biomarkers and drug-eluting stents (DES). Drug-eluting stents are scaffolds made of metal or polymers that are inserted into constricted arteries to preserve artery integrity while delivering antiproliferative drugs like paclitaxel or sirolimus locally. Through the inhibition of smooth muscle growth, the surface coating of the stent regulates sustained medication release, hence preventing restenosis. In order to reduce long-term inflammation and do away with the necessity for permanent implant, advanced DES platforms now include bioresorbable polymers that break down beyond the therapeutic window.

Biosensors for cardiac indicators including troponin, myoglobin, and C-reactive protein offer early detection of myocardial infarction and ischemic episodes in conjunction with interventional therapy. Rapid diagnosis in emergency situations is made possible by the capacity of lab-on-a-chip devices and electrochemical biosensors to detect troponin at nanomolar quantities in a matter of minutes [59, 60]. New smart cardiovascular implants combine sensing and medication release capabilities. One example of closed-loop vascular therapy is the use of stents equipped with pressure sensors and microtransmitters to monitor arterial conditions and release anti-inflammatory medications in response to localized changes. The shift from passive medical devices to intelligent, feedback-driven cardiovascular therapies is symbolized by these multifunctional systems.

6.6.4 Neurological Disorders

The problems of delivering treatments across the blood–brain barrier (BBB) and accomplishing long-term neural activity monitoring are addressed in the field of neurology by DDS and biosensors [61, 62]. Leading the way in this breakthrough are brain biosensors and implantable medication reservoirs. Bypassing the blood-brain barrier and delivering medications straight into the cerebrospinal fluid, implantable microreservoirs like the Ommaya reservoir allow for the regulated release of neuroprotective, analgesic, or chemotherapy medicines. More sophisticated reservoirs based on microelectromechanical systems (MEMS) provide customizable drug delivery using microvalves that are activated by biological or electrical signals. Neural biosensors, meanwhile, track electrophysiological activity, ions, and neurotransmitters to investigate brain pathology and function. For example, glutamate sensors evaluate excitotoxicity in traumatic brain damage, while electrochemical dopamine sensors aid in the detection of Parkinson's disease progression.

Closed-loop neural interfaces systems that can identify abnormal brain signals and respond by providing neuroactive medications or electrical stimulation are enabling the convergence of sensing and delivery. This type of technology is being investigated for the treatment of epilepsy, where biosensors identify the onset of seizures and initiate the release of targeted anticonvulsants, providing accurate and responsive control over neurological disorders.

6.6.5 *Infectious Disease Monitoring*

The global rise of infectious diseases and antibiotic resistance has accelerated the development of biosensors and drug-releasing surfaces that prevent, detect, and respond to microbial threats. To stop biofilm formation, antimicrobial coatings on catheters, wound dressings, and medical implants emit bactericidal agents such nitric oxide, silver ions, or antibiotics in a regulated way. Under light activation, nanostructured coatings with photothermal or photocatalytic qualities (such as titanium dioxide doped with graphene oxide or silver) improve microbial death, offering dual protection and sterilizing benefits. Real-time infection monitoring and quick diagnosis are made possible by pathogen-detecting biosensors. For instance, surface plasmon resonance (SPR) sensors detect antigen–antibody interactions without labeling, whereas electrochemical DNA biosensors may identify bacterial or viral genetic material in a matter of minutes. Point-of-care biosensors using graphene-based transducers and CRISPR-Cas detection made it possible to do ultrasensitive, portable viral testing during the COVID-19 epidemic with outcomes similar to PCR assays [63, 64].

Integration of biosensing with localized antimicrobial delivery such as smart wound dressings that sense infection markers (e.g., pH or protease levels) and release antibiotics in response illustrates a promising approach toward autonomous infection management systems.

6.6.6 *Clinical Case Studies Highlighting the Convergence of Sensing and Therapeutic Delivery*

The successful integration of drug delivery with biosensing technology is demonstrated by several clinical case studies. Targeted cytotoxicity with little collateral damage was achieved in a clinical experiment in oncology that used theranostic gold nanoshells to simultaneously image, photothermal ablate, and release medication in patients with head and neck cancer. Glycemic variability in Type 1 and Type

2 diabetes has been significantly reduced by artificial pancreas systems that include insulin pumps with CGMs. Preclinical models of wireless stents with real-time drug delivery and pressure sensing in cardiology have shown promise for adaptive vascular treatment. For the closed-loop treatment of epilepsy and Parkinson's disease, neuroprosthetic devices that combine electrophysiological sensors with micro-reservoirs are presently being researched. These examples illustrate the clinical potential of integrated sensing–delivery platforms to transform conventional treatment into data-driven, self-regulating medical care.

From diabetes and cancer to cardiovascular and neurological disorders, drug delivery systems and biosensors are used in almost every area of contemporary medicine. Each example shows how biosensing feedback and controlled release mechanisms can work together to improve safety, efficacy, and precision. A significant development in biomedical technology is the move toward theranostic systems, in which diagnosis and treatment are inextricably connected. The combination of sensing, delivery, and feedback will revolutionize clinical practice such as nanotechnology, AI, and smart materials develop further. This will present a new paradigm of intelligent, personalized, and adaptive healthcare systems that react dynamically to the body's needs [65].

6.7 Recent Advances and Innovations

When nanotechnology, microengineering, computational modeling, and materials science come together, the field of drug delivery systems (DDS) and biosensors is radically different. By facilitating real-time monitoring and adaptive feedback, these advancements seek to enhance treatment precision, sensing sensitivity, and patient-specific personalization. Now, the discipline is shifting toward intelligent, integrated systems that can diagnose and treat problems on their own, changing the way biomedical technology interacts with the human body. Key developments in six areas nanotechnology, microfluidics, wearable technology, smart materials, artificial intelligence (AI), and bioprinting that are all influencing the development of next-generation customized healthcare solutions are examined in this section.

6.7.1 Nanotechnology in DDS and Biosensors

Nanotechnology's capacity to modify materials at the molecular level, providing previously unheard-of control over drug release, surface area, and signal sensitivity, has transformed both DDS and biosensors. This advancement is demonstrated by quantum dots (QDs), carbon nanotubes (CNTs), and nanowires, each of which offers distinct physicochemical benefits. Because of their remarkable fluorescence stability and adjustable optical characteristics, quantum dots semiconductor nanocrystals are perfect for optical biosensing and real-time drug distribution imaging.

By adjusting particle size, their emission wavelength can be customized, enabling multiplexed detection of several biomarkers [66]. QDs have been functionalized with ligands or antibodies for targeted theranostic platforms in drug delivery, allowing imaging and therapy to occur at the same time.

High electrical conductivity, a huge surface area, and mechanical toughness are all provided by carbon nanotubes (CNTs) and graphene derivatives. With the use of these materials, electrochemical biosensors can detect analytes like glucose, dopamine, or cardiac biomarkers with extreme sensitivity. Functionalized surfaces on CNTs enhance their solubility and biocompatibility, enabling the regulated release of chemotherapeutics straight into tumor microenvironments. CNTs have also been developed as drug nanocarriers. Similarly, label-free biosensing is made possible by nanowires, which are metallic or semiconducting structures that convert chemical interactions into quantifiable electrical impulses. Their nanoscale size enables single-molecule sensitivity detection, improving implanted sensor platforms and point-of-care diagnostics. All of these nanomaterials are working together to advance the accuracy, responsiveness, and integration of DDS and biosensors with real-time monitoring systems.

6.7.2 Microfluidic and Lab-on-a-Chip Systems

Lab-on-a-chip (LOC) and microfluidic technologies mark a paradigm change toward automated, high-throughput, and miniature biomedical systems. These platforms enable precise control of fluids and chemicals for diagnostic and therapeutic applications by integrating several laboratory functions sample processing, detection, and delivery within micro-scale channels. Microfluidic devices in medication delivery minimize systemic side effects by enabling localized and on-demand therapeutic administration [67]. Pneumatic and electrokinetic pumps manage flow according to physiological feedback, whereas microreservoir-based systems can deliver medications in controlled pulses. For instance, microfluidic sensors that adjust release in response to observed glucose levels have been used in the construction of glucose-sensitive insulin delivery systems.

LOC systems enable real-time biochemical monitoring for biosensing with small sample volumes. Rapid detection of proteins, nucleic acids, and metabolites is made possible by integrated platforms that combine microchannels with optical or electrochemical sensors. Translational research is accelerated by the physiologically realistic conditions that microfluidic organ-on-chip models offer for in vitro testing of DDS behavior and immunological interactions. These devices' scalability and mobility have fueled their use in point-of-care diagnostics, especially for metabolic monitoring and infectious disorders. LOC systems are developing into self-regulating bioelectronic platforms that use wireless communication and AI-driven analytics to combine precise treatments and diagnostics into a single device.

6.7.3 4D and Smart Systems

A new frontier in biomaterial innovation has been opened by the development of 4D materials, which change over time in response to outside stimuli. 4D DDS and biosensors, in contrast to static systems, are able to dynamically adjust to physiological changes, guaranteeing intelligent response and temporal control. These intelligent systems incorporate stimuli-responsive materials that respond to mechanical stress, pH, temperature, enzymes, and shape-memory polymers, hydrogels, and nanocomposites. For example, temperature-responsive carriers like poly(*N*-isopropylacrylamide) allow regulated release based on body heat or localized hyperthermia, while pH-sensitive hydrogels can release medications selectively in acidic tumor microenvironments.

By regenerating after fouling or self-regulating their surface states, smart materials in biosensing increase sensitivity and durability. Continuous monitoring without saturation or deterioration is made possible by dynamic sensing membranes that open or close in response to biomolecular recognition events. By combining 4D printing with intelligent materials, it is possible to create devices that can self-heal, fold, or change shape, improving the functionality of implantable systems [68]. For instance, shape-memory stents can expand after implantation without the need for outside assistance, and 4D-printed microvalves can independently modify flow rates in DDS. The development of autonomous biomedical systems that can interact adaptively with the body's changing physiological environment is represented by these technologies.

6.7.4 Wearable and Implantable Devices

Healthcare is changing from reactive to proactive, continuous monitoring through the integration of drug delivery platforms with wearable and implantable biosensors. These gadgets gather physiological data in real time, such as heart rate, blood sugar levels, or inflammatory indicators, and modify the way that treatments are administered in response. For conformal skin contact, flexible, elastic materials like silicone elastomers and conductive polymers are used in wearable technology, such as epidermal patches or smart textiles. More sophisticated examples include microneedle patches for painless transdermal medicine delivery and electrochemical sweat sensors for electrolyte and metabolite monitoring. Smart insulin patches, which automatically release insulin in response to detected hyperglycemia, are an example of closed-loop therapeutic systems, which are created by combining sensing and delivery functions.

Higher precision is available for long-term internal parameter monitoring using implantable biosensors [69]. They allow for chronotherapeutic administration, which releases medications based on metabolic or circadian rhythms, when used in conjunction with microreservoir drug release systems. Clinicians can remotely monitor and modify treatment plans thanks to integration with wireless telemetry. New platforms eliminate the need for surgical extraction by using biodegradable electronics that decompose innocuously after use. Wearable and implantable technologies are moving toward seamless integration within personalized healthcare ecosystems thanks to the combination of biocompatibility, downsizing, and intelligent feedback control.

6.7.5 AI and Machine Learning Integration

The analysis, interpretation, and application of data from DDS and biosensors for individualized therapy are being revolutionized by artificial intelligence (AI) and machine learning (ML). The accuracy and effectiveness of biomedical systems are improved by these computational techniques, which make predictive modeling, pattern recognition, and adaptive control possible. AI systems evaluate pharmacokinetic and pharmacodynamic data in medication delivery to forecast drug interactions, improve dosing regimens, and customize release patterns based on patient reactions. Reinforcement learning algorithms can autonomously modify delivery parameters in real time, maintaining therapeutic amounts within a specific range. For example, to avoid hypoglycemia or hyperglycemia, AI-powered insulin pumps can learn a patient's metabolic habits.

ML improves signal processing and lowers noise for biosensors, increasing detection accuracy even in intricate biological matrices. Predictive health warnings or early disease detection are made possible by algorithms' ability to identify minute variations in sensor output that occur before pathological alterations. Additionally, AI enables multimodal data fusion, which creates comprehensive patient profiles by combining data from several sensors, including optical, electrical, and biochemical ones. Additionally, medication distribution and immunological reactions can be simulated using digital twins, which are virtual representations of biological systems, speeding up the development of DDS and biosensors. Healthcare is shifting toward closed-loop, intelligent systems that can operate autonomously and optimize for individual needs thanks to the combination of AI analytics and real-time biosensor input [70, 71].

6.7.6 Bioprinting and Personalized Systems

A revolutionary method for developing biosensors and customized medication delivery systems based on each person's unique anatomy, physiology, and disease profile is bioprinting. Biomaterials, cells, and bioactive chemicals are carefully deposited using additive manufacturing techniques to create three-dimensional (3D) or four-dimensional (4D) architectures that closely resemble natural tissue environments. Drug distribution in DDS can be spatially controlled thanks to bioprinting, allowing for targeted or gradient delivery inside intricate tissue structures. Growth factors or nanoparticles that release medications in response to mechanical stress or cellular activity can be included into 3D-printed hydrogel scaffolds. Biocompatible polymers and ceramics that meet specific mechanical and biological needs can be used to print customized implants, such as vascular stents or patient-specific bone grafts.

Bioprinting makes it easier to integrate microelectrodes, bioreceptors, and microfluidic networks into flexible substrates for biosensors. This method makes it possible to create implantable sensors or personalized diagnostic patches that closely match the geometry of the tissue. Precision medicine, in which devices are customized not just to disease but also to each patient's particular biological landscape, is supported by bioprinting in conjunction with patient-specific data from AI and imaging technologies [72]. To provide dynamic, self-healing systems with ongoing sensing and therapeutic feedback, future advances are investigating multi-material and cell-laden printing. Bioprinting is redefining the frontier of adaptable, configurable biomedical systems by fusing technical precision with biological complexity.

Medicine is moving toward intelligent, integrated, and patient-centric solutions as a result of the quick development of DDS and biosensor technologies. While wearable, AI-integrated, and bioprinted systems allow for continuous, individualized care, nanotechnology improves sensitivity and control, while microfluidics and 4D materials offer flexibility and automation [73]. The future of regenerative and precision medicine will be redefined by these convergent technologies, which have the potential to transform biomedical equipment from passive tools into active, responsive, and adaptive healthcare companions. They will also change diagnosis, monitoring, and therapy.

6.8 Challenges and Limitations

Drug delivery systems (DDS) and biosensors have advanced significantly, but there are still many ethical, technical, and scientific obstacles to their widespread clinical application. The goal of these technologies is to deliver accurate, regulated, and responsive diagnostic and therapeutic results. However, their full potential is frequently hampered by the intricacy of biological systems, constraints in materials engineering, and challenges in guaranteeing long-term effectiveness as shown in Fig. 6.2. With emphasis on control accuracy, biocompatibility, energy management, immunological interactions, manufacturing scalability, and regulatory oversight, this section critically analyzes the main obstacles impeding the development and implementation of integrated DDS and biosensor platforms.

6.8.1 Complexity in Achieving Precise Spatiotemporal Control of Drug Release

Accurate spatiotemporal control over drug release is one of the main issues in DDS design. The objective is to administer therapeutic molecules at the appropriate time, location, and dosage a challenge made more difficult by the human body's

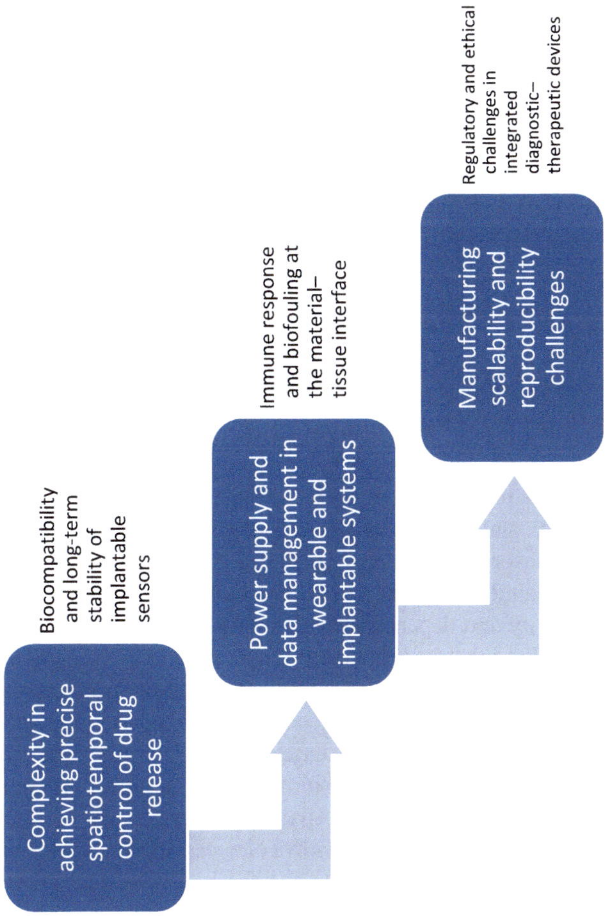

Fig. 6.2 Overview of the major challenges and limitations affecting drug delivery systems and biosensors, including issues related to precise release control, long-term biocompatibility, power and data management, immune responses, manufacturing scalability, and regulatory constraints

dynamic nature. Because of their diverse pH, enzymatic activity, and mechanical pressures, most biological surroundings have unpredictable effects on release kinetics. Systems that respond to stimuli, diffusion, and degradation frequently display non-linear or burst-release behavior, which can result in initial overdose and subsequent subtherapeutic levels [74, 75]. Predictability is further complicated by the milieu surrounding sick tissues; for example, tumors' hypoxic and acidic circumstances may prematurely activate pH-sensitive carriers. Similarly, real-time medication release and biological feedback synchronization is a challenge for pulsatile or feedback-controlled systems, which are designed to replicate physiological rhythms.

Furthermore, 4D biomaterials that are intended to adjust to external stimuli still have trouble being consistent over extended periods of time. Although release predictability has increased with computational models and AI-based simulations, intricate immunological, enzymatic, or mechanical interactions sometimes cause in vivo validation to differ. Thus, attaining precise, repeatable control over release dynamics continues to be a challenge in the development of DDS.

6.8.2 Biocompatibility and Long-Term Stability of Implantable Sensors

A significant challenge for biosensors, especially implanted ones, is guaranteeing their biocompatibility and long-term operating stability. Inflammation, fibrotic encapsulation, and sensor component degradation are examples of foreign body reactions that are frequently brought on by the introduction of foreign materials into the body. The sensitivity and dependability of the sensor may be reduced by these biological responses that insulate it from the target analyte. For example, denaturation, fouling, or leaching of bioactive components causes a progressive loss of catalytic performance in enzyme-based glucose biosensors. Likewise, electrochemical sensors experience drifting in signal baselines or electrode deterioration over time. Additionally, prolonged exposure to biofluids encourages fouling, oxidation, and corrosion, all of which shorten the lifespan of devices.

Although biocompatible coatings like hydrogel encapsulation, zwitterionic polymers, and PEGylation have been used to lessen these effects, total immunological tolerance is still elusive. Additionally, encapsulation frequently impairs analyte diffusion, which lowers sensitivity. Although the creation of bioinspired, degradable, or self-healing sensor materials is showing promise, real-world performance stability for more than a few months is still uncommon [76]. Thus, long-term sensor integration remains a challenge of preserving functional biostability without compromising responsiveness.

6.8.3 *Power Supply and Data Management in Wearable and Implantable Systems*

Power supply and data management present special difficulties as wearable and implantable biosensing-delivery platforms get smaller and more integrated. Reliable, durable, and secure energy sources are necessary for continuous operation; traditional battery technologies struggle to meet these demands. Size, biocompatibility, and the requirement for energy harvesting or wireless recharging pose significant challenges for implantable systems. Although partial answers are provided by inductive coupling, piezoelectric, and thermoelectric energy harvesting techniques, their power densities are still constrained and frequently insufficient for real-time sensing and actuation. Additionally, there are hazards of electromagnetic interference and tissue heating when using wireless charging.

Data handling presents additional difficulties. Massive datasets are produced by wearable biosensors' continuous data streams, which need to be safely analyzed, stored, and transferred [77]. Cybersecurity flaws, latency, and data loss are still major issues, especially when devices are connected over wireless or Internet of Things-based networks. Efficient on-device processing is also necessary for real-time analytics to lessen reliance on remote computers. Therefore, a major technological constraint for next-generation smart biomedical systems continues to be the integration of energy-efficient microelectronics, secure data pipelines, and self-powered designs.

6.8.4 *Immune Response and Biofouling at the Material–Tissue Interface*

The interaction between biomaterials and host immune responses at the material–tissue interface has a significant impact on device performance. The body starts an immunological cascade after implantation, which can affect drug release dynamics and sensor accuracy. This cascade includes protein adsorption, macrophage activation, and fibrous capsule construction. The buildup of proteins, cells, and microorganisms on device surfaces, known as biofouling, has two risks: it reduces the fidelity of sensor signals and blocks the passage of therapeutic drugs. These deposits may eventually result in inflammatory conditions that hasten deterioration or physical obstacles to analyte delivery.

Surface modification techniques like hydrophilic coatings, zwitterionic polymers, and nanostructured topographies that inhibit protein attachment attempts to lessen these effects. Furthermore, the goal of immunomodulatory materials that contain cytokine inhibitors or anti-inflammatory compounds is to balance the interactions between the device and the tissue. Even with these developments, there is still a problem with striking a dynamic balance between immunological tolerance and device operation, especially in long-term or chronic applications [78].

Additionally, biofilm formation and bacterial colonization increase the risk of infection and device failure. Although cytotoxicity and antimicrobial resistance are still issues, antimicrobial nanocoatings can lower infection rates. Thus, it is still a multifactorial materials problem to design interfaces that resist fouling, infection, and immunological rejection all at once.

6.8.5 Manufacturing Scalability and Reproducibility Challenges

Significant manufacturing hurdles arise when converting laboratory-scale DDS and biosensor prototypes into commercially viable solutions. These devices frequently use precision microfabrication, multi-layered composites, and intricate nanostructures all of which are challenging to consistently create at industrial sizes. Inconsistent drug loading, release kinetics, or sensor sensitivity may result from batch-to-batch variations in the production of nanoparticles, polymer crosslinking, or microfluidic channel construction. Manufacturing is made more difficult by the need to maintain sterility, stability, and calibration throughout high production volumes. Furthermore, regulatory-grade materials must adhere to strict Good Manufacturing Practice (GMP) guidelines, which raise the complexity and cost of manufacture.

Customization and accuracy have increased because of 3D printing and microfabrication but expanding these processes without sacrificing resolution or biocompatibility is still difficult [3]. Because living cells and biomolecules are extremely sensitive to processing conditions, their incorporation into DDS and biosensors introduces even more complexity. As a result, maintaining scalability, cost effectiveness, and repeatability continues to be a major obstacle to broad clinical adoption.

6.8.6 Regulatory and Ethical Challenges in Integrated Diagnostic Therapeutic Devices

Complicated ethical and regulatory issues arise when sensing and delivery are combined into a single diagnostic-therapeutic (theranostic) device. These methods make it difficult to distinguish between drugs and medical devices, raising questions regarding the best regulatory frameworks. For pharmaceuticals and devices, agencies like the FDA and EMA have different approval procedures, but integrated platforms sometimes call for hybrid evaluations, which delay clinical approval. The dual nature of these systems raises safety concerns because the embedded electronics, sensors, and data transmission components must all adhere to medical device safety regulations in addition to the medication formulation's need to be biocompatible and efficacious.

Furthermore, processing patient data from biosensing devices is subject to stringent restrictions under data privacy laws including the Health Insurance Portability and Accountability Act (HIPAA) and the General Data Protection Regulation (GDPR).

Autonomous or AI-powered DDS raise ethical concerns around decision-making transparency, accountability, and patient consent. Closed-loop systems that automatically modify drug dosage in response to sensor feedback, for instance, need to strike a balance between algorithmic control and human supervision. Inequalities in access to cutting-edge bio-integrated technology also raise issues of equity and accessibility to healthcare worldwide. As theranostic technologies advance toward clinical maturity, it will be crucial to develop strong ethical standards and flexible regulatory frameworks to guarantee safety, trust, and equity [79, 80].

Significant scientific, technological, and regulatory barriers have limited the development of drug delivery systems and biosensors, despite their remarkable potential to advance customized and adaptive healthcare. There is still ongoing research into achieving accurate spatiotemporal control, guaranteeing long-term biocompatibility, preserving steady power and data management, and resolving manufacturing and immunological issues. To overcome these complex constraints, interdisciplinary cooperation involving materials science, computer modeling, bioengineering, and ethics will be essential to the future development of these technologies. The final integration of integrated diagnostic–therapeutic systems into standard medical practice will depend on how well innovations balance performance, safety, and accessibility [81].

6.9 Future Directions

One of the most exciting areas of biomedical engineering is the junction of drug delivery systems (DDS) with biosensors. Achieving intelligent, flexible, and long-lasting platforms that smoothly combine tests and treatments will be essential to future advancement. The combination of materials science, nanotechnology, bioinformatics, and artificial intelligence (AI) will revolutionize the way diseases are identified, tracked, and treated as healthcare moves toward personalized and data-driven paradigms [21, 82]. This talks about new developments that will influence the next generation of intelligent biomedical systems, with a focus on sustainability, autonomy, integration, and personalization.

6.9.1 Integration of Biosensing and Controlled Drug Delivery into Unified Smart Platforms

Fully integrated "theranostic" platforms systems that can concurrently sense physiological indicators and deliver therapeutic drugs in a regulated, feedback-driven manner are the direction that the next generation of biomedical devices is headed.

These technologies allow for autonomous treatment modification and real-time monitoring by bridging the gap between diagnosis and therapy. Without the help of a clinician, a biosensor that recognizes inflammatory cytokines, for instance, can cause the release of localized anti-inflammatory medication, preserving homeostasis [83]. This integration is supported by recent developments in nanotechnology and microfluidics, which provide fine-grained control over micro-scale surroundings. For example, hydrogel-based systems can contain drug reservoirs and biosensing elements, releasing therapeutic payloads in response to mechanical or biochemical stimuli. Likewise, implantable devices may employ optical and electrochemical biosensors to monitor parameters such as pH or glucose, thereby autonomously adjusting medication release profiles for cancer or diabetic patients.

To guarantee quick reaction, stability, and biocompatibility, the sensor and delivery subsystems must communicate as efficiently as possible. Improvements in signal transduction efficiency and bioelectronic interfaces will be essential. Essentially, integrated smart platforms of the future will provide ongoing, individualized therapy by moving away from passive monitoring and toward active, closed-loop patient health regulation.

6.9.2 *Development of Biodegradable and Self-Powered Biosensors*

Concerns about sustainability and long-term safety are driving the creation of transitory and biodegradable biosensors, which are intended to function for a predetermined amount of time before dissolving naturally in the body. By doing away with the necessity for surgical removal, these next-generation devices lower the risk of infection and patient pain. Polylactic acid (PLA), magnesium, and silk fibroin are among the materials being developed to decompose gradually while retaining mechanical and electrical performance over the course of their useful lives. The limits of traditional batteries are being overcome at the same time by advancements in self-powered biosensors. Emerging as viable long-term substitutes are devices that capture biological energy sources, such as body heat, glucose oxidation, or mechanical motion. Continuous sensing or medication release functionalities can be maintained by using biofuel cells and piezoelectric nanogenerators, which can transform chemical or kinetic energy into electrical power.

Transient yet intelligent biosensing systems are made possible by combining energy autonomy and biodegradability; these platforms are especially helpful for wound healing, post-operative monitoring, and short-term medication delivery [84]. Maintaining sensor accuracy throughout deterioration and making sure that byproducts are non-toxic and bioresorbable are still difficult tasks, nevertheless. To create completely self-sustaining medical microsystems, future research will concentrate on striking a balance between performance, biodegradation kinetics, and environmental safety.

6.9.3 Use of AI-Driven Adaptive Systems for Personalized Medicine

By facilitating adaptive, predictive, and customized healthcare, artificial intelligence (AI) has the potential to completely transform both biosensing and DDS. Real-time anomaly detection, dosing schedule optimization, and illness trend identification are all made possible by AI algorithms that can evaluate complicated biological data from wearable and implanted sensors. Unmatched drug delivery precision can be achieved by using machine learning (ML) to continuously improve therapy regimens depending on the reactions of specific patients. AI-integrated insulin pumps, for example, currently exhibit closed-loop glycemic management, automatically adjusting insulin infusion based on data from continuous glucose monitors. By extending this idea, AI may make it possible for multi-analyte monitoring systems to concurrently monitor biomarkers for neurological, metabolic, and cardiovascular health, allowing for the coordination of focused interventions across systems [85, 86].

AI also makes it easier to model drug kinetics, degradation behavior, and tissue interactions in silico, which speeds up design optimization and lessens the need for animal testing. Precision diagnostics may be further supported by combining real-time biosensor data with bioinformatics databases to find patient-specific molecular signatures and adjust treatments accordingly. Future advancements will prioritize regulatory frameworks that guarantee safe algorithmic decision-making in conjunction with explainable AI (XAI) to improve transparency and clinical trust. Static medication regimens will give way to dynamic, learning-based therapeutic ecosystems as a result.

6.9.4 Advances in Wireless, Real-Time, and Closed-Loop Therapeutic Feedback Systems

For continuous, autonomous operation, next-generation DDS and biosensors will depend more on wireless and closed-loop feedback designs. Real-time physiological data transfer to smartphones and cloud databases has already been made possible by developments in miniaturized electronics, Bluetooth Low Energy (BLE), and near-field communication (NFC). These advancements open the door to networked medical ecosystems, in which implanted or wearable technology works together to concurrently monitor, diagnose, and treat illnesses. Wireless biosensors, for instance, can identify changes in blood pressure or troponin and initiate response drug release from implanted stents or micro-reservoirs in the treatment of cardiovascular disease. In a similar vein, wearable skin patches can maintain homeostatic control by delivering transdermal medications and detecting metabolic changes.

Future systems will make use of closed-loop algorithms that directly combine drug release mechanisms and sensor data, creating intelligent networks that may dynamically modify therapeutic actions. Technologies like energy harvesting and wireless power transfer will increase device lifespans, save maintenance costs, and improve patient comfort [87]. It is still technically difficult to guarantee data security, minimal latency, and biocompatibility of wireless components. Strong cybersecurity protocols and encryption standards will be necessary to protect patient privacy and clinical dependability as devices become more networked.

6.9.5 Sustainable Materials and Green Manufacturing for Biomedical Devices

One increasingly important aspect of biomedical innovation is environmental sustainability. Toxic solvents, rare metals, and energy-intensive fabrication techniques are frequently used in the traditional production of DDS and biosensors, raising ethical and environmental issues. Biomedical engineering is in line with more general environmental stewardship objectives because of the move toward sustainable production and green materials. For the creation of devices, scientists are investigating biopolymers made from renewable resources like chitosan, cellulose, and alginate. These materials offer intrinsic biocompatibility and degradability in addition to reducing ecological effect. Developments in solvent-free microfabrication methods and additive manufacturing (3D/4D printing) significantly reduce waste and make it possible to produce complicated structures quickly.

Furthermore, the long-term viability of biomedical technology will depend heavily on the adoption of circular economy concepts, which call for materials that can be recycled or safely disintegrate. The need for life-cycle assessments (LCAs) to examine environmental effect in addition to therapeutic performance will grow in regulatory frameworks [88]. Thus, eco-innovative biomedical systems that strike a balance between ecological responsibility and therapeutic efficacy are the way of the future.

6.9.6 Interdisciplinary Convergence of Materials Science, Nanotechnology, and Bioinformatics

The ongoing multidisciplinary convergence of several scientific and engineering fields will be crucial to the development of DDS and biosensors. Nanotechnology offers precise control at the molecular scale for targeting and sensing; materials science lays the groundwork for creating nanostructured coatings, biocompatible polymers, and hybrid composites; and bioinformatics connects systems biology and computational prediction with biological data analysis [89, 90]. For instance, by expanding the number of reaction sites, nanostructured surfaces increase the sensitivity of biosensors, and nanoencapsulation methods increase medication solubility and safeguard delicate biomolecules. In the meanwhile, researchers can model intricate biological interactions using bioinformatics and systems-level modeling, which helps them choose materials and develop functionalization plans.

New partnerships are combining knowledge in soft robotics, microfluidics, regenerative medicine, and quantum sensing to create integrated innovation ecosystems. It is anticipated that this convergence would result in multifunctional, adaptable platforms that learn and adapt to biological systems in addition to sensing and reacting. Such interdisciplinary collaboration will eventually make it possible for patient-centered, holistic healthcare systems devices that not only identify and treat illnesses but also predict their course, maximize treatment, and reduce their environmental impact.

The development of intelligent, sustainable, and adaptable biomedical ecosystems is key to the future of drug delivery systems and biosensors. Precision medicine will be redefined by combining sensing and delivery capabilities, biodegradable and self-powered materials, AI-driven personalization, and wireless closed-loop control. Meanwhile, interdisciplinary convergence and green manufacturing will guarantee that innovation stays morally and ecologically responsible. An era where biology and technology coevolve toward human well-being will be ushered in by the next generation of biomedical devices, which will represent a move away from reactive treatment and toward proactive, autonomous, and regenerative healthcare [91].

6.10 Conclusion

One of the most revolutionary developments in contemporary biomedical engineering is the combination of biomaterials, drug delivery systems (DDS), and biosensors. These technologies have developed over the past few decades from static and compartmentalized platforms to dynamic, cooperative systems that can perform targeted therapy, real-time diagnosis, and ongoing physiological monitoring. This convergence is indicative of a larger medical paradigm change away from reactive care and toward proactive, individualized, and flexible healthcare. Innovation in materials, interdisciplinary cooperation, and the smooth integration of technical and biological complexity are essential to the success of this transition.

6.10.1 Summary of Biomaterial-Based Drug Delivery and Biosensor Integration

Drug delivery systems and biosensors are both structurally and functionally based on biomaterials. They offer localized localization, regulated release kinetics, and biocompatible interfaces in DDS, which maximizes therapeutic results while reducing adverse effects. Biomaterials create biointerfaces in biosensors, which convert biological reactions into electrical or physical signals that may be measured with high selectivity and sensitivity. Theranostic platforms multifunctional systems that can diagnose, monitor, and treat patients at the same time are the result of the merging of these two disciplines.

Hydrogels and polymeric nanoparticles, for instance, are increasingly used as both sensing matrices and drug carriers, identifying biomarkers that control their own release processes. Electrochemical biosensors integrated into implanted delivery systems can monitor drug concentrations or metabolic states and promptly adjust dosages. Traditional therapeutic approaches are transformed into closed-loop systems by this combination of sensing and delivery, guaranteeing responsive, self-regulated treatment that is adapted to the patient's physiological state. This kind of integration emphasizes how crucial biomaterials are to the developing area of precision medicine not just as passive scaffolds, but also as active, intelligent elements.

6.10.2 Emphasis on Precision, Responsiveness, and Biocompatibility in Design

The fundamental design tenets of contemporary DDS and biosensor technologies are accuracy, responsiveness, and biocompatibility. By ensuring that therapeutic drugs are administered at the right time and dose to their intended target, precision lowers systemic toxicity. This is accomplished by designing materials at the micro and nanoscales, enabling control over surface functions, degradation rates, and porosity. A dynamic dimension is added by responsiveness, which allows materials to change their structural or chemical states in response to environmental cues like pH, temperature, glucose content, or enzyme activity. These stimuli-responsive devices, which mimic the adaptive complexity of biological systems, allow for real-time feedback and on-demand release.

The fundamental design tenets of contemporary DDS and biosensor technologies are accuracy, responsiveness, and biocompatibility. By ensuring that therapeutic drugs are administered at the right time and dose to their intended target, precision lowers systemic toxicity. This is accomplished by designing materials at the micro and nanoscales, enabling control over surface functions, degradation rates, and porosity. A dynamic dimension is added by responsiveness, which allows materials to change their structural or chemical states in response to environmental cues like pH, temperature, glucose content, or enzyme activity. These stimuli-responsive devices, which mimic the adaptive complexity of biological systems, allow for real-time feedback and on-demand release.

6.10.3 Recognition of Interdisciplinary Progress Bridging Diagnostics and Therapy

The advancements made in this area are a result of the convergence of several scientific fields, including computer science, chemistry, materials science, nanotechnology, and bioengineering, all of which are working toward the development of intelligent biological systems. Microfluidics and lab-on-a-chip technologies have made it possible for small, multipurpose devices for simultaneous detection and delivery, while developments in nanomaterials have improved sensor sensitivity and drug encapsulation effectiveness. In the meantime, predicted insights into drug kinetics, patient-specific reactions, and long-term device performance are now possible thanks to artificial intelligence (AI) and machine learning (ML).

A new generation of intelligent theranostic devices has been created because of this interdisciplinary collaboration. These devices can precisely carry out therapeutic actions, analyze biological signals, and make decisions on their own. By enabling predictive design and lowering reliance on trial-and-error testing, the partnership between computer modeling and experimental validation spurs innovation. Furthermore, translating laboratory prototypes into clinically viable technology is facilitated by cross-disciplinary research, which closes the hitherto unachievable gap between diagnosis and therapy.

Additionally, discipline benefits from developments in bioprinting and additive manufacturing, which enable the customisation of devices that meet the unique physiological and anatomical needs of each patient. A vital step toward precision and regenerative medicine, this personalization improves therapeutic efficacy and lowers problems. This kind of integration highlights the value of system-level thinking, in which treatment and diagnosis are integrated into a single biomedical framework rather than existing as distinct procedures.

6.10.4 Outlook Toward Intelligent, Patient-Specific, and Sustainable Biomedical Systems

The creation of intelligent, flexible, and sustainable biomedical platforms is key to the future of biomaterial-based DDS and biosensor systems. In addition to diagnosing and treating illnesses, these systems will also adapt to the physiology of their patients. Predictive, self-regulating therapeutic interventions that reduce human error and increase clinical efficiency will be made possible by the integration of AI-driven control systems with real-time data analytics. New developments in self-healing materials and biodegradable electronics will improve sustainability even further by lowering environmental impact and doing away with the need for invasive removal techniques.

The trend toward eco-friendly and patient-specific design also emphasizes how crucial it is to have legal and ethical frameworks that guarantee accessibility, safety, and reproducibility. Clinical translation will depend on the creation of common criteria for assessing the performance of integrated biosensors and DDSs, considering factors like degradation behavior, long-term biostability, and data privacy. Furthermore, biomedical innovation is in line with international environmental goals when sustainability principles are incorporated into the synthesis of biomaterials and the production of devices. The goal is the development of bioresponsive, flawlessly integrated systems that work in unison with the human body devices that can provide precise therapies, identify early pathological changes, and continuously provide feedback to preserve homeostasis. An era of adaptive, personalized, and sustainable medicine is being ushered in by these next-generation platforms, which represent the meeting point of biological intelligence, engineering precision, and digital connectivity.

To sum up, the integration of biosensors and drug delivery based on biomaterials are essential components of the upcoming biomedical science revolution. Their development represents a shift from passive medical equipment to intelligent, networked systems that combine therapy and diagnosis into a single, cohesive whole. Researchers are establishing groundwork for technologies that not only restore health but also foresee and prevent disease by placing a strong emphasis on accuracy, biocompatibility, and interdisciplinary cooperation. The future of really customized, responsive, and regenerative healthcare will be determined by the convergence of materials innovation, data-driven intelligence, and patient-centered design as the field develops.

References

1. Stielow, M., Witczyńska, A., Kubryń, N., Fijałkowski, Ł., Nowaczyk, J., Nowaczyk, A.: The bioavailability of drugs—the current state of knowledge. Molecules. **28**(24), 8038 (2023)
2. Zorkina, Y., Abramova, O., Ushakova, V., Morozova, A., Zubkov, E., Valikhov, M., Melnikov, P., Majouga, A., Chekhonin, V.: Nano carrier drug delivery systems for the treatment of neuropsychiatric disorders: advantages and limitations. Molecules. **25**(22), 5294 (2020)
3. Alzoubi, L., Aljabali, A.A., Tambuwala, M.M.: Empowering precision medicine: the impact of 3D printing on personalized therapeutic. AAPS PharmSciTech. **24**(8), 228 (2023)
4. Dave, S., Dave, A., Radhakrishnan, S., Das, J., Dave, S.: Biosensors for healthcare: an artificial intelligence approach. In: Biosensors for Emerging and Re-Emerging Infectious Diseases, pp. 365–383. Elsevier (2022)
5. Szunerits, S., Boukherroub, R., Kleber, C., Knoll, W., Yunda, J., Rumipamba, J., et al.: Biosensors integrated within wearable devices for monitoring chronic wound status. APL Bioeng. **9**(1) (2025)
6. Zeng, Q., Huang, C., Zhu, J.: AI-driven transformation of precision medicine: a comprehensive narrative review of key application areas, emerging paradigms, and future directions. Front. Public Health. **13**, 1656603 (2025)
7. Alowais, S.A., Alghamdi, S.S., Alsuhebany, N., Alqahtani, T., Alshaya, A.I., Almohareb, S.N., Aldairem, A., Alrashed, M., Bin Saleh, K., Badreldin, H.A., Al Yami, M.S.: Revolutionizing healthcare: the role of artificial intelligence in clinical practice. BMC Med. Educ. **23**(1), 689 (2023)

8. Rehan, H.: Artificial intelligence and machine learning: the impact of machine learning on predictive analytics in healthcare. Innov. Comput. Sci. J. **9**(1), 1–20 (2023)
9. Singh, S., Rai, S., Bandopadhyay, A., Das, M.: From detection to drug delivery: innovations in cancer biosensors from concept to clinical impact. Biotechnol. Sustain. Mater. **2**(1), 17 (2025)
10. Jarosinski, M.A., Dhayalan, B., Rege, N., Chatterjee, D., Weiss, M.A.: 'Smart' insulin-delivery technologies and intrinsic glucose-responsive insulin analogues. Diabetologia. **64**(5), 1016–1029 (2021)
11. Caballero, D., Abreu, C.M., Reis, R.L., Kundu, S.C.: Emerging microfluidic and biosensor technologies for improved cancer theranostics. In: Microfluidics and Biosensors in Cancer Research: Applications in Cancer Modeling and Theranostics, pp. 461–495. Springer International Publishing, Cham (2022)
12. Sharma, A.K.: Current trends in nanotheranostics: a concise review on bioimaging and smart wearable technology. Nanotheranostics. **7**(3), 258–269 (2023)
13. Adepu, S., Ramakrishna, S.: Controlled drug delivery systems: current status and future directions. Molecules. **26**(19), 5905 (2021)
14. Ezike, T.C., Okpala, U.S., Onoja, U.L., Nwike, C.P., Ezeako, E.C., Okpara, O.J., Okoroafor, C.C., Eze, S.C., Kalu, O.L., Odoh, E.C., Nwadike, U.G.: Advances in drug delivery systems, challenges and future directions. Heliyon. **9**(6), e17488 (2023)
15. Martinek, R., Ladrova, M., Sidikova, M., Jaros, R., Behbehani, K., Kahankova, R., Kawala-Sterniuk, A.: Advanced bioelectrical signal processing methods: past, present and future approach—part II: brain signals. Sensors. **21**(19), 6343 (2021)
16. Koide, H.: Design of functional nanoparticles for intractable disease therapy. Biol. Pharm. Bull. **44**(1), 1–6 (2021)
17. Su, C.J., Murugan, A., Linton, J.M., Yeluri, A., Bois, J., Klumpe, H., Langley, M.A., Antebi, Y.E., Elowitz, M.B.: Ligand-receptor promiscuity enables cellular addressing. Cell Syst. **13**(5), 408–425 (2022)
18. Jones, S.J., Taylor, A.F., Beales, P.A.: Towards feedback-controlled nanomedicines for smart, adaptive delivery. Exp. Biol. Med. **244**(4), 283–293 (2019)
19. Wells, C.M., Harris, M., Choi, L., Murali, V.P., Guerra, F.D., Jennings, J.A.: Stimuli-responsive drug release from smart polymers. J. Funct. Biomater. **10**(3), 34 (2019)
20. Zhu, X., Chen, J., Zhao, J., Zhang, Z., Wang, C.: Nanomaterials for theranostic management of oral cancer: advances in imaging, biosensing, targeted delivery, and multimodal synergistic therapy. Int. J. Nanomedicine. **20**, 13689–13719 (2025)
21. Hassan, J.Z., Raza, A., Babar, Z.U.D., Qumar, U., Kaner, N.T., Cassinese, A.: 2D material-based sensing devices: an update. J. Mater. Chem. A. **11**(12), 6016–6063 (2023)
22. McLamore, E.S., Datta, S.P.: A connected world: system-level support through biosensors. Annu. Rev. Anal. Chem. **16**(1), 285–309 (2023)
23. Badiceanu, M., Anghel, S., Mihailescu, N., Visan, A.I., Mihailescu, C.N., Mihailescu, I.N.: Coatings functionalization via laser versus other deposition techniques for medical applications: a comparative review. Coatings. **12**(1), 71 (2022)
24. Huang, Q., Li, N., Zhang, H., Che, C., Sun, F., Xiong, Y., Canady, T.D., Cunningham, B.T.: Critical review: digital resolution biomolecular sensing for diagnostics and life science research. Lab Chip. **20**(16), 2816–2840 (2020)
25. Paramshetti, S., Angolkar, M., Al Fatease, A., Alshahrani, S.M., Hani, U., Garg, A., Ravi, G., Osmani, R.A.M.: Revolutionizing drug delivery and therapeutics: the biomedical applications of conductive polymers and composites-based systems. Pharmaceutics. **15**(4), 1204 (2023)
26. Visan, A.I., Popescu-Pelin, G., Socol, G.: Degradation behavior of polymers used as coating materials for drug delivery—a basic review. Polymers. **13**(8), 1272 (2021)
27. Farooque, F., Wasi, M., Mughees, M.M.: Liposomes as drug delivery system: an updated review. J. Drug Deliv. Ther. **11**, 149–158 (2021)
28. Pande, S.: Liposomes for drug delivery: review of vesicular composition, factors affecting drug release and drug loading in liposomes. Artif. Cells Nanomed. Biotechnol. **51**(1), 428–440 (2023)

29. Kim, M.W., Kwon, S.H., Choi, J.H., Lee, A.: A promising biocompatible platform: lipid-based and bio-inspired smart drug delivery systems for cancer therapy. Int. J. Mol. Sci. **19**(12), 3859 (2018)
30. Naziris, N., Demetzos, C.: Lipid nanoparticles as platforms for theranostic purposes: recent advances in the field. J. Nanotheranostics. **3**(2), 86–101 (2022)
31. Fobian, S.F., Cheng, Z., Ten Hagen, T.L.: Smart lipid-based nanosystems for therapeutic immune induction against cancers: perspectives and outlooks. Pharmaceutics. **14**(1), 26 (2021)
32. Hao, Y., Ji, Z., Zhou, H., Wu, D., Gu, Z., Wang, D., Ten Dijke, P.: Lipid-based nanoparticles as drug delivery systems for cancer immunotherapy. MedComm. **4**(4), e339 (2023)
33. Herrmann, A., Haag, R., Schedler, U.: Hydrogels and their role in biosensing applications. Adv. Healthc. Mater. **10**(11), 2100062 (2021)
34. Gato-Diaz, U., Concheiro, A., Alvarez-Lorenzo, C., Blanco-Fernandez, B.: 4D printed hydrogels for precision delivery of bioactive molecules in cancer. Expert Opin. Drug Deliv. **22**(10), 1565–1581 (2025)
35. Zhang, Y.S., Haghiashtiani, G., Hübscher, T., Kelly, D.J., Lee, J.M., Lutolf, M., McAlpine, M.C., Yeong, W.Y., Zenobi-Wong, M., Malda, J.: 3D extrusion bioprinting. Nat. Rev. Methods Primers. **1**(1), 75 (2021)
36. Cicha, I., Priefer, R., Severino, P., Souto, E.B., Jain, S.: Biosensor-integrated drug delivery systems as new materials for biomedical applications. Biomolecules. **12**(9), 1198 (2022)
37. Lim, Y.Y., Zaidi, A.M.A., Miskon, A.: Composing on-program triggers and on-demand stimuli into biosensor drug carriers in drug delivery systems for programmable arthritis therapy. Pharmaceuticals. **15**(11), 1330 (2022)
38. García-Estrada, P., García-Bon, M.A., López-Naranjo, E.J., Basaldúa-Pérez, D.N., Santos, A., Navarro-Partida, J.: Polymeric implants for the treatment of intraocular eye diseases: trends in biodegradable and non-biodegradable materials. Pharmaceutics. **13**(5), 701 (2021)
39. Kunjiappan, S., Pavadai, P., Vellaichamy, S., Ram Kumar Pandian, S., Ravishankar, V., Palanisamy, P., Govindaraj, S., Srinivasan, G., Premanand, A., Sankaranarayanan, M., Theivendren, P.: Surface receptor-mediated targeted drug delivery systems for enhanced cancer treatment: a state-of-the-art review. Drug Dev. Res. **82**(3), 309–340 (2021)
40. Yadav, S., Saini, A., Devi, R., Lata, S.: Transducers in biosensors. In: Biomaterials-Based Sensors: Recent Advances and Applications, pp. 101–125. Springer Nature Singapore, Singapore (2023)
41. Manickam, P., Mariappan, S.A., Murugesan, S.M., Hansda, S., Kaushik, A., Shinde, R., Thipperudraswamy, S.P.: Artificial intelligence (AI) and internet of medical things (IoMT) assisted biomedical systems for intelligent healthcare. Biosensors. **12**(8), 562 (2022)
42. Qureshi, R., Irfan, M., Ali, H., Khan, A., Nittala, A.S., Ali, S., Shah, A., Gondal, T.M., Sadak, F., Shah, Z., Hadi, M.U.: Artificial intelligence and biosensors in healthcare and its clinical relevance: a review. IEEE Access. **11**, 61600–61620 (2023)
43. Kashyap, B.K., Singh, V.V., Solanki, M.K., Kumar, A., Ruokolainen, J., Kesari, K.K.: Smart nanomaterials in cancer theranostics: challenges and opportunities. ACS Omega. **8**(16), 14290–14320 (2023)
44. Lim, E.K., Kim, T., Paik, S., Haam, S., Huh, Y.M., Leec, K.: Nanomaterials for theranostics: recent advances and future challenges. In: Nanomaterials and Neoplasms, pp. 587–775. Jenny Stanford Publishing (2021)
45. Ibegbulam, C.M., Olowonubi, J.A., Fatounde, S.A., Oyegunwa, O.A.: Artificial intelligence in the era of 4IR: drivers, challenges and opportunities. Eng. Sci. Technol. J. **4**(6), 473–488 (2023)
46. Rajan, A.B.K., Dhavamani, C.: Principles of Nanoscience and Nanotechnology. Academic Guru Publishing House (2023)
47. Chenthamara, D., Subramaniam, S., Ramakrishnan, S.G., Krishnaswamy, S., Essa, M.M., Lin, F.H., Qoronfleh, M.W.: Therapeutic efficacy of nanoparticles and routes of administration. Biomater. Res. **23**(1), 20 (2019)

48. Yang, C., Lin, Z.I., Chen, J.A., Xu, Z., Gu, J., Law, W.C., Yang, J.H.C., Chen, C.K.: Organic/inorganic self-assembled hybrid nano-architectures for cancer therapy applications. Macromol. Biosci. **22**(2), 2100349 (2022)
49. Herdiana, Y., Wathoni, N., Shamsuddin, S., Muchtaridi, M.: Drug release study of the chitosan-based nanoparticles. Heliyon. **8**(1), e08674 (2022)
50. Vlachopoulos, A., Karlioti, G., Balla, E., Daniilidis, V., Kalamas, T., Stefanidou, M., Bikiaris, N.D., Christodoulou, E., Koumentakou, I., Karavas, E., Bikiaris, D.N.: Poly(lactic acid)-based microparticles for drug delivery applications: an overview of recent advances. Pharmaceutics. **14**(2), 359 (2022)
51. Naresh, V., Lee, N.: A review on biosensors and recent development of nanostructured materials-enabled biosensors. Sensors. **21**(4), 1109 (2021)
52. Patel, M., Agrawal, M., Srivastava, A.: Signal amplification strategies in electrochemical biosensors via antibody immobilization and nanomaterial-based transducers. Mater. Adv. **3**(24), 8864–8885 (2022)
53. Gao, N., Li, X.J.: Controlled drug delivery using microdevices. In: Microfluidic Devices for Biomedical Applications, pp. 205–223. Woodhead Publishing (2021)
54. Williams, D.F.: Assessing the triad of biocompatibility, medical device functionality and biological safety. Med. Devices Sens. **4**(1), e10150 (2021)
55. Hsueh, P.Y.S.: Ecosystem of patient-centered research and information system design. In: Personal Health Informatics: Patient Participation in Precision Health, pp. 329–351. Springer International Publishing, Cham (2022)
56. Morrison, M., Prainsack, B.: Responsible Personalised Medicine: Exploring the Ethical, Legal, Social, Political and Economic Issues of Manufacturing, Distribution, Access and Reimbursement. A Report by the Future Targeted Healthcare Manufacturing Hub (2022)
57. Song, F.X., Xu, X., Ding, H., Yu, L., Huang, H., Hao, J., Wu, C., Liang, R., Zhang, S.: Recent progress in nanomaterial-based biosensors and theranostic nanomedicine for bladder cancer. Biosensors. **13**(1), 106 (2023)
58. Saha, T., Del Caño, R., Mahato, K., De la Paz, E., Chen, C., Ding, S., Yin, L., Wang, J.: Wearable electrochemical glucose sensors in diabetes management: a comprehensive review. Chem. Rev. **123**(12), 7854–7889 (2023)
59. Biswas, G.C., Choudhury, S., Rabbani, M.M., Das, J.: A review on potential electrochemical point-of-care tests targeting pandemic infectious disease detection: COVID-19 as a reference. Chemosensors. **10**(7), 269 (2022)
60. Zida, S.I., Lin, Y.D., Khung, Y.L.: Current trends on surface acoustic wave biosensors. Adv. Mater. Technol. **6**(6), 2001018 (2021)
61. Bors, L.A., Erdő, F.: Overcoming the blood–brain barrier. Challenges and tricks for CNS drug delivery. Sci. Pharm. **87**(1), 6 (2019)
62. Hivare, P., Panda, C., Gupta, S., Bhatia, D.: Programmable DNA nanodevices for applications in neuroscience. ACS Chem. Neurosci. **12**(3), 363–377 (2021)
63. Erdem, O., Es, I., Saylan, Y., Inci, F.: Unifying the efforts of medicine, chemistry, and engineering in biosensing technologies to tackle the challenges of the COVID-19 pandemic. Anal. Chem. **94**(1), 3–25 (2021)
64. Qin, J., Wang, W., Gao, L., Yao, S.Q.: Emerging biosensing and transducing techniques for potential applications in point-of-care diagnostics. Chem. Sci. **13**(10), 2857–2876 (2022)
65. Malik, S., Muhammad, K., Waheed, Y.: Emerging applications of nanotechnology in healthcare and medicine. Molecules. **28**(18), 6624 (2023)
66. Mitchell, K.R., Esene, J.E., Woolley, A.T.: Advances in multiplex electrical and optical detection of biomarkers using microfluidic devices. Anal. Bioanal. Chem. **414**(1), 167–180 (2022)
67. Jia, F., Gao, Y., Wang, H.: Recent advances in drug delivery system fabricated by microfluidics for disease therapy. Bioengineering. **9**(11), 625 (2022)
68. Farid, M.I., Wu, W., Guiwei, L., Yu, Z.: Research on imminent enlargements of smart materials and structures towards novel 4D printing (4DP: SMs-SSs). Int. J. Adv. Manuf. Technol. **126**(7), 2803–2823 (2023)

69. Argun, A.A., Rana, M., Rather, H.A., Dar, M.A.: Implantable biosensors for long-term monitoring of cardiac health. Biosens. Nanotheranostics. **1**(1), 1–14 (2022)
70. Haick, H., Tang, N.: Artificial intelligence in medical sensors for clinical decisions. ACS Nano. **15**(3), 3557–3567 (2021)
71. Sagdic, K., Eş, I., Sitti, M., Inci, F.: Smart materials: rational design in biosystems via artificial intelligence. Trends Biotechnol. **40**(8), 987–1003 (2022)
72. Bax, M., Thorpe, J., Romanov, V.: The future of personalized cardiovascular medicine demands 3D and 4D printing, stem cells, and artificial intelligence. Front. Sens. **4**, 1294721 (2023)
73. Ma, X., Guo, G., Wu, X., Wu, Q., Liu, F., Zhang, H., Shi, N., Guan, Y.: Advances in integration, wearable applications, and artificial intelligence of biomedical microfluidics systems. Micromachines. **14**(5), 972 (2023)
74. Abbasnezhad, N., Kebdani, M., Shirinbayan, M., Champmartin, S., Tcharkhtchi, A., Kouidri, S., Bakir, F.: Development of a model based on physical mechanisms for the explanation of drug release: application to diclofenac release from polyurethane films. Polymers. **13**(8), 1230 (2021)
75. AlSawaftah, N.M., Paul, V., Awad, N.S., Husseini, G.: Modeling of Drug Release Kinetics from Stimuli-Responsive Micelles and Liposomes: A Review (2021)
76. Shen, S.C., Khare, E., Lee, N.A., Saad, M.K., Kaplan, D.L., Buehler, M.J.: Computational design and manufacturing of sustainable materials through first-principles and materiomics. Chem. Rev. **123**(5), 2242–2275 (2023)
77. Rumbut, J., Fang, H., Carreiro, S., Smelson, D., Boyer, E.: An overview of wearable biosensor systems for real-time substance use detection. IEEE Internet Things J. **9**(23), 23405–23415 (2022)
78. Paramithiotis, E., Varaklis, C., Pillet, S., Shafiani, S., Lancelotta, M.P., Steinhubl, S., Sugden, S., Clutter, M., Montamat-Sicotte, D., Chermak, T., Crawford, S.Y.: Integrated antibody and cellular immunity monitoring are required for assessment of the long term protection that will be essential for effective next generation vaccine development. Front. Immunol. **14**, 1166059 (2023)
79. Chianumba, E.C., Ikhalea, N., Mustapha, A.Y., Forkuo, A.Y.: Developing a framework for using AI in personalized medicine to optimize treatment plans. J. Front. Multidiscip. Res. **3**(1), 57–71 (2022)
80. Goldmann, N., Skalicky, S.E., Weinreb, R.N., Guedes, R.A.P., Baudouin, C., Zhang, X., van Gestel, A., Blumenthal, E.Z., Kaufman, P.L., Rothman, R., Vasquez, A.M.: Defining functional requirements for a patient-centric computerized glaucoma treatment and care ecosystem. J. Med. Artif. Intell. **6**, 3 (2023)
81. He, J., Baxter, S.L., Xu, J., Xu, J., Zhou, X., Zhang, K.: The practical implementation of artificial intelligence technologies in medicine. Nat. Med. **25**(1), 30–36 (2019)
82. Eskandar, K.: Artificial intelligence in healthcare: explore the applications of AI in various medical domains, such as medical imaging, diagnosis, drug discovery, and patient care. Series Med. Sci. **4**, 37–53 (2023)
83. Shekhar, S., Yadav, A.K., Khosla, A., Solanki, P.R.: Interleukins profiling for biosensing applications: possibilities and the future of disease detection. ECS Sens. Plus. **1**(4), 041601 (2022)
84. Zhai, Z., Du, X., Long, Y., Zheng, H.: Biodegradable polymeric materials for flexible and degradable electronics. Front. Electron. **3**, 985681 (2022)
85. Kny, E., Reiner-Rozman, C., Dostalek, J., Hassel, A.W., Nöhammer, C., Pfaffeneder-Mantai, F., Szunerits, S., Weber, V., Knoll, W., Kleber, C.: State of the art of chemosensors in a biomedical context. Chemosensors. **10**(6), 199 (2022)
86. Pohlman, A.W., Moudgalya, H., Jordano, L., Lobato, G.C., Gerard, D., Liptay, M.J., Seder, C.W., Borgia, J.A.: The role of IGF-pathway biomarkers in determining risks, screening, and prognosis in lung cancer. Oncotarget. **13**, 393–407 (2022)
87. Roy, S., Azad, A.W., Baidya, S., Alam, M.K., Khan, F.: Powering solutions for biomedical sensors and implants inside the human body: a comprehensive review on energy harvesting

units, energy storage, and wireless power transfer techniques. IEEE Trans. Power Electron. **37**(10), 12237–12263 (2022)

88. Lichter, K.E., Charbonneau, K., Sabbagh, A., Witztum, A., Chuter, R., Anand, C., Thiel, C.L., Mohamad, O.: Evaluating the environmental impact of radiation therapy using life cycle assessments: a critical review. Int. J. Radiat. Oncol. Biol. Phys. **117**(3), 554–567 (2023)
89. Asdaq, S.M.B., Ikbal, A.M.A., Sahu, R.K., Bhattacharjee, B., Paul, T., Deka, B., Fattepur, S., Widyowati, R., Vijaya, J., Al Mohaini, M., Alsalman, A.J.: Nanotechnology integration for SARS-CoV-2 diagnosis and treatment: an approach to preventing pandemic. Nanomaterials. **11**(7), 1841 (2021)
90. Kasture, K., Shende, P.: Amalgamation of artificial intelligence with nanoscience for biomedical applications. Arch. Comput. Methods Eng. **30**(8), 4667–4685 (2023)
91. Timmermans, J., Zhao, Y., van den Hoven, J.: Ethics and nanopharmacy: value sensitive design of new drugs. In: The Ethical Challenges of Emerging Medical Technologies, pp. 139–153. Routledge (2020)

Chapter 7
Orthopedic, Cardiovascular, Dental, and Ophthalmic Applications

Abstract In the fields of orthopedic, cardiovascular, dental, and ophthalmic medicine, where exact integration of mechanical, biological, and chemical properties is necessary for the restoration of form and function, biomaterials are revolutionary. Biomaterials like titanium alloys, hydroxyapatite, and biodegradable polymers are used in orthopedic applications for bone fixation devices, scaffolds that promote osteogenesis, and joint replacements. The creation of patient-specific implants that replicate the architecture of natural bone while encouraging cellular adhesion and vascularization is now possible because to advancements in 3D printing and surface modification. In cardiovascular medicine, devices like heart valves, vascular grafts, and stents where long-term hemocompatibility, elasticity, and resistance to thrombosis are crucial and are supported by biocompatible polymers, metals, and hybrid composites. One significant breakthrough in restoring vascular integrity without the risk of chronic inflammation is the development of bioresorbable stents and endothelialized scaffolds. Bioactive ceramics, glass ionomers, and polymer composites are examples of dental biomaterials that have developed to achieve higher mechanical strength, remineralization capability, and aesthetic appeal. From guided bone regeneration to restorative fillings and implants, they facilitate applications by providing improved periodontal tissue integration and less bacterial colonization. Hydrogels, collagen matrices, and biodegradable polymers are used in ophthalmology as intraocular lenses, corneal substitutes, and drug-eluting contact devices that preserve optical clarity and encourage epithelial healing. Nanostructured surfaces and sophisticated biomimetic coating enhance comfort, lower the risk of infection, and promote regenerative repair in sensitive ocular environments. When taken as a whole, these uses demonstrate how material science, biomechanics, and regenerative engineering come together to advance precision medicine by using multipurpose, adaptable biomaterials. By combining intelligent, biodegradable, and patient-specific designs, these systems' ongoing development promises to revolutionize therapeutic results and improve the robustness and physiological compatibility of biomedical implants and devices in several vital healthcare areas.

M. Adeoba, T. Pandelani, *Application of Biomaterials in Biomedical Engineering*, Series in BioEngineering,
https://doi.org/10.1007/978-3-032-34477-9_7

7.1 Introduction

The development of biomaterials has had a significant impact on contemporary medicine by making it possible to replace, repair, and regenerate tissues and organs in a variety of clinical settings. Biomaterials are the cornerstone of biomedical innovation, from cardiovascular devices that preserve hemodynamic stability to orthopedic implants that restore skeletal integrity, and from dental prosthesis that enhance oral function to ocular systems that restore eyesight [1, 2]. Their ability to maintain mechanical and biochemical performance while integrating with biological systems has made them essential for enhancing therapeutic results and patient quality of life. These applications are supported by the dynamic junction of clinical medicine, tissue biology, and materials science, which promotes the development of next-generation biomaterials with lifespan, precision, and flexibility [3, 4].

7.1.1 Overview of Biomedical Applications Across Major Clinical Fields

Biomaterials are essential in many important clinical areas, each with its own set of mechanical, physiological, and biochemical requirements. Metals like cobalt-chromium and titanium alloys, ceramics like hydroxyapatite, and polymeric scaffolds are used in orthopedics to heal bones and joints. These materials must support controlled biodegradation and osseointegration while offering enough load-bearing capacity. Stents, heart valves, and vascular grafts are made of polymers, metallic alloys, and composites; in cardiovascular medicine, these materials' elasticity, hemocompatibility, and resistance to corrosion are essential for preventing thrombosis and immunological rejection. Dental biomaterials combine strength, aesthetic quality, and bioactivity to restore both function and beauty [5]. Examples of these materials include zirconia and titanium implants, resin composites, and bioactive glass. Transparent hydrogels, silicone elastomers, and biodegradable matrices are utilized in ophthalmology for intraocular lenses, corneal substitutes, and ocular medication administration; these materials must have high optical clarity, low immunogenicity, and no toxicity [6, 7]. When taken as a whole, these therapeutic areas show how versatile biomaterials are in addressing structural, regenerative, and functional issues throughout the human body.

7.1.2 Importance of Material–Tissue Interaction in Functional Restoration and Regeneration

The relationship between the implanted material and the surrounding biological environment is fundamental to all effective biomaterial applications. Whether integration, encapsulation, or rejection takes place depends on the host response. Modulation of immunological activity, protein adsorption, and cellular adhesion at the material interface is necessary for the best results [8]. For instance, orthopedic implants require surfaces that facilitate osteoblast attachment and extracellular matrix formation, while cardiovascular devices must minimize platelet adhesion and complement activation. Similarly, ophthalmic materials must maintain ocular compatibility without inducing inflammatory reactions, and dental implants rely on efficient osseointegration for long-term durability. In order to ensure that implanted systems actively support tissue regeneration and homeostasis rather than just coexisting with them, biomaterial design must balance mechanical functioning with biological compatibility, as demonstrated by these examples. Advances in surface modification, nanostructuring, and biofunctionalization have further refined these interactions, enabling materials that direct specific cellular behaviors and tissue-specific healing processes.

7.1.3 *Rationale for Selecting Biomaterials in Orthopedic, Cardiovascular, Dental, and Ophthalmic Systems*

A complex interaction of mechanical characteristics, degradation kinetics, biological response, and clinical context determines which biomaterials are best suited for clinical usage [9]. The great tensile strength, fatigue resistance, and corrosion stability of metals like titanium or stainless steel, along with ceramic coatings that improve bioactivity, are what drive their selection in orthopedics. Since compliance and hemocompatibility are crucial in dynamic blood flow conditions, flexible polymers and corrosion-resistant metals like nitinol are recommended for cardiovascular systems. Materials like zirconia or glass-ceramics that can tolerate masticatory pressures and moisture exposure while maintaining biocompatibility and aesthetics are necessary for dental systems. However, transparency, oxygen permeability, and delicate tissue interaction achievable through hydrogels and silicone-based polymers must be given top priority in ophthalmic biomaterials. The balance between engineering performance and clinical practicality is highlighted by the consideration of sterilizing compatibility, manufacturability, and regulatory compliance in addition to physical and chemical factors while choosing materials. This selection process is also being impacted by the push for personalized medicine, which promotes the use of additive manufacturing and patient-specific materials to create customized mechanical and biological features [10, 11].

7.1.4 *Cross-Disciplinary Significance Engineering, Biology, and Clinical Sciences Convergence*

By combining the concepts of materials engineering, molecular biology, and clinical research, the subject of biomaterials is a prime example of multidisciplinary integration. Biologists clarify the cellular and molecular mechanisms governing host response and tissue regeneration. Engineers help synthesize, characterize, and optimize materials with desired structural and functional traits, and clinicians offer the translational insight required to guarantee that biomaterials function well in actual therapeutic settings. This convergence makes it easier to create cutting-edge materials with dynamic biological interaction capabilities, like smart polymers that react to physiological stimuli or bioactive ceramics that encourage osteogenesis [12, 13]. Additionally, collaborative research has sped up the development of hybrid materials that combine biological signaling ability with mechanical resilience. For instance, bioresorbable polymers combined with microelectronics are revolutionizing cardiovascular and ophthalmology treatments, while nanocomposites combining polymeric flexibility with ceramic bioactivity have found uses in bone and tooth healing. A systems-level approach to regenerative design is reflected in this integration, where each field helps to maximize material–tissue harmony for improved clinical results.

7.1.5 Scope and Organization of the Chapter

With a focus on the ways that material characteristics affect biological response and functional recovery, this chapter offers a thorough examination of biomaterial applications in the orthopedic, cardiovascular, dental, and ocular systems. It starts by going over the fundamental ideas and terms that underlie biomedical applications. Next, it looks at how biomaterials have evolved historically within each sector. The section on material kinds and qualities discusses the benefits and drawbacks of metallic, polymeric, ceramic, and composite systems. The following sections examine the cellular and molecular interactions that govern integration and healing, delving into mechanisms and processes. The design considerations discuss how to balance biocompatibility, mechanical optimization, and surface modification to meet performance objectives. While current developments span cutting-edge technologies like nanotechnology, bioactive coatings, and patient-specific design, applications and case studies offer empirical insights into the usage of biomaterials in actual clinical contexts. The section on problems and future directions concludes by outlining the possible advancement toward adaptable, regenerative, and intelligent biomaterials as well as the obstacles to clinical translation.

By connecting scientific fields and clinical requirements, biomaterials are positioned in this introduction as essential components in the restoration of human health. By integrating into dental, ophthalmology, cardiovascular, and orthopedic systems, biomaterials have expanded the potential of regenerative medicine. An era of customized, multipurpose, and sustainable biomedical technologies is set to dawn with the continued development of material–tissue engineering, which promises to produce next-generation implants and devices that are both structurally compatible and biologically active [14, 15].

7.2 Key Concepts and Definitions

Biomaterials bridge the gap between engineered materials and biological tissues, providing the basis for contemporary implants and medical devices. The particular clinical application domain, the mechanical and biological needs of the target tissues, and the demand for long-term integration within the body's physiological environment all influence their design, selection, and functionality. To advance functional and regenerative medicine, it is essential to comprehend the fundamental ideas that characterize the behavior of biomaterials in a variety of applications, including cardiovascular stents, dental restorations, ophthalmic lenses, and orthopedic load-bearing systems [16, 17]. The conceptual framework supporting biomaterial applications is further explained here, with a focus on functional classifications, biocompatibility standards, performance metrics, and the fusion of mechanical and biological principles for long-term usefulness.

7.2.1 Definition of Biomaterial Application Domains in Relation to Tissue Function and Mechanics

The physiological function and mechanical requirements of the tissue that biomaterials are intended to support, replace, or regenerate determine their application domains. The performance requirements of the corresponding biomaterial are determined by the unique mechanical, chemical, and biological characteristics of each tissue type, including bone, cartilage, myocardium, tooth enamel, and corneal epithelium [18, 19].

Biomaterials, for example, must endure severe mechanical loads, cyclic stresses, and fatigue for extended periods of time in orthopedic applications. Materials like titanium alloys, stainless steel, or reinforced composites that provide high stiffness, strength, and wear resistance are the focus. On the other hand, in pulsatile flow circumstances, cardiovascular implants, such as heart valves and stents, need materials that retain their hemodynamic compatibility, flexibility, and resistance to corrosion [20, 21]. Dental fillings, crowns, and implants require materials that mimic enamel's hardness and longevity while fending off microbial and salivary deterioration. Ophthalmic biomaterials, on the other hand, including intraocular lenses and corneal substitutes, place a higher value on surface smoothness, optical transparency, and biostability in aqueous conditions.

Therefore, mechanical-physiological congruence the capacity of a material to replicate the dynamic and structural responsibilities of the tissue it replaces rather than anatomical location alone determines the application areas of biomaterials. The interdisciplinary integration of biology, materials science, and mechanics is highlighted by this idea, which guarantees that performance is in line with the biochemical and mechanical environment of host tissues.

7.2.2 Functional Classification of Biomedical Implants: Structural, Regenerative, and Diagnostic

Based on its main function in a clinical setting, biomedical implants can be functionally divided into three categories: structural, regenerative, and diagnostic systems. The purpose of structural implants is to give diseased or injured tissues their mechanical stability and physical integrity back. Cardiovascular stents, dental implants, fixation plates, and orthopaedic joint replacements are a few examples. To provide long-lasting support under physiological loads, these materials mainly prioritize mechanical strength, fatigue resistance, and corrosion stability.

In contrast, regenerative implants are bioactive devices designed to promote tissue repair and regeneration. They frequently include hydrogels, composite scaffolds, or biodegradable polymers that break down in tandem with the growth of new tissue. These systems are designed to release biological signals that control cell migration, differentiation, and the deposition of extracellular matrix (ECM), such as growth factors or peptides. Both mechanical compliance and biochemical signaling are essential for the success of regenerative implants because they work together to promote functional tissue restoration.

Biosensors, microelectronic probes, and implantable monitoring devices that provide real-time physiological data are all included in diagnostic implants. Electrophysiological electrodes, pressure transducers, and glucose sensors are a few examples. For these systems to remain accurate over long periods of time, biocompatibility, signal quality, and interface stability are given top priority. The distinction between functional categories is becoming increasingly hazy with the emergence of theranostic systems, which combine therapeutic administration and diagnostic sensing, demonstrating how biology and engineering are combining to create contemporary biomaterials [22, 23].

7.2.3 Criteria for Biocompatibility, Mechanical Integrity, and Degradation Behavior in Application-Specific Contexts

Aligning biocompatibility, mechanical integrity, and degradation behavior in the context of therapeutic applications is a fundamental tenet of biomaterials science. The capacity of a material to carry out its intended function without causing unfavorable immunological, inflammatory, or toxic reactions is known as biocompatibility. This characteristic is dynamic and changes depending on the tissue type and implantation site. For instance, because of varying cellular and metabolic reactions, a polymer that is thought to be biocompatible in soft tissue may cause fibrosis in bone or brain settings.

Implants with mechanical integrity are guaranteed to withstand physiological pressures without experiencing structural failure. Materials used in dentistry or orthopedic applications need to be able to withstand fatigue, wear, and fracture under repeated loads. Viscoelastic damping and elastic compliance are equally important for cardiovascular and soft tissue implants in order to handle dynamic strain. The necessity for mechanically biomimetic materials is highlighted by the fact that mechanical mismatch between the implant and host tissue frequently results in stress shielding, implant loosening, or mechanical fatigue [24–26].

Another crucial factor is degradation behavior, especially for bioresorbable implants. While avoiding premature loss of function, controlled deterioration allows for the gradual transfer of mechanical load to regenerative tissues. To prevent inflammatory or immunogenic effects, breakdown by-products must, however, continue to be non-toxic and readily metabolized. For these applications, polymers like PLA, PGA, and PCL are widely utilized. Their specific molecular weights and copolymer ratios allow for fine-grained control over the rate of degradation. Metallic systems, such as magnesium alloys, on the other hand, are designed to corrode slowly to balance mechanical endurance and resorption. Thus, the fundamental paradigm directing the design of biomaterials tailored to specific applications is the triad of biocompatibility, mechanical integrity, and degradation control.

7.2.4 Overview of Performance Parameters Load-Bearing Capacity, Corrosion Resistance, and Optical Transparency

Application-relevant metrics that measure the physical and functional characteristics of biomaterials are used to evaluate their performance. The variety of requirements across medical professions is demonstrated by three universal parameters: load-bearing capability, corrosion resistance, and optical transparency. The ability of a material to tolerate mechanical stresses without deforming or failing is measured by its load-bearing capacity. Orthopedic implants, such knee and hip replacements, require fatigue lifetimes of millions of cycles and a high load tolerance [27]. High Young's modulus, yield strength, and fracture toughness materials are needed for this, and these are frequently attained by alloy optimization and surface treatments that improve wear resistance. Zirconia-toughened alumina is one of the advanced ceramics that minimize wear detritus while offering excellent compressive strength for articulating surfaces.

For metallic biomaterials exposed to physiological fluids that contain proteins and chlorides, corrosion resistance is essential. In addition to compromising mechanical integrity, corrosion releases metal ions that have the potential to cause systemic or local toxicity. Electrochemical stability is improved by self-healing barriers formed by passive oxide layers on titanium and stainless steel. Ion leaching is reduced and resistance is further increased by surface modification methods such anodization, ion implantation, and ceramic coatings. Controlled corrosion is no longer a failure mode but rather a design parameter for degradable systems, guaranteeing that dissolution coincides with healing processes.

The appropriateness of materials for ophthalmic applications, such as intraocular lenses and corneal replacements, is determined by their optical transparency. Long-term photostability, low light scattering, and excellent refractive clarity are necessary for these materials. Hydrogels like PHEMA (polyhydroxyethyl methacrylate) and polymers like PMMA (polymethyl methacrylate) combine biocompatibility and optical accuracy to provide clarity while thwarting calcification and protein deposition. To incorporate sensing without optical distortion, optoelectronic biosensors in developing applications require transparency in both the visible and infrared bands. When taken as a whole, these many factors guarantee that materials attain functional harmony with their operating environments.

7.2.5 Integration of Biological Cues and Mechanical Design for Long-Term Functionality

The incorporation of biological cues that facilitate active communication between the implant and surrounding tissue is a key component of contemporary biomaterial design, which goes beyond static mechanical performance [28, 29]. The realization that long-term success depends on biological adaptation and tissue remodeling in addition to mechanical stability is reflected in this paradigm shift. At the cellular level, protein adsorption, cell adhesion, and differentiation are controlled by surface chemistry, topography, and stiffness. For example, endothelial cells prefer smooth, elastic substrates with anti-thrombogenic coatings, whereas osteoblasts prefer rough, hydrophilic titanium surfaces with nanoscale characteristics that encourage focal adhesion formation [30, 31]. This calls for surfaces that are micro- and nano-engineered such that they can use biochemical and physical cues to control cell behavior.

Integration and tissue-specific regeneration are promoted by the incorporation of bioactive compounds, such as peptides, growth factors, or ECM-mimetic ligands, into material surfaces. Long-term compatibility is supported by dynamic systems, such as shape-memory polymers and stimuli-responsive hydrogels, which modify their mechanical or biochemical characteristics in reaction to environmental changes. In the meanwhile, methods for computational and finite element modeling help anticipate interface stability under physiological stresses and optimize stress distribution.

Additionally, the significance of matching material stiffness to tissue mechanics is highlighted by mechanotransduction, the cellular process that transforms mechanical impulses into biochemical responses. While overly compliant materials run the danger of mechanical failure, implants that are too rigid may prevent natural remodeling. To provide sustained functionality across a variety of clinical applications, the rising frontier of biomaterial design is defined by the integration of mechanical flexibility and biological responsiveness [32, 33].

Tissue mechanics, material functioning, and biological integration interact to provide the conceptual foundation of biomaterial science. Through the establishment of application domains, functional classifications, and performance requirements, scientists can create materials that balance physiological contexts with mechanical needs. The success of biomaterials continues to depend on striking a balance between mechanical stability, controlled degradation, and biocompatibility. Biomaterials evolve from passive structural supports into active, regenerative, and intelligent systems as engineering tactics change to include bioactive signaling and adaptive design. This change reflects a conceptual reinterpretation of biomaterials as living interfaces that can sense, react, and change in tandem with the tissues they serve, in addition to technological progress.

7.3 Historical Background

A remarkable journey from the empirical use of natural and metallic materials to the intricate design of bioactive, regenerative, and patient-specific systems that characterize modern medicine can be seen in the historical development of biomaterials for orthopedic, cardiovascular, dental, and ophthalmic applications. From crude alternatives intended for structural repair to dynamic interfaces encouraging integration, regeneration, and homeostasis, advancements in materials science, surface engineering, and biological knowledge have revolutionized the biomaterials landscape over the past century [34, 35]. This charts the significant turning points and paradigm changes that have influenced the development of biomaterials in these important clinical areas.

7.3.1 Early Use of Metals and Ceramics in Orthopedic and Dental Reconstruction

The use of biomaterials in dentistry and orthopedics has its roots in the early 1900s, when metals like gold, silver, and platinum were first employed for dental restorations and bone fixation because of their inertness and resistance to corrosion. Since its introduction in the 1930s, stainless steel has been the mainstay of orthopedic hardware, such as screws, plates, and hip prostheses, due to its relative biocompatibility and mechanical strength. But allergic reactions and ion release brought on by corrosion quickly made it clear that more stable alloys were required. Significant progress was made in the 1950s with the development of titanium and cobalt-chromium alloys, which were perfect for long-term implantation due to their favorable mechanical-to-weight ratio and exceptional corrosion resistance.

Ceramics like zirconia (ZrO_2) and alumina (AlO_3) were investigated concurrently due to their high compressive strength, wear resistance, and bioinertness, which led to their application in femoral heads, orthopedic joint bearings, and dental crowns. The idea of osseointegration of the direct structural and functional bond between living bone and the implant surface was first proposed in the 1970s with the introduction of hydroxyapatite (HA), a calcium phosphate ceramic that chemically resembles genuine bone material. Per-Ingvar Brånemark made this groundbreaking discovery, which revolutionized dentistry and orthopedic implantology by shifting the focus from inert replacement materials to physiologically integrated systems.

By proving that biological interaction and host acceptance were just as important for clinical success as mechanical compatibility, these early attempts laid the groundwork for contemporary biomaterial science [36, 37].

7.3.2 Evolution of Cardiovascular Prostheses from Mechanical Valves to Tissue-Engineered Grafts

The development of surgical innovation and materials technology is reflected in the history of cardiovascular biomaterials. Pioneers like Hufnagel and Starr-Edwards created the first mechanical heart valves in the 1950s using Teflon, silicone rubber, and stainless steel. Despite being successful in regaining hemodynamic function, these devices' lack of hemocompatibility led to problems like thrombosis and hemolysis. Patients thus needed anticoagulant medication for the rest of their lives, highlighting the need for better materials.

Polymeric materials like expanded polytetrafluoroethylene (ePTFE) and polyethylene terephthalate (Dacron) became the norm for vascular grafts by the 1970s because of their mechanical resilience, porosity, and flexibility. But problems including infection, intimal hyperplasia, and chronic patency limits continued. Similar advancements in biological prosthesis, which were modeled after pig valves or the pericardium of cows, provided improved hemodynamic performance and decreased thrombogenicity; but, durability was still an issue [38, 39].

A paradigm shifts toward tissue-engineered cardiovascular grafts and bioresorbable stents was brought about by the late twentieth century. These devices combined surface-modified metals and biodegradable polymers, such as poly-L-lactic acid (PLLA), to encourage endothelialization, or the vascular lining's natural regeneration. These developments mark a shift from passive mechanical support to regenerative and biologically active cardiovascular devices that can change and respond to physiological situations. The field is moving closer to completely functional, patient-specific grafts that can restore tissue over the long term without causing chronic inflammation or thrombosis thanks to the continuous integration of stem cell biology, growth hormones, and nanotechnology.

7.3.3 Development of Synthetic Polymers in Contact Lenses and Intraocular Lenses

Beginning in the middle of the twentieth century with the creation of polymethyl methacrylate (PMMA), a transparent, stiff polymer that transformed vision correction, ophthalmic biomaterials developed in tandem with developments in polymer chemistry. Harold Ridley originally employed PMMA for intraocular lenses (IOLs) after cataract surgery in the 1940s. He did this after seeing how well pilots tolerated PMMA particles stuck in their eyes during World War II. Although its rigidity restricted its usage in some applications, its optical clarity, stability, and non-toxicity made it perfect for permanent implantation.

Soft contact lenses consisting of hydrophilic polymers, like poly(2-hydroxyethyl methacrylate) (PHEMA), were developed in the 1970s and 1980s to increase comfort and oxygen permeability. Additional advancements included silicone hydrogels, which combine oxygen transfer and flexibility to enhance eye health over time. Since then, these materials have been modified for cutting-edge uses that combine therapeutic delivery and optical correction, such as drug-eluting contact lenses and biointegrative corneal implants. In a same vein, contemporary IOLs use flexible silicone and acrylic polymers to minimize posterior capsule opacification and enable less invasive insertion. The shift in biomaterials from robust and safe to adaptable and biologically interacting designs is reflected in the development of smart, hydrophilic, and functionalized ophthalmic polymers from inert PMMA [40, 41].

7.3.4 Key Milestones in Biomaterial Regulation and Standardization

Regulation and standardization became necessary when biomaterials became a crucial part of clinical practice to guarantee their safe, effective, and moral use. The 1970s and 1980s saw the establishment of stringent preclinical and clinical testing procedures by the U.S. Food and Drug Administration (FDA) and other organizations throughout the world, classifying devices according to risk levels. Testing frameworks for mechanical performance, sterilizing techniques, and biocompatibility (ISO 10993) were created by standards groups including the International Organization for Standardization (ISO) and ASTM International.

To guarantee reproducibility, quality control, and traceability in the manufacture of biomaterials, the Good Manufacturing Practices (GMP) concept was created [42]. These regulatory developments reduced the dangers of immunogenicity, toxicity, or device failure while offering an organized avenue for innovation. Lately, the emphasis has moved to ethical procurement of biological elements, long-term performance research, and post-market surveillance. As a reflection of the complexity of modern biomaterials in personalized healthcare, emerging rules are also adjusting to new paradigms, such as 3D-printed implants, combination products (device–drug hybrids), and AI-assisted medical systems.

7.3.5 Transition from Inert to Bioactive and Regenerative Material Paradigms

The idea of moving from inertness to bioactivity and regeneration has been the most revolutionary development in biomaterials. At first, materials were made to be passive substitutes with as little biological reaction as possible. But this method frequently resulted in long-term failure, mechanical mismatch, and fibrous encapsulation. The ability of materials to create chemical interactions with soft tissue and bone was shown by the discovery of bioactive materials, especially Larry Hench's creation of bioactive glass in 1969. The creation of materials that interact positively with the biological environment was sparked by this discovery.

Regenerative biomaterials systems that can direct cellular activity and tissue remodeling began to take shape in the 1990s with the introduction of biodegradable polymers, cell-responsive coatings, and growth factor-loaded scaffolds. Control over protein adsorption, cell adhesion, and immunological regulation was further improved by developments in tissue engineering, surface modification, and nanotechnology. Since then, patient-specific structures that replicate the dynamics and architecture of natural tissue have been made possible by the fusion of stem cell biology with biofabrication technologies, such as 3D bioprinting.

Adaptive and smart biomaterials systems that react dynamically to physiological stimuli like pH, temperature, or enzyme activity have been the focus of modern biomedical engineering. These materials represent a mature paradigm where the line between synthetic and biological becomes increasingly hazy, since they are not only made to be compatible but also to communicate and work in tandem with living tissues.

The development of biomaterials over time shows a steady shift from simple structural stand-ins to sophisticated, bioactive systems incorporated into live physiology. Advanced, multipurpose biomaterials that support healing, control immunological response, and adjust to biological settings have replaced the early reliance on metallic and ceramic materials for mechanical function [43, 44]. The transition from mechanical prostheses to regenerative tissue constructs highlights the collaboration of biological knowledge, therapeutic insight, and material innovation. A new era of customized and regenerative medicine is anticipated as regulatory frameworks and fabrication technology develop, leading to the development of biomaterials that actively coordinate regeneration in addition to replacing lost function.

7.4 Material Types and Properties

The material's composition, structure, mechanical qualities, and interaction with the biological environment all have a significant impact on how well biomedical devices and implants work. Materials are selected and designed to meet certain functional, mechanical, and biological needs in the fields of orthopedics, cardiovascular disease, dentistry, and ophthalmology. Under physiological conditions, these materials must preserve mechanical integrity, corrosion resistance, biocompatibility, and suitable degradation or stability profiles [45]. This offers a thorough examination of the various kinds of materials and their characteristics that are pertinent to different clinical domains, highlighting the ways in which composition and structure impact mechanical behavior, biological performance, and clinical results.

7.4.1 Orthopedic Materials

Orthopedic biomaterials must withstand high loads, cyclic stresses, and biological environments without failure. The primary categories include metals, ceramics, and polymers/composites, each tailored to specific biomechanical and biological demands.

Orthopedic applications are dominated by metals like cobalt-chromium (Co–Cr) alloys, stainless steel (316 L), and titanium alloys (Ti-6Al-4 V) because of their exceptional strength, durability, and fatigue resistance. A persistent titanium oxide (TiO_2) layer that prevents corrosion and encourages osseointegration forms in titanium and its alloys, giving them remarkable biocompatibility. Although titanium has a lower elastic modulus ($\approx$110 GPa) than stainless steel ($\approx$200 GPa), it is more in line with cortical bone ($\approx$20 GPa), which reduces bone resorption and stress shielding [46, 47]. Co-Cr alloys are frequently utilized for articulating surfaces in hip and knee replacements because of their exceptional hardness and wear resistance. However, issues with long-term biocompatibility and systemic exposure are brought up by their high stiffness and possible ion release (Co^{2+}, Cr^{3+}).

Ceramics are perfect for bearing surfaces and bone-interfacing components because of their exceptional hardness, wear resistance, and chemical stability. Zirconia (ZrO_2) and alumina (AlO_3) are distinguished by their low friction coefficients, strong compressive strengths, and little production of wear debris. The transformation toughening mechanism of zirconia increases the lifespan of hip joint components by imparting fracture resistance. By enabling direct chemical contact with bone tissue, hydroxyapatite (HA), a calcium phosphate ceramic that shares chemical similarities with bone mineral, encourages osseointegration. On metallic implants, HA coatings improve bioactivity without sacrificing mechanical stability.

Composites and polymers provide customizable degradation behavior, flexibility, and decreased weight. Although oxidative deterioration is still a concern, ultra-high molecular weight polyethylene (UHMWPE), which is utilized in joint replacement liners, offers exceptional wear resistance and reduced friction. High-performance thermoplastic polyether ether ketone (PEEK) is a prominent substitute for metals due to its chemical inertness, radiolucency for imaging, and strength and stiffness comparable to cortical bone. In scaffolds and fracture fixation devices, bioresorbable polymers like polylactic acid (PLA), polyglycolic acid (PGA), and polycaprolactone (PCL) are used. They break down gradually to permit tissue reconstruction. Copolymerization or blending can be used to modify their mechanical behavior and rate of degradation, guaranteeing mechanical support in the early stages of healing.

Together, these materials establish a foundation for orthopedic implant design, balancing mechanical strength, fatigue resistance, and bioactivity with long-term biocompatibility and integration.

7.4.2 Cardiovascular Materials

In order to maintain mechanical resilience, flexibility, and hemocompatibility, cardiovascular biomaterials must function in dynamic fluidic environments under pulsatile stress. They can be generically classified as metals or polymers, and they are frequently altered with bioactive surfaces or antithrombogenic coatings to promote endothelialization. Vascular grafts, heart valves, and blood-contacting devices all make substantial use of polymers like polytetrafluoroethylene (PTFE) and polyurethane (PU). Because of its exceptional chemical inertness, low friction, and porosity control, PTFE more specifically, expanded PTFE, or ePTFE allows tissue ingrowth while preventing thrombosis. Polyurethane reduces flow disturbances at the graft interface by combining durability and elasticity with mechanical qualities that can be adjusted to replicate native vessel compliance [48]. However, long-term stability may be restricted by calcification and oxidative breakdown.

The production of stents is dominated by metals like stainless steel and nitinol (a nickel-titanium alloy) because of their great strength and tolerance to fatigue. The superelastic nature of nitinol, a shape-memory alloy, makes it perfect for self-expanding stents that adjust to vascular dynamics. Electropolishing and surface passivation improves its biocompatibility and corrosion resistance. Although stainless steel (316 L) is inexpensive and mechanically robust, it lacks the flexibility needed in dynamic situations and is prone to ion release. Cobalt-chrome and platinum-chromium alloys have therefore become more popular for thinner, high-radial-strength stents.

Antithrombogenic coatings, such as phosphorylcholine, heparin, or nitric oxide (NO)-releasing layers, are used to reduce platelet adherence and coagulation and increase hemocompatibility. Endothelialization-promoting surfaces that have fixed cell-adhesive peptides (such RGD motifs) or micro- and nanoscale topographies help to quickly create a stable endothelium layer, which lowers inflammation and restenosis. An example of the synergy between structural and therapeutic activities in cardiovascular biomaterials is the development of drug-eluting stents (DES), which combine metal scaffolds with polymeric coatings for localized drug delivery (e.g., sirolimus, paclitaxel).

7.4.3 Dental Materials

High compressive pressures, chemical stability in the oral environment, and aesthetic balance with the native teeth are all requirements for dental biomaterials. Ceramics, composites/cements, and metallic implants are the three primary groups. Ceramics, especially porcelain and zirconia, offer a special harmony between translucency and mechanical robustness. Yttria-stabilized zirconia (YSZ) exhibits remarkable resistance to corrosion and wear, as well as excellent compressive strength (~1200 MPa) and fracture toughness. It is perfect for crowns, bridges, and abutments because of its inherent tooth-like hue and visual characteristics. Although thermal expansion mismatch may cause delamination, porcelain-fused-to-metal (PFM) systems combine the robustness of metallic substructures with the beauty of ceramic coverings.

Resin matrices supplemented with inorganic fillers like glass, zirconia, or silica make up dental composites and cement. These materials have exceptional adhesion, polishability, and wear resistance, making them ideal for restorative applications. Fluoride ions released by glass ionomer cements (GICs), which are made of fluoroaluminosilicate glass and polyacrylic acid, promote remineralization and guard against secondary caries. Nano-fillers used to hybrid composites increase mechanical qualities and decrease polymerization shrinkage, prolonging the life of restorations.

Osteointegration, a direct structural and functional bond between the implant surface and bone, is how titanium implants, which are frequently used to replace tooth roots, merge into alveolar bone. By increasing roughness and surface energy, surface modification methods like sandblasting, acid etching, plasma spraying, and anodization encourage osteoblast adhesion and differentiation [49]. Long-term stability and load transfer are ensured by bioactive coatings, such as hydroxyapatite and biofunctional peptides, which further strengthen the bone–implant contact.

7.4.4 Ophthalmic Materials

Soft tissue compatibility, biocompatibility, optical clarity, and refractive stability are all necessary for ophthalmic biomaterials [50]. For devices like corneal scaffolds, intraocular lenses (IOLs), and contact lenses, these characteristics are essential. The production of soft contact lenses is dominated by hydrogels and silicone elastomers because of their high-water content and oxygen permeability, which guarantee ocular comfort and hydration. The traditional hydrogel used in lenses is poly(2-hydroxyethyl methacrylate) (PHEMA), which is prized for its mechanical flexibility and clarity. By adding siloxane groups, modern silicone hydrogels increase oxygen transmissibility (Dk value) while retaining hydration with hydrophilic monomers.

The main components of intraocular lenses that are implanted following cataract surgery are acrylics and polymethyl methacrylate (PMMA). PMMA offers outstanding stability and visual clarity, but because of its rigidity, larger surgical incisions are required. Because they are made of hydrophobic or hydrophilic copolymers, foldable acrylic lenses allow for quicker recuperation after surgery and smaller incisions. The incidence of posterior capsule opacification (PCO), a frequent surgical complication, is decreased by surface changes that minimize cellular adherence and protein adsorption.

Biocompatible polymers like collagen hydrogels, polycaprolactone, and PEG-based copolymers are used in emerging ophthalmic technologies for drug-eluting contact lenses and corneal tissue scaffolds. These technologies provide controlled medication delivery and cell integration by fusing biodegradability and mechanical flexibility. These intelligent materials highlight the intersection of material science and regenerative ophthalmology by reacting to physiological cues, releasing medications on-demand, and promoting epithelial regeneration [51, 52].

7.4.5 Correlation Between Chemical Composition, Mechanical Behavior, and Clinical Application

A material's therapeutic appropriateness and biological response are directly influenced by the relationship between its mechanical behavior and chemical composition. Elastic modulus, hardness, corrosion resistance, and rate of deterioration are important material qualities that are determined by the atomic structure, bonding type, and microstructural organization.

Superior load-bearing capability is offered by metals because of their metallic bonding and crystalline structures, but if alloyed or handled incorrectly, they run the risk of ion release and corrosion. Although alloying elements (such as aluminum and vanadium in Ti-6Al-4 V) increase strength, they may also have an impact on cytocompatibility, therefore careful compositional control is required. Ceramics have a high compressive strength and hardness due to their ionic and covalent bonding, however they are fragile [53]. They are perfect for articulating surfaces and inert settings because of their chemical stability, which guarantees less degradation. Covalently bound molecular chains make up polymers, which provide processability, flexibility, and adjustable degradation. Although they may experience oxidative or hydrolytic breakdown in vivo, their viscoelastic nature makes them ideal for soft tissue applications. These materials are purposefully combined in composites to produce synergistic qualities, such as the flexibility of polymers, the stiffness of ceramics, and the toughness of metals, enabling application-specific tuning.

Biomaterials' clinical efficacy ultimately rests on their ability to match physiological needs with their composition, structure, and function. In order to ensure mechanical compatibility, cellular integration, and long-term safety across a variety of biomedical applications, the new trend places an emphasis on bioactive and multifunctional materials that can change dynamically.

7.5 Mechanisms and Processes

The complex interaction of material characteristics, biological environment, and mechanical performance is essential for the success of biomaterials in orthopedic, cardiovascular, dental, and ophthalmic applications. Whether a biomaterial promotes healing and regeneration or causes negative reactions depends on integration, remodeling, and functional compatibility at the cellular and molecular levels. Different physiological obstacles are presented by each clinical domain, such as ocular correction, dental reconstruction, vascular restoration, or bone regeneration, necessitating specific methods of interaction and adaptation [54, 55]. This investigates the mechanisms underlying the performance of biomaterials in these organ systems.

7.5.1 Orthopedic Integration and Remodeling

Orthopedic biomaterial success is based on bone–implant osseointegration and bioresorption processes. As soon as the biomaterial surface is implanted, it interacts with blood proteins like fibronectin and fibrinogen to create a temporary matrix that promotes osteoblast adhesion and growth. Favored for their corrosion resistance and mechanical compatibility, titanium and its alloys accomplish osseointegration by forming a stable layer of titanium oxide (TiO_2) that promotes bone adhesion and calcium phosphate nucleation. Similarly, by releasing calcium and phosphate ions, hydroxyapatite (HA) and bioactive glasses cause direct chemical interaction with bone, encouraging the development of a physiologically active apatite layer [56, 57].

Controlled degradation is essential in bioresorbable systems, such magnesium alloys or polymeric scaffolds (like poly-L-lactic acid, or PLLA), in order to coordinate the production of new bones with structural support. Implants made of magnesium slowly dissolve into magnesium ions, which can promote osteogenic differentiation but need to be carefully managed to avoid alkalization and excessive hydrogen evolution. In contrast, polymeric scaffolds undergo hydrolytic breakdown, with the rate of degradation being influenced by the molecular weight, crystallinity, and composition of the polymer.

Osteoblasts, osteoclasts, and mesenchymal stem cells (MSCs) work in concert to promote cellular signaling in bone remodeling and regeneration. Bone morphogenetic proteins (BMPs) and vascular endothelial growth factor (VEGF) are examples of cytokines that control angiogenesis, differentiation, and cell recruitment. Through mechanotransduction pathways, mechanical loading further activates osteocytes, improving bone remodeling surrounding the implant. Successful orthopedic integration is characterized by the dynamic reciprocity between biomaterial surfaces and host cells, which is highlighted by several mechanisms.

7.5.2 Cardiovascular Performance

Hemostasis, endothelialization, and flow dynamics are the main factors influencing the mechanisms controlling the performance of cardiovascular biomaterials. Stents, heart valves, and vascular grafts are examples of blood-contacting devices that need to preserve hemostatic equilibrium in order to facilitate tissue integration and avoid inflammation and thrombosis. Plasma proteins like albumin and fibrinogen quickly adsorb when blood comes into touch with a foreign surface, influencing platelet adhesion and activation later. In general, hydrophilic and negatively charged surfaces improve thromboresistance by reducing platelet activation and protein denaturation.

The development of endothelial cells across the surfaces of biomaterials, or endothelialization processes, is natural protection against thrombosis. To improve endothelial cell adherence and decrease clot formation, biomaterials intended for cardiovascular implants frequently include surface coatings of extracellular matrix (ECM) proteins, nitric oxide (NO)-releasing polymers, or heparinization [58, 59]. For example, the goal of bioresorbable stents composed of magnesium alloys or PLLA is to restore normal vascular function by allowing native endothelium tissue to regrow while offering temporary mechanical support.

The success of the device is largely dependent on flow dynamics and thromboresistance. In contrast to turbulent flow, which can cause thrombosis and neointimal hyperplasia, laminar flow conditions reduce shear stress-induced platelet activation. Graft shape and surface design are increasingly optimized using computational fluid dynamics (CFD) models to preserve physiological shear rates. Furthermore, it has been demonstrated that microtopographical patterns and nanostructured coatings affect endothelial cell alignment in the blood flow direction, imitating native vessel organization and enhancing long-term patency. The mechanistic foundation for cardiovascular device performance is defined by the combination of hemodynamic compatibility, mechanical compliance, and biomaterial surface chemistry.

7.5.3 Dental Bonding and Mineralization

Adhesion processes between tooth tissues and restorative materials are essential for mechanical integrity and lifespan in dental applications. Both chemical coupling and mechanical interlocking are used in the bonding process to enamel and dentin.

By causing microporosities in enamel, etching chemicals (such phosphoric acid) facilitate the entry of resin monomers, which then polymerize to form a robust adhesive surface. A micromechanical bond that is resistant to debonding under stress is created in dentin by the formation of hybrid layers made of collagen fibrils infiltrated with resin.

By promoting chemical adhesion through ionic exchange with tooth mineral components, glass ionomer cements (GICs) and bioactive composites further improve bonding. These materials release calcium and phosphate ions, which can remineralize nearby dentin and promote stability and resistance to microleakage over the long run. The interaction between dental implants and bone is based on the principles of biomineralization; the surfaces of titanium or zirconia encourage the deposition of hydroxyapatite and guide osseointegration. By increasing osteoblast activity and ECM mineralization, surface roughness, nanostructuring, and chemical changes (such as anodization and calcium phosphate coating) quicken this process.

Non-collagenous proteins that control crystal nucleation and orientation, such as osteocalcin and dentin phosphoprotein, orchestrate the biological mechanism of biomineralization. By simulating these natural mediators with controlled ion release or peptide-functionalized surfaces, synthetic materials can actively promote the creation of mineralized tissue. Therefore, the mechanistic basis of dental biomaterial performance is defined by the combination of biochemical signaling and mechanical adhesion.

7.5.4 Ophthalmic Transparency and Biomechanics

The context in which ophthalmic biomaterials function requires surface compatibility with sensitive ocular tissues, optical clarity, and biomechanical stability. By preserving homogenous refractive indices and reducing light dispersion, transparency and refractive stability are attained. Materials designed to preserve optical homogeneity and fend off degradation-induced opacity include silicone, polymethyl methacrylate (PMMA), and hydrogels like poly(2-hydroxyethyl methacrylate) (PHEMA).

The biocompatibility of contact lenses and intraocular lenses (IOLs) is determined by the surface wetting and protein adsorption processes. Maintaining adequate hydration minimizes discomfort and hypoxia by ensuring lubrication and oxygen diffusion across the cornea. However, surface fouling, reduced transparency, and microbial colonization can result from protein adsorption, particularly with lysozyme and albumin. Hydrophilic coatings, zwitterionic polymers, or surface-grafted polyethylene glycol (PEG) chains that prevent protein binding and biofilm formation are used in contemporary ophthalmic materials to combat this.

Another important consideration is biomechanical flexibility, since ocular devices need to adapt to the curvature of the tissue without causing inflammation or mechanical stress. Adaptive lenses and corneal implants that replicate the behavior of natural tissue are now possible thanks to developments in hydrogel elasticity, tear-film compatibility, and shape-memory polymers. The efficacy of ophthalmic biomaterials in preserving ocular health and visual clarity is determined by the mechanistic balance among tissue tolerance, surface chemistry, and optical performance [6, 60].

7.5.5 Cellular and Molecular Interactions Driving Tissue Response

The success or failure of biomaterials is determined by cellular and molecular interactions in all application fields. Integrins, which are transmembrane receptors, mediate adhesion to material surfaces at the cellular level by recognizing ligands produced from extracellular matrix (ECM), such as RGD (arginine-glycine-aspartic acid) patterns. The focal adhesion kinase (FAK) and MAPK pathways are two examples of intracellular signaling cascades that are activated by this binding and control cell survival, differentiation, and proliferation. The main mediator of these interactions is the adsorbed protein layer on the surfaces of biomaterials, which modifies cell activity by altering its composition and conformation.

The polarization of macrophages is essential for long-term tissue integration. Whether the host response results in fibrosis or constructive remodeling depends on the balance between pro-inflammatory (M1) and pro-regenerative (M2) phenotypes. Beneficial M2 polarization can be promoted by biomaterials that control oxidative stress and cytokine release, improving the results of healing. Further connecting material degradation to regenerative signaling is the regulated release of ions or molecules from degradable biomaterials, such as calcium, magnesium, or silicate ions, which can promote angiogenesis and stem cell recruitment.

Coordination of tissue growth is ensured by molecular interactions among endothelial, osteogenic, and fibroblastic cells, especially in hybrid systems such as periodontal regeneration or bone–vascular interfaces. Bioactive chemicals can now be spatially patterned thanks to developments in biomaterial chemistry, creating gradient cues that replicate natural developmental processes. Together, these interconnected molecular and cellular processes support biomaterials' dynamic adaptation to their host surroundings.

The integration of structural design with biological functionality is a common topic among the mechanisms and processes controlling biomaterial behavior in the dental, ophthalmic, cardiovascular, and orthopedic systems. The interaction between material characteristics and cellular response determines therapeutic effectiveness, ranging from bone remodeling and endothelialization to biomineralization and optical transparency [61, 62]. Gaining an understanding of these processes not only makes it possible to optimize existing devices but also directs the creation of next-generation biomaterials, which are systems that can seamlessly integrate with the human body and are adaptive and regenerative.

7.6 Design Considerations

A complex balancing act between mechanical performance, biological compatibility, and environmental adaptation is necessary when designing biomaterials for therapeutic purposes. The specific functional limitations and biophysical requirements imposed by each application ophthalmic, dental, cardiovascular or orthopaedic determine the methods for surface modification, processing, and material selection. In addition to mechanical and biological optimization, design feasibility is governed by safety and regulatory considerations, which guarantee patient safety and long-term clinical success. The basic design principles that underpin the development of biomaterials in the main biomedical domains are critically examined in this section, with a focus on the multidisciplinary integration of biology, engineering, and clinical requirements.

7.6.1 Mechanical, Biological, and Environmental Constraints Unique to Each Application

Understanding the unique mechanical and biological environment in which the implant or device will operate is the first step in the design of biomaterials. Materials used in orthopedic systems must withstand compressive forces, torsional stress, and cyclic mechanical loads that are similar to those found in cortical or cancellous bone. High yield strength, fatigue resistance, and the right amount of stiffness are necessary in these conditions to prevent stress shielding, which can lead to bone resorption [63, 64]. Corrosion-resistant metals and coatings are required because bodily fluids and enzymes cause oxidative and corrosive stress.

Shear stress, pulsatile flow, and continuous exposure to blood components define the dynamic environment found in cardiovascular devices. In this case, surface smoothness, hemocompatibility, and elastic compliance are crucial for preventing hemolysis and thrombosis. Materials used in dentistry must be aesthetically pleasing and biocompatible while withstanding masticatory stresses, pH changes, enzymatic breakdown, and microbial colonization. Ophthalmic devices, on the other hand, work in sensitive, delicate tissues that need to be flexible, bioinert, and optically clear to avoid irritation or immunological reaction. Biochemical reactivity, sterilization resistance, and temperature stability are all aspects of the environment [65, 66]. To ensure performance under a variety of physiological and environmental situations, a successful design balances mechanical integrity with biochemical stability.

7.6.2 Surface Modification for Improved Cell Adhesion, Corrosion Resistance, and Biofunctionality

The way biomaterials interact with the biological systems around them is determined by their surface characteristics. Changes to the energy, topography, and surface chemistry can have a significant impact on bacterial colonization, cell adhesion, and protein adsorption. Sandblasting or acid etching the surface of orthopedic implants encourages osteoblast adhesion and development, which improves osseointegration. Nanostructured oxide coatings produced by plasma treatment, anodization, and ion implantation boost surface energy and bioactivity while offering corrosion resistance.

Antithrombogenic coatings such as phosphorylcholine, heparin, or nitric oxide-releasing layers, reduce platelet adherence and stop coagulation in cardiovascular devices. Hydrophilic coatings on stents and catheters also lessen tissue damage and friction during insertion. Biofunctional coatings for dental implants, including hydroxyapatite or peptide layers, promote soft tissue integration while preventing the growth of bacterial biofilms. Surface treatments in ophthalmic materials increase hydrophilicity, which ensures proper tear film compatibility and improves wettability and comfort. UV grafting and plasma polymerization increase oxygen permeability without sacrificing optical clarity. In the end, surface modification acts as a link between biological function and material performance, enabling precise adjustment of interfacial characteristics for the best possible integration [67, 68].

7.6.3 Design for Load-Bearing Performance and Fatigue Resistance in Orthopedic Systems

The mechanical behavior of natural bone must be replicated in orthopedic implant design while avoiding long-term issues like wear, fracture, and implant loosening. The chosen material's mechanical characteristics, such as its elastic modulus, strength, and fatigue resistance, must meet physiological and anatomical requirements as shown in Fig. 7.1. Because of its high specific strength and biocompatibility, titanium and its alloys continue to be the industry standard for load-bearing implants; however, they must be designed to prevent excessive stiffness. Modulus mismatch is decreased and osseointegration is improved by innovations like porous titanium scaffolds made through additive manufacturing.

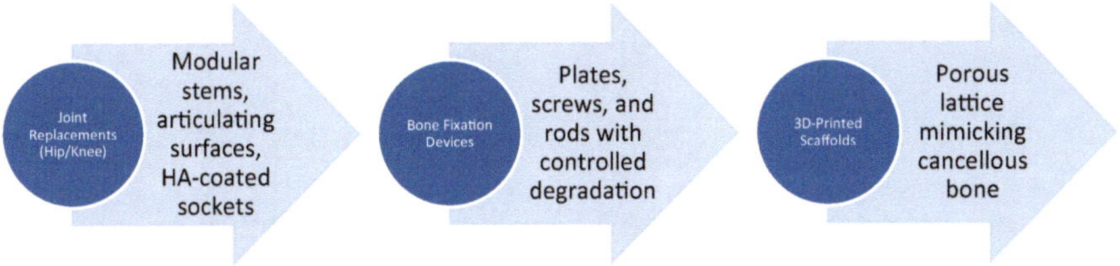

Fig. 7.1 Illustration of the typical components of an orthopedic implant system, including load-bearing metallic structures, fixation elements, and bioactive surface coatings designed to enhance osseointegration and mechanical stability

Under repeated motion, polymeric components like UHMWPE liners in joint replacements must withstand oxidative deterioration and wear. By reducing the production of wear particles, which would otherwise cause osteolysis, crosslinking and antioxidant stabilization procedures increase lifetime. In hip replacements, ceramic-on-ceramic bearing pairs reduce wear but need to be precisely designed to avoid fracture because of their brittleness. To guarantee mechanical stability over many years of cyclic loading, orthopedic device design must include fatigue testing, finite element analysis, and microstructural optimization.

7.6.4 Optimization of Hemodynamics and Flexibility in Cardiovascular Devices

The mechanical and surface design of cardiovascular implants, including heart valves, grafts, and stents, must guarantee compatibility with the body's dynamic circulatory system as shown in Fig. 7.2. Optimizing hemodynamics preserving laminar flow, reducing turbulence, and avoiding thrombogenesis is one of the main objectives. Blood flow patterns and endothelial cell responses are directly impacted by the geometry, surface finish, and expansion mechanics of stent struts. Nitinol stents, for example, use superelastic behavior to adapt to vessel walls, allowing for pulsatile motion while preserving radial strength.

Vascular grafts, usually composed of polyurethane or PTFE, must be as compliant as native arteries to prevent intimal hyperplasia and flow disruptions. Mechanical flexibility and tissue in-growth are influenced by porosity and wall thickness. Nitric oxide donors or endothelial cell adhesion peptides added to surface coatings improve hemocompatibility and encourage vascular regeneration. Leaflet geometry and flexibility are improved in artificial heart valves to balance biocompatibility and longevity by minimizing shear stress on blood components. To simulate flow profiles and forecast in vivo performance, computational fluid dynamics (CFD) has emerged as a key technology that facilitates iterative design optimization [69, 70].

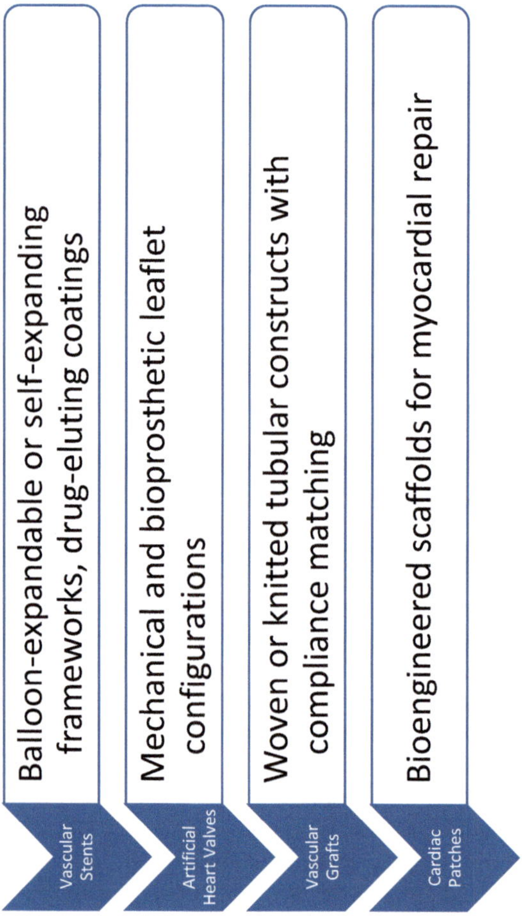

Fig. 7.2 Illustration representative of cardiovascular implant systems showing including stents, vascular grafts and artificial heart valves designed to optimize hemodynamics, enhance hemocompatibility, and maintain long-term vascular function

7.6.5 Aesthetic and Structural Balance in Dental Restorations

Designing dental biomaterials demands combining mechanical strength, biocompatibility, and cosmetic integrity. Ceramics made of zirconia and lithium disilicates are designed to be both strong and translucent, much like natural enamel. Mechanical toughness and optical scattering are determined by the composition of the crystalline phase and the microstructure. Hardness and flexibility must be balanced for restorations to be both fracture-resistant and gentle on neighboring teeth.

In the chemically demanding oral environment, resin composites used for fillings must preserve dimensional stability, color matching, and wear resistance. Surface polishability and mechanical qualities are controlled by silane coupling, matrix crosslinking, and filler particle size [71]. Additionally, dentin and enamel can be chemically and micromechanically interlocked with adhesives and bonding agents to preserve marginal integrity and stop microleakage. Dental materials must, from an engineering standpoint, accomplish the double objectives of regaining both beauty and functioning while guaranteeing durability under heat cycling and masticatory stress.

7.6.6 Transparency, Comfort, and Oxygen Permeability in Ophthalmic Materials

The design of ophthalmic biomaterials is dictated by the concepts of mechanical comfort, physiological compatibility, and optical clarity. Intraocular lenses (IOLs) and contact lenses must continue to be transparent, refractively stable, and non-irritating to the tissues of the eyes. In order to attain high oxygen permeability (Dk value), which is necessary for corneal metabolism and preventing hypoxia, materials like silicone hydrogels mix hydrophobic and hydrophilic domains. Lens comfort is guaranteed by mechanical flexibility, and proper tear film distribution is maintained by surface hydrophilicity. Surface alterations that improve wettability and prevent protein or lipid deposition include plasma treatment and the grafting of hydrophilic polymers [72, 73].

In order to enable minimally invasive implantation, acrylic and PMMA formulations for IOLs are designed for low light scattering, UV resistance, and foldability. To guarantee compatibility and clarity over time, the water content, optical index, and mechanical modulus are all carefully adjusted. Drug-eluting lenses and corneal scaffolds are becoming more and more common in future designs, combining regenerative and therapeutic purposes. Therefore, the foundation of ophthalmic material design is the interaction of mechanical robustness, oxygen permeability, and transparency.

7.6.7 *Regulatory and Safety Design Frameworks for Implantable Devices*

Designing biomaterials is not just an engineering problem; it also involves ethical and legal obligations. International standards including FDA/EMA approval frameworks, ISO 13485 (quality management systems), and ISO 10993 (biological evaluation of medical devices) must be followed by implantable medical devices. The cytotoxicity, sensitization, genotoxicity, degradation product analysis, and sterilization validation requirements are set out in these standards.

It is the responsibility of designers to guarantee material traceability, manufacturing process reproducibility, and mechanical and biological testing documentation. To verify long-term safety and functionality, biocompatibility evaluations are supplemented by in vitro, in vivo, and clinical validation. To avoid property alteration, environmental considerations including packaging stability and sterilizing techniques (such as ethylene oxide and gamma irradiation) must be incorporated early in the design process. Furthermore, ethical issues are becoming increasingly important in biomedical innovation, including patient-specific tailoring, post-market surveillance, and data transparency.

A multifaceted approach is necessary for the design of biomaterials, balancing biological response, mechanical performance, environmental durability, and regulatory compliance. Orthopedic systems emphasize fatigue resistance and load carrying; cardiovascular devices require hemodynamic optimization; dental materials combine structural integrity with aesthetics; and ocular devices concentrate on oxygen delivery and transparency. While clinical safety is ensured by regulatory control, surface modification is still a universal method to improve biocompatibility and function [74]. As computer modeling, nanotechnology, and bioactive design continue to be integrated, biomedical solutions will become more adaptable, patient-specific, and durable.

7.7 Applications and Case Studies

The integration of clinical medicine, cellular biology, materials science, and orthopedic, cardiovascular, and dental systems is exemplified using biomaterials. Materials that combine functionality and biocompatibility are needed for the unique physiological, mechanical, and biochemical problems that each domain provides. The therapeutic potential of biomaterials has been greatly increased by developments in material synthesis, surface modification, and bioactive design, allowing for patient-specific solutions and long-term performance as shown in Table 7.1. Following case studies and comparative analyses across application domains, this part looks at the real-world applications of biomaterials in key therapeutic areas.

Table 7.1 Biomaterials used in each application area

	Application area	Primary devices/systems	Representative biomaterials used	Key functional properties
Orthopedic	Joint replacements	Hip, knee, and shoulder prostheses	Titanium alloys (Ti-6Al-4 V), co–Cr alloys, UHMWPE, hydroxyapatite coatings	High mechanical strength, wear resistance, osseointegration capability
	Bone grafts and scaffolds	Structural and injectable graft substitutes	Calcium phosphates (HA, TCP), bioactive glass, collagen–PCL composites	Osteoconductive and osteoinductive; biodegradable with controlled resorption
	Bioresorbable fixation systems	Screws, plates, and pins	PLGA, PLLA, Mg-based alloys	Biodegradability, gradual load transfer to healing tissue
Cardiovascular	Stents	Coronary and peripheral vascular stents	Stainless steel, nitinol, PLGA–drug coatings, Mg alloys	High radial strength, fatigue resistance, controlled drug elution
	Artificial valves	Mechanical and bioprosthetic valves	Pyrolytic carbon, bovine pericardium, polyurethane	Hemocompatibility, fatigue resistance, anti-calcification
	Vascular grafts	Synthetic or hybrid vascular conduits	ePTFE, Dacron, collagen–elastin composites	Compliance matching, thromboresistance, biointegration
	Cardiac patches	Regenerative scaffolds for myocardium	Decellularized ECM, PEG hydrogels, graphene–polymer composites	Electrical conductivity, elasticity, bioactivity
Dental	Dental implants	Root-form and zygomatic implants	Titanium and Ti–Zr alloys, bioactive ceramic coatings	Osseointegration, corrosion resistance, biocompatibility
	Crowns and bridges	Restorative and aesthetic dental prostheses	Zirconia, alumina, lithium disilicate	High hardness, translucency, aesthetic stability
	Restorative composites	Fillings and bonding systems	Bis-GMA, UDMA resins with nano-silica fillers	Optical clarity, wear resistance, adhesive strength
	Guided tissue regeneration (GTR) membranes	Periodontal regeneration barriers	Collagen, chitosan, PLA membranes	Biodegradable, cell-selective barrier function
Ophthalmic	Intraocular lenses (IOLs)	Cataract replacement lenses	PMMA, hydrophobic acrylics, silicone elastomers	Optical transparency, refractive stability, biocompatibility

(continued)

Table 7.1 (continued)

	Application area	Primary devices/systems	Representative biomaterials used	Key functional properties
	Corneal implants	Artificial corneas and scaffolds	PHEMA hydrogels, collagen–PEG composites	Oxygen permeability, transparency, biointegration
	Biosensing contact lenses	Continuous glucose or pressure monitoring	Hydrogel–graphene composites, silicone elastomers with embedded sensors	Flexibility, biocompatibility, electrochemical responsiveness
Translational case studies	Nanostructured orthopedic coatings	Nanoscale HA–TiO_2 coatings on implants	Enhanced bone–implant integration, reduced infection risk	Demonstrated 30% faster osseointegration in clinical trials.
	Drug-eluting cardiovascular implants	PLGA-based drug reservoirs	Dual therapy: Mechanical support + local pharmacologic action	Reduced thrombosis and inflammation in >10-year follow-ups.
	Hybrid dental–bone regenerative systems	Nano-HAp–collagen scaffolds for jaw reconstruction	Combined osteoconductive and soft tissue regeneration	Successful translation to clinical reconstruction of maxillofacial defects.
Comparative performance metrics	Longevity and biostability	Orthopedic > cardiovascular > dental > ophthalmic	Controlled degradation and fatigue performance critical to clinical lifespan	Orthopedic implants show the highest durability; ophthalmic devices emphasize optical clarity and comfort.
	Regulatory and translational readiness	Dental and ophthalmic devices achieve fastest approval cycles	Preclinical biocompatibility, ISO 10993, and ISO 13485 compliance essential	Cardiovascular and orthopedic devices face most stringent regulatory pathways.

7.7.1 Orthopedic Applications: Joint Replacements, Bone Grafts, and Bioresorbable Fixation Systems

With uses in bone grafting, joint replacements, and bioresorbable anchoring systems, orthopedic biomaterials have completely transformed musculoskeletal medicine. Because of their remarkable strength, resistance to corrosion, and ability to support weight, metallic biomaterials specifically titanium (Ti) alloys, cobalt-chromium (Co–Cr) alloys, and stainless steel dominate joint arthroplasty. Modular designs with ultra-high molecular weight polyethylene (UHMWPE) acetabular cups for reduced friction articulation and titanium alloy stems for osseointegration are used in hip and knee replacements [75, 76]. Bioactive glass or hydroxyapatite surface coatings improve bone-implant bonding even more.

Both natural and synthetic materials are used in bone grafts and scaffolds to promote osteoconduction and osteoinduction. Because of their inherent osteogenic potential, autografts are still the gold standard, but synthetic alternatives including calcium phosphate ceramics, bioactive glass, and polymer–ceramic composites provide scalable and adaptable options. For example, mesenchymal stem cell-seeded β-tricalcium phosphate (β-TCP) scaffolds have shown faster bone synthesis in critical-size defects.

Bioresorbable fixation systems, which are made of magnesium alloys, poly-L-lactic acid (PLLA), or poly-D,L-lactide (PDLLA), offer short-term mechanical support that breaks down as natural bone grows back. These solutions avoid long-term metal residual dangers and lessen the requirement for follow-up procedures. By combining structural integrity with progressive degradation that complements the healing process, the MAGNEZIX® magnesium screw's clinical performance serves as an example of the translational potential of bioresorbable fixation.

7.7.2 Cardiovascular Applications: Stents, Artificial Valves, Vascular Grafts, and Cardiac Patches

In dynamic circulatory conditions, cardiovascular biomaterials need to be biologically integrated, mechanically flexible, and hemocompatible. One of the most effective cardiovascular devices is a stent, which is an inflatable tubular scaffold. Next-generation drug-eluting stents (DES), which were first made of stainless steel, use biocompatible coatings that release antiproliferative drugs like paclitaxel or sirolimus to stop restenosis. The development of bioresorbable vascular scaffolds (BVS) from magnesium alloys or PLLA in more recent times has reduced the danger of long-term thrombosis while maintaining artery patency.

Mechanical, bioprosthetic, or hybrid designs are used in artificial heart valves. Although they require lifelong anticoagulation, mechanical valves composed of titanium or pyrolytic carbon offer long-lasting endurance. On the other hand, tissue-engineered valves intended to attain native-like hemodynamics and regeneration capabilities are made from decellularized xenografts or polymer scaffolds seeded with endothelial cells [77]. Although small-diameter vascular grafts frequently experience thrombosis, expanded polytetrafluoroethylene (ePTFE) and polyethylene terephthalate (Dacron®) vascular grafts continue to be the industry standard for large-diameter replacements. In order to recreate natural vascular compliance and stop intimal hyperplasia, endothelialized grafts and elastin-mimetic polymers are being developed.

Cardiac patches use biodegradable scaffolding of collagen, alginate, or polycaprolactone (PCL) with cardiac stem cells or growth factors included to restore the myocardium following an infarction. Case studies show that they can encourage angiogenesis and restore contractility, which is a big step toward regenerative cardiac treatments.

7.7.3 Dental Applications: Implants, Crowns, Restorative Composites, and Guided Tissue Regeneration Membranes

Biomaterials are used in dentistry to promote both aesthetic reconstruction and practical restoration. Osteointegration provides long-term stability for dental implants, which are attached directly into the jawbone and are primarily made of titanium or zirconia. Surface alteration, like anodization, acid etching, or sandblasting, promotes bone cell adhesion and speeds up the healing process [78]. Zirconia is a ceramic substitute that is perfect for anterior restorations because of its excellent appearance, reduced plaque buildup, and chemical inertness. Ceramics (such as alumina and lithium disilicate) and resin-based composites are used in dental crowns and restorative composites to provide strength, translucency, and resistance to wear. Improvements in filler dispersion and interfacial bonding brought forth by nanocomposite technology advancements have increased polish retention and mechanical durability.

Collagen, polylactic acid, or expanded PTFE-based guided tissue regeneration (GTR) membranes serve as physical barriers that prevent epithelial migration, enabling bone and periodontal ligament cells to repopulate deficiencies. Tissue integration and regeneration are further supported by bioactive GTR systems that release growth factors or incorporate hydroxyapatite nanoparticles. These dental biomaterials have demonstrated the efficacy of surface-engineered materials in fostering consistent osseointegration and long-term performance by enabling over 90% success rates for implant-supported prostheses over a 10-year period.

7.7.4 Ophthalmic Applications: Intraocular Lenses, Corneal Implants, and Biosensing Contact Lenses

The environment in which ophthalmic biomaterials function requires surface biocompatibility, biostability, and optical clarity. Following cataract surgery, intraocular lenses (IOLs) are constructed of hydrophilic acrylics, silicone, or polymethyl methacrylate (PMMA). Aspheric and UV-blocking features are used in modern IOLs to reduce optical aberrations and improve visual performance. Hydrogels that are compatible with fragile ocular tissues, including poly(2-hydroxyethyl methacrylate) (PHEMA), offer flexibility and precise refractive index. Corneal scaffolds and implants, made of collagen or artificial polymers such as poly(ethylene glycol) (PEG), imitate the extracellular matrix found in the cornea and promote the adherence of epithelial cells. In preclinical and clinical experiments, bioengineered corneal substitutes have shown good integration and clarity, providing alternatives to donor transplants.

One of the newest developments in ocular biomaterials is biosensing contact lenses. These devices use hydrogel-based biosensors or microelectronics to continuously monitor indicators like intraocular pressure or glucose. Permeability, flexibility, and sensor stability must all be balanced in the silicon hydrogels with embedded conductive polymers that are employed in these systems [79]. Although it is still in the early stages of development, Google's experimental glucose-sensing lens is a prime example of how ophthalmic materials are combining ongoing health monitoring with diagnoses.

7.7.5 Case Studies of Successful Translational Innovations and Long-Term Clinical Outcomes

The practical effects of biomaterial innovation are demonstrated by several translational milestones. With survival rates above 95% over a 20-year period, porous-coated titanium hip implants set a standard for permanent osseointegration when they were first introduced in the 1980s. Comparing the Cypher® drug-eluting stent to bare-metal stents, the former showed a 70% decrease in restenosis rates, revolutionizing the results of cardiovascular interventions. Hydrophobic acrylic IOLs have reduced posterior capsule opacification, one of the most frequent post-operative problems in ophthalmology, whereas titanium-zirconia hybrid implants have demonstrated greater stability and soft tissue integration in dentistry. Every example shows how surface engineering and material selection result in quantifiable increases in patient happiness and clinical lifespan.

7.7.6 Comparative Analysis of Performance Metrics Across Application Domains

In contrast, cardiovascular systems place a higher priority on hemocompatibility and dynamic compliance, whereas orthopedic biomaterials prioritize mechanical durability and load transmission. In high-load settings, dental applications require precise bonding and biointegration, whereas ophthalmic materials prioritize surface biocompatibility and optical transparency. All disciplines agree on three crucial performance determinants: adaptation, stability, and biocompatibility, although having different functional measurements.

Although bioceramics are excellent in osteogenic applications, their brittleness in dynamic systems limits their use. Although polymers are flexible and degradable, they must be modified to reduce inflammatory reactions. Bioactive composites and metal–polymer hybrids are becoming ubiquitous platforms that integrate processability, biological signaling, and strength. Biomaterials have changed clinical practice from simple repair to functional regeneration in the orthopedic, cardiovascular, dental, and ocular systems [80]. The case studies presented demonstrate how developments in bioactive modification, materials engineering, and regenerative design concepts result in long-lasting, patient-centered solutions. The next generation of biomaterials will incorporate intelligence, adaptability, and personalization as these domains continue to converge, making it harder to distinguish between biological and artificial systems.

7.8 Recent Advances and Innovations

The design, production, and functionalization of biomaterials for orthopedic, cardiovascular, dental, and ophthalmic applications have advanced at an unparalleled rate in the last 10 years. The precision, effectiveness, and personalization of biomedical implants and devices have been revolutionized by the convergence of emerging technologies including artificial intelligence (AI), regenerative medicine, nanotechnology, and additive manufacturing [81]. Better biocompatibility, better mechanical and biological integration, and dynamic performance catered to the physiological and anatomical needs of individual patients have all been made possible by these advancements. This highlights the multidisciplinary character of recent achievements by examining significant developments across the four primary application sectors.

7.8.1 *Orthopedic Advances: 3D-Printed Bone Scaffolds, Bioactive Coatings, and Smart Implants*

Additive manufacturing, or 3D printing, has revolutionized implant design in orthopedics by making it possible to precisely replicate bone porosity and geometry. Bone scaffolds made of titanium, hydroxyapatite, or bioresorbable polymers can be customized to improve both mechanical and biological performance at the same time. Finite element analysis (FEA) and computer-aided design (CAD) are used to simulate native trabecular architecture, guarantee mechanical stability, and encourage vascular infiltration and osteointegration.

Another significant advancement is represented by bioactive coatings, especially when calcium phosphate, graphene oxide, and biofunctional peptides are added to improve bone–implant integration. These coatings promote osteoblast proliferation and differentiation by releasing osteogenic ions and biomolecules in a regulated manner. Real-time monitoring of load distribution, strain, and healing progress is now possible thanks to smart orthopedic implants that include sensors and wireless communication modules. Piezoelectric titanium implants, which combine materials science with digital health, can even promote bone remodeling by means of electrical microcurrents [82]. When taken as a whole, these developments point to the development of intelligent, flexible orthopaedic systems that can provide therapeutic feedback and self-evaluation.

7.8.2 Cardiovascular Innovations: Biodegradable Stents, Tissue-Engineered Valves, and Self-Healing Coatings

The development of cardiovascular biomaterials has greatly improved physiological compatibility and decreased long-term problems. The problems with permanent metallic stents, like chronic inflammation and late thrombosis, have been solved by biodegradable stents derived from magnesium alloys, poly-L-lactic acid (PLLA), and zinc-based composites. During vascular healing, these stents offer short-term mechanical support before resorbing gradually to reveal a natural lumen. Concurrent developments in tissue-engineered heart valves (TEHVs) combine decellularized matrices seeded with endothelium obtained from stem cells or autologous cells to produce living, adaptable valves. These systems have the capacity to expand and remodel, which is especially advantageous for patients who are young adults and children. Self-healing polymeric coatings that imitate endothelium repair mechanisms are another example of surface innovation in progress. These coatings utilize dynamic covalent bonds or embedded nanoparticles to restore functionality after mechanical or oxidative damage.

Computational fluid dynamics (CFD) modeling has improved hemodynamic optimization, enabling accurate graft and stent design to reduce shear stress and turbulence. Another example of how cardiovascular biomaterials are progressing toward multifunctional therapeutic platforms that integrate mechanical and pharmacological interventions is the incorporation of nanocarriers into vascular grafts for targeted delivery of anti-thrombotic or pro-endothelial drugs.

7.8.3 Dental Developments: Nanocomposite Restoratives, Antimicrobial Coatings, and Laser-Assisted Bonding

The field of dental biomaterials has progressed toward materials that support remineralization, prevent microbial colonization, and restore structure and aesthetics. When it comes to mechanical strength, wear resistance, and translucency, nanocomposite restorative materials that contain nanoparticles like silica, zirconia, or hydroxyapatite have outperformed conventional composites. The clinical longevity of restorations is increased by their nanoscale fillers, which also improve stress distribution and polish retention.

Another important development that tackles the ongoing problem of biofilm production is antimicrobial surface coatings. To prevent bacterial adherence and metabolic activity, silver nanoparticles, zinc oxide, and quaternary ammonium compounds are included into resin matrix or coated as surface coatings [83]. Additionally, dentin remineralization and recurrent caries can be actively promoted by bioactive glass composites that release calcium and phosphate ions.

By improving micromechanical interlocking and decreasing microleakage, laser-assisted bonding methods like erbium:YAG laser etching have improved adhesive dentistry. It can now be used in conjunction with CAD/CAM machining and digital intraoral scanning to create dental restorations with micron-level accuracy. All of these advancements point to a shift toward biomimetic, minimally invasive dentistry that performs better biologically and lasts longer.

7.8.4 Ophthalmic Progress: Drug-Eluting Contact Lenses, Corneal Regeneration Scaffolds, and Biosensing Lenses

Recent developments in ophthalmology have extended the use of biomaterials from passive vision correction to platforms for active therapy and diagnosis. The limits of traditional eye drops are overcome by drug-eluting contact lenses made of hydrogel matrices, which provide prolonged release of drugs for ailments like glaucoma, dry eye, and allergic conjunctivitis. Direct, extended medication administration to the ocular surface is made possible via molecular imprinting and the inclusion of nanoparticles. The creation of biocompatible scaffolds from collagen, gelatin methacrylate (GelMA), and decellularized corneal matrices has also advanced corneal tissue engineering. These materials preserve mechanical toughness and optical transparency while promoting epithelium regeneration. Additionally, as an alternative to donor transplants, bioengineered corneal replacements utilizing keratocytes produced from stem cells are being investigated.

The biosensing contact lens, an intelligent interface that may track tear biomarkers, intraocular pressure, or glucose levels, is arguably the most futuristic advancement. These devices demonstrate the increasing confluence of materials science, microelectronics, and customized healthcare by integrating wireless transmitters and microelectronic sensors into transparent polymer matrices. With real-time input, these technologies could improve patient outcomes by providing continuous, non-invasive monitoring of systemic and ocular disorders.

7.8.5 Interdisciplinary Integration with Nanotechnology, Regenerative Medicine, and Digital Fabrication

The combination of digital fabrication, regenerative medicine, and nanotechnology has spurred previously unheard-of innovation across all application disciplines. At the molecular level, nanostructured surfaces have been designed to affect immunological response, cell behavior, and protein adsorption. By imitating the structure of the extracellular matrix (ECM), nanofibrous scaffolds and nanotopographical cues promote angiogenesis, osteogenesis, and neuronal regeneration. By adding stem cells, growth factors, and gene delivery vectors to scaffold systems, regenerative medicine has further increased the utility of biomaterials. Orthopedic and cardiovascular scaffolds, for instance, are being used as platforms for regulated gene expression, which encourages tissue regeneration in specific areas [84]. In the meanwhile, digital fabrication methods like bioprinting and multi-material 3D printing allow cells and biomolecules to be patterned spatially, accurately reproducing the heterogeneity of original tissue. The integration of these technologies underscores a paradigm shift from passive implants to active, regenerative systems capable of interacting dynamically with biological environments.

7.8.6 Role of AI and Computational Modeling in Personalized Implant Design and Performance Prediction

Computational modeling and artificial intelligence (AI) are now essential technologies in the creation of biomaterials. To forecast the best material formulas and geometries, machine learning algorithms examine massive datasets that include mechanical performance, degradation trends, and clinical results. Based on anatomical information unique to each patient, AI-driven generative design enables the autonomous optimization of scaffold porosity, load distribution, and biological interactions. Extensive animal and clinical testing is no longer necessary thanks to in silico modeling of biological reactions, including inflammation, cell migration, and tissue remodeling, which offers predictive insights into long-term implant effectiveness. Computational models, when combined with imaging modalities like MRI or CT, make it easier to design implants that are unique to each patient and have specialized mechanical and biological characteristics.

Furthermore, AI is increasingly integrated into the manufacturing and quality assurance processes of biomaterials, ensuring consistency, scalability, and compliance with regulatory standards. This computational synergy enables not only predictive precision but also adaptive feedback control in "smart" implants devices capable of sensing mechanical stress or biochemical signals and autonomously modulating their function.

A revolutionary era marked by intelligence, integration, and personalization is heralded by recent developments in biomaterial science. Innovations are bridging the gap between biological systems and materials engineering, from biodegradable stents and 3D-printed bone scaffolds to biosensing lenses and nanocomposite restoratives. Biomaterials that are not only structurally strong but also biologically dynamic and functionally responsive are now possible because of the combination of nanotechnology, regenerative biology, and AI-driven modeling [85]. The next generation of biomedical devices adaptive, patient-specific, and seamlessly linked into the intricate physiological networks of the human body is anticipated as these technologies advance.

7.9 Challenges and Limitations

One outstanding accomplishment of contemporary biomedical science is the translation of biomaterials into orthopedic, cardiovascular, dental, and ocular applications. However, a number of difficulties and restrictions still exist despite improvements in clinical performance, design, and production. These include immunological compatibility, microbiological infection, optical stability, reproducibility in production, material degradation, and socioeconomic constraints. To create biomaterial-based treatments that are safer, more durable, and easier to obtain, it is imperative to comprehend these constraints.

7.9.1 Material Fatigue, Wear, and Corrosion in Load-Bearing Systems

Implants and prostheses used in orthopedic and dental applications are subjected to constant mechanical loading, friction, and environmental stressors, which can cause wear, corrosion, and fatigue. Despite their extreme durability, metals like titanium (Ti) and cobalt-chromium (Co–Cr) alloys are susceptible to long-term microstructural degradation. In joint replacements, cyclic stress can cause debris production, fretting corrosion, and microcrack formation, all of which can lead to osteolysis and implant loosening. Similarly, periprosthetic bone resorption and inflammatory reactions are triggered by polyethylene wear particles from tibial inserts or acetabular cups.

Metal ions like nickel, chromium, and cobalt are released when metallic implants corrode, especially near modular junctions or interfaces. These ions may cause systemic toxicity or hypersensitivity, which could lead to implant failure. Galvanic corrosion between dissimilar metals in the oral cavity speeds up the deterioration of dental prosthesis, changing their mechanical and aesthetic results. In high-stress areas such as the hips, knees, and dental occlusal zones, long-term fatigue performance is still a limiting concern, even though surface coatings, anodization, and ceramic barriers increase corrosion resistance. By fusing the durability of ceramics or polymers with the strength of metals, emerging composite and hybrid materials aim to address these problems [86]. However, maintaining mechanical compatibility across many material stages remains a difficulty for structural stability over the long term.

7.9.2 Immune and Inflammatory Responses Leading to Implant Rejection

Host immune response remains a critical determinant of implant success or failure. Even protein adsorption, macrophage activation, or fibrotic encapsulation are some of the ways that highly biocompatible materials can cause chronic inflammation. The foreign body response (FBR), which is typified by fibrous tissue deposition and macrophage fusion into multinucleated giant cells, can separate implants from the surrounding tissue, hence compromising their functionality [87]. Surface wear particles or corrosion byproducts in orthopedic and cardiovascular devices worsen inflammation, whereas bacterial leaking around the abutment in dental implants can cause peri-implantitis. The regenerative or degenerative nature of the response depends on the interaction of surface roughness, material chemistry, and immune cell signaling. It is still difficult to achieve a healthy immunological equilibrium, even with advancements in immunomodulatory coatings and bioactive surface treatments.

Preclinical evaluation is made more difficult by species- and patient-specific heterogeneity, since animal models frequently fall short in predicting human immune responses. The creation of next-generation biomaterials that actively control immunological pathways, such as by modifying macrophage polarization or releasing anti-inflammatory drugs, shows potential but adds complexity to long-term safety validation and regulatory approval.

7.9.3 Biofilm Formation and Infection Management in Oral and Cardiovascular Implants

Major reasons for implant-associated failure, especially in the cardiovascular, orthopedic, and oral systems, are microbial colonization and biofilm formation. Once formed, biofilms dense microbial populations covered in extracellular polymers show significant resistance to both host defenses and antibiotics. Porphyromonas gingivalis and Streptococcus mutans can cause peri-implant mucositis or peri-implantitis in dental implants, which can impair osseointegration. Similarly, biofilms of *Pseudomonas aeruginosa* and *Staphylococcus epidermidis* can cause endocarditis or device-related sepsis in cardiovascular stents and grafts.

Bacterial adhesion is significantly influenced by material surface characteristics such as charge, hydrophobicity, and roughness. Although hydrophilic coatings and nanoscale topographies lessen microbial colonization, total protection is still unattainable. Antimicrobial coatings that contain peptide-based compounds, silver nanoparticles, or chlorhexidine provide localized protection but run the risk of becoming toxic or developing resistance. Furthermore, bioactive layers may be broken down by sterilization processes, reducing their effectiveness. Clinically, implant removal and systemic antibiotic therapy are frequently required for infection control, which raises morbidity and medical expenses. Therefore, a continuous area of biomaterial innovation is the creation of self-sterilizing surfaces and intelligent antimicrobial systems that can detect and neutralize pathogens on demand [88].

7.9.4 Optical Degradation and Long-Term Biostability in Ophthalmic Materials

In the delicate ocular environment, ophthalmic biomaterials in particular, intraocular lenses (IOLs), contact lenses, and corneal implants must preserve optical clarity, refractive stability, and biostability for years or decades. Nonetheless, there are ongoing difficulties with optical degradation brought on by protein adsorption, calcification, and photodegradation. For example, although being well-liked for their mechanical stability, hydrophobic acrylic IOLs can produce glistening, which are small water microvacuoles that scatter light and reduce image clarity. Similarly, prolonged usage of hydrogel-based contact lenses may cause lipids, proteins, and microbes to foul the surface, decreasing comfort and oxygen permeability. For corneal scaffolds, where transparency and integration are jeopardized by polymer opacification or degradation, biostability is especially important.

Degradation processes are accelerated by the special microenvironment of the eye, which is defined by exposure to UV radiation, enzyme activity, and mechanical blinking. Predicting decades-long optical stability is still challenging, even though resistance is increased by UV-absorbing compounds and plasma surface treatments. The difficulty of creating long-lasting ophthalmic materials appropriate for long-term implantation is highlighted by the trade-off between mechanical flexibility, water content, and refractive precision.

7.9.5 Manufacturing Reproducibility, Sterilization, and Quality Assurance Challenges

For clinical-grade biomaterials to be safe and effective, manufacturing uniformity is essential. However, differences in surface treatment homogeneity, nanoparticle dispersion, or polymerization conditions frequently result in reproducibility issues. Small variations in porosity or coating thickness can significantly change mechanical and biological results in cardiovascular and orthopedic systems [89]. Another level of difficulty is introduced by sterilization. Methods including autoclaving, ethylene oxide, and gamma irradiation can change surface chemistry, denature bioactive compounds, and break down polymers. It is especially difficult to achieve sterility without sacrificing functioning in composite or hybrid biomaterials that combine biological, ceramic, and polymer components.

Beyond technical challenges, the adoption of advanced biomaterials faces ethical, economic, and accessibility constraints. The high costs associated with development, testing, and regulatory approval restrict widespread clinical implementation, particularly in low-resource settings. Personalized implants or tissue-engineered constructs, while promising, demand specialized equipment and expertise that elevate treatment expenses.

Ethical considerations include equitable access, data privacy in personalized design, and the use of animal-derived or genetically modified materials. In ophthalmic and cardiovascular applications, the use of xenografts raises concerns regarding cross-species disease transmission and public acceptance. Similarly, the incorporation of nanomaterials introduces uncertainties about long-term toxicity and environmental impact upon disposal.

7.9.6 Ethical and Cost-Related Barriers in Adopting Next-Generation Biomaterials

Beyond technological difficulties, there are accessibility, financial, and ethical barriers to the use of sophisticated biomaterials. Widespread clinical adoption is hampered by the high expenses of research, testing, and regulatory approval, especially in environments with limited resources. Although promising, customized implants or tissue-engineered structures require specific tools and knowledge, which raise treatment costs. Fair access, data privacy in customized design, and the usage of materials obtained from animals or genetically engineered organisms are all ethical issues. Concerns about public acceptance and cross-species disease transmission are raised by the use of xenografts in cardiovascular and ocular applications. Likewise, the use of nanomaterials raises questions over their long-term toxicity and disposal's effects on the environment.

Balancing innovation with affordability and ethical responsibility requires collaborative frameworks between industry, regulators, and healthcare systems [90]. Emerging models such as open source biomanufacturing and tiered pricing strategies could enhance accessibility without compromising safety or quality.

Long-standing issues with mechanical durability, immunocompatibility, infection control, optical stability, and manufacturing repeatability limit the therapeutic success of biomaterials in the orthopedic, cardiovascular, dental, and ophthalmic domains. Addressing these limitations is becoming more important as technology develops toward adaptive and bioresponsive systems. Future research must concentrate on creating multipurpose, standardized, and morally sound biomaterials that are accessible to a range of patient populations and can endure physiological demands [91]. The future of biomaterials will be shaped by overcoming these obstacles, not only as useful tools but also as sustainable, integrated elements of human regeneration and healing.

7.10 Future Directions

From inert mechanical supports to multipurpose, bioresponsive systems that interact dynamically with biological surroundings, biomaterials have advanced in evolution. Future directions in the discipline focus on sustainability, intelligence, and adaptability as it moves toward precision and regenerative medicine. With the goal of creating next-generation implants and technologies that can continuously interact, mend, and communicate within the human body, these developments represent an interdisciplinary convergence of materials science, computational biology, and clinical engineering. The main trends influencing the development of biomaterials for orthopedic, cardiovascular, dental, and ophthalmic applications are covered in the ensuing subsections.

7.10.1 Development of Multifunctional and Adaptive Biomaterials Integrating Sensing, Regeneration, and Actuation

It is envisaged that next-generation biomaterials would play an active role in physiological regulation rather than just playing static mechanical roles. To react instantly to mechanical or biological inputs, multifunctional devices that include sensing, regeneration, and actuation capabilities are being created. Orthopedic implants that have strain or pressure sensors built in, for instance, can track the development of bone repair and identify early indications of infection or implant loosening. Anticoagulants can also be dynamically released via cardiovascular stents equipped with biosensors and drug reservoirs in response to endothelial signals.

It is envisaged that next-generation biomaterials would play an active role in physiological regulation rather than just playing static mechanical roles. To react instantly to mechanical or biological inputs, multifunctional devices that include sensing, regeneration, and actuation capabilities are being created. Orthopedic implants that have strain or pressure sensors built in, for instance, can track the development of bone repair and identify early indications of infection or implant loosening [92]. Anticoagulants can also be dynamically released via cardiovascular stents equipped with biosensors and drug reservoirs in response to endothelial signals.

7.10.2 Regenerative and Bioinspired Materials Mimicking Native Tissue Architecture

Creating biomaterials that closely resemble organic tissues' hierarchical, anisotropic, and adaptable properties is a crucial future direction. To direct tissue-specific regeneration, bioinspired materials take inspiration from natural architectures, such as the cornea's layered transparency or bone's composite structure of collagen and hydroxyapatite. Extracellular matrix (ECM) microenvironments that support cell adhesion, migration, and differentiation can be replicated thanks to developments in molecular self-assembly, 3D bioprinting, and decellularization procedures.

Biomimetic mineralized scaffolds that mimic osteon microstructures enhance osteointegration and mechanical compatibility in orthopedics. Elastin-mimetic and enamel-like composites offer strength and flexibility for dental and cardiovascular applications. Hydrogels with nanofibrillar alignment in ophthalmology replicate the corneal stroma, preserving transparency while promoting the proliferation of epithelial cells. Furthermore, pharmacological signaling cues including growth factors, peptides, and gene vectors are increasingly combined with regenerative materials to promote endogenous repair pathways. The growing concept of regenerative implants that may coordinate self-healing processes inside host tissues is supported by this confluence of biological functionality and structural biomimicry [93].

7.10.3 Use of AI-Driven Predictive Modeling for Performance Optimization and Failure Prevention

The clinical assessment and predictive design of biomaterials are undergoing a revolution because of computer modeling and artificial intelligence (AI). The effects of composition, structure, and surface characteristics on biological performance and degradation can be predicted by machine learning algorithms that have been trained on large materials and clinical datasets. By allowing virtual screening of material candidates prior to experimental validation, this data-driven technique speeds up discovery.

Scaffold structures are further optimized for the intended mechanical and biological results using AI-driven generative design algorithms, which guarantee the optimal ratio of porosity, strength, and mass transfer. While computational fluid dynamics (CFD) simulations in cardiovascular implants forecast shear stress and flow behavior to prevent thrombosis, predictive models aid in evaluating fatigue resistance under cyclic loading in orthopedic applications [45, 94]. Furthermore, digital twins virtual implants combined with real-time patient data allow for predictive maintenance and ongoing monitoring of implanted equipment. By enabling early identification of inflammatory reactions, infections, or mechanical failure, this combination of AI and sensor technology turns biomaterials from reactive to proactive medical systems.

7.10.4 Expansion of 4D Printing for Dynamic, Self-Adjusting Implants

Although patient-specific implant creation has already been transformed by 3D printing, the development of 4D printing adds a time dimension, allowing implants to alter their stiffness, shape, or functionality in reaction to external stimuli. Stimuli-responsive polymers, shape-memory alloys, and hydrogel networks that adjust to physiological parameters like pH, temperature, or mechanical pressure are all included in 4D-printed biomaterials. 4D-printed scaffolds in orthopedics can stiffen to offer mechanical support after expanding or contracting to match defect geometries during surgery. Shape-memory polymer-made cardiovascular devices can self-deploy inside blood vessels, doing away with the necessity for invasive delivery methods. Curvature may soon be dynamically adjusted in ophthalmology by contact lenses or corneal scaffolds to improve medicine administration or visual function.

When 4D printing and multi-material bioprinting are combined, cells, extracellular matrix (ECM) mimics, and bioactive chemicals can be patterned both spatially and temporally. This makes it easier to create tissue constructions at the organ level that can regenerate adaptively. A new generation of intelligent, self-regulating biomedical devices that are suited to dynamic biological conditions are anticipated to be powered by this technology as it develops.

7.10.5 Sustainable Manufacturing and Circular Material Approaches for Biomedical Devices

Sustainability is increasingly recognized as a fundamental pillar in the future of biomaterials Sustainability is becoming more widely acknowledged as a key component of biomaterials research and manufacturing in the future. The biomedical industry must reduce waste, energy consumption, and ecological impact across the material life cycle in response to increasing ethical and environmental requirements. Green chemistry, bio-based polymers, and recyclable or biodegradable products are therefore becoming more popular. Biopolymers made from renewable resources, like cellulose, chitosan, and polylactic acid (PLA), provide good substitutes for petroleum-based polymers in temporary scaffolds and disposable medical devices [95]. Furthermore, where it is safe and practical, circular design principles promote the reuse, recycling, and remanufacturing of medical components.

Chemical emissions and material waste are further decreased by advanced production methods including solvent-free processing and additive manufacturing. Biomaterial development pipelines are incorporating life cycle assessment (LCA) technologies to measure environmental effect and direct environmentally conscious design. In addition to supporting global environmental goals, the shift to sustainable biomedical engineering also improves social responsibility and regulatory acceptance in the healthcare sector.

7.10.6 Enhanced Clinical Translation Pipelines through Interdisciplinary Collaboration

Many biomaterial breakthroughs still encounter obstacles in clinical translation despite impressive laboratory advancements because of intricate regulatory requirements, limited scalability, and a lack of knowledge regarding long-term biocompatibility. Strengthening multidisciplinary cooperation between material scientists, bioengineers, physicians, data scientists, and regulatory agencies will be essential for future success. Preclinical validation can be streamlined by establishing standardized testing frameworks that incorporate in vitro, in vivo, and in silico approaches. While working with physicians guarantees that gadget design meets practical clinical objectives, collaborating with computational experts allows for more accurate predictive modeling of biological outcomes. Additionally, by coordinating safety standards and production procedures, collaborations between industry and regulatory bodies can hasten product approval.

Global innovation ecosystems will be fostered by the establishment of open-access biomaterial databases and cooperative research networks, which will further improve transparency and reproducibility. In order to improve patient outcomes and healthcare efficiency, integrative solutions like these are crucial for bridging the gap between bench-top discovery and bedside application. The development of intelligent, flexible, and sustainable systems that blend in perfectly with human physiology is the key to the future of biomaterials. Implants that can perceive, react, and heal dynamically are promised by developments in multifunctional design, bioinspired regeneration, AI-driven modeling, and 4D printing. Growing dedications to sustainability and interdisciplinary cooperation are equally significant, as they will guarantee that these technologies are not only cutting edge but also morally and ecologically sound and clinically applicable [96].

By uniting computational intelligence, regenerative biology, and eco-conscious engineering, the next generation of biomaterials will redefine the interface between synthetic systems and living tissues heralding an era of personalized, adaptive, and life-sustaining biomedical innovation.

7.11 Conclusion

By facilitating the replacement, regeneration, and repair of intricate tissues, the incorporation of biomaterials into orthopedic, cardiovascular, dental, and ocular applications has completely transformed contemporary medicine. Material selection, surface modification, and structural design strategies are determined by the distinct mechanical, chemical, and biological needs of each of these domains. Biomaterials are the vital link between artificial structures and living tissues in everything from load-bearing orthopedic implants to optically transparent corneal substitutes, affecting patient outcomes and clinical success. The main ideas are summarized in this conclusion, which places special emphasis on biocompatibility, usefulness, interdisciplinary collaboration, and the path toward intelligent regenerative systems.

7.11.1 Summary of Application-Specific Material Requirements and Design Strategies

The ability to adapt material qualities to certain anatomical and physiological situations is critical to the success of biomedical implants and devices. Porous titanium scaffolds, bioactive ceramics, and biodegradable fixation systems are examples of materials used in orthopedics that combine high compressive strength, fatigue resistance, and osseointegrative potential. On the other hand, under dynamic flow circumstances, cardiovascular implants like stents and grafts require flexibility, corrosion resistance, and hemocompatibility. Performance is directly impacted by material design, as demonstrated by surface engineering and polymer coatings that minimize thrombosis and encourage endothelialization.

Mechanical hardness, chemical inertness, and aesthetic compatibility are important factors in dental applications. When paired with directed tissue regeneration membranes or calcium phosphate coatings, titanium and zirconia implants form a strong link with soft tissue and bone. Hydrogels and silicone-based materials are meticulously designed to preserve oxygen permeability and comfort without sacrificing optical clarity, while ophthalmic biomaterials demand remarkable optical transparency, refractive accuracy, and long-term biostability. To combine biological integration with mechanical and functional stability, rational design solutions for these systems optimize porosity, degradation rate, and surface energy. Additionally, patient-specific designs with spatially controlled architecture and drug-release capabilities are made possible by the convergence of additive manufacturing and computer modeling.

7.11.2 Emphasis on Biocompatibility, Functionality, and Patient-Centered Design

Biocompatibility, or a material's capacity to carry out its intended function without causing unfavorable biological reactions, is the foundation of all biomedical material development. This characteristic goes beyond inertness; it also includes immunomodulation, bioactivity, and the capacity to blend in with the surrounding tissues. This paradigm change toward dynamic interaction rather than passive cohabitation is reflected in the development of bioactive and bioresorbable systems from bioinert metals and ceramics.

Functionality is just as important. Dental restorations must withstand masticatory stresses; cardiovascular stents must expand consistently and prevent restenosis; orthopedic implants must facilitate mechanical load transfer and encourage bone remodeling; and ophthalmic lenses must retain optical integrity throughout many years of use. A sensitive but crucial design objective is still striking a balance between these functional requirements and biological performance. Patient-centered design, which matches material functionality with individual needs, anatomy, and lifestyle, is another focus of contemporary biomaterial development. Anatomical matching is possible with customized implants made using digital imaging and 3D printing, and surface modification methods can customize cellular and molecular reactions to biological settings unique to each patient. In ophthalmology and cardiology, smart biomaterials capable of real-time feedback or therapeutic release further reflect the shift toward interactive and adaptive systems designed around patient well-being and long-term comfort.

7.11.3 Recognition of the Synergy Between Materials Science, Tissue Biology, and Clinical Innovation

A natural synergy between materials science, tissue biology, and clinical innovation propels the development of biomedical materials. Developments in polymer synthesis, surface chemistry, and nanostructuring have made it possible to precisely regulate cellular behavior, such as adhesion, proliferation, and differentiation. Bioinspired and biomimetic materials that mimic natural extracellular matrix

(ECM) cues have been inspired by molecular biology discoveries on how cells perceive and react to micro- and nanoscale characteristics.

Clinicians are essential in putting these technologies into use and making sure that scientific discoveries are applied to actual medical problems. Cross-disciplinary cooperation can result in revolutionary outcomes, as demonstrated by the clinical success of hydrogel-based corneal implants, drug-eluting cardiovascular stents, and osseointegrated dental implants. Additionally, machine learning, imaging technology, and computer modeling have made it possible to predict biological response and material performance, bridging the gap between bench and bedside. This partnership encourages iterative innovation, which speeds up safe and efficient deployment by incorporating clinical feedback into material redesign and engineering improvement.

7.11.4 Outlook Toward Next-Generation, Intelligent, and Regenerative Biomedical Systems

The development of intelligent, adaptive, and regenerative systems is key to the future of biomaterials in the domains of orthopedics, cardiovascular disease, dentistry, and ophthalmology. These next-generation materials will actively interact, react, and heal inside the body rather than just replacing damaged tissues. In order to react dynamically through controlled drug release or structural adaptation, intelligent biomaterials are created that can sense local biochemical changes, such as pH, oxygen tension, or inflammatory indicators. Personalized treatment regulation, reduced complications, and improved long-term functionality are all promised by such intelligent systems.

A new era of precision medicine is being ushered in by the combination of nanotechnology, 4D printing, and artificial intelligence (AI). While 4D-printed materials will change their stiffness or geometry in response to physiological cues, AI-driven predictive modeling will make it possible to create patient-specific implants with optimal mechanical compatibility and degradation rates. Simultaneously, regenerative strategies that make use of growth factors, stem cells, and bioinspired scaffolds will encourage endogenous repair as an alternative to permanent implants.

The next stage of the development of biomaterials will also be influenced by sustainability and ethical responsibility. The emphasis will move toward environmentally benign, recyclable, and resource-efficient materials that reduce their negative effects on the environment as manufacturing technologies develop. Additionally, to guarantee fair access and uniform safety standards across various healthcare systems, international cooperation and regulatory harmonization will be crucial.

In orthopedic, cardiovascular, dental, and ocular applications, biomaterials form the basis of restorative and regenerative medicine. Their success hinges on the careful matching of structural design, biological compatibility, and material composition with therapeutic function. Medical materials are changing from static prosthesis to dynamic, responsive, and patient-tailored systems because of the ongoing interaction between biological understanding, clinical translation, and technical innovation. The idea of a smooth transition between artificial materials and live tissues is becoming more real as research advances toward intelligent and regenerative paradigms, portending a time when biomaterials would not only preserve but also improve and prolong human life.

References

1. Aslam, M., McClintock, S., Harber, I., Nadeem, D. and Varani, J.. LPS and Cytokines-Induced Pro-Inflammatory Insult: Upregulation of Barrier Proteomic Expression in Human Colonoids (2023)
2. Di Vizio, D., Erdbruegger, U., Lötvall, J.: ISEV2023 abstract book. J. Extracell. Vesicl. **12**, 1 (2023)
3. Kantaros, A., Ganetsos, T.: From static to dynamic: smart materials pioneering additive manufacturing in regenerative medicine. Int. J. Mol. Sci. **24**(21), 15748 (2023)
4. Rastogi, P., Kandasubramanian, B.: Review of alginate-based hydrogel bioprinting for application in tissue engineering. Biofabrication. **11**(4), 042001 (2019)
5. Dhingra, P., Kumar, A., Raj, P.M., Patel, P., Sahu, K.K., Das Kurmi, B.: Salivary protein macromolecules as diagnostic and therapeutic biomarkers linking oral health and neurodegenerative diseases-emerging mechanisms and future perspectives. Inflammopharmacology, 1–16 (2026)
6. Ferraz, M.P.: Biomaterials for ophthalmic applications. Appl. Sci. **12**(12), 5886 (2022)
7. Karayilan, M., Clamen, L., Becker, M.L.: Polymeric materials for eye surface and intraocular applications. Biomacromolecules. **22**(2), 223–261 (2021)
8. Batool, F., Özçelik, H., Stutz, C., Gegout, P.Y., Benkirane-Jessel, N., Petit, C., Huck, O.: Modulation of immune-inflammatory responses through surface modifications of biomaterials to promote bone healing and regeneration. J. Tissue Eng. **12**, 20417314211041428 (2021)
9. Minotti, M.: Recent progress in materials for biomedical implants: a concise review. Med. Mater. **5**(3), 161–168 (2025)
10. Franssen, F.M., Alter, P., Bar, N., Benedikter, B.J., Iurato, S., Maier, D., Maxheim, M., Roessler, F.K., Spruit, M.A., Vogelmeier, C.F., Wouters, E.F.: Personalized medicine for patients with COPD: where are we? Int. J. Chron. Obstruct. Pulmon. Dis. **14**, 1465–1484 (2019)
11. Strianese, O., Rizzo, F., Ciccarelli, M., Galasso, G., D'Agostino, Y., Salvati, A., Del Giudice, C., Tesorio, P., Rusciano, M.R.: Precision and personalized medicine: how genomic approach improves the management of cardiovascular and neurodegenerative disease. Genes. **11**(7), 747 (2020)
12. Alavi, S.E., Gholami, M., Shahmabadi, H.E., Reher, P.: Resorbable GBR scaffolds in oral and maxillofacial tissue engineering: design, fabrication, and applications. J. Clin. Med. **12**(22), 6962 (2023)
13. Sumathy, B., Nair, L.V., Vijayan, V.M., Anil Kumar, P.R., Velayudhan, S., Thomas, V.: Additive manufacturing of smart bionanomaterials for fabrication of medical implants. In: Nanotechnology-Based Additive Manufacturing: Product Design, Properties and Applications, vol. 2, pp. 455–494. Wiley (2023)
14. Ashammakhi, N., GhavamiNejad, A., Tutar, R., Fricker, A., Roy, I., Chatzistavrou, X., Hoque Apu, E., Nguyen, K.L., Ahsan, T., Pountos, I., Caterson, E.J.: Highlights on advancing frontiers in tissue engineering. Tissue Eng. Part B Rev. **28**(3), 633–664 (2022)
15. Cho, S., Discher, D.E., Leong, K.W., Vunjak-Novakovic, G., Wu, J.C.: Challenges and opportunities for the next generation of cardiovascular tissue engineering. Nat. Methods. **19**(9), 1064–1071 (2022)

16. Goyal, A.S.: Biomaterials in Biomedical Engineering. Aditya Sandeep Goyal (2023)
17. Oladele, I.O., Onuh, L.N., Agbeboh, N.I., Alewi, D.D., Lephuthing, S.S.: The relationship and functional links between human age, growth, and biomedical implants: a review on the application of bulk and nanomaterials. Nano Select. **4**(7), 419–441 (2023)
18. Abraham, A.M., Venkatesan, S.: A review on application of biomaterials for medical and dental implants. Proc. Inst. Mech. Eng. L J. Mater. Des. Appl. **237**(2), 249–273 (2023)
19. Kim, Y., Zharkinbekov, Z., Raziyeva, K., Tabyldiyeva, L., Berikova, K., Zhumagul, D., Temirkhanova, K., Saparov, A.: Chitosan-based biomaterials for tissue regeneration. Pharmaceutics. **15**(3), 807 (2023)
20. Cavallo, A., Gasparotti, E., Losi, P., Foffa, I., Al Kayal, T., Vignali, E., Celi, S., Soldani, G.: Fabrication and in-vitro characterization of a polymeric aortic valve for minimally invasive valve replacement. J. Mech. Behav. Biomed. Mater. **115**, 104294 (2021)
21. Seidman, M.A., Padera, R.F., Schoen, F.J.: Cardiovascular medical devices: stents, grafts, stent-grafts and other endovascular devices. In: Biomaterials Science, pp. 1033–1050. Academic (2020)
22. Lim, E.K., Kim, T., Paik, S., Haam, S., Huh, Y.M., Leec, K.: Nanomaterials for theranostics: recent advances and future challenges. In: Nanomaterials and Neoplasms, pp. 587–775. Jenny Stanford Publishing (2021)
23. Vallabhajosula, S.: Molecular Imaging and Targeted Therapy. Springer International Publishing (2023)
24. Carotenuto, F., Politi, S., Ul Haq, A., De Matteis, F., Tamburri, E., Terranova, M.L., Teodori, L., Pasquo, A., Di Nardo, P.: From soft to hard biomimetic materials: tuning micro/nano-architecture of scaffolds for tissue regeneration. Micromachines. **13**(5), 780 (2022)
25. Cruz, M.B., Silva, N., Marques, J.F., Mata, A., Silva, F.S., Caramês, J.: Biomimetic implant surfaces and their role in biological integration—a concise review. Biomimetics. **7**(2), 74 (2022)
26. Kishore, R.N., Kaliamoorthy, S., Uddarraju, S.R., Kameswari, N.: The role of bioactive molecules in enhancing bone healing in oral and maxillofacial surgery: a review of current approaches and future directions. Oral Maxillofac. Surg. **30**(1), 97 (2026)
27. Campanelli, L.C.: A review on the recent advances concerning the fatigue performance of titanium alloys for orthopedic applications. J. Mater. Res. **36**(1), 151–165 (2021)
28. Montoya, C., Du, Y., Gianforcaro, A.L., Orrego, S., Yang, M., Lelkes, P.I.: On the road to smart biomaterials for bone research: definitions, concepts, advances, and outlook. Bone Res. **9**(1), 12 (2021)
29. Xie, W., Wei, X., Kang, H., Jiang, H., Chu, Z., Lin, Y., Hou, Y., Wei, Q.: Static and dynamic: evolving biomaterial mechanical properties to control cellular mechanotransduction. Adv. Sci. **10**(9), 2204594 (2023)
30. Viana de Carvalho, T.C., Menezes Lima, A., Brito Jalil da Fonseca, W., Alberto Senna, C., Prioli Menezes, R., Huguenin Maia da Costa, M.E., Balestra, M.R., Antunes Ribeiro, A.: Titanium surfaces coated with alginate/hydroxyapatite composites by dip-coating technique. J. Sol-Gel Sci. Technol. **118**(3), 68 (2026a)
31. Viana de Carvalho, T.C., Lima, A.M., da Fonseca, W.B.J., Senna, C.A., Menezes, R.P., da Costa, M.E.H.M., Balestra, R.M., Ribeiro, A.A.: Titanium surfaces coated with alginate/hydroxyapatite composites by dip-coating technique. J. Sol-Gel Sci. Technol. **118**(3), 68 (2026b)
32. Guimarães, C.F., Marques, A.P., Reis, R.L.: Pushing the natural frontier: Progress on the integration of biomaterial cues toward combinatorial biofabrication and tissue engineering. Adv. Mater. **34**(33), 2105645 (2022)
33. Xu, X., Jia, Z., Zheng, Y., Wang, Y.: Bioadaptability of biomaterials: aiming at precision medicine. Matter. **4**(8), 2648–2650 (2021)
34. Huang, H., Feng, W., Chen, Y.: Two-dimensional biomaterials: material science, biological effect and biomedical engineering applications. Chem. Soc. Rev. **50**(20), 11381–11485 (2021)
35. Marin, E., Boschetto, F., Pezzotti, G.: Biomaterials and biocompatibility: an historical overview. J. Biomed. Mater. Res. A. **108**(8), 1617–1633 (2020)

36. Crawford, L., Wyatt, M., Bryers, J., Ratner, B.: Biocompatibility evolves: phenomenology to toxicology to regeneration. Adv. Healthc. Mater. **10**(11), 2002153 (2021)
37. Dawson, K.A., Yan, Y.: Current understanding of biological identity at the nanoscale and future prospects. Nat. Nanotechnol. **16**(3), 229–242 (2021)
38. Celi, S., Cioffi, M., Capellini, K., Fanni, B.M., Gasparotti, E., Vignali, E., Positano, V., Haxhiademi, D., Costa, E., Landini, L., DASKALOPOULOS, E.: Advanced Non-animal Models in Biomedical Research. JRC Publications (2022)
39. Sazzad, F., Kollengode, R., Beverly, C.L.X., Kiat, T.Y., Ganesh, G., Kofidis, T.: Preclinical large animal in-vivo experiments for surgically implanted atrioventricular valve: reappraisal and systematic review. Curr. Cardiol. Rev. **19**(1), 100–110 (2023)
40. Uwaezuoke, O.J., Kumar, P., Pillay, V., Choonara, Y.E.: Fouling in ocular devices: implications for drug delivery, bioactive surface immobilization, and biomaterial design. Drug Deliv. Transl. Res. **11**(5), 1903–1923 (2021)
41. Vacalebre, M., Frison, R., Corsaro, C., Neri, F., Santoro, A., Conoci, S., Anastasi, E., Curatolo, M.C., Fazio, E.: Current state of the art and next generation of materials for a customized intraocular lens according to a patient-specific eye power. Polymers. **15**(6), 1590 (2023)
42. Seet, W.T., Mat Afandi, M.A., Shamsuddin, S.A., Lokanathan, Y., Ng, M.H., Maarof, M.: Current good manufacturing practice (cGMP) facility and production of stem cell. In: Stem Cell Production: Processes, Practices and Regulations, pp. 37–68. Springer Singapore, Singapore (2022)
43. Kumar, R., Pattanayak, I., Dash, P.A., Mohanty, S.: Bioceramics: a review on design concepts toward tailor-made (multi)-functional materials for tissue engineering applications. J. Mater. Sci. **58**(8), 3460–3484 (2023)
44. Vaiani, L., Boccaccio, A., Uva, A.E., Palumbo, G., Piccininni, A., Guglielmi, P., Cantore, S., Santacroce, L., Charitos, I.A., Ballini, A.: Ceramic materials for biomedical applications: an overview on properties and fabrication processes. J. Funct. Biomater. **14**(3), 146 (2023)
45. Alaneme, K.K., Kareem, S.A., Olajide, J.L., Sadiku, R.E., Bodunrin, M.O.: Computational biomechanical and biodegradation integrity assessment of Mg-based biomedical devices for cardiovascular and orthopedic applications: a review. Int. J. Lightweight Mater. Manuf. **5**(2), 251–266 (2022)
46. Bandyopadhyay, A., Mitra, I., Avila, J.D., Upadhyayula, M., Bose, S.: Porous metal implants: processing, properties, and challenges. Int. J. Extreme Manuf. **5**(3), 032014 (2023)
47. Teshager, F.K.: Master of Science in Mechanical Design (2021)
48. Zia, A.W., Liu, R., Wu, X.: Structural design and mechanical performance of composite vascular grafts. Bio-Des. Manuf. **5**(4), 757–785 (2022)
49. Stoilov, M., Stoilov, L., Enkling, N., Stark, H., Winter, J., Marder, M., Kraus, D.: Effects of different titanium surface treatments on adhesion, proliferation and differentiation of bone cells: an in vitro study. J. Funct. Biomater. **13**(3), 143 (2022)
50. Prasathkumar, M., Dhrisya, C., Lin, F.H., Sadhasivam, S.: The design and developments of protein-polysaccharide biomaterials for corneal tissue engineering. Adv. Mater. Technol. **8**(15), 2300171 (2023)
51. Gao, Q., Lee, J.S., Kim, B.S., Gao, G.: Three-dimensional printing of smart constructs using stimuli-responsive biomaterials: a future direction of precision medicine. Int. J. Bioprint. **9**(1), 638 (2022)
52. Khalilov, R.: A comprehensive review of advanced nano-biomaterials in regenerative medicine and drug delivery. Adv. Biol. Earth Sci. **8**(1) (2023)
53. Bai, R., Sun, Q., He, Y., Peng, L., Zhang, Y., Zhang, L., Lu, W., Deng, J., Zhuang, Z., Yu, T., Wei, Y.: Ceramic toughening strategies for biomedical applications. Front. Bioeng. Biotechnol. **10**, 840372 (2022)
54. Latimer, J.M., Maekawa, S., Yao, Y., Wu, D.T., Chen, M., Giannobile, W.V.: Regenerative medicine technologies to treat dental, oral, and craniofacial defects. Front. Bioeng. Biotechnol. **9**, 704048 (2021)

55. Roberts, W.E.: Bone physiology, metabolism, and biomechanics. In: Misch's Contemp Implant Dent E-Book, vol. 10, p. 69 (2020)
56. Filip, D.G., Surdu, V.A., Paduraru, A.V., Andronescu, E.: Current development in biomaterials—hydroxyapatite and bioglass for applications in biomedical field: a review. J. Funct. Biomater. **13**(4), 248 (2022)
57. Radulescu, D.E., Vasile, O.R., Andronescu, E., Ficai, A.: Latest research of doped hydroxyapatite for bone tissue engineering. Int. J. Mol. Sci. **24**(17), 13157 (2023)
58. Feng, L.A., Shi, J., Guo, J.Y., Wang, S.F.: Recent strategies for improving hemocompatibility and endothelialization of cardiovascular devices and inhibition of intimal hyperplasia. J. Mater. Chem. B. **10**(20), 3781–3792 (2022)
59. Yao, S., Cui, J., Chen, S., Zhou, X., Li, J., Zhang, K.: Extracellular matrix coatings on cardiovascular materials—a review. Coatings. **12**(8), 1039 (2022)
60. Suhag, D.: Ophthalmic biomaterials. In: Handbook of Biomaterials for Medical Applications, Volume 2: Applications, pp. 205–234. Springer Nature Singapore, Singapore (2024)
61. Levin, A., Hakala, T.A., Schnaider, L., Bernardes, G.J., Gazit, E., Knowles, T.P.: Biomimetic peptide self-assembly for functional materials. Nat. Rev. Chem. **4**(11), 615–634 (2020)
62. Niu, Y., Chen, L., Wu, T.: Recent advances in bioengineering bone revascularization based on composite materials comprising hydroxyapatite. Int. J. Mol. Sci. **24**(15), 12492 (2023)
63. Safavi, S., Yu, Y., Robinson, D.L., Gray, H.A., Ackland, D.C., Lee, P.V.: Additively manufactured controlled porous orthopedic joint replacement designs to reduce bone stress shielding: a systematic review. J. Orthop. Surg. Res. **18**(1), 42 (2023)
64. Savio, D., Bagno, A.: When the total hip replacement fails: a review on the stress-shielding effect. PRO. **10**(3), 612 (2022)
65. Tang, Z., Fan, X., Chen, Y., Gu, P.: Ocular nanomedicine. Adv. Sci. **9**(15), 2003699 (2022)
66. Wang, X., Li, F., Liu, X., Zhang, H.: Applications and recent developments of hydrogels in ophthalmology. ACS Biomater Sci. Eng. **9**(11), 5968–5984 (2023)
67. Drobota, M., Ursache, S., Aflori, M.: Surface functionalities of polymers for biomaterial applications. Polymers. **14**(12), 2307 (2022)
68. Jafarzadeh, S., Forough, M., Kouzegaran, V.J., Zargar, M., Garavand, F., Azizi-Lalabadi, M., Abdollahi, M., Jafari, S.M.: Improving the functionality of biodegradable food packaging materials via porous nanomaterials. Compr. Rev. Food Sci. Food Saf. **22**(4), 2850–2886 (2023)
69. Schoenborn, S., Pirola, S., Woodruff, M.A., Allenby, M.C.: Fluid-structure interaction within models of patient-specific arteries: computational simulations and experimental validations. IEEE Rev. Biomed. Eng. **17**, 280–296 (2022)
70. Schwarz, E.L., Pegolotti, L., Pfaller, M.R., Marsden, A.L.: Beyond CFD: emerging methodologies for predictive simulation in cardiovascular health and disease. Biophys. Rev. **4**(1) (2023)
71. Sabri, B.A., Meenaloshini, S., Abreeza, N.M., Abed, A.N.: A review study on coupling agents used as ceramic fillers modifiers for dental applications. Mater. Today Proc. **80**, 2315–2326 (2023)
72. Bhatt, P., Kumar, V., Subramaniyan, V., Nagarajan, K., Sekar, M., Chinni, S.V., Ramachawolran, G.: Plasma modification techniques for natural polymer-based drug delivery systems. Pharmaceutics. **15**(8), 2066 (2023)
73. Ma, C., Nikiforov, A., Hegemann, D., De Geyter, N., Morent, R., Ostrikov, K.: Plasma-controlled surface wettability: recent advances and future applications. Int. Mater. Rev. **68**(1), 82–119 (2023)
74. Thakur, A., Kumar, A., Kaya, S., Marzouki, R., Zhang, F., Guo, L.: Recent advancements in surface modification, characterization and functionalization for enhancing the biocompatibility and corrosion resistance of biomedical implants. Coatings. **12**(10), 1459 (2022)
75. Said, A.: Ultra-high-molecular-weight-polyethylene (UHMWPE) as desired polymer material for biomedical. Khalij-Libya J. Dent. Med. Res., 11–16 (2022)
76. Savin, L., Pinteala, T., Mihai, D.N., Mihailescu, D., Miu, S.S., Sirbu, M.T., Veliceasa, B., Popescu, D.C., Sirbu, P.D., Forna, N.: Updates on biomaterials used in total hip arthroplasty (THA). Polymers. **15**(15), 3278 (2023)

77. Fioretta, E.S., Motta, S.E., Lintas, V., Loerakker, S., Parker, K.K., Baaijens, F.P., Falk, V., Hoerstrup, S.P., Emmert, M.Y.: Next-generation tissue-engineered heart valves with repair, remodelling and regeneration capacity. Nat. Rev. Cardiol. **18**(2), 92–116 (2021)
78. Kazimierczak, P., Przekora, A.: Osteoconductive and osteoinductive surface modifications of biomaterials for bone regeneration: a concise review. Coatings. **10**(10), 971 (2020)
79. Liu, D., Huyan, C., Wang, Z., Guo, Z., Zhang, X., Torun, H., Mulvihill, D., Xu, B.B., Chen, F.: Conductive polymer based hydrogels and their application in wearable sensors: a review. Mater. Horiz. **10**(8), 2800–2823 (2023)
80. Todros, S., Todesco, M., Bagno, A.: Biomaterials and their biomedical applications: from replacement to regeneration. PRO. **9**(11), 1949 (2021)
81. Alzoubi, L., Aljabali, A.A., Tambuwala, M.M.: Empowering precision medicine: the impact of 3D printing on personalized therapeutic. AAPS PharmSciTech. **24**(8), 228 (2023)
82. Carter, A., Popowski, K., Cheng, K., Greenbaum, A., Ligler, F.S., Moatti, A.: Enhancement of bone regeneration through the converse piezoelectric effect, a novel approach for applying mechanical stimulation. Bioelectricity. **3**(4), 255–271 (2021)
83. Sun, Q., Zhang, L., Bai, R., Zhuang, Z., Zhang, Y., Yu, T., Peng, L., Xin, T., Chen, S., Han, B.: Recent progress in antimicrobial strategies for resin-based restoratives. Polymers. **13**(10), 1590 (2021)
84. Shende, P., Trivedi, R.: 3D printed bioconstructs: regenerative modulation for genetic expression. Stem Cell Rev. Rep. **17**(4), 1239–1250 (2021)
85. Ejeian, F., Razmjou, A., Nasr-Esfahani, M.H., Mohammad, M., Karamali, F., Ebrahimi Warkiani, M., Asadnia, M., Chen, V.: ZIF-8 modified polypropylene membrane: a biomimetic cell culture platform with a view to the improvement of guided bone regeneration. Int. J. Nanomedicine. **15**, 10029–10043 (2020)
86. Ince, J.C., Peerzada, M., Mathews, L.D., Pai, A.R., Al-Qatatsheh, A., Abbasi, S., Yin, Y., Hameed, N., Duffy, A.R., Lau, A.K., Salim, N.V.: Overview of emerging hybrid and composite materials for space applications. Adv. Compos. Hybrid Mater. **6**(4), 130 (2023)
87. Noskovicova, N., Hinz, B., Pakshir, P.: Implant fibrosis and the underappreciated role of myofibroblasts in the foreign body reaction. Cells. **10**(7), 1794 (2021)
88. Balaure, P.C., Grumezescu, A.M.: Recent advances in surface nanoengineering for biofilm prevention and control. Part II: active, combined active and passive, and smart bacteria-responsive antibiofilm nanocoatings. Nano. **10**(8), 1527 (2020)
89. Lee, C.Y., Hu, S.M., Christy, J., Chou, F.Y., Ramli, T.C., Chen, H.Y.: Biointerface coatings with structural and biochemical properties modifications of biomaterials. Adv. Mater. Interfaces. **10**(10), 2202286 (2023)
90. Lescrauwaet, L., Wagner, H., Yoon, C., Shukla, S.: Adaptive legal frameworks and economic dynamics in emerging tech-nologies: navigating the intersection for responsible innovation. Law Econom. **16**(3), 202–220 (2022)
91. Hunckler, M.D., Levine, A.D.: Navigating ethical challenges in the development and translation of biomaterials research. Front. Bioeng. Biotechnol. **10**, 949280 (2022)
92. Veletic, M., Apu, E.H., Simic, M., Bergsland, J., Balasingham, I., Contag, C.H., Ashammakhi, N.: Implants with sensing capabilities. Chem. Rev. **122**(21), 16329–16363 (2022)
93. Yang, B., Chen, Y., Shi, J.: Exosome biochemistry and advanced nanotechnology for next-generation theranostic platforms. Adv. Mater. **31**(2), 1802896 (2019)
94. Mulder, M.P., Fresiello, L., Donker, D.W.: Computational models for hemodynamic management in critically ill patients: a systematic review. In: Virtual physiological human conference, VPH 2022: digital twins for personalized treatment development and clinical trials (2022, September)
95. Gowthaman, N.S.K., Lim, H.N., Sreeraj, T.R., Amalraj, A., Gopi, S.: Advantages of biopolymers over synthetic polymers: social, economic, and environmental aspects. In: Biopolymers and their Industrial Applications, pp. 351–372. Elsevier (2021)
96. Nwulu, E.O., Elete, T.Y., Omomo, K.O., Akano, O.A., Erhueh, O.V.: The importance of interdisciplinary collaboration for successful engineering project completions: a strategic framework. World J. Eng. Technol. Res. **2**(3), 48–56 (2023)

Chapter 8
Neural Biomaterials and Advanced Therapies

Abstract A revolutionary development in biomedical engineering, neural biomaterials bridge the fields of neuroscience, materials science, and regenerative medicine to tackle the intricate problems of nervous system modulation and repair. Designing biomaterials that can direct axonal growth, restore synapse function, and modify neuronal activity is a crucial scientific endeavor because the central and peripheral nervous systems have limited intrinsic regenerative potential. Neural biomaterials are engineered to interact intimately with neurons, glial cells, and extracellular matrices, offering both structural support and biochemical cues for regeneration and functional recovery. Biocompatible polymers, hydrogels, carbon-based nanomaterials, and bioactive scaffolds that mimic the mechanical softness and conductivity of brain tissue are the main topics of current study. To encourage cell adhesion, differentiation, and survival, these materials can be functionalized with neurotrophic factors, peptides, or extracellular matrix constituents. Engineered scaffolds and brain circuits can communicate electrically thanks to electrically conductive and responsive materials like graphene, polypyrrole, and PEDOT: PSS. This allows for precise stimulation, signal recording, and neuromodulation. These characteristics are essential for brain-machine integration, neural interfaces, and the management of neurodegenerative illnesses like Alzheimer's and Parkinson's. Advanced therapeutic approaches, including gene delivery systems, optoelectronic interfaces, and scaffolds loaded with stem cells, increase the potential of neural biomaterials beyond passive healing and toward active functional restoration. Real-time monitoring and adaptive reactions to physiological inputs are made possible by hybrid bioelectronic implants and 3D bioprinted brain structures, which promote long-term integration and dynamic feedback in vivo. Furthermore, neural interface design optimization and material performance prediction are now aided by computational modeling and artificial intelligence. A new age of customized neurological repair is being ushered in by the combination of biofabrication, nanotechnology, and neuroengineering. In the quest for adaptive, regenerative, and intelligent nervous system medicines, neural biomaterials and cutting-edge therapies work together to restore lost function, reorganize damaged neural networks, and ultimately redraw the lines between biology and technology.

M. Adeoba, T. Pandelani, *Application of Biomaterials in Biomedical Engineering*, Series in BioEngineering,
https://doi.org/10.1007/978-3-032-34477-9_8

8.1 Introduction

Sensory perception, muscular control, cognition, and homeostatic regulation are all functions of the human nervous system, which is a complex network made up of the central nervous system (CNS) and peripheral nervous system (PNS). With billions of neurons and glial cells forming highly specialized, interconnected circuits that transfer electrical and chemical information with astounding precision, it represents one of the most sensitive and complicated biological systems. But because of its intricacy, the nervous system is extremely susceptible to harm and illness. Because of restrictive microenvironments, scar formation, and inadequate axonal guidance after damage, brain tissues have a restricted intrinsic regenerating capacity in contrast to other tissues like bone or skin. Accordingly, spinal cord injuries, traumatic brain injuries, and neurodegenerative diseases (such as Alzheimer's, Parkinson's, and amyotrophic lateral sclerosis) continue to rank among the most difficult clinical issues in medicine [1, 2]. Since these disorders frequently cause irreversible functional losses, there is an urgent need for novel approaches that can repair, regenerate, or replace damaged brain structures.

8.1.1 Overview of the Nervous System's Complexity and Challenges in Repair and Regeneration

Although the blood–brain barrier (BBB) protects the central nervous system (CNS), which includes the brain and spinal cord, it also restricts the delivery of therapeutic medicines while preserving homeostasis. Although the PNS, which controls motor and sensory communication between the central nervous system and the rest of the body, has a somewhat higher capacity for regeneration, in extreme situations, recovery is still not complete. A complex series of cellular and molecular processes, such as inflammation, glial scarring, axonal sprouting, and synaptic reconnection, are involved in neural tissue repair [3, 4]. However, regeneration is hampered by chronic inflammation, loss of extracellular matrix (ECM) components, and post-injury inhibitory molecules (including Nogo-A and chondroitin sulfate proteoglycans). Biomaterial-based approaches that can replicate a permissive milieu to direct axonal development, regulate immunological responses, and restore electrophysiological function are necessary to address these issues.

8.1.2 Importance of Biomaterials in Neural Tissue Engineering, Neuroprosthetics, and Regenerative Medicine

Through their ability to bridge the gap between biology and engineering, biomaterials have become essential tools for neuronal repair and functional restoration. Biomaterials serve as scaffolds in neural tissue engineering, offering structural support for cell adhesion, proliferation, and differentiation. By imitating the structure and molecular characteristics of the extracellular matrix, they make it possible to recreate a regenerative environment that promotes synaptogenesis and axonal guidance [5, 6]. Biomaterials serve as the foundation for interfaces between biological tissues and electronic components, including electrodes, sensors, and stimulators, in neuroprosthetics. This ensures bioelectrical connection that is stable and long-lasting with no immunological reaction. Biomaterials facilitate localized and sustained release at target areas by acting as delivery systems for growth factors, medications, and stem cells in regenerative medicine. These applications underscore the versatility of neural biomaterials, which must be biocompatible, mechanically compliant, electrically conductive, and functionally adaptable to the unique demands of neural tissues.

8.1.3 The Multidisciplinary Nature of Neural Biomaterials

Neural biomaterials design and use are intrinsically multidisciplinary, combining materials science, bioengineering, and neuroscience. Materials science offers tools for surface modification, molecular design, and characterization; neuroscience contributes knowledge of neural development, injury mechanisms, and electrophysiology; and bioengineering converts these ideas into useful devices and therapeutic systems. To mimic the neuronal microenvironment and encourage electrochemical communication, the research makes use of conductive polymers, carbon-based nanomaterials, polymeric hydrogels, and hybrid composites. Furthermore, complex designs that promote neuronal alignment and connectivity can be created using sophisticated fabrication techniques such 3D bioprinting, electrospinning, and microfabrication [7, 8]. This convergence of disciplines allows for the creation of dynamic, interactive biomaterials capable of not only supporting neural regeneration but also monitoring and modulating neural activity in real time.

8.1.4 Scope of Neural Biomaterials in Addressing Neurodegenerative Diseases, Spinal Cord Injury, and Brain–Machine Interfaces

Neural biomaterials have a wide range of potential uses in both medicinal and technological fields. Biomaterial-based delivery systems help reduce or reverse neuronal death in neurodegenerative illnesses by facilitating the controlled release of therapeutic medicines and neurotrophic factors. Engineered scaffolds facilitate axonal bridging across lesion locations in spinal cord damage, while conductive polymers help restore electrophysiological continuity. Bioresorbable conduits derived from collagen, chitosan, or polylactic acid direct axon regrowth in peripheral nerve regeneration while reducing immunological rejection. Biomaterials support flexible neural probes and implantable electrodes that accurately record and stimulate neural activity in the field of brain–machine interfaces (BMIs). New designs combine drug delivery and biosensing to create closed-loop devices that instantly adjust to changes in the brain. Such innovations promise to enhance patient outcomes, improve prosthetic control, and enable bidirectional communication between the nervous system and external devices, heralding a new era of intelligent, adaptive neural therapeutics [9, 10].

8.1.5 Objectives and Structure of the Chapter

With a focus on their scientific underpinnings, material design approaches, and clinical applications, this chapter seeks to offer a thorough examination of brain biomaterials and advanced therapies. A review of the main material types and their physicochemical and biological characteristics comes first, then a look at the mechanisms and processes that underline brain tissue contact, including signal transduction, cell adhesion, and neuroinflammatory regulation. The chapter next looks at design factors including mechanical compliance, electrical conductivity, and biodegradability that are important for creating functioning brain interfaces and regenerative scaffolds. Additionally, it looks at case studies and applications in important clinical contexts, including retinal regeneration, neuroprosthetic integration, and spinal cord restoration, illustrating both translational achievements and difficulties [11, 12]. Lastly, the conversation moves on to new developments and potential paths, such as the incorporation of bioelectronic systems, 3D bioprinting, and artificial intelligence in next-generation neurological therapies.

Neural biomaterials are essentially the nexus of biology and technology, revolutionizing the fields of medicine and neuroscience. In the age of precision neuroengineering, these materials have the potential to not only restore lost function but also augment and enhance neural capabilities by mimicking neural microenvironments and seamlessly integrating with living tissue. This opens the door to patient-specific, adaptive, and intelligent interventions.

8.2 Key Concepts and Definitions

The brain, spinal cord, and peripheral nerves make up the human nervous system, which is the most complex organ network in biology. It is distinguished by complicated electrochemical communication, high sensitivity, and a limited capacity for regeneration. Serious clinical problems arise when brain tissues are damaged, whether because of ischemia injury, neurodegenerative illness, or trauma. By facilitating neuronal regeneration, function restoration, and interface between biological and electronic systems, neural biomaterials have become essential instruments in closing this therapeutic gap [13, 14]. By outlining material attributes, functional categories, and the metrics used to assess their performance, this outlines the core ideas that support the field.

8.2.1 Definition of Neural Biomaterials Materials Designed for Interaction with Neural Tissues

Specialized materials known as neural biomaterials are designed to interact physically, chemically, and functionally with nervous system components. Through protective, communicative, or supporting mechanisms, they primarily maintain, replace, or modify the function of brain tissue. These materials cover a wide range, from conductive composites that allow electrical interfacing in brain–machine applications to biopolymers that direct axonal regeneration [15, 16].

Neural biomaterials must fundamentally meet three interconnected design requirements: mechanical compliance, which should match the soft modulus of neural tissue (roughly 0.1–10 kPa); biocompatibility, which guarantees the absence of cytotoxicity or chronic inflammation; and functional responsiveness, which permits the transmission of electrical or biochemical signals. The ability of materials like graphene, polypyrrole, and poly(3,4-ethylenedioxythiophene) (PEDOT) to carry brain impulses while remaining stable in physiological settings has been the subject of much research. The ultimate objective of neural biomaterials is to provide a smooth, long-lasting interface that makes it easier for biological neurons and artificial devices to communicate.

8.2.2 Concepts of Neurocompatibility, Neuroconductivity, and Neuroinductivity

The functional success of neural biomaterials is determined by three interrelated characteristics: neurocompatibility, neuroconductivity, and neuroinductivity. By highlighting a material's capacity to cohabit with neurons, glia, and extracellular matrix without causing unfavorable immunological or glial scarring reactions, neurocompatibility expands the idea of biocompatibility to the neurological setting. It includes prolonged cellular viability, little cytotoxicity, and little activation of astrocytes or microglia. The ability of a substance to promote or enable the passage of electrical signals as the primary means of neural communication is referred to as neuroconductivity. To facilitate bidirectional communication between brain circuits and electronic devices, conductive polymers, carbon-based nanomaterials, and metallic microelectrodes are essential components of neuroprosthetic and electrophysiological systems [17, 18].

The ability of a material to stimulate neuronal differentiation, axonal extension, and synaptic network creation is referred to as neuroinductivity, a relatively new word. Usually, topographical features that direct neurite development or biochemical signals (such as adhesion peptides or neurotrophic factors) mediate this ability. These three characteristics work together to create next-generation neural interfaces that facilitate real tissue regeneration in addition to recording or stimulating it.

8.2.3 Overview of Neural Repair Strategies: Regeneration, Protection, and Modulation

Three main techniques regeneration, protection, and modulation are used in neural repair strategies, which seek to restore lost or compromised nervous system function. Each of these approaches requires unique material functions. The goal of regenerative techniques is to promote synaptic reconnection and axonal development after injury. In addition to supplying bioactive chemicals to promote axonal extension, biomaterial scaffolds, hydrogels, and conduits offer physical guidance pathways that support guided neuron regeneration. Collagen-based nerve guides and fibrin hydrogels enhanced with neurotrophic factors like brain-derived neurotrophic factor (BDNF) or nerve growth factor (NGF) are two examples [19].

Protective measures, which frequently involve antioxidative, anti-inflammatory, or neuroprotective coatings, focus on stopping more neuronal injury or secondary degeneration. In this situation, materials that scavenge reactive oxygen species or produce anti-inflammatory compounds are essential, especially after ischemia or traumatic injury. Controlled electrical or pharmacological stimulation is used in modulatory methods to alter synaptic activity and neuronal excitability. This strategy is demonstrated by neural biomaterials incorporated into deep brain stimulators or vagus nerve interfaces, which allow for precise neuromodulation to cure ailments including Parkinson's disease, epilepsy, and chronic pain [20, 21]. Collectively, these tactics demonstrate the range of neural biomaterial uses, from active, feedback-driven neural network regulation to passive scaffolding and protection.

8.2.4 Classification of Neural Interfaces

Based on how they interact with neural circuits, neural interfaces can be broadly divided into passive and active systems. The main purpose of passive neural interfaces is to capture bioelectrical activity, which includes action potentials and local field potentials, without modifying the behavior of neurons directly. Flexible electrocorticography (ECoG) grids and microelectrode arrays (MEAs) are two examples. These gadgets use biostable, highly conductive materials that reduce tissue discomfort and signal noise. On the other hand, active neural interfaces modulate brain activity by delivering electrical, chemical, or visual stimuli. These consist of optogenetic interfaces, spinal cord stimulators, deep brain stimulators, and cochlear implants. Under repeated stimulation cycles, the materials must guarantee accurate charge transfer, electrochemical stability, and long-term durability.

At the forefront of neural device design are hybrid systems that combine passive and active functionalities, like closed-loop brain–machine interfaces. By integrating sensing and stimulation into a single feedback circuit, they enable real-time brain function regulation in response to physiological signals that are detected [22]. The path for autonomous, self-regulating neuroprosthetic devices with adaptive therapeutic capabilities is being paved by this convergence.

8.2.5 Advanced Therapeutic Concepts

Numerous cutting-edge therapeutic paradigms, including neuroprosthetics, neural tissue engineering, and neuromodulation, are based on contemporary neural biomaterials. The deliberate modification of brain activity by electrical, magnetic, or pharmacological techniques is referred to as neuromodulation. Recent developments in biomaterials for neuromodulatory systems include soft, flexible electrodes that adapt to neuronal surfaces without mechanical mismatch, enabling localized and selective stimulation. This idea is furthered by neuroprosthetics, which use electronic interfaces to replace or enhance sensory or motor function. Retinal implants for vision restoration, brain-controlled robotic limbs, and aural prostheses are a few examples. Biomaterials serve as vital bridges between biological tissue and electronics in these systems, guaranteeing both biocompatibility and steady electrical contact.

To repair or replace damaged brain tissue, neural tissue engineering uses a combination of cells, scaffolds, and signaling molecules. Three-dimensional structures that resemble the extracellular environment are offered by hydrogels, aligned nanofibers, and bioactive conduits, which promote axonal development and synapse formation. The treatment of spinal cord injuries, stroke, and neurodegenerative disorders like Alzheimer's or amyotrophic lateral sclerosis (ALS) could be greatly enhanced by the combination of neural tissue engineering, stem cell therapy, and gene editing [23, 24]. The development of neural biomaterials from static implants to dynamic living systems with the ability to communicate and repair is best illustrated by these therapeutic fields.

8.2.6 Metrics for Assessing Neural Biomaterials

For neural biomaterials to be quantitatively evaluated, a multidisciplinary analysis that considers electrical, biological, and structural factors is necessary. A material's electrical conductivity dictates how well it delivers stimulation or sends neurological signals. Reliable neural interfacing requires high signal-to-noise ratios and low impedance, which are guaranteed by high-conductivity materials (such as graphene, gold, and PEDOT: PSS). Measured by electrode impedance, material stability, and tissue encapsulation, signal fidelity quantifies the precision and repeatability of recorded or transmitted data. For more sophisticated neuroprosthetic control, enhanced fidelity makes it possible to precisely decode brain activity.

The ability of the material to form functional, structural, and biochemical connections with surrounding neural tissue, including alignment of neural fibers, formation of synaptic contacts, and stable adhesion without micromotion-induced damage, is referred to as integration. Advanced imaging and electrophysiological techniques, such as impedance spectroscopy and two-photon microscopy, are used to monitor these interactions over time. Together, these metrics define the holistic performance of neural biomaterials, ensuring that they meet the dual demands of functional efficacy and biological safety in long-term neural interfacing [14, 25]. Biocompatibility is still a key metric, which includes the absence of glial scarring, minimal inflammation, and prevention of glial scarring, as well as the prevention of glial scarring, and the maintenance of stable interfaces without fibrotic encapsulation that can insulate electrodes from neurons.

With the goal of developing intelligent systems that can sense, communicate, and regenerate inside the nervous system, the topic of neural biomaterials represents the nexus of materials science, neurobiology, and bioengineering. Numerous applications in regeneration, neuromodulation, and prosthetic integration are based on fundamental ideas that encompass neurocompatibility, neuroconductivity, and neuroinductivity. Neural biomaterials have the potential to redefine therapeutic frontiers and close the gap between biological cognition and artificial intelligence as evaluation criteria and interdisciplinary collaboration advance.

8.3 Material Types and Properties

One of the most cutting-edge and multidisciplinary areas of biomedical engineering and regenerative medicine is neural biomaterials. To effectively interface with the delicate architecture of the nervous system, materials used in neural applications must meet a wide range of characteristics, including mechanical compliance,

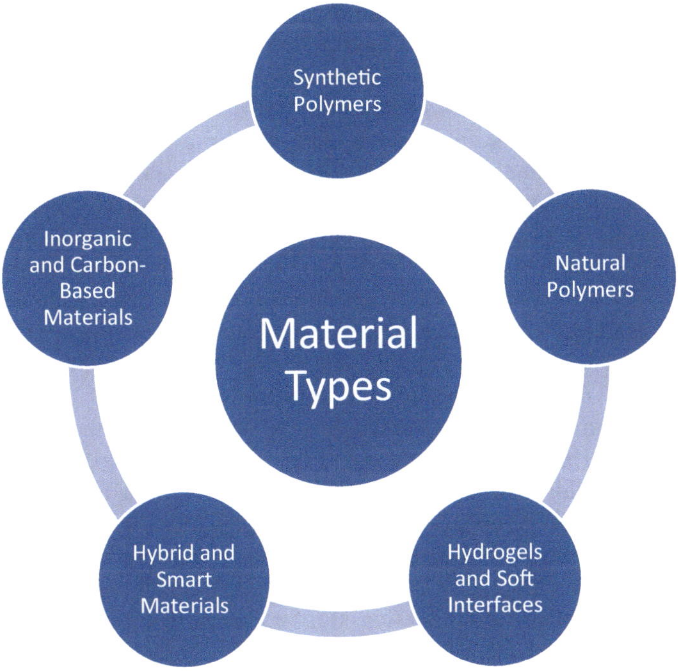

Fig. 8.1 Overview of biomaterial categories used in neural engineering

electrical conductivity, biocompatibility, biodegradability, and neuroinductivity. They serve as functional platforms for bioelectrical communication, drug transport, and biochemical signaling in addition to provide structural support for cell attachment and axonal development [26, 27]. Brain biomaterials have advanced from just structural scaffolds to bioactive and intelligent materials that can interact with brain cells dynamically and change their function. This explores the main classes of materials used in neural repair and interface systems natural polymers, synthetic polymers, inorganic and carbon-based materials, hydrogels, and hybrid smart materials highlighting their properties, mechanisms of action, and applications in neuroregeneration and neuroprosthetics as shown in Fig. 8.1.

8.3.1 Natural Polymers

Natural polymers' inherent biocompatibility, biodegradability, and bioactivity make them one of the most popular materials in neural tissue engineering. Originating from biological sources, they closely resemble the extracellular matrix (ECM) and offer a favorable milieu for axonal development, cell adhesion, and proliferation. The most prevalent protein in the extracellular matrix, collagen plays a crucial structural role in neural scaffolds. In addition to providing biochemical cues necessary for cell–matrix interactions, its fibrillar architecture stimulates neurite development. Collagen-based scaffolds have been effectively used in spinal cord regeneration and peripheral nerve conduits. To improve neuroinduction, they are frequently coupled with neurotrophic factors like brain-derived neurotrophic factor (BDNF) or nerve growth factor (NGF).

A polysaccharide made from chitin, chitosan has outstanding biocompatibility and biodegradability and can be chemically modified to adjust its mechanical and biological characteristics. It is appropriate for peripheral nerve repair and drug delivery systems that target the central nervous system (CNS) because it promotes Schwann cell proliferation and axonal regeneration. Derived from the cocoons of silkworms, silk fibroin provides a combination of mechanical strength, delayed disintegration, and low immunological response [28]. It can be processed into films, sponges, or electrospun fibers to guide axonal alignment because of its nanofibrous structure, which resembles the extracellular matrix.

The glycosaminoglycan hyaluronic acid (HA), which is abundant in neural extracellular matrix (ECM), is especially important for CNS applications because of its hydrophilicity and capacity to regulate inflammation and cell migration. HA-based hydrogels are utilized in injectable formulations for minimally invasive brain repair and promote the development of neural progenitor cells. When taken as a whole, natural polymers offer crucial physiological signals and structural models for tissue integration and cell adhesion. But because of their poor mechanical control, fast deterioration, and batch variability, they may need to be combined with synthetic materials for best results.

8.3.2 Synthetic Polymers

Because of their processing adaptability, tunability, and reproducibility, synthetic polymers are preferred in the design of neural biomaterials. Customized methods for neural healing and device manufacture are made possible by the ability to carefully tune their qualities to control electrical behavior, mechanical stiffness, and degradation rate. Depending on the ratio of lactic to glycolic acid, the biodegradable copolymer poly(lactic-co-glycolic acid) (PLGA) has adjustable degradation kinetics. It offers mechanical stability during initial tissue regeneration and progressively resorbs to permit new tissue ingrowth, making it a popular choice for controlled drug delivery and nerve guidance conduits.

A hydrophilic polymer with a reputation for being biocompatible and resistant to proteins, polyethylene glycol (PEG) is frequently utilized to create hydrogels and surface coatings for neural interfaces. PEGylation improves the long-term durability of implanted devices and decreases immunological recognition. Polycaprolactone (PCL) is perfect for long-term implants and 3D-printed neural scaffolds because it degrades more slowly and is more flexible than PLGA [29]. When combined with natural polymers like collagen or gelatin, it enhances biocompatibility and cell adhesion.

Furthermore, neural interface technology has been transformed by conductive polymers as poly(3,4-ethylenedioxythiophene) (PEDOT) and polypyrrole (PPy).

By combining mechanical flexibility and electrical conductivity, these materials enable efficient brain signal transmission without creating mechanical mismatches with soft neural tissue. They allow for two-way communication with neurons and are utilized in electrodes, biosensors, and brain probes. Synthetic polymers can attain precise control over degradation rate, electrical responsiveness, and drug release behavior by adjusting polymer composition, molecular weight, and surface chemistry. This is necessary for synchronized neuronal regeneration and regulation.

8.3.3 Inorganic and Carbon-Based Materials

The development of electrically active brain interfaces and sensors heavily relies on inorganic and carbon-based materials. They are essential in neuroprosthetic and neuroelectronic applications due to their remarkable electrical conductivity, mechanical robustness, and chemical stability. A novel material for neural interfaces is graphene, which is made up of a single layer of carbon atoms organized in a hexagonal lattice. Its conductivity, flexibility, and large surface area facilitate effective neural recording and stimulation, and its atomic thinness reduces tissue injury after implantation. It has been demonstrated that graphene coatings enhance synaptic activity and neural adhesion, providing a route for high-fidelity brain–machine interfaces [17, 30].

Similar benefits are offered by carbon nanotubes (CNTs), which have a tubular nanostructure that improves mechanical reinforcement and electrochemical performance. For nerve healing and signal transduction, CNTs can be added to polymer matrices to create conductive composites that enhance scaffold conductivity and promote charge transfer. Neural microelectrode arrays (MEAs) and biosensors continue to rely on silicon, a material that has historically been employed in microelectronic production. Despite their rigidity, silicon-based devices can be precisely microfabricated at the nanoscale to target certain populations of neurons. To increase biocompatibility and lessen inflammatory reactions, recent developments have concentrated on softening silicon surfaces or combining them with polymers.

The nanostructured surfaces of these materials also promote synaptic connection, cell anchoring, and protein adsorption, which improves electrical coupling and the long-term functionality of brain interfaces. To guarantee safe long-term implantation, cautious surface modification and encapsulating techniques are necessary because of their restricted biodegradability and possible cytotoxicity.

8.3.4 Hydrogels and Soft Interfaces

For drug administration and neural regeneration, hydrogels three-dimensional, water-rich networks of polymers are perfect because they replicate the mechanical and biochemical properties of neural tissue. Their structure can be modified to regulate stiffness, disintegration, and bioactivity, and their softness and high permeability promote cell viability and nutrition transfer. For the repair of brain or spinal cord injuries, injectable hydrogels provide a minimally invasive method. They can be loaded with growth agents, stem cells, or nanoparticles for dynamic remodeling and localized delivery. The viscoelastic characteristics of neural tissue (elastic modulus 0.1–10 kPa) can be matched by hydrogels based on PEG, HA, or gelatin methacrylate (GelMA), reducing inflammatory response and mechanical strain.

Similar benefits are offered by carbon nanotubes (CNTs), which have a tubular nanostructure that improves mechanical reinforcement and electrochemical performance. For nerve healing and signal transduction, CNTs can be added to polymer matrices to create conductive composites that enhance scaffold conductivity and promote charge transfer. Neural microelectrode arrays (MEAs) and biosensors continue to rely on silicon, a material that has historically been employed in microelectronic production. Despite their rigidity, silicon-based devices can be precisely microfabricated at the nanoscale to target certain populations of neurons. To increase biocompatibility and lessen inflammatory reactions, recent developments have concentrated on softening silicon surfaces or combining them with polymers [31].

8.3.5 Hybrid and Smart Materials

The cutting edge of neural biomaterials research is represented by hybrid and smart materials, which combine electrical performance, mechanical compliance, and bioactivity to create multipurpose systems. By combining the benefits of both organic and inorganic components, these materials frequently create layered structures or nanocomposites with complementary qualities. Graphene–polymer and CNT–hydrogel systems are examples of hybrid composites that provide enhanced conductivity, flexibility, and biocompatibility. They preserve strong electrical connection for neurological stimulation or recording while promoting neuronal attachment and guidance.

Conversely, smart materials behave in a stimulus-responsive manner, altering their characteristics in reaction to external stimuli like electrical fields, pH, temperature, or enzyme activity. For instance, thermosensitive polymers can change from liquid to gel at body temperature, allowing for precise distribution and spatial control, while electroresponsive hydrogels can release neuroactive chemicals in response to electrical stimulation. These flexible materials pave the way for new developments in dynamic brain modulation, where biomaterials actively contribute to signal processing and neural repair. These systems' ability to react intelligently to cerebral activity is further enhanced by the addition of biosensing and feedback loops, opening the door for autonomous, self-regulating neuroprosthetics.

The variety of material platforms used in neural biomaterials highlights the complex needs of interface and brain healing technology. Each material class makes a distinct contribution to the advancement of neural engineering, ranging from synthetic and carbon-based materials that provide electrical conductivity to natural polymers that offer biological affinity, from soft hydrogels that mimic brain tissue to hybrid smart systems that allow adaptive interactions. In order to bridge the gap between living tissues and engineered systems for truly regenerative and functional neural therapies, next-generation neural biomaterials are shaped by the continuous integration of bioactivity, mechanical compliance, and intelligent responsiveness [13, 32].

8.4 Mechanisms and Processes

The processes and mechanisms that control neural biomaterials involve a complex interaction between physiological signal transmission, cellular reactions, and material characteristics. In addition to integrating physically and physiologically with neural tissue, effective neural interfaces and scaffolds must maintain and improve the electrochemical communication that is essential to the nervous system's operation [33, 34]. Through five interrelated domains cell–material interactions, neural regeneration, electrical and chemical transmission, neural stimulation and recording, and drug and gene delivery this investigates the biological, molecular, and biophysical concepts that underlie neural biomaterials.

8.4.1 Cell–Material Interactions

The dynamic interaction between cells glia and neurons and the material interface is the cornerstone of neural biomaterials. Since neural tissue is electrically active, physically soft, and extremely sensitive to environmental stimuli, biomaterials must offer substrates that are both supportive and non-disruptive for cell survival and function. A key component of this relationship is mechanotransduction, which is how cells perceive and react to mechanical stresses. Through cytoskeletal remodeling and focal adhesions, neurons and glial cells are able to detect changes in substrate stiffness and topography, which affects network creation and differentiation. Hydrogels and other materials with elastic moduli between 0.1 and 10 kPa, which are similar to those of native brain tissue, can improve the viability and functional maturation of neurons.

Electrical cues have an equal impact. By facilitating charge transfer across the cell membrane, electroactive materials such as conductive polymers like polypyrrole (PPy) and poly(3,4-ethylenedioxythiophene) (PEDOT) promote synaptic activity and neurite elongation. For instance, by preserving low impedance and high charge storage capacity, doped PEDOT surfaces promote neurite development and improve neural cell adhesion. Furthermore, to support cellular adhesion and differentiation processes, biomaterials can be functionalized with bioactive ligands like nerve growth factor (NGF) or laminin-derived peptides. The long-term biocompatibility and functionality of brain implants and scaffolds are determined by the combined regulation of cell–material communication by these biochemical and biophysical signals.

8.4.2 Neural Regeneration Processes

Unlike regeneration in many other tissues, neural regeneration has inherent limitations because of restricted neuronal growth and inhibitory molecular environments. Therefore, favorable microenvironments that direct axonal regrowth, inhibit scar formation, and regulate inflammation must be established by biomaterials intended for brain repair. In this situation, biochemical and topographical clues are crucial. It has been demonstrated that micro- and nanoscale surface patterns, including microgrooves or aligned electrospun fibers, can mimic the natural guiding of extracellular matrix (ECM) fibers by directing axonal elongation along certain paths. To improve directed regeneration, these physical signals are frequently coupled with biochemical gradients of neurotrophic factors, such as glial cell line-derived neurotrophic factor (GDNF) or brain-derived neurotrophic factor (BDNF).

Inhibiting glial scarring, which is mostly brought on by reactive astrocyte proliferation and the deposition of chondroitin sulfate proteoglycans, is a major problem in brain repair. Hydrogels containing heparin or interleukin-10 are examples of biomaterials with immunomodulatory or anti-inflammatory qualities that can reduce the foreign body reaction and encourage a regenerative healing pathway as opposed to a fibrotic one [35, 36]. Furthermore, intelligent biomaterials with on-demand breakdown enable long-term tissue integration without persistent inflammation by releasing therapeutic compounds in response to environmental cues (such as pH or enzymatic activity). Together, these processes show how neural biomaterials can coordinate the intricate biological processes required for functional recovery and axonal regeneration.

8.4.3 Electrical and Chemical Signal Transmission

Neural biomaterials are distinguished by their ability to communicate with the brain's electrochemical signaling network. Rapid ionic and electrical fluxes across membranes are necessary for neuronal communication, hence biomaterials must facilitate effective charge transport while preserving biocompatibility. To simulate the electrical conductivity of neural tissue (usually 0.1–1.0 S/m), conductive polymers, carbon-based materials (such as graphene and carbon nanotubes), and doped ceramics are being used more and more. These substances improve the accuracy of stimulation and the fidelity of recorded data by lowering impedance at the electrode–tissue interface.

The effectiveness of electrochemical coupling is determined by ion transport and charge transfer mechanisms at the material–cell contact. In response to electrical stimulation, conductive polymers can store and release charge through reversible redox processes while retaining chemical stability. By promoting electrochemical capacitance mechanisms, these materials reduce the likelihood of tissue injury from faradaic reactions. Furthermore, ionically conductive hydrogels and electrically conductive scaffolds are combined to create bioelectronic interfaces that improve electrical communication and biocompatibility while bridging the gap between artificial and biological systems. Chemical signaling is equally important as electrical transmission. Bioactive coatings that release neurotransmitters or signaling molecules can alter neuronal excitability and synaptic function; this is an emerging field in hybrid electrochemical biomaterials [6, 37].

8.4.4 Neural Stimulation and Recording Mechanisms

At the cutting edge of neuroengineering is the incorporation of neural biomaterials into functional stimulation and recording devices. Action potentials and local field potentials must be captured with the least amount of signal loss for electrophysiological sensing to function. High signal-to-noise ratios, low impedance, and consistent long-term performance are required for these interfaces. Excellent electrical properties are provided by materials like graphene electrodes and PEDOT:PSS, which also minimize tissue damage and retain flexibility. Signal quality and tissue compatibility are further influenced by the shape and microarchitecture of the electrodes, which can be microneedles, meshes, or flexible films.

Controlled electrical, optical, or magnetic fields are used in stimulation devices to alter the activity of neurons. While electrical pulses are used in traditional deep brain stimulation (DBS) to reduce Parkinson's disease symptoms, newer multimodal stimulation techniques like optogenetics and magnetoelectric stimulation have higher specificity. To accomplish cell-type-specific activation, optogenetic devices, for instance, integrate biocompatible optical fibers or photoconductive materials with light-responsive ion channels (channelrhodopsins). On the other hand, magnetoelectric materials enable wireless neuromodulation without the need for physical connectors by converting external magnetic fields into local electrical impulses. These processes signify a move toward closed-loop, less invasive neural interfaces that integrate real-time stimulation and sensing.

8.4.5 Drug and Gene Delivery

Targeted medication and gene delivery is essential for regulating brain plasticity, preventing neuronal degeneration, and fostering neural repair. Growth factors, anti-inflammatory medications, and genetic payloads are examples of neuroactive chemicals that can be released under regulated conditions using biomaterials. Diffusion through polymer matrices, degradation-controlled systems, or responsive hydrogels are examples of controlled release methods that allow for prolonged therapeutic activity with less systemic toxicity. For example, in spinal cord damage models, PLGA-based microspheres loaded with nerve growth factors have been utilized to preserve targeted delivery, improving axonal regeneration.

Apart from small chemicals, gene delivery techniques that use non-viral nanoparticles or viral vectors (like lentivirus or adeno-associated virus) can also change the expression of certain genes in neural tissues. By integrating these vectors into biomaterial scaffolds, transgene release can be controlled both spatially and temporally, promoting the long-term expression of neuroprotective or regenerative proteins. Through receptor-mediated transport, nanostructured carriers like liposomes, dendrimers, and polymeric nanoparticles can pass through the blood–brain barrier (BBB), opening systemic delivery pathways for treatments affecting the central nervous system. Modern neuroengineering's mechanistic sophistication is further demonstrated by the combination of brain biomaterials with theranostic systems, which can both detect pathogenic alterations and provide therapeutic drugs [38].

The biological, electrical, and chemical characteristics of the nervous system are closely related to the systems and procedures that support neuronal biomaterials. Every step of neural repair depends on carefully designed interfaces, from cell–material interactions that determine biocompatibility and the creation of neural networks to regeneration processes that get beyond restrictive surroundings. While stimulation and recording techniques are moving toward adaptive, wireless, and multimodal configurations, advances in electrical and chemical signal transmission have increased the potential for smooth integration between biological tissues and electronic equipment. Lastly, by combining diagnosis, therapy, and regeneration onto a single platform, the use of medication and gene delivery systems highlights the therapeutic potential of neural biomaterials [39, 40]. Together, these processes define the mechanistic landscape of neural biomaterials and lay the foundation for next generation neurotechnologies capable of restoring, enhancing, and interfacing with the human nervous system.

8.5 Design Considerations

Given the remarkable structural delicacy, electrochemical sensitivity, and restricted regenerative capacity of the nervous system, designing biomaterials for neural applications is an exceptionally difficult task. To guarantee safety and effectiveness in long-term applications, neural biomaterials and devices must strike the ideal balance between mechanical, electrical, biological, and ethical requirements. Neurons, glial cells, extracellular matrix (ECM), and interstitial fluid make up the neural environment as shown in Fig. 8.2. This environment is electrically active, physically soft (with an elastic modulus of 0.1–10 kPa), and extremely susceptible to inflammation or foreign body incursion. Neural biomaterials must therefore blend in perfectly with this setting in order to facilitate effective signal transmission, encourage

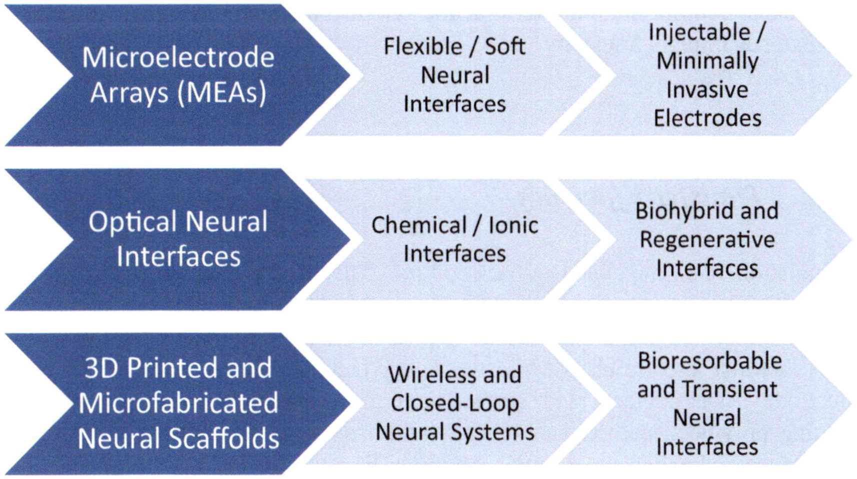

Fig. 8.2 Neural interface designs

regeneration, and reduce immunological responses. This key design considerations shaping the development of neural biomaterials and devices, including mechanical compliance, electrical conductivity, biocompatibility, surface engineering, functional integration, stability, and ethical aspects, emphasizing their roles in advancing next generation neurotechnologies.

8.5.1 Matching Mechanical Compliance with Soft Neural Tissues

One of the most important design factors for neural scaffolds and implants is mechanical compatibility. Chronic inflammation, neuronal loss, and glial scarring can result from the mechanical mismatch between soft neural tissue and stiff implant materials (such as silicon or metals). Materials must have elastic moduli that closely resemble those of brain or spinal tissue to avoid such effects. Because of their adjustable elasticity and viscoelastic properties, flexible polymers like hydrogels, poly(ethylene glycol) (PEG), and poly(dimethylsiloxane) (PDMS) are widely employed. To reduce damage caused by micromotion, hydrogels, in particular, can achieve moduli in the kilopascal range, which enables them to deform synchronously with surrounding tissue.

Stretchable brain probes and electrodes that retain electrical integrity under deformation have been made possible by recent developments in soft electronics and microfabrication [41]. PEDOT:PSS, graphene sheets, and elastomer composites are examples of materials that bridge the gap between biological softness and device functioning by offering both conductivity and flexibility. By striking this mechanical equilibrium, long-term neural interfacing maintains signal consistency and extends implant longevity.

8.5.2 Optimization of Electrical Conductivity and Charge Transfer Efficiency

Stimulation, recording, and feedback control all depend on effective electrical communication between neural devices and tissues. In order to prevent electrochemical side reactions that could harm tissue or deteriorate the electrode, neural interfaces must facilitate precise charge transfer. A key factor in charge transmission is the electrode–tissue contact. High surface area and conductivity materials, like conducting polymers, carbon nanotubes, iridium oxide, and platinum black, lower impedance and enhance capacitive coupling. Because they can combine ionic and electrical conductivity, conductive polymers like PEDOT and polypyrrole (PPy) have gained popularity. This allows for smooth signal transduction in the moist brain environment.

By expanding the effective contact area, nanostructuring the electrode surface using methods like chemical vapor deposition, electrospinning, or nanopatterning can further improve charge injection capability. Hybrid systems that use gold or graphene nanostructures also lower power consumption and enhance charge stability. Optimizing energy efficiency, temporal resolution, and signal fidelity while preserving a safe electrochemical environment is the aim. Cytotoxicity can result from ion buildup or local heating brought on by very high current densities. Therefore, to guarantee safe and effective neural interfacing, careful design of the material composition, electrode shape, and charge density parameters is necessary.

8.5.3 Biocompatibility and Immunomodulation to Prevent Glial Encapsulation

One of the key factors limiting the lifetime of brain implants is the foreign body response (FBR). When the material is implanted, the body perceives it as alien, which causes astrocytes and microglia to become activated, pro-inflammatory cytokines to be secreted, and ultimately the device to be encapsulated by glia [42, 43]. The implant is electrically isolated by this fibrous capsule, which reduces its capacity for stimulation and recording.

Materials must be highly biocompatible and ideally have immunomodulatory qualities to reduce FBR. Surface coatings that prevent protein adsorption and lower immunological activation include PEG, hyaluronic acid, and zwitterionic polymers. Bioactive compounds, including cytokine modulators (like interleukin-10) or anti-inflammatory medications (like dexamethasone), can be incorporated to promote a regenerative immune response instead of a destructive one and locally reduce inflammation. Recent Brain–Computer Interface (BCI) focused evidence confirms that poor biocompatibility and mechanical mismatch remain major causes of immune activation, scar-tissue formation, reduced recording quality and shortened implant lifetime in chronic neural electrodes [44]. Using pharmacological or topographical signals, emerging techniques target macrophage polarization and encourage a change from pro-inflammatory (M1) to pro-healing (M2) phenotypes. Furthermore, neural ECM-inspired coverings that contain collagen or laminin fragments can promote neuronal adhesion while inhibiting glial proliferation.

Through careful material selection and surface functionalization, it is possible to design neural interfaces that not only minimize adverse immune reactions but also actively participate in maintaining homeostasis within the neural microenvironment.

8.5.4 Microscale and Nanoscale Surface Engineering for Improved Neurite Guidance

Neural biomaterials' surface architecture has a significant impact on synaptic connection, neurite alignment, and cell activity. The morphology and functional organization of neurons can be influenced by microscales and nanoscale characteristics, to which they are extremely sensitive. Topographical cues that direct axonal extension are produced using methods including laser ablation, nanoimprinting, and microcontact printing. Electrospun aligned nanofibers provide channels for targeted nerve regeneration by imitating the anisotropic nature of native neural tissue [45].

Protein adsorption and focal adhesion formation can be modulated at the nanoscale by surface roughness and pattern shape, which can affect cell signaling cascades including integrin-mediated mechanotransduction. For instance, gradient topographies can trigger chemotactic or haptotactic responses that direct cell migration, whereas nanogrooved or nanopillar surfaces encourage neurite elongation. Furthermore, cellular adhesion and differentiation are impacted by surface charge and wettability. Moderate hydrophilicity encourages balanced protein adsorption that supports neural growth, while positively charged surfaces improve neuron attachment. Thus, obtaining spatial control over neural network development and interface performance requires the merging of such bioinspired and topography-engineered surfaces.

8.5.5 Integration of Biosensing and Stimulation Functionalities in Hybrid Systems

More next-generation brain biomaterials are being created as multipurpose hybrid systems that include drug delivery, stimulation, and sensing. Real-time brain activity monitoring and regulation are made possible by this integration, which results in more accurate and flexible therapeutic approaches. By identifying biological markers (such as neurotransmitters, ions, or metabolites), biosensing components can guide stimulation techniques and provide information about local tissue conditions. Modules for electrical or optical stimulation can simultaneously alter how neurons fire or encourage tissue repair. For example, high spatial resolution simultaneous signal recording and photostimulation are made possible by graphene-based electrodes and optogenetic interfaces.

In reaction to sensor feedback, drug-eluting coatings or microfluidic channels integrated with brain devices enable the on-demand release of neuroprotective or anti-inflammatory medicines. An important step toward brain prostheses that are adaptable and self-regulating is represented by such closed-loop devices. Within small, biocompatible platforms, the design challenge is to seamlessly integrate a variety of capabilities, including mechanical flexibility, electrical performance, biochemical sensing, and controlled release. These multipurpose hybrid structures need the use of sophisticated production processes like soft lithography and 3D microprinting.

8.5.6 Long-Term Stability, Miniaturization, and Data Interface Considerations

Neural biomaterials and devices must exhibit remarkable long-term stability in the demanding physiological environment to be used for chronic implantation. Over time, corrosion, delamination, or performance drift may result from mechanical stress, enzymatic degradation, and ongoing exposure to ionic fluids. To prevent deterioration of delicate components while preserving their flexibility and clarity, protective coatings like silicon carbide, parylene-C, or ultrathin oxides are frequently used. Miniaturization is also necessary to enhance spatial resolution in brain recording and lessen tissue damage after implantation. Microneedle arrays and flexible neural meshes that adapt to the topography of the brain have been developed as a result of the miniaturization trend. Smaller devices still need to make sure they have enough power and data transfer, though. Consequently, wireless power transfer, energy harvesting, and telemetry systems have become integral to modern neural interface design.

Data interface design, or the capacity to rapidly process and transfer massive amounts of brain data while reducing noise and delay, is equally critical. Enhancing interpretability through integration with AI-driven signal analysis allows for adaptive therapeutic control in brain-machine systems [46].

8.5.7 Ethical and Safety Design Aspects for Neural Implants and Brain–Machine Systems

Safety and ethical issues become critical as neural biomaterials and interfaces move closer to therapeutic and cognitive integration. Concerns about autonomy, privacy, and informed permission are brought up by neural implants that record or alter brain activity. Just as important as the technological design of neurodevices is making sure that the data they acquire is safely stored and used in an ethical manner. Long-term tissue change, infection risk, and implant-induced toxicity are among biomedical safety issues. Before clinical translation, active implanted medical devices (AIMDs) must pass stringent biocompatibility testing, sterility validation, and failure analysis, according to regulatory frameworks like the FDA and ISO standards.

Designers must also account for reversibility the ability to safely remove or deactivate devices if adverse effects occur and equitable access, ensuring that emerging neurotechnologies do not exacerbate socioeconomic disparities in healthcare.

The smooth integration of mechanical compliance, electrical accuracy, biological harmony, and ethical responsibility is necessary for the creation of neural biomaterials. Researchers can design devices that naturally communicate with neurons while reducing negative reactions by integrating immune-modulatory and topographical aspects, maximizing charge transmission, and matching material stiffness with neural tissue. A new era of intelligent, adaptable neurointerfaces is being ushered in by hybrid systems that combine biosensing, stimulation, and medication delivery functions. However, long-term stability, data integration, and adherence to safety and ethical standards are all as important to their success. The creation of human-centered, secure, and responsive systems that improve, restore, and respectfully interact with the human nervous system is ultimately what will shape neural biomaterial design in the future [47].

8.6 Applications and Case Studies

A key component of contemporary neuroengineering, neural biomaterials allow materials science, biotechnology, and clinical neurology to come together to preserve, improve, and restore neuronal function as shown in Table 8.1. Their uses range from sophisticated neuromodulatory and neuroprotective devices to regenerative scaffolds and neuroprosthetic systems. To demonstrate how biomaterials convert basic mechanisms into concrete therapeutic results, this part examines six important domains: neural tissue engineering, neuroprosthetics, neuromodulation, neuroprotective medication delivery, retinal and cortical implants, and clinical case studies [13, 48].

8.6.1 Neural Tissue Engineering

By fusing biomaterials with cells and biochemical cues to encourage regeneration, neural tissue engineering aims to replace or repair damaged neural structures. In damage to the spinal cord and peripheral nerves, where scarring and inhibitory molecules frequently prevent axonal regrowth, three-dimensional (3D) scaffolds offer a biochemical and structural environment that is like the extracellular matrix (ECM).

Table 8.1 Biomaterials for neural applications

	Application area	Representative biomaterials	Design features/functional mechanisms	Clinical or experimental case studies	Outcomes/performance metrics
Neural tissue engineering	3D scaffolds for spinal cord regeneration	Collagen, chitosan, hyaluronic acid (HA), PLGA, graphene–gelatin composites	Porous 3D scaffolds supporting axonal alignment, neurotrophic factor loading, and controlled degradation	Collagen–chitosan conduits implanted in rat spinal cord lesions promoted axon bridging and partial motor recovery	Enhanced axonal elongation, glial scar reduction, and improved locomotor function in vivo
	Peripheral nerve regeneration conduits	Polycaprolactone (PCL), silk fibroin, polypyrrole (PPy), conductive hydrogels	Tubular or aligned fiber structures guiding Schwann cell migration and electrical stimulation	FDA-approved NeuraGen® collagen nerve guide and experimental PPy–PCL conduits for sciatic nerve repair	Functional reconnection across 10–20 mm nerve gaps; restoration of muscle innervation within 12 weeks
Neuroprosthetics and brain–machine interfaces (BMI)	Electrode arrays for motor control	Platinum–iridium, gold, silicon, polyimide, graphene	High-density microelectrode arrays (Utah Array, NeuroGrid) enabling cortical signal acquisition	BrainGate clinical trials using intracortical microelectrodes for prosthetic arm control	Real-time translation of motor cortex signals to robotic movement with millisecond precision
	Sensory feedback interfaces	Carbon nanotube (CNT) composites, PEDOT:PSS coatings, soft parylene-C electrodes	Flexible electrodes interfacing with sensory cortices or peripheral nerves for bidirectional communication	Peripheral nerve interfaces restoring tactile feedback in upper-limb amputees (cuff electrodes, EPFL studies)	Users achieved object discrimination through artificial tactile input; reduced phantom limb pain
Neuromodulation devices	Deep brain stimulation (DBS)	Titanium–silicone casings, Pt–Ir electrodes, polyurethane insulation	Implanted pulse generators delivering electrical impulses to basal ganglia regions	Medtronic® DBS systems for Parkinson's disease and essential tremor	Tremor reduction up to 80%; improved motor control and quality of life
	Vagus nerve stimulation (VNS)	Silicone-encapsulated platinum electrodes	Modulation of parasympathetic tone via cervical vagus nerve stimulation	Cyberonics® VNS therapy for refractory epilepsy and depression	50–60% seizure reduction; improved mood regulation and cortical excitability

	Application area	Representative biomaterials	Design features/functional mechanisms	Clinical or experimental case studies	Outcomes/performance metrics
	Cochlear implants	Silicone arrays, platinum contacts, titanium housing	Converts acoustic signals into electrical impulses transmitted to cochlear nerve	Cochlear™ nucleus and MED-EL implants widely used clinically	Restored speech perception in >90% of pediatric implant users; stable long-term function over decades
Neuroprotective drug delivery systems	Targeted and sustained drug release	Liposomes, PLGA nanoparticles, PEG hydrogels, lipid–polymer hybrids	Blood–brain barrier (BBB) crossing via receptor-mediated transport or intranasal delivery	PEG–PLGA nanoparticles delivering neurotrophic factors (BDNF, NGF) to injured cortex	Prolonged neurop

Guided axonal extension and cellular infiltration are facilitated by scaffolds made of biodegradable polymers like poly(lactic-co-glycolic acid) (PLGA), polycaprolactone (PCL), and natural hydrogels like collagen and alginate. Neurite growth may be directed along regulated orientations by using aligned nanofibers, which can be created by electrospinning or 3D bioprinting. This is important for functional reconnection in both the central and peripheral neural systems.

Neuronal survival and differentiation are further supported by the inclusion of bioactive substances, such as glial cell line-derived neurotrophic factor (GDNF), brain-derived neurotrophic factor (BDNF), and nerve growth factor (NGF) [49]. Scaffolds can dynamically change their stiffness or geometry in response to environmental stimuli thanks to emerging biofabrication techniques like 4D bioprinting, which further facilitates integration with host tissue. In spinal cord repair models, for instance, composite scaffolds made of graphene oxide and gelatin methacrylate have shown improved conductivity and neurocompatibility, underscoring the translational potential of multipurpose 3D systems. Recent experimental work on injectable double-network conductive hydrogels shows that such materials can support multidimensional spinal cord repair by reducing glial scar formation, promoting remyelination, protecting neurons and improving electrophysiological recovery [50].

8.6.2 Neuroprosthetics and Brain–Machine Interfaces (BMI)

By directly connecting neural signals with external devices, neuroprosthetics and brain–machine interfaces (BMIs) restore lost motor or sensory functions. These applications of neural biomaterials are revolutionary. Electrode arrays with excellent spatial and temporal resolution that can record brain activity and provide electrical stimulation are the basis of these systems. Conventional electrode arrays composed of metals like iridium oxide and platinum have good conductivity but are mechanically mismatched with soft brain tissues, which causes scarring and inflammation. Flexible biopolymer-based electrodes with components including PEDOT:PSS, PDMS, and polyimide have been created to address these problems. Long-term stability and decreased immune activation are made possible by these bioelectronic materials' combination of tissue-like flexibility and low impedance.

In clinical settings, intracortical BMIs have allowed tetraplegic patients to use thought-driven commands to manipulate computer cursors or robotic limbs. By electrically microstimulating the somatosensory brain or peripheral nerves, advanced closed-loop systems now incorporate sensory feedback, allowing amputees to regain touch perception [51]. Neuralink's flexible polymer threads and the Utah Electrode Array, for instance, are important advancements in chronic neural interfacing that move BMIs closer to fully bidirectional and less invasive setups.

8.6.3 Neuromodulation Devices

To control aberrant brain activity linked to neurological illnesses, neuromodulation devices use controlled electrical, magnetic, or optical stimulation. Biomaterial interfaces that guarantee accurate, reliable, and biocompatible contact with neural circuits are crucial to these devices. A gold-standard treatment for movement disorders like Parkinson's disease is deep brain stimulation (DBS), which entails implanting microelectrodes into brain nuclei (such as the subthalamic nucleus). Both biostability and electrical performance are guaranteed by materials like titanium encasements and platinum-iridium. In order to reduce side effects and increase therapeutic efficacy, recent advancements have concentrated on adaptive DBS systems that use biosensors to modify stimulation parameters in real time [52, 53].

Flexible cuff electrodes composed of conductive polymers and silicone elastomers are used in vagus nerve stimulation (VNS) devices, which affect autonomic and cerebral pathways and have shown promise in the treatment of depression and epilepsy. By translating sound into electrical impulses that directly stimulate auditory neurons, electrode arrays placed into the cochlea enable cochlear implants to restore auditory function. To survive the ionic environment of inner ear fluids, these devices are made of materials that are hermetically sealed and resistant to corrosion. When taken as a whole, these neuromodulation platforms demonstrate how neural biomaterials allow for long-term, safe stimulation.

8.6.4 Neuroprotective Drug Delivery Systems

The blood-brain barrier's (BBB) repressive properties and the requirement for long-term, targeted therapy make the introduction of neuroprotective drugs extremely difficult. Through regulated medication delivery systems that release therapeutic compounds at precise locations and rates, neural biomaterials provide novel treatments. Neuroprotective substances like growth factors, anti-inflammatory medications, and antioxidants are encapsulated in biodegradable microspheres, hydrogels, and nanoparticles made of PLGA, PEG, or chitosan. In order to ensure extended bioavailability in the injury microenvironment, these materials can be modified for diffusion-controlled or degradation-controlled release. Injectable hydrogel systems that release erythropoietin and BDNF, for instance, have been shown to improve neuronal survival after ischemic stroke.

Targeting ligands, such as transferrin or apolipoprotein E peptides, are included into advanced designs to allow nanoparticles to traverse the blood-brain barrier by receptor-mediated transport. Additionally, medication release can be precisely timed and spaced with stimuli-responsive delivery devices that are activated by pH, enzyme concentration, or electric fields. In order to halt the progression of neurodegenerative disorders like Alzheimer's and amyotrophic lateral sclerosis (ALS), where localized neuroprotection is crucial, such technologies are being used more and more.

8.6.5 Retinal and Cortical Implants

One of the most impressive uses of neural biomaterials is the restoration of sensory function via retinal and cortical implants. In order to transform visual signals from an external camera into electrical stimulation patterns that activate the remaining retinal ganglion cells, retinal prosthesis, like the Argus II system, use arrays of microelectrodes positioned on or beneath the retina. These implants' materials need to be biocompatible, electrically conductive, and optically transparent. Platinum-black coatings, PEDOT:PSS, and indium tin oxide (ITO) thin-film electrodes offer low-impedance interfaces without sacrificing visual field clarity. Flexible substrates, such as PDMS and parylene-C, minimize mechanical discomfort by enabling conformal contact with curved retinal surfaces.

In addition to retinal systems, cortical visual prosthesis stimulates the visual cortex directly in an attempt to completely avoid the optic nerve. To convert visual data into brain activity patterns, these devices need high-resolution electrode arrays and accurate signal processing. Concurrent developments in bioelectronic nanomaterials, like graphene sheets and carbon nanotube networks, provide enhanced durability and charge transfer, advancing the long-term objective of helping blind people regain functional vision [54].

8.6.6 Case Studies in Spinal Cord Repair, Parkinson's Treatment and Epilepsy Control

Clinical and preclinical case studies are the best example of neural biomaterials' translational potential [55]. Collagen-chitosan scaffolds implanted with neural stem cells have partially restored motor function in animal models of spinal cord regeneration, and injectable hydrogel therapies are currently being investigated in human studies. The synergy between cellular and material techniques was highlighted in a noteworthy example from China that showed enhanced sensory and motor outcomes in paraplegic patients treated with olfactory ensheathing cells placed within a collagen matrix. For more than 20 years, DBS with platinum-iridium electrodes has been the clinical standard for treating Parkinson's disease, providing long-lasting symptom alleviation. Real-time stimulation intensity modulation has been demonstrated in recent trials of adaptive DBS systems using dopamine sensors, which is a step toward closed-loop neuromodulation.

For epilepsy management, VNS and responsive neurostimulation (RNS) devices exemplify bioelectronic precision medicine. The RNS system monitors cortical activity and delivers targeted electrical pulses to prevent seizure onset, integrating biosensing and stimulation within a single implant. These examples demonstrate how advances in neural biomaterials and interface design directly translate into improved patient outcomes and quality of life.

Neural biomaterials' range of applications, from intelligent prosthetics to regenerative scaffolds, demonstrates the revolutionary potential of materials innovation in neuroscience. Neuromodulation devices control abnormal brain activity, bioelectronic interfaces restore sensory and motor function, and 3D-engineered scaffolds direct neural regeneration. In the meantime, retinal implants and neuroprotective drug delivery systems expand the therapeutic application of biomaterials into intricate disease domains [56]. Neural biomaterials are quickly making the transition from experimental research to ordinary clinical practice, as demonstrated by clinical case studies in epilepsy, Parkinson's disease, and spinal cord damage. The combination of neurobiology, materials science, and digital technology holds the potential to completely transform neurological healing and augmentation in the twenty-first century as the field moves toward multifunctional, adaptable, and patient-specific systems.

8.7 Recent Advances and Innovations

The combination of biotechnology, materials science, nanotechnology, and artificial intelligence has led to revolutionary advancements in the field of neural biomaterials in recent years. The way that researchers and medical professionals approach the replacement, repair, and modification of brain tissues has been completely transformed by these developments. The objective is to develop biointegrated technologies that seamlessly integrate with the complex circuitry of the brain while also restoring lost neuronal function. Bioelectronics, nanomaterial-based treatments, optogenetic interfaces, 3D bioprinting, hydrogel–electrode hybrids, AI-driven models, and regenerative neurotherapies are examples of emerging approaches. When taken as a whole, these advancements represent a paradigm shift away from passive implants and toward intelligent, adaptive, and regenerative brain systems that can monitor and repair in real time.

8.7.1 Bioelectronic Medicine

One of the most fascinating areas of neural engineering is bioelectronic medicine, which combines electronic control with neurophysiology to modify biological processes via electrical stimulation. Closed-loop bioelectronic devices continuously monitor physiological inputs and modify stimulation parameters in real time, in contrast to typical neuroprosthetics that function in an open-loop fashion. Contemporary systems incorporate miniature sensors, electrodes, and microcontrollers that can identify biochemical or neurological activity and react by stimulating specific areas. One treatment for Parkinson's disease is closed-loop deep brain stimulation (DBS), which uses neural feedback to dynamically modify dopaminergic circuits to minimize side effects and reduce tremors. In a similar vein, feedback-based control is used by vagus nerve stimulation (VNS) devices to treat inflammatory diseases, depression, and epilepsy. Recent research on bio-inspired neural interfaces is advancing from passive electrodes to soft, biohybrid, and living interfaces that integrate biomaterials, cells, and electronics to enhance tissue integration and long-term functionality [57].

These bioelectronic systems can form intimately with soft neural tissues thanks to developments in soft electronics and biocompatible materials, such as flexible PEDOT:PSS conductors and graphene-based arrays. Chronic implantation has also been made easier by untethered operation made possible by wireless power transfer and data tracking [58]. A major step toward adaptive neuromodulation, in which devices become active participants in the management of neural health, is the incorporation of bioelectronic medicine into clinical practice.

8.7.2 Nanotechnology in Neural Repair

With the use of nanotechnology, neuronal microenvironments may now be manipulated at the molecular level with unparalleled control over localized drug delivery, synaptic connection, and axon guidance. Nanostructured materials can mimic the extracellular matrix (ECM) and guide neuronal regeneration because of their high surface area-to-volume ratios and adjustable surface chemistry. In spinal cord injury models, aligned topographical cues from electrospun nanofibers derived from polymers like collagen, silk fibroin, or polycaprolactone (PCL) promote neurite proliferation and directed axonal healing. High-fidelity electrical connection with neurons is made possible by carbon nanotubes (CNTs) and nanowires, which enhances the effectiveness of neural transmission and signal transduction.

Simultaneously, nanoparticles function as precise delivery systems for nucleic acids, growth hormones, and anti-inflammatory medications across the blood–brain barrier (BBB). Selective attachment to neuronal or glial cells is made possible by functionalization with targeted ligands (such as transferrin or peptides). To encourage neuronal survival and plasticity, for instance, nerve growth factor (NGF) or brain-derived neurotrophic factor (BDNF) have been delivered using liposomal carriers and gold nanoparticles. Thus, incorporating nanotechnology into brain repair techniques allows for a multimodal strategy that combines biochemical modulation, electrical integration, and structural guiding to improve neural interface performance and regeneration.

8.7.3 Optogenetic and Photothermal Interfaces

By providing precise, light-driven control over genetically altered neurons that express light-sensitive ion channels, such channelrhodopsins and halorhodopsins, optogenetics has completely redesigned neuromodulation [59]. The spatial precision of conventional electrical stimulation is surpassed by this technique, which provides cell-type specificity and millisecond-scale temporal resolution. Implantable optoelectronic interfaces made of flexible, transparent, and biocompatible materials that allow light to enter neural tissue directly without inflicting thermal damage have been the focus of recent advancements. Minimally invasive probes for cerebral and spinal stimulation have been developed that use micro-LED arrays and optical waveguides made of silicon carbide or polymers.

Similar to optogenetics, photothermal stimulation uses nanomaterials to depolarize neuronal membranes. Examples of these materials include graphene, carbon nanotubes, and gold nanorods. These techniques have been utilized to excite neurons in both central and peripheral neural tissues without requiring genetic alteration. Thus, optical neuromodulation offers a non-electrical and less invasive method of regulating brain circuits, creating opportunities for the unparalleled precision treatment of neuropsychiatric illnesses, chronic pain, and sensory deficiencies.

8.7.4 3D Bioprinting and Microfabrication

Highly customized neural scaffolds that mimic the structure and mechanical characteristics of natural brain tissues can now be created because of the development of 3D bioprinting and microfabrication technology. Researchers may create intricate three-dimensional structures with regulated porosity and composition by using bio-inks made of hydrogels, extracellular matrix proteins, and living cells. Personalized healing of spinal cord injuries or cortical deficiencies is possible with 3D bioprinted neural scaffolds that can be tailored to each patient's anatomy based on MRI or CT data. These structures are further refined by microfabrication techniques like soft lithography and microfluidic templating, which allow for exact spatial control of implanted electrodes, gradients, and channels.

The possibility of functional neural tissue replacement has been suggested by recent research showing bioprinted constructions with neuronal and glial co-cultures that promote axon extension and synaptic activation. Additionally, adding electrical and optical activity to printed scaffolds through the incorporation of conductive or photoresponsive materials turns static biomaterials into active, bioelectronic constructs that can interface with the nervous system. Recent two-photon lithography work has demonstrated 3D micropatterned PEDOT:PSS/gelatin conductive hydrogels with reduced impedance and soft mechanical properties, supporting improved electrical and mechanical integration at the cell–electrode interface [60]. Neural biomaterials are therefore being advanced toward patient-specific, multifunctional implants that combine biological fidelity with device intelligence thanks to the confluence of bioprinting and microengineering [61].

8.7.5 Hydrogel–Electrode Hybrids

Hydrogels' high water content, biocompatibility, and mechanical resemblance to brain tissue have made them the perfect choice for soft, flexible neural interfaces. Hydrogels by themselves, however, don't have enough electrical conductivity to facilitate brain interfaces. Hydrogel–electrode hybrids, which combine the mechanical softness of hydrogels with the electrochemical performance of conductive materials, have been developed as a solution to this problem. Strong charge transport channels are provided by hybrid systems that integrate PEDOT, polypyrrole, graphene, or metallic nanostructures within hydrogel matrices while still adhering to brain tissue. These composites improve long-term stability in vivo, lower impedance, and increase charge injection capacity.

For minimally invasive delivery, injectable hydrogel–electrode systems have also been created. In these systems, the material is injected as a liquid and polymerizes in situ to create a conductive, conformal network surrounding brain regions. These biointerfaces are especially useful for long-term uses such as cortical recording, neuroprosthetic control, and epidural stimulation. Hydrogel–electrode hybrids offer a significant step forward for the development of next-generation, tissue-mimetic brain implants by fusing mechanical comfort, conductivity, and biointegration.

8.7.6 AI and Computational Modeling

The design, testing, and optimization of neural biomaterials and interfaces have been completely transformed by artificial intelligence (AI) and computational modeling. Researchers can now forecast how particular material compositions or structures will function within neural tissues by using machine learning algorithms that have been trained on massive datasets of material attributes, neural activity, and biological responses. For instance, prior to experimental testing, AI-driven modeling can forecast glial encapsulation processes, optimize charge transfer properties, and simulate electrode–tissue interactions. Inverse design, in which optimal material characteristics or device geometries are inferred from desired functional results (such as signal strength or selectivity), is also supported by computational frameworks [62].

The design, testing, and optimization of neural biomaterials and interfaces have been completely transformed by artificial intelligence (AI) and computational modeling. Researchers can now forecast how particular material compositions or structures will function within neural tissues by using machine learning algorithms that have been trained on massive datasets of material attributes, neural activity, and biological responses. For instance, prior to experimental testing, AI-driven modeling can forecast glial encapsulation processes, optimize charge transfer properties, and simulate electrode–tissue interactions. Inverse design, in which optimal material characteristics or device geometries are inferred from desired functional results (such as signal strength or selectivity), is also supported by computational frameworks.

8.7.7 *Regenerative Neurotherapies*

Regenerative neurotherapies, which attempt to restore lost brain tissue and functional connection, are the result of the fusion of stem cell biology with biomaterial science. Biomaterials function as three-dimensional scaffolding that facilitate axonal extension, differentiation, and cell adhesion. They also enable the local administration of morphogens and growth factors. In order to treat spinal cord injuries, for instance, scaffolds loaded with neural stem cells (NSCs) and BDNF or NGF have demonstrated potential in promoting remyelination and reestablishing synaptic connections. The controlled release of these bioactive chemicals is made possible by hydrogel systems that contain microspheres or nanoparticles, maintaining a pro-regenerative milieu for long periods of time.

Recent research has shown that stem cell–biomaterial composites can transfer electrical impulses and enhance behavioral recovery in animal models by functionally integrating with host brain circuitry. Additionally, gene-edited stem cells that express anti-inflammatory or neuroprotective molecules have even more therapeutic potential refinement. By combining biological self-healing processes with specially designed scaffolds, these regenerative neurotherapies take a comprehensive approach to functional restoration as opposed to symptom management. The increasing overlap between manufactured systems and living life is demonstrated by recent developments in brain biomaterials. Neural engineering has been reshaped by innovations like bioelectronic medicine, nanotechnology-enabled repair, optogenetic modulation, and AI-driven design. Regenerative techniques that combine stem cells, bioactive substances, and 3D-printed structures, on the other hand, hold out the possibility of repairing damaged brain networks and regaining cognitive and physical abilities.

An era of adaptive, self-healing, and morally guided neurotechnologies aimed at repairing, enhancing, and balancing with the human nervous system will be ushered in by the next generation of neural biomaterials, which will further blur the boundaries between biological and artificial intelligence as these technologies advance [13, 63].

8.8 Challenges and Limitations

The full development of restorative and augmentative neural technologies is hampered by several scientific, technological, and ethical issues, despite the impressive advancements in neural biomaterials and neuroengineering. Implants, regeneration scaffolds, and neural interfaces must work in the brain and peripheral nervous system, which are highly immunoreactive, physically delicate, and electrically active tissues. These systems must meet strict ethical and regulatory requirements while maintaining long-term biocompatibility, steady electrical performance, and dependable brain circuit integration. The main drawbacks of neural biomaterials and technologies are discussed in this section. These include material stability, immunological reactions, regeneration restrictions, power and data management, and the socioethical context of brain–computer interfaces (BCIs).

8.8.1 Achieving Long-Term Biocompatibility and Stability in the Neural Environment

One of the most enduring problems in neuroengineering is the long-term functionality of brain biomaterials. High ionic concentration, metabolic activity, and sensitivity to external substances are characteristics of the brain environment. The introduction of implants like electrodes, scaffolds, or drug reservoirs exposes them to oxidation, corrosion, and enzymatic degradation, which over time may jeopardize their structural soundness and electrical functionality.

Despite being extremely conductive, conventional electrode materials like tungsten and platinum-iridium can undergo chemical instability and mechanical delamination after prolonged implantation. Furthermore, insulation failure may result from hydrolytic breakdown or microcracking of polymer coatings like polyimide and parylene-C. Therefore, the creation of hybrid materials that combine strong conductivity with surfaces that are resistant to corrosion and fatigue is necessary to provide long-term biostability.

Neural tissues also change their metabolic environment in response to external things. Neurointegration, or the material's capacity to sustain functional interaction with neurons and glia without causing long-term inflammation or gliosis, is just as important to long-term biocompatibility as inertness. To maintain harmonic tissue–device interactions, future advancements will depend on bioinspired materials that mimic the elasticity, chemistry, and signaling characteristics of the extracellular matrix (ECM) [64, 65].

8.8.2 Balancing Conductivity with Mechanical Softness in Implant Materials

A significant design challenge in neural biomaterials is balancing mechanical softness, which is essential for reducing tissue injury, with electrical conductivity, which is necessary for signal transmission and stimulation. Traditional conductors like metals or doped polymers are orders of magnitude stiffer than the brain and peripheral nerves, which have an elastic modulus of ~0.1–1 kPa. This discrepancy causes shear stress brought on by micromotion, which damages neuronal membranes and results in fibrosis, cell death, and loss of recording quality.

Soft conductive polymers (such PEDOT:PSS and polypyrrole) and nanocomposite materials that contain carbon nanotubes, graphene, or gold nanowires scattered across elastic matrices have been developed in an attempt to overcome this difficulty. These substances offer a modifiable balance between conductivity and flexibility. Furthermore, transitory or biodegradable conductors, like composites made of magnesium or zinc, present the possibility of short-term cerebral stimulation or recording without long-term mechanical interference. Stable electrical performance over long periods of time is still challenging to achieve, though, because soft materials might change their impedance due to mechanical creep or water absorption. As a result, the field must constantly balance mechanical compliance with long-term signal stability, which calls for interdisciplinary methods that combine neural interface optimization, polymer chemistry, and nanostructured design.

8.8.3 Minimizing Immune Response and Foreign Body Encapsulation

A series of immunological reactions brought on by the installation of neural implants can seriously impede function. The central nervous system's (CNS) resident immune and support cells, microglia and astrocytes, quickly move in the direction of foreign objects and start the inflammatory encapsulation process, creating a thick glial scar surrounding the implant. This procedure physically separates the gadget from neighboring neurons, raises impedance, and reduces signal transmission. Surface functionalization with anti-inflammatory coatings like polyethylene glycol (PEG), dexamethasone-releasing films, and zwitterionic polymers that thwart protein adsorption are some of the current methods to lower immune reactivity [66]. Moreover, glial cell adhesion and polarization can be altered by nanotopographical signals on implant surfaces, which can change immune responses to pro-healing characteristics.

Even materials that are extremely soft and bioresorbable can cause mild inflammatory reactions over time, thus total immunological tolerance is still elusive despite these advancements. Therefore, attaining long-lasting neural integration requires a greater comprehension of neuroimmunomodulation of how materials affect glial and neuronal signaling.

8.8.4 Limited Regeneration Potential in Central Nervous System Tissues

The limited ability of the central nervous system to regenerate itself is one of the most significant biological constraints on neural regeneration. In contrast to peripheral nerves, which can partially regenerate under the direction of Schwann cells,

CNS neurons are unable to do so because of inhibitory chemicals (such Nogo-A and MAG) and glial scarring. Collagen, chitosan, and conductive hydrogels are examples of biomaterials that can release neurotrophic factors and provide scaffolding, but they are unable to completely get past inherent molecular barriers. While some progress has been made in promoting regeneration using gene therapy, stem cell transplantation, or the regulated release of inhibitory antagonists, complete functional connection has still not been restored.

Furthermore, there are biological and geographical difficulties in incorporating biomaterial scaffolds into the highly structured structure of the brain or spinal cord. It takes sophisticated construction techniques, such 3D bioprinting with microscale guide channels and local control of biochemical gradients, to precisely align axons and synapses across damaged regions.

8.8.5 *Complexities in Data Transmission and Power Management for Implantable Devices*

The growing complexity of implanted neural systems, including closed-loop stimulators, biosensors, and brain–machine interfaces, necessitates effective power management and data transfer in constrained biological settings. While wireless communication has problems with signal attenuation, latency, and battery consumption, conventional connected connections present mechanical stress and infection hazards. Wireless energy transfer has been enhanced by inductive coupling and miniature electronics, but it is still difficult to maintain steady power flow without producing tissue-heating effects. Biocompatible energy harvesters that turn chemical gradients or body motion into electrical power, like triboelectric or biofuel cells, are examples of emerging solutions. These technologies are still in their infancy, though, and have limitations with regard to durability and power density.

Moreover, managing data in real time from multichannel brain recordings creates enormous datasets that call for sophisticated on-chip signal processing and compression techniques. One major engineering challenge in the design of neural devices is integrating these electrical components into flexible, biocompatible substrates while maintaining signal integrity [67].

8.8.6 *Ethical and Privacy Concerns in Brain–Computer Interface Technologies*

As neural biomaterials allow for more personal interactions between humans and machines, ethical and privacy concerns are becoming more pressing in addition to technical and biological difficulties. The ability of brain-computer interfaces (BCIs) to decode intentions, feelings, or ideas raises concerns over data ownership, autonomy, and mental privacy. There is a serious risk to society from the possible misuse of neurological data for commercial exploitation or monitoring. Furthermore, the distinction between therapy and augmentation is blurred by therapies that change behavior or cognition, such as mood or memory enhancement. As a result, these technologies need to be created within strong ethical frameworks that guarantee fair access, transparency, and informed consent. As neural interfaces grow more common, bioethicists and neuroscientists support the creation of "neuro-rights" to safeguard cognitive liberty and the right to mental integrity.

8.8.7 *Translational and Regulatory Barriers for Clinical Neural Therapies*

The process of converting brain biomaterials into clinically authorized treatments is still difficult and sluggish, despite promising preclinical and laboratory results. Development timetables for neural implants are frequently prolonged by decades due to the regulatory environment, which includes extensive biocompatibility testing, long-term safety research, and functional validation. Additional challenges include manufacturing repeatability, especially for nanostructured and composite materials where even little changes in surface chemistry or microarchitecture might result in unanticipated biological reactions. Preclinical validation is further complicated by the fact that animal models frequently fall short in reproducing human neurophysiology.

The FDA, EMA, and other regulatory bodies need detailed information on the stability, degradation, and systemic toxicity of materials. However, multifunctional and adaptable systems that blur the lines between biologics and medical devices, like drug-releasing electrodes or bioelectronic scaffolds, are frequently poorly suited to current frameworks [68, 69]. It will be essential to expedite clinical translation while preserving safety and efficacy by streamlining approval processes through adaptive regulation and uniform testing procedures.

At the nexus of tremendous potential and unfathomable intricacy lies the frontier of brain biomaterials and neuroengineering. Maintaining implant performance continues to depend on achieving long-term biocompatibility, mechanical–electrical balance, and immunological acceptance. In the meantime, actual deployment is limited by the biological limitations of CNS regeneration as well as engineering difficulties in power management and data processing. The translational gap is further exacerbated by ethical quandaries pertaining to cognitive privacy and regulatory inertia. However, continuous advancements in immunomodulatory coatings, hybrid regeneration systems, and soft bioelectronics keep pushing the envelope for more patient-specific and adaptable treatments [70]. To overcome these obstacles, materials scientists, physicians, ethicists, and legislators must work closely together to ensure that brain technologies maintain the integrity of the human body and mind while simultaneously restoring function.

8.9 Future Directions

A new generation of intelligent, adaptable, and regenerative systems that go beyond conventional implantable devices is the direction that neural biomaterials and cutting-edge neurotechnologies are taking. A major future direction is the integration of living biomaterials into neuroelectronic systems, where cells, spheroids or organoid-derived components may help devices adapt to the host environment, establish bidirectional interfaces, conform to living tissue and support repair [71]. The goal of current research is to develop biohybrid systems that can sense, interpret, and react to complex neurological environments by seamlessly combining materials science, neuroengineering, and artificial intelligence. In the quest to restore and enhance neuronal function, these future directions place an emphasis on long-term functionality, biocompatibility, customisation, and ethical design. Self-healing interfaces, AI-integrated neuromodulation, hybrid living-electronic materials, non-invasive technologies, bioprinted neural constructions, and translational approaches toward neuroregeneration and cognitive restoration are the main development avenues.

8.9.1 Development of Adaptive, Self-Healing Neural Interfaces for Continuous Function

It is anticipated that next-generation neural interfaces will be self-healing and adaptive, guaranteeing dependable performance and long-term stability in the ever-changing neurological environment. Damage, gliosis, and signal deterioration are frequently caused by the mechanical mismatch between brain tissue and traditional electrodes. By using dynamic covalent connections and self-repairing polymers, which may restore microstructural integrity following mechanical stress or biological degradation, future materials seek to address these problems.

For example, hydrogel-based interfaces with supramolecular assemblies or reversible cross-linking chemistries can self-heal microcracks while preserving electrical performance. Furthermore, elastomeric composites and shape-memory polymers might allow adaptive deformation that takes tissue movement into account. Conductive pathways may potentially possess self-healing qualities, guaranteeing continuous brain signal transmission for years after implantation. These developments will signal a move toward sustainable, self-sustaining neural implants that act as genuine extensions of the nervous system and will be essential to the lifespan of neuroprosthetics and chronic monitoring systems.

8.9.2 Integration of AI-Driven Neuromodulation Systems with Real-Time Feedback

Precision neurotherapy is undergoing a paradigm shift with the incorporation of artificial intelligence (AI) into neuromodulation devices. AI systems that have been trained on large neural datasets are able to decipher intricate electrical and biochemical signals and dynamically adjust stimulation parameters. In response to changing brain states, future systems will have closed-loop feedback mechanisms that continually modify the location, frequency, and strength of stimulation [72, 73]. In Parkinson's disease, for instance, adaptive deep brain stimulation (DBS) systems are now able to identify abnormal oscillations and automatically adjust electrical output to reduce tremors. This idea could be expanded by using AI-driven neuromodulators to evaluate multimodal data, such as metabolic markers, electrophysiological signals, and behavioral feedback, to customize treatments for depression, chronic pain, or epilepsy.

On-device learning will be made possible by developments in edge computing and low-power neural processors, which will lessen latency and reliance on outside computation. Long-term goals call for self-governing neurodevices that may learn from each patient's responses, guaranteeing individualized treatment while reducing adverse effects. A new field of cognitive bioelectronics will emerge because of these intelligent interfaces, which will close the gap between human neurophysiology and machine accuracy.

8.9.3 Hybrid Living–Electronic Materials Combining Biological Cells with Synthetic Networks

The development of hybrid living-electronic materials that combine synthetic conductive matrices and live cells is a revolutionary path in neural biomaterials. The goal of these biohybrids is to combine the resilience and programmability of constructed systems with the computational power of living neural tissue. Researchers are creating materials that can do bioelectronic computation, self-organization, and adaptive learning by incorporating neuronal or glial cells into nanostructured carbon networks or conducting polymer scaffolds. As biologically derived computer units, neural organoids interfaced with microelectrode arrays, for instance, can process and transmit electrical impulses. Similarly, live feedback networks that may dynamically change conductivity in response to neural activity are provided by cell-seeded conductive hydrogels. These materials pave the door for symbiotic bioelectronics, in which artificial circuits and biological neurons coevolve to improve long-term integration and signal fidelity.

Achieving synthetic–biological co-interfaces that smoothly interact with native neural tissue and provide bidirectional information flow is the ultimate objective.

These hybrid systems have potential applications in biohybrid computing, neuroprosthetics, adaptive cognitive systems, and brain–machine interfaces.

8.9.4 Advances in Bioprinted Neural Networks for Personalized Therapy

An unparalleled chance to create patient-specific neural architectures that mimic the structural and functional complexity of the nervous system is presented by the use of 3D and 4D bioprinting in neural tissue engineering. Researchers can now create pathway-guided scaffolds and functioning neural networks that are customized to each patient's needs by using bioinks made of neural stem cells, extracellular matrix proteins, and conductive hydrogels. Vascular channels, growth factor gradients, and electrode components can now all be included in a single construct thanks to recent advancements in multi-material bioprinting. These printed neural tissues can be used as drug screening platforms, customized grafts for spinal cord or cortical repair, and in vitro disease models.

Going forward, time-responsive bioinks that can self-morph or adjust to physiological stimuli after implantation are made possible by 4D bioprinting. Future bioprinted neural constructs will go from static scaffolds to dynamic, living systems that actively contribute to neural circuit development and regeneration by combining genetic engineering, optogenetics, and smart biomaterials [74, 75]. Personalized neurotherapies that combine clinical accuracy and biological fidelity will be supported by such technology.

8.9.5 Expansion of Non-Invasive and Wireless Neural Devices

The goal of the push toward wireless and non-invasive neuromodulation is to preserve great spatiotemporal control over brain activity while reducing the risk of surgery. Therapeutic modulation without invasive implants is now possible thanks to technologies like transcranial magnetic stimulation (TMS), targeted ultrasonic neuromodulation, and optogenetic stimulation using external light sources. To provide continuous monitoring and control, future wireless systems will make use of biotelemetry, energy harvesting techniques, and ultra-thin flexible electronics. Technological developments in near-field communication (NFC), optical communication, and radiofrequency (RF) power transfer will further improve device autonomy and make closed-loop systems completely untethered.

These advancements also apply to wearable neurointerfaces, like e-skin patches or smart headbands, which use microfluidic components to dispense medications, deliver neuromodulation, or detect brain activity. To democratize neurological health technologies and introduce individualized therapy and real-time neurofeedback into clinical and home-care settings, non-invasive, wireless platforms are essential.

8.9.6 Translational Focus on Neuroregeneration and Cognitive Restoration

Restoring both functional cognition and physical connectivity is the key to the future of neural biomaterials. After neurological injury or degeneration, translational research is increasingly focused on boosting axon regrowth, synaptic plasticity, and circuit reformation. To produce settings that are favorable for regeneration, biomaterial scaffolds, stem cell therapies, and the delivery of bioactive molecules must come together. To direct axonal alignment and promote remyelination, emerging regenerative neurotherapies include hydrogels loaded with growth factors, gene-activated matrices, and constructions loaded with stem cells. Functional reintegration making sure that regenerated circuits contribute significantly to sensory and cognitive processing is becoming more important in addition to structural healing [76, 77].

Additionally, to bridge the gap between biological and computational restoration, neuroregenerative techniques are being combined with cognitive prostheses and AI-enhanced rehabilitation tools. One day, recovery from stroke, severe brain damage, and neurodegenerative diseases like Parkinson's and Alzheimer's may be made possible by this all-encompassing method of brain repair.

8.9.7 Convergence of Materials Science, Neuroengineering, and Regenerative Biology for Next-Generation Therapies

A growing interdisciplinary convergence between materials science, neuroengineering, and regenerative biology defines the future of neural biomaterials. Biologists are discovering the mechanics of cellular communication and regeneration, neuroengineers are improving microelectronic and computational interfaces, and materials scientists are creating bioinspired and adaptive polymers. These domains are coming together to form an ecosystem of sophisticated, multipurpose neural systems. The goal of next-generation medicines is to improve neuronal resilience and flexibility rather than to replace lost functions. Devices will develop into symbiotic systems that can communicate with the nervous system continuously and are driven by self-sustaining or biologically produced energy sources. To guarantee the safe and fair implementation of these revolutionary technologies, ethical frameworks and regulatory norms will also be essential.

In the end, these fields' convergence portends a time when neural augmentation and healing will be combined into adaptive processes that allow people to transcend neurological constraints and develop their cognitive capacities in a way that is compatible with their biology. With their capacity for self-healing, AI-driven control, and living-synthetic integration, future neural biomaterials are moving toward adaptable, intelligent, and regenerative paradigms. By enabling previously unheard-of degrees of brain regeneration, monitoring, and cognitive augmentation, these advancements will make it harder to distinguish between biological and technology systems. The next era of personalized neuroengineering will be defined by the convergence of advanced materials, computational intelligence, and regenerative medicine. This will provide hope for millions of people suffering from neurological disorders and pave the way for a future in which humans and machines coexist in a symbiotic relationship [78, 79].

8.10 Conclusion

From the initial application of inert metallic electrodes, the field of neural biomaterials has progressed to a time characterized by bioactive, intelligent, and adaptable devices that can easily interface with the human nervous system. From the simple repair of lost neuronal function to the active manipulation, regeneration, and augmentation of neural networks, this evolution represents a major change in biomedical engineering. Neural biomaterials are revolutionizing the way scientists study and work with the brain, spinal cord, and peripheral nerves as materials science, neurobiology, and digital technology come together.

8.10.1 Summary of the Evolution and Impact of Neural Biomaterials

Early twentieth-century neuroprosthetic research, which employed stiff iron electrodes for stimulation and data recording, are where the development of neural biomaterials got its start. These early interfaces had short-term functioning, mechanical mismatch, and poor biocompatibility. Chronic neural interfacing began in the late twentieth century with the introduction of polymeric insulating materials like polyimide and parylene. Passive tolerance gradually gave way to active biointegration. Soft, tissue-like interfaces that preserved high-fidelity electrical communication while reducing inflammation were made possible by the development of conductive polymers, hydrogels, and nanocomposites. At the same time, developments in microfabrication, 3D bioprinting, and neuroelectronic design have enabled the creation of accurate structures that replicate the extracellular matrix and neural circuits.

These developments have an impact on rehabilitation, neuroscience, and medicine. Deep brain stimulation for movement disorders, peripheral nerve conduits for damage repair, and brain–computer interfaces (BCIs) that give paralyzed people back control and communication have all been made possible by neural biomaterials. This interdisciplinary advancement highlights how materials innovation can revolutionize the field of neural augmentation and repair.

8.10.2 Reinforcement of Neurocompatibility, Conductivity, and Adaptability as Key Design Pillars

Three fundamental concepts neurocompatibility, conductivity, and adaptability remain essential to the development of brain interfaces as they get more complicated. To minimize inflammation and gliosis and maintain neuronal health, neurocompatibility guarantees that implanted materials coexist peacefully with neural tissue. Reliable stimulation and recording depend on the effective passage of electrical signals between the synthetic and biological domains, which conductivity makes possible. Materials with adaptability can react quickly to changes in the neuronal environment's mechanical, chemical, and physiological components.

The development of soft, bioelectronic materials that can adapt to neuronal surfaces without impairing their functionality is the result of the synthesis of these design pillars. Implants can also withstand physiological motion and deterioration over time because of developments in ionic conductors, stretchy electrodes, and self-healing polymers. Furthermore, a novel class of responsive therapies is represented by adaptive interfaces that integrate closed-loop control systems to sense and modify brain activity in real time. The development of neural biomaterials toward devices that function as living extensions of the nervous system rather than as alien objects is guided by these design concepts taken together.

8.10.3 Recognition of Interdisciplinary Synergy Among Engineering, Neuroscience, and Clinical Practice

Collaboration between several disciplines is essential for the successful transition of brain biomaterials from the lab to the clinic. Neuroscience offers insights into neuronal coding, plasticity, and cellular connections; clinical medicine grounds innovation in therapeutic relevance and patient safety; and engineering supplies the means for material synthesis, microfabrication, and device downsizing. Cross-disciplinary integration has advanced because of collaborative frameworks like translational research centers and neuroengineering consortia, which promote iterative design based on clinical results and biological feedback. For example, real-time electrophysiological investigations direct the adjustment of electrode impedance and signal selectivity, while knowledge of glial responses has influenced surface modification tactics. Bridging the ongoing gap between benchtop discovery and human application requires this interaction between materials innovation and empirical neurology.

Additionally, the use of artificial intelligence (AI) and computer modeling into neural biomaterials research has improved predictive capacities, enabling the customization of implant parameters, optimization of material geometries, and simulation of tissue responses. The future of neuroscience as a biological and technical field, bound together by the pursuit of repairing and expanding neuronal function, is exemplified by such cooperative intersections.

8.10.4 Outlook Toward Intelligent, Regenerative, and Patient-Responsive Neural Systems

Neural biomaterials of the future will be intelligent, regenerable, and responsive. AI-driven algorithms will be used by intelligent systems to decipher neurological signals, forecast disease occurrences, and independently modify drug delivery or stimulation. Therapeutic approaches will go from compensation to full neurorestoration thanks to regenerative materials, which are designed to encourage axonal development and synaptic reconnection. New developments like self-healing hydrogels, bioprinted neural scaffolds, and hybrid living-electronic structures are concrete advances toward biomaterials that combine synthetic and biological functions. Furthermore, real-time physiological feedback will be used by patient-responsive technology to customize therapy outcomes and match brain modulation to specific requirements.

With the ability to learn from and adjust to the body's signals, these developments herald a paradigm change toward closed-loop neural therapies, in which the interface actively participates in brain homeostasis. Such development embodies the idea of regenerative and adaptive neurotechnology and improves treatment efficacy while also personalizing medicine.

8.10.5 Final Reflection: The Path Toward Restoring Neural Function and Enhancing Human–Machine Integration

Humanity's desire to comprehend, treat, and improve the nervous system is ultimately reflected in the search for neural biomaterials. From the first neuroprosthetics to the most advanced biohybrid systems, this discipline unprecedently connects the digital and biological realms. The way forward is to balance technical proficiency with moral obligation, making sure that advancements in neural interfaces strengthen rather than jeopardize human identity and autonomy. The line between augmentation and repair will become increasingly hazy as neural technologies advance. This convergence portends a time when human-machine integration will allow for new kinds of engagement, communication, and cognition in addition to assisting functions. However, the fundamental idea must not change technology should help people with neurological injury or disease regain their connection, dignity, and agency.

In essence, neural biomaterials stand at the frontier of a new biomedical paradigm one that unites biology, engineering, and ethics in the shared mission of reclaiming neural function and redefining human experience.

References

1. Ciurea, A.V., Mohan, A.G., Covache-Busuioc, R.A., Costin, H.P., Glavan, L.A., Corlatescu, A.D., Saceleanu, V.M.: Unraveling molecular and genetic insights into neurodegenerative diseases: advances in understanding Alzheimer's, Parkinson's, and Huntington's diseases and amyotrophic lateral sclerosis. Int. J. Mol. Sci. **24**(13), 10809 (2023)
2. Lamptey, R.N., Chaulagain, B., Trivedi, R., Gothwal, A., Layek, B., Singh, J.: A review of the common neurodegenerative disorders: current therapeutic approaches and the potential role of nanotherapeutics. Int. J. Mol. Sci. **23**(3), 1851 (2022)
3. Nicaise, A.M., D'Angelo, A., Ionescu, R.B., Krzak, G., Willis, C.M., Pluchino, S.: The role of neural stem cells in regulating glial scar formation and repair. Cell Tissue Res. **387**(3), 399–414 (2022)
4. Tsujioka, H., Yamashita, T.: Neural circuit repair after central nervous system injury. Int. Immunol. **33**(6), 301–309 (2021)
5. Chelyshev, Y.A., Kabdesh, I.M., Mukhamedshina, Y.O.: Extracellular matrix in neural plasticity and regeneration. Cell. Mol. Neurobiol. **42**(3), 647–664 (2022)
6. Yang, Z., Zou, Y., Wang, L.: Neurotransmitters in prevention and treatment of Alzheimer's disease. Int. J. Mol. Sci. **24**(4), 3841 (2023)
7. Mariano, A., Bovio, C.L., Criscuolo, V., Santoro, F.: Bioinspired micro-and nano-structured neural interfaces. Nanotechnology. **33**(49), 492501 (2022)
8. Yang, D.L., Faraz, F., Wang, J.X., Radacsi, N.: Combination of 3D printing and electrospinning techniques for biofabrication. Adv. Mater. Technol. **7**(7), 2101309 (2022)
9. Cutrone, A., Micera, S.: Implantable neural interfaces and wearable tactile systems for bidirectional neuroprosthetics systems. Adv. Healthc. Mater. **8**(24), 1801345 (2019)
10. Pasluosta, C., Kiele, P., Čvančara, P., Micera, S., Aszmann, O.C., Stieglitz, T.: Bidirectional bionic limbs: a perspective bridging technology and physiology. J. Neural Eng. **19**(1), 013001 (2022)
11. Alastra, G., Aloe, L., Baldassarro, V.A., Calzà, L., Cescatti, M., Duskey, J.T., Focarete, M.L., Giacomini, D., Giardino, L., Giraldi, V., Lorenzini, L.: Nerve growth factor biodelivery: a limiting step in moving toward extensive clinical application? Front. Neurosci. **15**, 695592 (2021)
12. Stewart, A.N., Gensel, J.C., Jones, L., Fouad, K.: Challenges in translating regenerative therapies for spinal cord injury. Top. Spinal Cord Inj. Rehab. **29**(Supplement), 23–43 (2023)
13. Sadeghi, A., Afshari, E., Hashemi, M., Kaplan, D., Mozafari, M.: Brainy biomaterials: Latest advances in smart biomaterials to develop the next generation of neural interfaces. Curr. Opin. Biomed. Eng. **25**, 100420 (2023)
14. Zeng, Q., Huang, Z.: Challenges and opportunities of implantable neural interfaces: From material, electrochemical and biological perspectives. Adv. Funct. Mater. **33**(32), 2301223 (2023)
15. Parashar, K., Prajapati, D., McIntyre, R., Kandasubramanian, B.: Advancements in biological neural interfaces using conducting polymers: a review. Indust. Eng. Chem. Res. **59**(21), 9707–9718 (2020)

16. Ziai, Y., Zargarian, S.S., Rinoldi, C., Nakielski, P., Sola, A., Lanzi, M., Truong, Y.B., Pierini, F.: Conducting polymer-based nanostructured materials for brain–machine interfaces. Wiley Interdiscip. Rev. Nanomed. Nanobiotechnol. **15**(5), e1895 (2023)
17. Alahi, M.E.E., Rizu, M.I., Tina, F.W., Huang, Z., Nag, A., Afsarimanesh, N.: Recent advancements in graphene-based implantable electrodes for neural recording/stimulation. Sensors. **23**(24), 9911 (2023)
18. Liu, Y., Xu, S., Yang, Y., Zhang, K., He, E., Liang, W., Luo, J., Wu, Y., Cai, X.: Nanomaterial-based microelectrode arrays for in vitro bidirectional brain–computer interfaces: a review. Microsyst. Nanoeng. **9**(1), 13 (2023)
19. Mukherjee, N., Adak, A., Ghosh, S.: Recent trends in the development of peptide and protein-based hydrogel therapeutics for the healing of CNS injury. Soft Matter. **16**(44), 10046–10064 (2020)
20. Borton, D.A., Dawes, H.E., Worrell, G.A., Starr, P.A., Denison, T.J.: Developing collaborative platforms to advance neurotechnology and its translation. Neuron. **108**(2), 286–301 (2020)
21. Chitrakar, C., Hedrick, E., Adegoke, L., Ecker, M.: Flexible and stretchable bioelectronics. Materials. **15**(5), 1664 (2022)
22. Zhao, C., Wang, Z., Tang, X., Qin, J., Jiang, Z.: Recent advances in sensor-integrated brain-on-a-chip devices for real-time brain monitoring. Colloids Surf. B Biointerfaces. **229**, 113431 (2023)
23. Puranik, N., Arukha, A.P., Yadav, S.K., Yadav, D., Jin, J.O.: Exploring the role of stem cell therapy in treating neurodegenerative diseases: challenges and current perspectives. Curr. Stem Cell Res. Ther. **17**(2), 113–125 (2022)
24. Sykova, E., Cizkova, D., Kubinova, S.: Mesenchymal stem cells in treatment of spinal cord injury and amyotrophic lateral sclerosis. Front. Cell Dev. Biol. **9**, 695900 (2021)
25. Roth, J.G., Huang, M.S., Li, T.L., Feig, V.R., Jiang, Y., Cui, B., Greely, H.T., Bao, Z., Paşca, S.P., Heilshorn, S.C.: Advancing models of neural development with biomaterials. Nat. Rev. Neurosci. **22**(10), 593–615 (2021)
26. McMillen, P., Oudin, M.J., Levin, M., Payne, S.L.: Beyond neurons: long distance communication in development and cancer. Front. Cell Dev. Biol. **9**, 739024 (2021)
27. Tian, B., Lieber, C.M.: Nanowired bioelectric interfaces: focus review. Chem. Rev. **119**(15), 9136–9152 (2019)
28. Umuhoza, D., Yang, F., Long, D., Hao, Z., Dai, J., Zhao, A.: Strategies for tuning the biodegradation of silk fibroin-based materials for tissue engineering applications. ACS Biomater. Sci. Eng. **6**(3), 1290–1310 (2020)
29. Kennedy, S.W., Choudhury, N.R., Parthasarathy, R.: 3D printing soft tissue scaffolds using Poly (caprolactone). Bioprinting. **30**, e00259 (2023)
30. Akbari, M.K., Lopa, N.S., Shahriari, M., Najafzadehkhoee, A., Galusek, D., Zhuiykov, S.: Functional two-dimensional materials for bioelectronic neural interfacing. J. Funct. Biomater. **14**(1), 35 (2023)
31. Faruq, O., Chien, P.N., Dönmez, N., Nam, S.Y., Heo, C.Y.: Functionalization of silicone surface with drugs and polymers for regulation of capsular contracture. Polymers. **13**(16), 2731 (2021)
32. Khan, H.M., Liao, X., Sheikh, B.A., Wang, Y., Su, Z., Guo, C., Li, Z., Zhou, C., Cen, Y., Kong, Q.: Smart biomaterials and their potential applications in tissue engineering. J. Mater. Chem. B. **10**(36), 6859–6895 (2022)
33. Cho, W., Yoon, S.H., Chung, T.D.: Streamlining the interface between electronics and neural systems for bidirectional electrochemical communication. Chem. Sci. **14**(17), 4463–4479 (2023)
34. Park, Y., Chung, T.S., Lee, G., Rogers, J.A.: Materials chemistry of neural interface technologies and recent advances in three-dimensional systems. Chem. Rev. **122**(5), 5277–5316 (2021)
35. Lebaudy, E., Fournel, S., Lavalle, P., Vrana, N.E., Gribova, V.: Recent advances in antiinflammatory material design. Adv. Healthc. Mater. **10**(1), 2001373 (2021)

36. Steen, E.H., Wang, X., Balaji, S., Butte, M.J., Bollyky, P.L., Keswani, S.G.: The role of the anti-inflammatory cytokine interleukin-10 in tissue fibrosis. Adv. Wound Care. **9**(4), 184–198 (2020)
37. Liang, Y., Offenhäusser, A., Ingebrandt, S., Mayer, D.: PEDOT: PSS-based bioelectronic devices for recording and modulation of electrophysiological and biochemical cell signals. Adv. Healthc. Mater. **10**(11), 2100061 (2021)
38. Ramasubramanian, B., Reddy, V.S., Chellappan, V., Ramakrishna, S.: Emerging materials, wearables, and diagnostic advancements in therapeutic treatment of brain diseases. Biosensors. **12**(12), 1176 (2022)
39. Li, R., Ng, T.S., Garlin, M.A., Weissleder, R., Miller, M.A.: Understanding the in vivo fate of advanced materials by imaging. Adv. Funct. Mater. **30**(37), 1910369 (2020)
40. Thenuwara, G., Curtin, J., Tian, F.: Advances in diagnostic tools and therapeutic approaches for gliomas: a comprehensive review. Sensors. **23**(24), p.9842 (2023)
41. Tringides, C.M., Mooney, D.J.: Materials for implantable surface electrode arrays: current status and future directions. Adv. Mater. **34**(20), 2107207 (2022)
42. Aral, L.A., Peker, G.Ö.: A NOVEL HYBRID: NEURO-IMMUNO-ENGINEERING. Nat. Appl. Sci. J. **3**(2), 1–12 (2020)
43. Sharon, A., Jankowski, M.M., Shmoel, N., Erez, H., Spira, M.E.: Significantly reduced inflammatory foreign-body-response to neuroimplants and improved recording performance in young compared to adult rats. Acta Biomater. **158**, 292–307 (2023)
44. Gao, W., Yan, Z., Zhou, H., Xie, Y., Wang, H., Yang, J., Yu, J., Ni, C., Liu, P., Xie, M., Huang, L., Ye, Z.: Revolutionizing brain–computer interfaces: overcoming biocompatibility challenges in implantable neural interfaces. J. Nanobiotechnol. **23**(1), 498 (2025)
45. Shi, S., Ou, X., Cheng, D.: How advancing is peripheral nerve regeneration using nanofiber scaffolds? A comprehensive review of the literature. Int. J. Nanomed. **18**, 6763–6779 (2023)
46. Contreras, L.F.H., Truong, N.D., Eshraghian, J.K., Xu, Z., Huang, Z., Nikpour, A. and Kavehei, O., 2023. Neuromorphic neuromodulation: Towards the next generation of on-device AI-revolution in electroceuticals. arXiv preprint https://arxiv.org/abs/2307.12471
47. Puchert, P., Poonam, P., van Onzenoodt, C. and Ropinski, T., 2023. LLMMaps—A Visual Metaphor for Stratified Evaluation of Large Language Models. arXiv preprint https://arxiv.org/abs/2304.00457
48. Doblado, L.R., Martínez-Ramos, C., Pradas, M.M.: Biomaterials for neural tissue engineering. Front. Nanotechnol. **3**, 643507 (2021)
49. Palasz, E., Wilkaniec, A., Stanaszek, L., Andrzejewska, A., Adamczyk, A.: Glia-neurotrophic factor relationships: possible role in pathobiology of neuroinflammation-related brain disorders. Int. J. Mol. Sci. **24**(7), 6321 (2023)
50. Yu, H., Liu, F., Hu, Y., Wan, W., Liu, Q., Zhou, S., Zhang, L., Li, L., Huang, F.: Injectable ion-coordinated double-network conductive hydrogel for spinal cord injury repair. Front. Bioeng. Biotechnol. **13**, 1618680 (2025)
51. Raspopovic, S., Valle, G., Petrini, F.M.: Sensory feedback for limb prostheses in amputees. Nat. Mater. **20**(7), 925–939 (2021)
52. Beudel, M., Heijmans, M., Habets, J.G., Kubben, P.L.: Future perspectives: adaptive deep brain stimulation. In: Fundamentals and Clinics of Deep Brain Stimulation: An Interdisciplinary Approach, pp. 49–65. Springer International Publishing, Cham (2020)
53. Krauss, J.K., Lipsman, N., Aziz, T., Boutet, A., Brown, P., Chang, J.W., Davidson, B., Grill, W.M., Hariz, M.I., Horn, A., Schulder, M.: Technology of deep brain stimulation: current status and future directions. Nat. Rev. Neurol. **17**(2), 75–87 (2021)
54. Cho, K.W., Sunwoo, S.H., Hong, Y.J., Koo, J.H., Kim, J.H., Baik, S., Hyeon, T., Kim, D.H.: Soft bioelectronics based on nanomaterials. Chem. Rev. **122**(5), 5068–5143 (2021)
55. Ozgun, A., Lomboni, D., Arnott, H., Staines, W.A., Woulfe, J., Variola, F.: Biomaterials-based strategies for in vitro neural models. Biomater. Sci. **10**(5), 1134–1165 (2022)
56. Tsung, T.H., Tsai, Y.C., Lee, H.P., Chen, Y.H., Lu, D.W.: Biodegradable polymer-based drug-delivery systems for ocular diseases. Int. J. Mol. Sci. **24**(16), 12976 (2023)

57. Boufidis, D., Garg, R., Angelopoulos, E., Cullen, D.K., Vitale, F.: Bio-inspired electronics: Soft, biohybrid, and "living" neural interfaces. Nat. Commun. **16**(1), 1861 (2025)
58. Yoo, S., Lee, J., Joo, H., Sunwoo, S.H., Kim, S., Kim, D.H.: Wireless power transfer and telemetry for implantable bioelectronics. Adv. Healthc. Mater. **10**(17), 2100614 (2021)
59. Tan, P., He, L., Huang, Y., Zhou, Y.: Optophysiology: Illuminating cell physiology with optogenetics. Physiol. Rev. **102**(3), 1263–1325 (2022)
60. Buzio, M., Gini, M., Schneider, T.C., Stajkovic, N., Ingebrandt, S., De Laporte, L., Santoro, F.: 3D micropatterning of PEDOT: PSS/Gelatin conductive hydrogels via two-photon lithography for soft bioelectronics. NPJ Flex. Electr. **10**, 19 (2026)
61. Antezana, P.E., Municoy, S., Ostapchuk, G., Catalano, P.N., Hardy, J.G., Evelson, P.A., Orive, G., Desimone, M.F.: 4D printing: The development of responsive materials using 3D-printing technology. Pharmaceutics. **15**(12), 2743 (2023)
62. Sullivan, J., Mirhashemi, A., Lee, J.: Deep learning-based inverse design of microstructured materials for optical optimization and thermal radiation control. Sci. Rep. **13**(1), 7382 (2023)
63. Anurogo, D., Hidayat, N.A.: The Art of Televasculobiomedicine 5.0. Nas Media Pustaka (2023)
64. Ciulla, M.G., Massironi, A., Sugni, M., Ensign, M.A., Marzorati, S., Forouharshad, M.: Recent advances in the development of biomimetic materials. Gels. **9**(10), 833 (2023)
65. Nitti, P., Narayanan, A., Pellegrino, R., Villani, S., Madaghiele, M., Demitri, C.: Cell-tissue interaction: the biomimetic approach to design tissue engineered biomaterials. Bioengineering. **10**(10), 1122 (2023)
66. Rodrigues, D., Barbosa, A.I., Rebelo, R., Kwon, I.K., Reis, R.L., Correlo, V.M.: Skin-integrated wearable systems and implantable biosensors: a comprehensive review. Biosensors. **10**(7), 79 (2020)
67. Song, E., Li, J., Won, S.M., Bai, W., Rogers, J.A.: Materials for flexible bioelectronic systems as chronic neural interfaces. Nat. Mater.s. **19**(6), 590–603 (2020)
68. Mohapatra, S., Mirza, M.A., Hilles, A.R., Zakir, F., Gomes, A.C., Ansari, M.J., Iqbal, Z., Mahmood, S.: Biomedical application, patent repository, clinical trial and regulatory updates on hydrogel: an extensive review. Gels. **7**(4), 207 (2021)
69. Rybak, D., Su, Y.C., Li, Y., Ding, B., Lv, X., Li, Z., Yeh, Y.C., Nakielski, P., Rinoldi, C., Pierini, F., Dodda, J.M.: Evolution of nanostructured skin patches towards multifunctional wearable platforms for biomedical applications. Nanoscale. **15**(18), 8044–8083 (2023)
70. Gori, M., Vadalà, G., Giannitelli, S.M., Denaro, V., Di Pino, G.: Biomedical and tissue engineering strategies to control foreign body reaction to invasive neural electrodes. Front. Bioeng. Biotechnol. **9**, 659033 (2021)
71. Hong, M., Ye, Y., Kim, J., Kim, J.I., Rah, J.C., Tchoe, Y.: Integrating living biomaterials into neuroelectronic systems. Biomed. Eng. Lett. **16**, 1–22 (2026)
72. Sorrell, E., Rule, M.E., O'Leary, T.: Brain–machine interfaces: Closed-loop control in an adaptive system. Ann. Rev. Control Robot. Autonom. Syst. **4**(1), 167–189 (2021)
73. Tanskanen, J.M., Ahtiainen, A., Hyttinen, J.A.: Toward closed-loop electrical stimulation of neuronal systems: a review. Bioelectricity. **2**(4), 328–347 (2020)
74. Menon, A., Vijayavenkataraman, S.: Novel vision restoration techniques: 3D bioprinting, gene and stem cell therapy, optogenetics, and the bionic eye. Artif. Organs. **46**(8), 1463–1474 (2022)
75. Zhu, H., Yao, C., Wei, B., Xu, C., Huang, X., Liu, Y., He, J., Zhang, J., Li, D.: 3D printing of functional bioengineered constructs for neural regeneration: a review. Int. J. Extreme Manufact. **5**(4), 042004 (2023)
76. Krucoff, M.O., Miller, J.P., Saxena, T., Bellamkonda, R., Rahimpour, S., Harward, S.C., Lad, S.P., Turner, D.A.: Toward functional restoration of the central nervous system: a review of translational neuroscience principles. Neurosurgery. **84**(1), 30–40 (2019)
77. Nagappan, P.G., Chen, H., Wang, D.Y.: Neuroregeneration and plasticity: a review of the physiological mechanisms for achieving functional recovery postinjury. Milit. Med. Res. **7**(1), 30 (2020)

78. Gupta, C., Chandrashekar, P., Jin, T., He, C., Khullar, S., Chang, Q., Wang, D.: Bringing machine learning to research on intellectual and developmental disabilities: taking inspiration from neurological diseases. J Neurodev. Disord. **14**(1), 28 (2022)
79. Wong, J.K., Deuschl, G., Wolke, R., Bergman, H., Muthuraman, M., Groppa, S., Sheth, S.A., Bronte-Stewart, H.M., Wilkins, K.B., Petrucci, M.N., Lambert, E.: Proceedings of the ninth annual deep brain stimulation think tank: advances in cutting edge technologies, artificial intelligence, neuromodulation, neuroethics, pain, interventional psychiatry, epilepsy, and traumatic brain injury. Front. Human Neurosci. **16**, 813387 (2022)

Chapter 9
Nanomaterials and Additive Manufacturing

Abstract Additive manufacturing (AM) and nanomaterials are two revolutionary foundations of contemporary biomaterials science that provide previously unheard-of control over the structure, functionality, and performance of materials. Materials with special physicochemical characteristics at the nanoscale, like increased surface area, reactivity, mechanical strength, and electrical conductivity, can be carefully adjusted to affect biological interactions. These nanoscale capabilities are enhanced by additive manufacturing, especially 3D and 4D printing, which makes it possible to fabricate intricate, personalized architectures layer by layer that are intended to resemble the organization of genuine tissue. From biosensors and medication delivery systems to implantable devices and regenerative scaffolds, these technologies collectively are revolutionizing biomedical engineering. Additive manufacturing (AM) and nanomaterials are two revolutionary foundations of contemporary biomaterials science that provide previously unheard-of control over the structure, functionality, and performance of materials. Materials with special physicochemical characteristics at the nanoscale, like increased surface area, reactivity, mechanical strength, and electrical conductivity, can be carefully adjusted to affect biological interactions. These nanoscale capabilities are enhanced by additive manufacturing, especially 3D and 4D printing, which makes it possible to fabricate intricate, personalized architectures layer by layer that are intended to resemble the organization of genuine tissue. From biosensors and medication delivery systems to implantable devices and regenerative scaffolds, these technologies collectively are revolutionizing biomedical engineering. Significant advancements like as patient-specific implants, intelligent prosthetics, and bioresponsive tissue structures that dynamically interact with their surroundings have resulted from the combination of nanotechnology with AM. Reproducibility, interface stability, nanomaterial dispersion, and regulatory approval for clinical translation are still issues, nevertheless. To enhance nanoscale design and production processes, future initiatives will focus on the creation of data-driven, bioinspired, and adaptive manufacturing systems that incorporate artificial intelligence and real-time monitoring. In the end, the combination of additive manufacturing and nanomaterials is causing a paradigm change in the direction of customized, multipurpose, and sustainable biomedical systems,

M. Adeoba, T. Pandelani, *Application of Biomaterials in Biomedical Engineering*, Series in BioEngineering,
https://doi.org/10.1007/978-3-032-34477-9_9

closing the gap between clinical impact and materials innovation in next-generation healthcare.

9.1 Introduction

One significant development in the history of biomaterials science and biomedical engineering is the combination of nanomaterials and additive manufacturing (AM). By providing an unparalleled level of control over structural, functional, and biological properties, both technologies have revolutionized conventional methods for material design, processing, and clinical application. Additive manufacturing works at the macro-to-microscale, creating complex, patient-specific architectures layer by layer, whereas nanomaterials work at the molecular and atomic scale, modifying matter to harness special mechanical, electrical, and biochemical properties [1, 2]. These developments collectively lay the groundwork for a new generation of regenerative and biofabrication systems that mimic, restore, or even improve physiological processes.

9.1.1 Overview of Nanomaterials and Additive Manufacturing as Transformative Technologies

Metal nanoparticles, carbon nanostructures, quantum dots, and polymeric nanocomposites are all examples of the large class of materials known as nanomaterials, which have structural characteristics smaller than 100 nm. At this size, unique mechanical strength, catalytic activity, and biological interactions not found in bulk materials are provided by the high surface-to-volume ratio and quantum confinement effects. These characteristics allow nanomaterials to enhance biocompatibility, bioactivity, and tailored functionality in the biomedical setting, hence facilitating applications in drug delivery, tissue engineering, biosensing, and diagnostics.

Metal nanoparticles, carbon nanostructures, quantum dots, and polymeric nanocomposites are all examples of the large class of materials known as nanomaterials, which have structural characteristics smaller than 100 nm. At this size, unique mechanical strength, catalytic activity, and biological interactions not found in bulk materials are provided by the high surface-to-volume ratio and quantum confinement effects. These characteristics allow nanomaterials to enhance biocompatibility, bioactivity, and tailored functionality in the biomedical setting, hence facilitating applications in drug delivery, tissue engineering, biosensing, and diagnostics [3, 4].

9.1.2 Importance of Nanoscale Engineering for Performance Enhancement

The nanoscale is the critical dimension where material properties and biological systems converge. Cells interact with their environment at the nanometer scale through receptors, adhesion sites, and extracellular matrix components making nanoscale features essential for regulating biological responses. Nanoscale engineering thus enables precise modulation of surface chemistry, topography, and energy, directly influencing protein adsorption, cell adhesion, and signaling pathways.

Mechanically, polymeric matrices are reinforced by nanomaterials like carbon nanotubes (CNTs), graphene, and nanoceramics, which improve hardness, elasticity, and fatigue resistance without sacrificing flexibility. Functionalization of nanomaterials chemically enhances therapeutic efficacy while reducing systemic toxicity by enabling the controlled release of bioactive molecules or medications [5, 6]. By biologically simulating natural extracellular habitats, nanoparticles can aid in stem cell development and facilitate tissue incorporation. By these improvements, nanoscale design closes the gap between live tissue and synthetic materials, enabling mechanical compatibility and biofunctionality that are essential for long-term biomedical performance.

9.1.3 Role of Additive Manufacturing in Complex and Patient-Specific Constructs

Additive manufacturing serves as the architectural counterpart to nanoscale control, enabling macroscopic realization of intricate biomedical constructs. Through digital modeling and computer-aided design (CAD), AM allows the fabrication of implants and scaffolds that replicate the patient's anatomy, derived from medical imaging data such as MRI or CT scans. This personalization reduces the risk of implant mismatch, improves functional restoration, and shortens recovery time.

In addition to personalization, AM makes it possible to precisely adjust porosity, pore size, and interconnectivity parameters that are essential for tissue in-growth, vascularization, and nutrition delivery. Methods including selective laser sintering (SLS), fused deposition modeling (FDM), and stereolithography (SLA) have been modified for use in biomedicine and may process metals, polymers, and ceramics in biocompatible ways [7, 8]. These techniques make it easier to create gradient and multi-material structures that simulate intricate tissue interfaces like tendon-ligament junctions and bone-cartilage interfaces by varying stiffness, bioactivity, and degradation rates spatially. AM offers a platform for hybrid creation that combines structural accuracy with nanoscale biofunctionality when combined with nanomaterial integration.

9.1.4 Synergy Between Nanotechnology and Additive Manufacturing in Precision Medicine

The convergence of nanotechnology and additive manufacturing has accelerated progress toward precision medicine, where treatment is tailored to the individual's genetic, physiological, and pathological profile. Nanomaterials enhance AM-fabricated structures by introducing stimuli-responsive and bioactive functionalities, transforming static implants into dynamic, "smart" systems [9, 10]. For instance, nanostructured coatings can enable controlled drug release, antimicrobial activity, or electrical conductivity, while embedded nanoparticles can act as biosensors for monitoring inflammation or pH fluctuations in situ.

From microscale vascular channels and macroscale anatomical frameworks to nanoscale ECM-mimetic cues, the combination of nanomaterials and AM in regenerative engineering enables hierarchical tissue development. Because of this integration, scientists may create artificial tissues that actively engage with cells and physiological signals in addition to replicating natural shape, encouraging genuine regeneration as opposed to passive repair. Furthermore, new paradigms for producing functional brain, cardiac, and bone tissues have been offered by the development of bioprinting, which uses living cells and biomaterial "inks," opening the door to customized organ replacement. Furthermore, the use of AI-driven design and computational modeling strengthens this synergy by anticipating material–cell interactions, improving scaffold geometries, and simulating long-term deterioration and mechanical performance. Artificial intelligence, AM, and nanotechnology work together to create a networked ecosystem that propels data-driven, flexible medicinal innovation.

9.1.5 Scope and Objectives of the Chapter

This chapter explores the interrelated domains of nanomaterials and additive manufacturing within the context of biomaterial science and clinical translation. It aims to elucidate how the unique physicochemical and biological properties of nanomaterials contribute to performance enhancement in biomedical applications, and how AM provides the structural and design flexibility needed to realize these materials in functional devices.

The discussion begins by classifying nanomaterials and their defining properties, emphasizing their roles in strengthening, bioactivation, and sensing. Subsequent sections examine additive manufacturing techniques and design principles, focusing on the integration of nanostructures into 3D and 4D printed architectures. The chapter also reviews mechanistic insights, where the interplay of nanoscale interactions and macroscopic design dictates performance in applications such as tissue scaffolds, drug delivery systems, orthopedic implants, and biosensors.

Lastly, it discusses the difficulties, restrictions, and potential paths forward, including scalability, reproducibility, moral considerations, and the legal frameworks controlling nanostructured AM devices. The ultimate goal is to demonstrate how the future of customized, intelligent, and regenerative biomedical systems is being shaped by the combination of additive manufacturing and nanoscale engineering [11, 12]. A new era of material-driven healthcare innovation is being ushered in by this convergence, which is transforming biomaterials from static, inert components to dynamic, interactive platforms that can sense, react, and adapt to complicated biological settings.

9.2 Key Concepts and Definitions

By bridging the gap between molecular accuracy and macroscopic functioning, the advent of nanomaterials and additive manufacturing (AM) has revolutionized the field of biomaterials science. Researchers and engineers may now create materials and structures that closely resemble biological systems in terms of composition and function thanks to these technologies. Comprehending their fundamental ideas and terminology lays the groundwork for understanding how digital manufacturing and nanoscale research combine to promote tissue regeneration, personalized medicine, and biomedical device engineering.

9.2.1 Definition of Nanomaterials

Materials with at least one exterior dimension or internal structural characteristic less than 100 nm (nm) are referred to be nanomaterials. Compared to their mass equivalents, these scales impart distinct physical, chemical, and biological features. Mechanical strength, optical absorption, and surface chemistry are all changed at the nanoscale by quantum confinement effects, higher surface energy, and improved reactivity. Nanomaterials' capacity to replicate natural extracellular matrix (ECM) structures, engage with cellular constituents, and alter biological responses makes them valuable in biomaterials research. Tissue–material interactions can be precisely controlled by the nanoscale roughness and topography of materials, which can affect protein adsorption, cell adhesion, and differentiation [13, 14]. For example, titanium implants with nanoscale surface features enhance osteointegration, while nanoparticle-based carriers enable targeted drug delivery. Consequently, the nanoscale has become the critical interface where materials meet biology, driving innovation across regenerative medicine, biosensing, and drug delivery platforms.

9.2.2 Definition of Additive Manufacturing (AM)

The term Additive Manufacturing (AM) describes a group of fabrication techniques that use digital design files to build three-dimensional (3D) structures layer by layer. Using computer-aided design (CAD) or medical imaging data as a guide, AM adds material in successive layers as opposed to traditional subtractive procedures, which remove material from a solid block. The development of tissue scaffolds, implants, and microstructured devices tailored to each patient is made possible by this method's unmatched geometric complexity freedom. AM covers a variety of techniques in the biomedical field, such as bioprinting living tissues with cell-rich bioinks and printing plastic and metal for load-bearing implants. Its benefits include quick prototyping, material efficiency, and design flexibility, all of which complement individualized and regenerative treatment approaches. The layer-by-layer approach also facilitates gradient structures, porous architectures, and multimaterial compositions, all essential for replicating the heterogeneity of biological tissues [15, 16]. In sum, AM represents the digital embodiment of precision manufacturing, translating computational models into functional biomedical constructs.

9.2.3 Classification of Nanomaterials

According to their morphology and dimensionality, nanomaterials can be categorized as follows: nanoparticles (0D), which are spherical or nearly spherical objects with a diameter of 1–100 nm that are employed for drug administration, imaging, and sensing as shown in Fig. 9.1. Polymeric and lipid nanoparticles act as controlled-release carriers for medications, whereas metallic nanoparticles (such as gold and silver) have surface plasmon resonance that is helpful for diagnostics. High aspect ratio, elongated structures created by electrospinning or self-assembly are known as nanofibers (1D). They are perfect for tissue scaffolds and wound dressings because of their fibrous architecture, which resembles collagen and elastin in the extracellular matrix. Nanotubes (1D), cylindrical nanostructures with remarkable strength and electrical conductivity, as carbon nanotubes (CNTs) or titanium dioxide nanotubes. They are used in reinforced composites, biosensors, and brain electrodes. 2D–3D nanocomposites are hybrid materials that combine nanoscale fillers with a matrix that might be metallic, polymeric, or ceramic. The addition of nanoparticles improves bioactivity, thermal stability, and mechanical strength. For example, in orthopedic applications, hydroxyapatite–polymer nanocomposites enhance bone integration. Thin surface layers known as nanocoatings (2D) are used to alter the chemical or physical characteristics of biomaterials [17]. Long-term implant effectiveness depends on the antibacterial, antifouling, or osteoconductive properties that nanostructured coatings can provide. This variation in structure and function demonstrates how the principles of nanoscale design can be applied to biomedical goals, ranging from improving biocompatibility to administering targeted medicine.

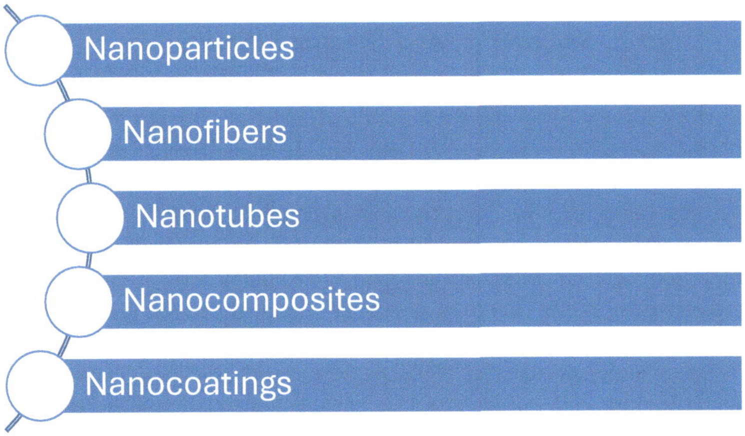

Fig. 9.1 Classification of nanomaterials based on dimensionality, ranging from zero-dimensional nanoparticles to one-dimensional nanofibers and nanotubes, two-dimensional nanocoatings, and three-dimensional nanocomposites used in biomedical applications

9.2.4 Classification of AM Processes: SLA, SLS, FDM, and Bioprinting

Stereolithography (SLA), which uses ultraviolet (UV) lasers to photopolymerize liquid resins layer by layer, is one of the fundamental methods of additive manufacturing. Each of these procedures has its own unique energy sources and material kinds. High-resolution production of complex microstructures is made possible by SLA and is frequently utilized in tissue scaffolds, dental prosthesis, and microfluidic devices. A laser beam is used in Selective Laser Sintering (SLS) to fuse powdered materials like metals, ceramics, and polymers. SLS manufactures mechanically strong, porous parts that are appropriate for orthopaedic implants and tailored prosthetics. Thermoplastic filaments are extruded through a heated nozzle in fused deposition modeling (FDM) to create successive layers. Biocompatible polymer structures, frequently supplemented with nanoparticles to improve mechanical or antibacterial qualities, are produced using FDM on a large scale [18]. Bioprinting, specialized AM technique that deposits cell-laden hydrogels (bioinks) in spatially controlled patterns to create living tissues. Bioprinting integrates biological, chemical, and mechanical cues to reproduce functional tissues, such as cartilage, skin, or vascularized grafts.

Each process offers trade-offs between resolution, material versatility, speed, and cell viability, and their selection depends on the desired application. The integration of nanoscale materials within these AM systems is expanding their potential, enabling multiscale architectures that couple structural precision with biofunctionality.

9.2.5 *Key Parameters: Surface-to-Volume Ratio, Precision Control, Scalability, and Biocompatibility*

A few factors influence how nanomaterials and AM-based systems are designed and function; Because of their incredibly large surface areas in relation to their volume, nanomaterials interact with biological molecules and cells more strongly. This improves protein adsorption, reactivity, and catalytic potential all of which are essential for drug delivery and tissue integration. Control over pore shape, surface roughness, and material composition is made possible by AM technologies' micron-to-nanometer resolution. This accuracy has a direct impact on mechanical performance, nutrition delivery, and cell adhesion. Despite its potential, scaling AM manufacturing and nanomaterial synthesis for clinical-grade applications continues to present difficulties [19]. Regulatory approval and translational success depend on reproducibility and consistency across large batches. AM-fabricated structures and nanomaterials must both steer clear of inflammatory and cytotoxic responses. Surface functionalization, sterilization, and degradation control are vital to achieving safe and predictable biological responses.

These parameters interact synergistically precision at the nanoscale enable improved biological compatibility, while scalable digital fabrication ensures clinical feasibility.

9.2.6 *Core Concepts*

Three fundamental scientific ideas underpin nanomaterials in additive manufacturing, defining their function in the development of biomaterials: The final success of biomaterials is determined by the interface between biological systems and nanoscale surfaces. Immune recognition, cell signaling, and protein corona formation are all impacted by interactions at this scale. It is possible to rationally create materials that trigger particular biological responses, such osteogenesis or angiogenesis, by comprehending and managing nano-biointeractions. From macroscopic bone trabeculae to nanofibrillar collagen, biological tissues are organized at several sizes. Materials that incorporate nanoscale characteristics into larger designs are needed to mimic this hierarchy. This bottom-up construction is made possible by AM technologies, which incorporate nanoscale cues into macroscale scaffolds to direct tissue creation and cell alignment [15, 20]. The convergence of nanotechnology and AM introduces a multiscale design paradigm, linking atomic-level material engineering with organ-level functionality. By coupling nanoscale reinforcement with macroscale form, researchers can create devices that are mechanically robust, biologically instructive, and functionally integrated.

Together, these concepts define the philosophy of modern biomaterial design where materials are not static entities but dynamic, biointeractive systems engineered across multiple dimensions.

In biomedical engineering, the combination of additive manufacturing and nanomaterials signifies a paradigm change. AM makes it possible to create accurate, patient-specific structures, whereas nanomaterials give molecular-level control over biological interactions. The foundation of next-generation biomaterials is defined by their classification, parameters, and guiding principles, which are focused on nano-biointeraction, hierarchical organization, and multiscale integration. The future of customized and precision medicine will be fueled by these technologies' potential to provide intelligent, regenerative, and adaptable systems that bridge the gap between artificial constructs and biological tissues.

9.3 Material Types and Properties

Nanoscale control of composition, structure, and surface characteristics is becoming more important in the development of sophisticated biomaterials because it enables previously unheard-of tuning of mechanical performance, chemical reactivity, and biological interaction. Nanomaterials offer the basis for improving biological response, endurance, and functional integration in the context of biomedical design and additive manufacturing as shown in Table 9.1. The main categories of

Table 9.1 Properties of nanomaterials vs. bulk materials

Property Category	Characteristic	Nanomaterials	Bulk Materials	Implications for Additive Manufacturing (AM)
Structural and dimensional	Scale and surface-to-volume ratio	Extremely high surface area (10–1000 m^2/g); quantum and interfacial effects dominate	Low surface area; bulk crystal and grain boundary effects dominate	Enables fine microstructural control and enhanced reactivity during AM powder sintering or nanoparticle-based printing
Mechanical	Strength and hardness	Enhanced yield strength, hardness, and fatigue resistance due to grain boundary strengthening (hall–Petch effect)	Lower mechanical strength; dislocation motion less constrained	Nanostructured AM parts show improved wear resistance and load-bearing capacity
	Elastic modulus	Tunable through nanostructure design (e.g., CNT networks, nanoceramic reinforcements)	Fixed by material composition and microstructure	Allows fabrication of gradient or functionally adaptive materials with tailored stiffness

(continued)

Table 9.1 (continued)

Property Category	Characteristic	Nanomaterials	Bulk Materials	Implications for Additive Manufacturing (AM)
Thermal	Melting point and thermal conductivity	Reduced melting temperature due to size effects; high phonon scattering limits conductivity	Stable melting point; predictable bulk thermal conductivity	Facilitates low-temperature AM processes and precise energy control in laser/e-beam sintering
Electrical	Conductivity and charge transport	Quantum confinement yields tunable electrical properties (semiconducting, metallic, or insulating)	Conductivity determined by atomic composition and impurity content	Supports fabrication of flexible electronics, sensors, and bioelectronic AM devices
Optical	Optical absorption and emission	Quantum size effects lead to color-tunable fluorescence and plasmonic resonance	Broad and fixed optical properties	Enables printing of photonic devices, biosensors, and optoelectronic implants
Chemical and surface	Reactivity and catalytic activity	High reactivity due to increased surface energy and active sites	Lower surface reactivity; slower reaction kinetics	Improves AM powder fusion, surface modification, and nanocomposite bonding
	Surface energy and wettability	Enhanced surface energy promotes adhesion and particle dispersion	Lower surface energy; reduced adhesion	Enhances powder bed cohesion and resin–nanoparticle interface quality in AM
Biological	Biocompatibility and cellular response	Nanotopography influences protein adsorption, cell adhesion, and differentiation	Limited control over biointerface behavior	Enables design of cell-instructive scaffolds and bioactive surfaces in bioprinting
Manufacturing and processing	Processability	Amenable to inkjet, aerosol jet, and stereolithography with nanosuspensions or colloidal inks	Requires melting, machining, or powder metallurgy	Expands AM to nanoscale precision and multifunctional hybrid fabrication
	Microstructural control	Self-assembly and nanoscale patterning achievable	Grain growth and defects limit fine control	Enables gradient, hierarchical, and metamaterial structures

(continued)

Table 9.1 (continued)

Property Category	Characteristic	Nanomaterials	Bulk Materials	Implications for Additive Manufacturing (AM)
Functional integration	Multi-functionality	Combines mechanical, electrical, optical, and biological functions within one platform	Typically single-function materials	Foundation for 4D printing, smart implants, and responsive medical devices

nanomaterial metallic, polymeric, ceramic, carbon-based, and hybrid nanofibrous or hydrogel systems are described in detail in the sections that follow. Additionally, the ways in which their nanoscale designs directly affect mechanical behavior and biological effects are examined.

9.3.1 Metallic Nanomaterials

Metallic nanomaterials, such as silver (Ag), gold (Au), and titanium (Ti) nanoparticles, are essential to biological innovation because of their superior surface reactivity, electrical conductivity, and mechanical strength. Because of their inherent biocompatibility and resistance to corrosion, titanium-based nanostructures particularly titanium dioxide (TiO_2) nanoparticles are frequently employed in orthopedic and dental applications. By improving protein adsorption, osteoblast adhesion, and mineralization at the bone–implant interface, nanoscale surface modification of titanium implants encourages osteointegration [21, 22].

Although chemically inert, gold nanoparticles (AuNPs) have plasmonic and electrical conductivity qualities that are advantageous for brain and biosensing applications. Site-specific delivery and diagnostic monitoring are made possible by coupling with peptides, antibodies, or medications because to their adjustable size and surface chemistry. Like this, silver nanoparticles (AgNPs) have strong antibacterial properties and break down bacterial membranes by releasing Ag^+ ions. Without sacrificing mechanical strength, AgNPs can be included into polymer or ceramic matrices to prevent infection in orthopedic devices, catheters, and wound dressings.

In composite systems, metallic nanostructures serve as mechanical reinforcing agents. For load-bearing biomedical components, the addition of nanoparticles or nanowires to polymers or ceramics can enhance wear performance, fatigue resistance, and tensile strength. Furthermore, conductivity and corrosion resistance are improved by nanoscale metallic coatings on additively created implants, opening the door for the creation of bioelectronic and electroactive scaffolds that can promote tissue regeneration.

9.3.2 Polymeric Nanomaterials

The adjustable chemistry, biodegradability, and biocompatibility of polymeric nanoparticles make them one of the most adaptable materials for biomedical applications. Polyethylene glycol (PEG), polycaprolactone (PCL), and poly(lactic-co-glycolic acid) (PLGA) are frequently utilized polymers that are used as scaffolds, coatings, and platforms for nanostructured drug delivery systems. Since their hydrolytic breakdown into lactic and glycolic acid permits predictable release kinetics, PLGA nanoparticles are widely used for controlled drug delivery. Long-term local delivery, cellular absorption, and biological barrier crossing are all made easier by the nanoscale size. To ensure synchronization with tissue healing timeframes, researchers can adjust mechanical stiffness and degradation rates by varying the lactide-to-glycolide ratio and molecular weight. PCL-based nanofibers and nanocomposites, on the other hand, exhibit mechanical flexibility and slow degradation, ideal for long-term scaffold applications. When fabricated through electrospinning or 3D printing, PCL nanostructures mimic the fibrous architecture of the extracellular matrix (ECM), guiding cell alignment and axonal growth in neural or musculoskeletal regeneration.

At the nanoscale, polymeric materials also allow mechanical property optimization such as adjusting stiffness and elasticity to match specific tissue types. Nanostructuring increases the surface area available for cell attachment and nutrient exchange, while chemical functionalization improves hydrophilicity and bioactivity, promoting effective host integration [23, 24].

9.3.3 Ceramic and Composite Nanomaterials

Silica nanoparticles, bioactive glass, and hydroxyapatite (HA) are examples of ceramic nanomaterials that are prized for their exceptional bioactivity and structural resemblance to real bone mineral. Because of their calcium-phosphate makeup, hydroxyapatite nanocrystals directly promote osteoblast adhesion, proliferation, and differentiation, which makes them essential for dental repair and bone tissue creation. When exposed to physiological fluids, their nanoscale shape promotes surface reactivity, speeding up ion exchange and the creation of apatite. When bioactive glasses, which are mostly made of SiO_2, CaO, NaO_2, and P_2O_5, meet biological fluids, they create a layer of hydroxycarbonate apatite that allows for chemical interaction with bone. These glasses have improved bioactivity and resorption at the nanoscale, which facilitates the regulated release of therapeutic ions like Ca2+ and Si2+ that promote osteogenesis and angiogenesis.

Within composite scaffolds, silica nanoparticles perform both structural and functional functions as carriers of proteins, growth factors, or medications. Diffusion-controlled release and effective molecular loading are made possible by their high porosity and pore size adjustability. Ceramics interact with metals or polymers to create nanocomposites that combine the hardness and bioactivity of inorganic phases with the flexibility and toughness of organic matrix. These hybrid nanocomposites provide a biomimetic balance between mechanical strength and biofunctionality, which is crucial for load bearing, bone, and dental applications. They also improve cellular adhesion, interfacial bonding, and fracture resistance.

9.3.4 Carbon-Based Nanomaterials

Graphene, carbon nanotubes (CNTs), and nanodiamonds are examples of carbon-based nanomaterials that have become ground-breaking platforms for improving biomedical devices' mechanical and electrical performance. A single sheet of carbon atoms organized in a hexagonal lattice, graphene combines remarkable surface area, electrical conductivity, and mechanical strength [25, 26]. Its distinct two-dimensional structure enables incorporation into hydrogel or polymeric matrices to produce electroconductive composites for cardiac scaffolds, biosensors, and neural interfaces. Selective cell interaction is made possible by functionalizing graphene's surface with biomolecules, peptides, or polymers to increase solubility and decrease cytotoxicity.

Both single-walled and multi-walled carbon nanotubes (CNTs) have comparable benefits, especially for applications like bioelectronic implants and smart scaffolds that call for electromechanical transduction. Their high aspect ratio and nanoscale size promote neurite outgrowth and cell alignment, promoting neural and muscle tissue regeneration. To reduce immunological reactivity, virgin CNTs must be modified on the surface with biocompatible coatings or oxygen-containing functional groups since they may cause oxidative stress or inflammatory reactions [27, 28].

Nanodiamonds are perfect for medication delivery and imaging applications because of their customizable surface chemistry and chemical inertness. While reducing cytotoxic effects, their surface can bind growth stimulants, antibiotics, or chemotherapeutics. Furthermore, in dental and orthopedic applications, nanodiamonds improve hardness and wear resistance by strengthening mechanical reinforcement in polymer matrices. All things considered, carbon-based nanomaterials allow materials to conduct, detect, and react dynamically in the biological environment by bridging the gap between structural integrity and bioelectronic functioning.

9.3.5 Hydrogels and Nanofibrous Scaffolds

The soft-matter domain of biomaterials based on nanomaterials is represented by hydrogels and nanofibrous scaffolds. Mechanical compliance, permeability, and cellular contact are governed by their nanoscale characteristics, including porosity, crosslinking density, and fiber orientation. Hydrogels made of natural or synthetic polymers (such gelatin, alginate, or PEG) offer hydrated, tissue-like conditions that are ideal for nutrition delivery and cell encapsulation. Researchers can adjust the diffusion rates of oxygen, metabolites, and signaling chemicals to maintain cell viability in three-dimensional structures by regulating nanoscale porosity. Furthermore, hydrogels can be functionalized with nanoparticles to add electrical or bioactive characteristics, such as conductive hydrogel composites for neurological stimulation or hydrogels that are magnetically sensitive.

Nanofibrous scaffolds, which are usually made by electrospinning, guide cell alignment, adhesion, and differentiation by imitating the fibrillar structure of native extracellular matrix. Gene expression and cellular morphology are influenced by nanofiber diameter, alignment, and surface chemistry. For instance, random orientations allow multidirectional tissue ingrowth, whereas aligned nanofibers encourage axonal extension and myogenic differentiation. When nanofibers and AM manufacturing are combined, hierarchical, multiscale scaffolds with biomimetic texture at the nanoscale and structural accuracy at the macro level are produced.

9.3.6 Relationship Between Nanoscale Architecture, Mechanical Behavior, and Biological Performance

A fundamental aspect of nanomaterial functionality is the connection between performance and structure. The way materials transfer stress, interact with cells, and deteriorate over time is determined by their nanoscale architecture. For example, nanoporous designs and smaller grain sizes preserve enough elasticity to match soft tissues while increasing mechanical strength through energy dissipation mechanisms and strengthening of grain boundaries. In biology, protein adsorption and integrin-mediated signaling are modulated by surface topography at the nanoscale, which controls subsequent processes like inflammation, differentiation, and proliferation. Multimodal interactions are facilitated by hierarchical architectures that combine micro- and nanoscale characteristics, facilitating biochemical communication as well as mechanical load transfer.

Additionally, synchronizing material resorption and tissue regeneration through nanoscale degradation control reduces inflammatory reactions and maintains structural integrity throughout the healing process. Therefore, the basis of next-generation biomaterials is the combination of mechanical and biological needs with nanoscale design. The core of nanomaterial science in additive manufacturing is the ability to design materials that are robust, flexible, biocompatible, and biofunctional all at once. This synergy makes it possible to move from passive implants to active, regenerative, and adaptive biomedical systems.

9.4 Mechanisms and Processes

A new generation of biomaterials with precision control, multifunctional performance, and hierarchical architecture has been produced by combining nanotechnology and additive manufacturing (AM) [29, 30]. Understanding the principles and procedures controlling the synthesis of nanomaterials, additive fabrication, and the interaction between nanoscale and macroscale architectures is crucial to achieving their full biological potential. This examines the fundamental engineering techniques and scientific ideas that guide the creation, modification, and performance and biocompatibility optimization of these cutting-edge materials.

9.4.1 Nanomaterial Synthesis Mechanisms

The synthesis of nanomaterials is generally categorized into two complementary strategies: **bottom-up** and **top-down** approaches.

Bottom-up approaches use chemical processes or self-assembly to create materials from atomic or molecule precursors. To attain homogeneity and order at the nanoscale, they depend on kinetic and thermodynamic control. Self-assembly, in which molecules or nanoparticles spontaneously arrange themselves into ordered structures under particular environmental conditions (such as pH or ionic strength), is one of the most notable examples. Lipid nanoparticles, micelles, and nanofibers employed in tissue scaffolding and drug delivery are formed by this method. Sol-gel synthesis creates nanostructured oxides (like silica or titania) by hydrolyzing and condensing metal alkoxides. These materials' adjustable porosity and bioactivity make them beneficial for biosensing and bone regeneration applications. Chemical vapor deposition (CVD), where gaseous precursors decompose and deposit as thin films or nanotubes on substrates. CVD enables the fabrication of conductive coatings and nanocarbon structures with controlled thickness and purity.

On the other hand, top-down approaches use lithographic or mechanical processes to reduce bulk materials to nanoscale dimensions. With shear and impact forces, mechanical milling (such as ball milling) produces nanoparticles or nanocomposites by reducing particle size. Nanoscale surface features are patterned using lithography, especially electron-beam and photolithography, which is essential to produce microelectronic and biological devices. There are trade-offs between cost, homogeneity, and scalability with each approach. While top-down approaches are better at patterning and maintaining structural integrity, bottom-up approaches typically provide more control over composition and morphology.

Importantly, surface modification and functionalization act as a link between the manufacture of nanomaterials and biological use. Nanoparticles can be engineered to improve protein adsorption behavior, cell-specific targeting, or biocompatibility via chemical grafting, plasma treatment, or ligand conjugation. Polyethylene glycol (PEG) coating of metallic nanoparticles, for example, decreases immunological recognition, whilst conjugating peptides or antibodies enables targeted delivery to particular cells or tissues [31]. Therefore, inert nanostructures are transformed into physiologically interacting elements essential to biomedical function through surface engineering.

9.4.2 Additive Manufacturing Processes

Additive manufacturing encompasses a range of techniques that fabricate 3D structures through **layer-by-layer deposition** of materials. Each process operates on distinct physical principles and material systems, influencing precision, porosity, and mechanical performance.

Extrusion-based AM creates continuous filaments by extruding hydrogels or fluid polymers through a nozzle; these filaments harden when cooled or crosslinked. It is frequently used in bioprinting, which produces living tissue constructions using inks loaded with cells. Cell survival, interlayer bonding, and pore shape are all influenced by extrusion factors like pressure, nozzle diameter, and extrusion rate. Using high-energy lasers, Powder Bed Fusion (PBF) processes including Selective Laser Sintering (SLS) and Selective Laser Melting (SLM) fuse powdered metals, polymers, or ceramics [32]. Porosity, surface roughness, and residual stress are influenced by the laser power, scan speed, and layer thickness. Orthopedic load-bearing implants with customized porosity for osseointegration can be made thanks to PBF.

Droplets of metallic, biological, or polymeric ink are deposited onto substrates via inkjet printing, which has a resolution of microns. Because the procedure is non-contact, gradient and multi-material deposition are possible. It is very helpful for microfluidic systems, medication delivery patches, and biosensors. Stereolithography (SLA) and two-photon polymerization are examples of laser-based fabrication, which uses light to cure photosensitive polymers. These techniques produce smooth surfaces and high precision (sub-micron), making them appropriate for optical devices and microstructured scaffolds.

Printing factors, including temperature, feed rate, and ambient conditions, control the behavior of materials during deposition in all AM systems. These elements affect porosity, dimensional precision, and interlayer adhesion all of which are essential for both biological and mechanical performance. By maximizing these variables, printed constructions for biomedical applications can attain the ideal ratio of permeability, mechanical strength, and cell compatibility.

9.4.3 Nano–Macro Integration

The integration of nanomaterials into additive manufacturing platforms to produce hierarchically organized composites that blend macroscale shape with nanoscale functionality is the real horizon of next-generation biomaterials. The benefits of both scales are combined in this nano–macro integration: AM guarantees spatial accuracy and design freedom, while nanoscale materials offer bioactivity and responsiveness [33, 34].

Performance can be greatly improved by adding nanomaterials to AM inks, resins, and powders. For example, incorporating graphene or carbon nanotubes improves electrical conductivity for brain or cardiac scaffolds, while adding hydroxyapatite nanoparticles to polymeric bioinks improves osteoconductivity. Likewise, silver nanoparticles give 3D-printed implants antibacterial qualities that lower the chance of infection.

The multiscale organization of the ECM can be replicated by layering nanofibrous mats inside printed scaffolds using hybrid fabrication techniques like electrospinning and 3D printing. This produces materials that can control the dynamics of tissue regeneration, promote nutrient diffusion, and guide cell alignment. Additionally, in situ synthesis, which creates nanoparticles during the AM process, has become a cutting-edge technique to enhance interfacial bonding and dispersion. These integrated systems are an example of a multiscale engineering paradigm, in which superior mechanical and biological results are achieved by smoothly integrating nanoscale cues into macroscale structures.

9.4.4 Interface and Bonding Mechanisms

Interface and bonding mechanisms that control stress transfer, degradation, and bioactivity are essential to the development of nanocomposites and hybrid biomaterials. How fillers or nanoparticles interact with the surrounding matrix at the nanoscale is determined by interfacial energy. Effective load transfer and the avoidance of microcrack start are guaranteed by good adhesion. In order to improve the bonding between inorganic fillers and polymer matrices, methods including surface functionalization, plasma treatment, and coupling agents (such silanes) are employed. Nanointerfaces also affect the distribution of stress and the rate of degradation in composite systems. While inadequate interfacial adhesion speeds up mechanical weakening and hydrolytic breakdown, a well-bonded interface can inhibit degradation by limiting fluid penetration. By adjusting the interfacial chemistry, biodegradable implants can synchronize their rates of degradation with the kinetics of tissue repair.

Protein adsorption and cellular response at the biointerface are determined by the surface characteristics of the materials. While reducing inflammatory signaling, nanostructured surfaces with regulated roughness and charge distribution encourage cell adhesion and proliferation. The significance of surface energy management in attaining both structural and biological performance is highlighted by these interfacial phenomena.

9.4.5 Post-Processing and Functionalization

Post-processing procedures improve durability, accuracy, and biocompatibility by refining structural and chemical characteristics after production. Thermal processes called annealing and sintering enhance the mechanical strength, interlayer adhesion, and crystallinity of AM-fabricated parts. Sintering densifies the material in ceramic and metal printing, improving fatigue resistance and decreasing porosity. In order to change surface chemistry without compromising bulk properties, plasma treatments are frequently employed. Functional groups added by oxygen or nitrogen plasma improve polymeric scaffolds' hydrophilicity and cell adhesion. Enhancing surface smoothness through laser polishing and mechanical finishing is essential for lowering bacterial colonization and enhancing implant wear resistance.

The biological extension of post-processing is called functionalization. It entails affixing growth factors, peptides, or bioactive compounds to material surfaces to alter biological reactions. For instance, grafting heparin or nitric oxide donors encourages the endothelialization of vascular implants, whereas immobilizing RGD peptides on scaffold surfaces improves integrin-mediated adhesion. Furthermore, ligand distribution can be spatially controlled by nanopatterning techniques, which can affect cell alignment and differentiation. Together, these processes specify the process by which materials evolve from mechanical prototypes to biomaterials with clinical functionality, guaranteeing the improvement of structural, chemical, and biological characteristics for specific medical uses.

Modern biomaterial engineering is based on the mechanisms and procedures that underline additive manufacturing and nanomaterial synthesis. Every step, from synthesis and integration to interface design and functionalization, helps to create adaptive, high-performance biomedical systems, from the atomic assembly of nanostructures to the digital stacking of complicated geometries. While additive manufacturing gives architectural control and patient-specific tailoring, nanomaterial synthesis processes provide the surface functionality and chemical accuracy required for biointeraction [35, 36]. Their combination, guided by interfacial research and improved by post-processing, produces materials that are both biologically informative and mechanically robust.

As research advances, understanding these multiscale processes will remain central to developing next-generation hybrid materials that bridge the nano–macro divide capable of dynamic response, seamless integration, and long-term functionality within the human body.

9.5 Design Considerations

The combination of additive manufacturing (AM) and nanomaterials in biomedical engineering necessitates a complex balancing act between biological compatibility, production accuracy, and material qualities. The AM–nanomaterial interface adds multiscale design complexity, ranging from atomic-level interactions to macroscopic geometries, in contrast to conventional production, where performance is determined by bulk materials. Optimization in the mechanical, thermal, and biological domains as well as sustainability and safety considerations are necessary for successful translation into clinical applications. The main design factors affecting the scalability, performance, and dependability of AM systems based on nanomaterials are examined in this section.

9.5.1 Material–Process Compatibility and Printability Optimization

For AM to succeed, material-process compatibility is essential. Direct ink writing (DIW), selective laser sintering (SLS), stereolithography (SLA), and fused deposition modeling (FDM) all place unique chemical, rheological, and thermal restrictions on the feedstock materials. It is very difficult to guarantee printability for systems based on nanomaterials without aggregation or degradation. In order to preserve mechanical integrity and prevent nozzle blockage or uneven energy absorption during sintering or curing, nanoparticles, nanofibers, and nanocomposites must be uniformly distributed inside polymeric or metallic matrices. Consistent extrusion and layer adhesion are ensured by rheological tuning, which can be accomplished by solvent optimization, surface modification, or binder addition [37, 38].

The addition of nanomaterials like graphene, hydroxyapatite, or gold nanoparticles to polymer-based AM changes its viscosity and thermal conductivity, which has an immediate impact on flow characteristics and layer bonding. Therefore, printability optimization entails balancing macroscale accuracy and nanoscale uniformity by modifying print temperature, speed, and layer height. Similarly, to prevent phase segregation or porosity problems in metal or ceramic AM, the laser power and scanning speed must match the melting or sintering thresholds of the nanoparticles. In the end, process–material compatibility is the cornerstone of the manufacturing of nanostructured biomaterials since it determines both geometric accuracy and functional performance.

9.5.2 Nanoscale Control for Tuning Mechanical, Thermal, and Biological Functions

The capacity to adjust material performance through nanoscale design is one of the distinguishing features of nanomaterial–AM systems. Grain refinement, nanoparticle reinforcement, or controlled porosity can all improve mechanical qualities including stiffness, tensile strength, and fatigue resistance. For instance, load transmission and dislocation pinning processes at the nanoscale result in greater yield strength in titanium or polymer–hydroxyapatite nanocomposites. Nanomaterials enhance thermal conductivity and dissipation, which is important in devices like neural implants and biosensors where tissue damage is avoided by thermal stability. As thermal and electrical bridges, carbon-based nanostructures such as graphene and carbon nanotubes (CNTs) evenly distribute current across printed electrodes.

From a biological perspective, cell adhesion, migration, and differentiation are regulated by nanoscale topography. Protein adsorption and integrin binding are improved by surface roughness in the 10–100 nm range, which also activates signaling pathways that support osteogenesis or angiogenesis. Immune compatibility and degradation kinetics are further influenced by tailoring the chemistry of nanoparticles, for as by changing surface charge or functional groups. Hierarchical structure, in which nanoscale elements are incorporated inside microscale geometries to replicate native extracellular matrices (ECM), is made possible by advanced AM techniques [39, 40]. Therefore, in addition to determining mechanical and thermal behavior, nanoscale control also coordinates biological reactions that are necessary for tissue integration and regeneration.

9.5.3 Layer Resolution, Geometric Fidelity, and Support Structure Management in AM

The structural and functional accuracy of printed structures is determined by AM's resolution and fidelity. When adding nanomaterials, high-resolution printing is often at the micrometer or sub-micrometer level because load distribution and bioactivity are directly impacted by layer alignment and interfacial bonding. Nozzle diameter, laser spot size, curing wavelength, and particle dispersion are process variables that affect layer resolution and the smallest feature size that may be achieved. Maintaining high fidelity in hydrogel-based AM or bioprinting necessitates precise viscosity control and quick crosslinking kinetics to avoid soft construct collapse or distortion.

Support structures are equally important for maintaining complex lattices and overhanging geometries. The choice of detachable or biodegradable supports that are compatible with biological habitats is crucial for systems that use nanomaterials. Cellular adhesion may be compromised by improper clearance, which may leave residues or change surface roughness. Additionally, to avoid phase separation or nanoparticle migration, dimensional stability during post-processing such as sintering or curing must be maximized. Mechanical anisotropy and porosity, which affect diffusion, vascularization, and cell infiltration in biomedical scaffolds, are defined by the interaction of resolution and geometry. Thus, careful coordination between material rheology, printer calibration, and support design is necessary to achieve geometric fidelity with nanoscale precision.

9.5.4 Biocompatibility and Cytotoxicity Evaluation of Nanomaterials

Although nanoparticles offer better functioning, there are still serious issues with their biocompatibility and even cytotoxicity. Because of their reactive surface chemistry and high surface area-to-volume ratio, materials interact with cells and proteins differently at the nanoscale. Unintended consequences including oxidative stress, DNA damage, or inflammatory reactions may result from this. Both in vitro and in vivo testing are used to assess biocompatibility, with an emphasis on immunological modulation, cytotoxicity, and hemocompatibility. Nonspecific protein adsorption is frequently decreased and immunological activation is avoided by surface coatings or functionalization with biopolymers such as collagen or PEG [41]. For instance, surface modification of graphene or silver nanoparticles is necessary to reduce macrophage activation and stop the production of reactive oxygen species (ROS).

The printing process itself can change the characteristics of materials in AM systems; if left unchecked, thermal degradation, leftover monomers, or unreacted photoinitiators can all be cytotoxic. Hence, sterilization and post-processing techniques (e.g., autoclaving, UV treatment, or solvent extraction) are crucial to assuring safety. Reproducibility and compliance are guaranteed when AM procedures are integrated with standardized ISO 10993 biocompatibility testing frameworks. Clinical translation of nanostructured AM biomaterials ultimately depends on striking a balance between biological safety and nanoscale functioning.

9.5.5 Scalability, Reproducibility, and Cost–Performance Balance

Despite achievements in the lab, scalability and repeatability issues hinder the industrial use of nanomaterial-based AM technologies. It might be challenging to maintain exact synthesis conditions and surface stability for nanomaterials on a big scale. Additionally, because agglomeration results in mechanical heterogeneity and uneven performance, homogeneous nanoparticle dispersion in bulk feedstocks continues to be a manufacturing bottleneck. Batch-to-batch uniformity in mechanical strength, porosity, and resolution is another requirement for additive manufacturing systems. These problems can be lessened by automated quality control using real-time imaging, sensor feedback, and AI-based mistake correction; nevertheless, these systems raise manufacturing costs.

Hybrid manufacturing techniques are required to balance cost and performance, combining traditional fabrication for bulk components with high-resolution AM for crucial sections. The high cost of creating nanoparticles and running a printer is partially mitigated by AM's intrinsic material economy, recyclability, and less waste. The commercial success of nanomaterial-enabled biomedical devices, such as drug delivery systems, tissue scaffolds, and orthopedic implants, will depend on their capacity to scale with regulated accuracy.

9.5.6 Integration of Computational Modeling and AI for Process Prediction and Defect Control

Artificial intelligence (AI) and computational modeling are now essential tools for improving nanomaterial–AM processes. By simulating heat gradients, stress distribution, and phase evolution during printing, finite element modeling (FEM) aids in the prediction of warping, delamination, or the production of microcracks. To create prediction connections between input variables and part quality, AI and machine learning (ML) algorithms examine large process datasets, such as print settings, sensor feedback, and post-print inspection [42, 43]. For instance, using laser energy density and nanoparticle dispersion uniformity, ML can forecast the establishment of porosity. Recent work on biomedical metal 3D printing shows that combining AI with nanomaterials can improve print-quality prediction, defect detection, material-property forecasting and patient-specific implant design, although standardised datasets and clearer regulatory pathways remain important barriers [44].

Computational material design frameworks can screen the best nanomaterial compositions for desired mechanical and biological properties at the design stage. Additionally, biomimetic structures that mimic vascular networks and tissue anisotropy are made possible by AI-driven generative design. Additionally, repeatability can be ensured by dynamically adjusting print parameters to remedy for faults with real-time adaptive control systems that integrate AI with sensor feedback. By combining experimental validation with computer prediction, researchers can increase performance and speed up development cycles.

9.5.7 Environmental and Safety Considerations in Nanomaterial and AM Handling

Workplace safety and environmental sustainability are becoming critical requirements in AM and nanomaterial processes. Particularly when handling, combining, or post-processing powders, nanoparticles can provide dangers for inhalation, skin contact, and environmental exposure. The use of personal protective equipment (PPE), enclosed chambers, and HEPA filtration reduces the discharge of airborne nanoparticles. Waste management is also important: solvents containing nanoparticles and polymer remnants need to be disposed of carefully to avoid contaminating the environment. Persistent metallic or carbon nanostructures have a larger long-term ecological impact than biodegradable nanomaterials like chitosan or PLGA.

From a sustainability standpoint, solvent-free manufacturing, recyclable feedstocks, and energy-efficient printing techniques lower operating expenses and carbon emissions. Data-driven decision-making for sustainable design is made possible by lifecycle assessment (LCA) technologies, which measure the environmental impact of the synthesis, processing, and disposal of nanomaterials. Furthermore, responsible management of nanomaterials during the production, testing, and clinical application phases is ensured by adherence to regulatory frameworks like REACH and ISO/TS 12901. The ethical and business basis of AM technologies based on nanomaterials is strengthened when environmental care and technological innovation are combined.

A multifaceted approach is required for designing nanomaterial-enabled additive manufacturing systems for biomedical applications, where printability, biological safety, and nanoscale precision converge with sustainability and computational optimization [45, 46]. The development of adaptive, high-performing, and ecologically friendly biomaterials is being made possible by the convergence of nanoscale material design, AM process control, and AI-driven modeling, which is revolutionizing the field of personalized medicine. In order to ensure that the next generation of nanostructured biomedical devices satisfies both technological and ethical standards for global healthcare innovation, future success in this field depends on striking a balanced balance between engineering precision, clinical efficacy, and ecological sustainability.

9.6 Applications and Case Studies

The combination of additive manufacturing (AM) with nanomaterials has made it possible to design, fabricate, and functionalize biomedical devices with previously unheard-of precision. By offering patient-specific, mechanically tuned, and physiologically integrated solutions, these technologies have revolutionized applications in the domains of soft tissue engineering, drug delivery, orthopedics, dentistry, cardiovascular disease, and biosensing. This examines the most recent uses as well as case studies that highlight clinical translation and regulatory issues.

9.6.1 Bone and Orthopedic Implants

Orthopedic reconstruction has been transformed by the additive fabrication of metallic nanostructured scaffolds, especially titanium and its alloys. By encouraging osteoblast adhesion, proliferation, and differentiation, nanoscale surface changes such as anodization, acid etching, and nanopatterning improve osseointegration [47,

48]. Stress shielding and long-term implant failure are decreased by 3D-printed porous titanium scaffolds with regulated lattice architecture, which offer mechanical characteristics matched to the surrounding bone. Recent scaffold-focused evidence confirms that biomaterial selection, composite design, biodegradability, biomimicry and porous architecture are decisive factors controlling cellular response and regenerative performance in AM-based tissue-engineering scaffolds [49].

In a clinical investigation, complicated tibial lesions were treated with patient-specific 3D-printed titanium scaffolds that had nanoscale surface roughness. When compared to traditional implants, the scaffolds showed improved integration and promoted early bone ingrowth; at 6 months, radiographic evidence of remodeling was seen. Regulatory approval relied on ASTM F2982–16 standards for AM metallic implants, highlighting the interplay of material characterization, biocompatibility, and mechanical testing in clinical translation.

9.6.2 Dental and Craniofacial Reconstruction

Dental and craniofacial prosthetics tailored to each patient with improved mechanical strength and bioactivity are made possible by nanoceramic-filled polymer composites, such as hydroxyapatite–polycaprolactone (HA–PCL). The incorporation of nanoceramics enhances osteoconductivity, wear resistance, and surface hardness, while AM enables tailored geometries that fit the anatomy of the patient. Selective laser sintering (SLS) was used to create nanoceramic-embedded PCL scaffolds for a few craniofacial restorations. Excellent structural fit, a shorter recovery period, and a low inflammatory response were all shown in the postoperative results. Regulatory compliance required mechanical examination under simulated masticatory stresses and biocompatibility testing in accordance with ISO 10993 standards. This illustration emphasizes how crucial it is to combine AM design freedom with nanoscale material qualities for functional restoration.

9.6.3 Cardiovascular Devices

Stents and biodegradable scaffolds are examples of cardiovascular implants with nanostructured surfaces that provide improved endothelialization, anti-thrombogenicity, and hemocompatibility. Platelet aggregation is decreased and endothelial cell adhesion is enhanced by nanotexturing and surface functionalization with bioactive coatings. For resorbable vascular devices, additive manufacturing offers exact control over the strut thickness, scaffold shape, and degradation patterns.

For coronary procedures, biodegradable polymeric stents with AM-controlled porosity and incorporated silver nanoparticles were tested. Over a 12-month period, in vivo experiments showed incremental bioresorption, decreased neointimal hyperplasia, and fast endothelialization. Comprehensive preclinical cardiovascular safety evaluations were part of the regulatory considerations, emphasizing the incorporation of data on nanomaterial cytotoxicity with AM manufacturing validation.

9.6.4 Drug Delivery and Biosensing

Highly accurate platforms for real-time biosensing and regulated medication release have been made possible by the combination of nanomaterials and AM microdevices. Within 3D-printed matrices, polymeric nanocarriers, liposomes, and nanoparticles offer adjustable release kinetics without sacrificing structural integrity. At the same time, biosensing electrodes can be integrated into AM-fabricated microchannels to provide multiplexed physiological parameter monitoring [10]. For targeted post-surgical treatment, a 3D-printed hydrogel implantable microdevice containing PLGA nanoparticles loaded with anti-inflammatory medications was tested. The apparatus enabled optical biosensing of local pH variations suggestive of inflammation and achieved sustained release over a period of six weeks. In accordance with ISO 13485 quality management systems, regulatory clearance placed a strong emphasis on both device functionality and material biocompatibility.

9.6.5 Soft Tissue Engineering

Skin, muscle, and peripheral nerve tissue regeneration are made possible by 3D bioprinting hydrogel-nanofiber composites. Recent reviews on 3D bioprinting highlight that bioink design, cell viability, vascularisation, maturation and reproducibility remain central requirements for translating printed tissues from laboratory constructs into functional tissues and organ-like systems [50]. Hydrogels sustain a moist, bioactive environment for cellular growth, while nanofibers such as silk fibroin or electrospun PCL offer topographical cues and mechanical support for cell alignment. AM makes it possible to replicate intricate tissue structures and gradient compositions by layer-by-layer deposition. Bioprinted dermal scaffolds with embedded nanofibers were used in a clinical pilot to treat persistent wounds. Four weeks later, histological examination showed minimal fibrotic encapsulation, improved vascularization, and ordered collagen deposition. To guarantee patient safety, regulatory channels mandated preclinical safety investigations, sterility validation, and ISO 10993 biocompatibility evaluations. The viability of incorporating nanoparticles into AM-based soft tissue constructions for functional repair is illustrated by this example. Recent regenerative-medicine literature emphasises that 4D printing extends conventional 3D bioprinting by introducing time-dependent responsiveness, allowing printed constructs to change shape, stiffness, porosity or drug-release behaviour under stimuli such as pH, temperature, light or humidity [51].

9.6.6 Clinical Translation and Regulatory Milestones

Reproducible fabrication, regulatory compliance, and thorough characterization are essential for the effective clinical use of nanomaterials in conjunction with additive manufacturing. Important standards are ISO 10993 for biocompatibility, ISO 13485 for quality management, and ISO/ASTM for AM. Examples from the fields of soft tissue, drug delivery, dentistry, orthopedics, and cardiovasculars show how nanoscale engineering improves mechanical performance, biological integration, and patient-specific personalization. Furthermore, establishing material traceability, producing clinical evidence to support preclinical investigations, and upholding strict post-market surveillance are all critical to translational success. In addition to AM's complexity in terms of reproducibility and process validation, nanomaterials provide special regulatory issues, such as cytotoxicity, biodistribution, and long-term safety [52, 53]. Collaborative engagement with regulatory authorities, clinicians, and patients is essential to ensure that advanced biomaterial devices meet both safety and efficacy requirements.

In a variety of biomedical fields, nanomaterials combined with additive manufacturing have shown revolutionary potential. Precision, customization, and improved biological performance are made possible by technologies ranging from bioresorbable vascular devices and responsive medication delivery systems to osseointegrating orthopedic scaffolds and patient-specific craniofacial implants. Successful clinical translation is demonstrated by case studies, underscoring the significance of exacting material characterization, AM process validation, and regulatory compliance. In order to create safe, efficient, and customized biomedical solutions, future research is probably going to concentrate on multifunctional hybrid systems, real-time biosensing integration, and the ongoing convergence of nanotechnology and additive manufacturing.

9.7 Recent Advances and Innovations

The design, manufacture, and functionalization of biomedical constructions are being revolutionized by the convergence of nanotechnology and additive manufacturing (AM), which is a frontier in contemporary biomaterials science. A new class of multifunctional materials and intelligent manufacturing systems that can replicate biological complexity at the micro- and nanoscale have emerged as a result of ongoing advancements in this field [54, 55]. From stimuli-responsive 4D printing to nanoscale bioprinting, hybrid inks, AI-driven design, sustainable additive manufacturing, and microfluidic-integrated systems, this examines recent developments that are revolutionizing biomedical engineering and leading to the development of nanorobotics for targeted medical intervention as shown in Fig. 9.2.

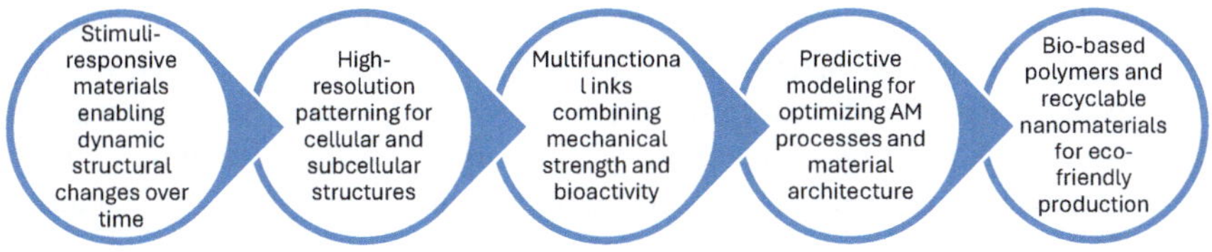

Fig. 9.2 Recent advances and innovations in the integration of nanotechnology and additive manufacturing, highlighting developments such as 4D printing, nanoscale bioprinting, hybrid nanocomposite inks, AI-driven design, sustainable additive manufacturing, microfluidic-integrated systems, and emerging nanorobotics

9.7.1 4D Printing Technologies: Stimuli-Responsive Materials for Dynamic Functionality

By adding time as a transformative parameter, 4D printing goes beyond conventional 3D printing. Stimuli-responsive nanomaterials allow printed structures to respond to external stimuli like light, pH, temperature, or magnetic fields by changing their shape, mechanical characteristics, or function on their own. 4D-printed scaffolds made of shape-memory polymers supplemented with nanofillers (such as graphene or carbon nanotubes) are being developed for use in biomedical applications. These scaffolds are intended to dynamically adapt to the morphology of the tissue throughout the healing or regeneration process. Self-folding implants for less invasive treatments are made possible by these materials, which also provide adaptive mechanical compliance. Additionally, by directing cell alignment, vascularization, and biointegration, nanoscale surface patterning in 4D constructions can improve regeneration results. Thus, patient-specific implants that change in tandem with biological processes are made possible by the combination of nanotechnology and 4D printing.

9.7.2 Nanoscale Bioprinting: Precision Fabrication of Cellular and Subcellular Architectures

Cells, biomolecules, and extracellular matrix (ECM)-mimetic materials can now be precisely positioned thanks to recent developments in nanoscale bioprinting technologies that have attained submicron precision. Techniques including laser-assisted bioprinting, electrohydrodynamic jet printing, and two-photon polymerization (TPP) have made it possible to create vascular microchannels, neural networks, and even organoid templates with cellular fidelity. The intricate microenvironments present in natural tissues can be replicated and cell–matrix interactions are improved by nanoscale regulation of spatial structure. Additionally, localized medication administration, biosensing, or photothermal therapy within engineered tissues are made possible by including nanoparticles such as silica nanospheres or gold nanorods into printed bioinks. A crucial first step toward the creation of functional tissue regeneration and organs is the development of bioprinting devices that can generate gradient structures and dynamic cell habitats [56, 57].

9.7.3 Hybrid Nanocomposite Inks: Multifunctional Materials for Mechanical and Biological Integration

The range of materials available for AM has been greatly expanded by the development of hybrid nanocomposite inks. These inks provide multifunctional biomaterials with exceptional mechanical, electrical, and biological qualities by combining polymers, ceramics, and metallic nanoparticles. For instance, hydroxyapatite nanoparticles added to polycaprolactone (PCL) matrices have improved compressive strength and osteoconductivity, which makes them perfect for creating bone scaffolds. Similarly, carbon nanotubes or PEDOT:PSS enhance conductivity for neurological and cardiac applications, while silver and copper nanoparticles provide antibacterial activity. In order to guarantee printability and structural integrity, recent research has concentrated on improving interfacial bonding, rheological control, and nanoparticle dispersion within inks. Additionally, gradient scaffolds where bioactivity or mechanical stiffness vary spatially can be used with hybrid inks to imitate diverse tissue architectures like vascularized bone or osteochondral interfaces.

9.7.4 AI-Driven Design and Simulation: Computational Intelligence in AM Optimization

Machine learning and artificial intelligence are becoming essential for developing AM enabled by nanomaterials. Researchers can forecast print quality, maximize material deposition, and reduce structural flaws by incorporating AI algorithms into process monitoring and design workflows. Relationships between printing settings, mechanical strength, porosity, and degradation rate, as well as nanoscale architecture, are now simulated by data-driven models. Additionally, biomimetic designs optimized for electrical conductivity, nutritional transport, or stress distribution can be automatically explored using generative design frameworks. Adaptive printing is also made possible by AI-enhanced control systems, where sensors offer real-time feedback to dynamically modify curing strength, laser power, or extrusion speed [58]. AI basically turns AM from a static fabrication process into an intelligent manufacturing ecosystem that corrects itself, speeding up clinical translation and regulatory compliance.

9.7.5 Green and Sustainable Additive Manufacturing: Eco-Responsibility in Material Innovation

In AM and nanomaterials research, sustainability has become a crucial design requirement. To reduce its influence on the environment, Green AM promotes the use of solvent-free processes, bio-based polymers, and biodegradable nanofillers. For example, renewable-source cellulose nanocrystals (CNCs) and polylactic acid (PLA) are being used to create environmentally acceptable scaffolds. In biomedical manufacturing, recyclable metallic nanoparticles and carbon-based nanostructures further advance the concepts of the circular economy. Additionally, by only generating the necessary number of components, AM's digital production method naturally minimizes material waste. Nanocomposite materials' energy consumption, emissions, and end-of-life biodegradation are being evaluated using life-cycle analysis (LCA) frameworks more and more. Thus, the combination of AM and green chemistry maintains performance criteria necessary for clinical safety while bringing biomedical innovation into line with global sustainability goals.

9.7.6 Microfluidic-Integrated Printing

A revolutionary development in the creation of lab-on-chip and organ-on-chip systems for tissue engineering, disease modeling, and drug testing is microfluidic-integrated AM. This method creates perfusable conduits that resemble physiological microenvironments by combining nanoscale patterning with microscale fluid manipulation. Through direct printing of nanocomposite hydrogels and biopolymers into microfluidic architectures, scientists have created biomimetic structures that facilitate cellular activity monitoring in real time, endothelialization, and nutrition transfer. For example, brain and cardiac chips with incorporated nanosensors can simultaneously capture biochemical indicators and electrical impulses. Rapid prototyping of multi-organ systems connected by vascular-like channels is made possible by integration with 3D printing, which speeds up personalized treatment and lessens the need for animal testing [59, 60]. Fully automated, AI-controlled platforms that can simulate intricate organ-level operations on demand are the key to the future of microfluidic-AM convergence.

9.7.7 Nanorobotics and Autonomous Systems

One of the most exciting results of fusing AM technology with nanomaterials is nanorobotics. For targeted medication administration, biosensing, and microsurgery, nanoscale actuators, sensors, and propulsion systems often made using high-precision additive techniques are being developed. These nanorobots can navigate biological fluids and deliver therapeutic payloads to specific cellular sites with previously unheard-of precision thanks to magnetic, acoustic, or chemical propulsion methods. Functionalization with stimuli-responsive nanoparticles and biocompatible coatings guarantees minimum immunogenicity and regulated release. Autonomous nanosystems are expected to carry out tissue regeneration, microfluidic construction, and brain regulation via mechanical or electrical stimulation in addition to medication delivery. The combination of nanorobotics and AM-driven fabrication represents a revolutionary step toward autonomous, intelligent, and customized healthcare systems, despite ongoing issues with scalability, control, and regulatory approval [61].

A new era of precision biomaterial engineering marked by sustainability, intelligence, and adaptability has been brought about by the combination of nanotechnology and additive manufacturing. The limits of biomedical design and function are being redefined by recent advancements, ranging from AI-driven optimization and nanorobotics to 4D printing and nanoscale bioprinting. Implants, scaffolds, and other devices that more closely resemble living systems can be made possible by the nanoscale engineering of hierarchical designs, dynamic materials, and integrated sensing capabilities. The next generation of biomedical manufacturing is expected to include autonomous treatment systems, self-healing implants, and responsive tissue interfaces as multi-modal production, green materials, and computer intelligence continue to progress. Together, these developments represent a paradigm shift away from passive biomaterials and toward active, regenerative, and intelligent platforms that have the potential to revolutionize clinical care and personalized medicine [62, 63].

9.8 Challenges and Limitations

Significant advancements in biomedical engineering, including high-performance implants, drug delivery systems, and tissue scaffolds, have been made possible by the combination of nanomaterials with additive manufacturing (AM). Notwithstanding these groundbreaking successes, the industry still faces a number of biological, technical, and legal obstacles that restrict clinical translation, scalability, and reproducibility. These difficulties are brought on by the intricacy of controlling at the nanoscale, the delicate nature of biological systems, and the changing state of digital manufacturing technology. Comprehending these constraints is essential for streamlining manufacturing procedures, guaranteeing patient security, and directing forthcoming advancements.

9.8.1 High Production Cost and Scalability Issues of Nanomaterial Synthesis

The high cost and limited scalability of synthesis techniques are two of the most enduring problems in the biomedical manufacturing of nanomaterials. Methods like electrospinning, sol-gel synthesis, and chemical vapor deposition (CVD) call for specialized equipment, costly precursors, and well regulated conditions.

Large-scale, repeatable production is challenging due to these characteristics, especially for intricate hybrid nanostructures. Although bottom-up synthesis techniques can produce homogeneous nanoparticles with exacting characteristics, they frequently have poor yields and protracted reaction times. On the other hand, top-down techniques like lithography or milling can create more, but they sacrifice structural accuracy [64, 65]. It is still very difficult to achieve industrial-level throughput while preserving nanoscale uniformity.

Additionally, problems with batch variability, contamination risk, and process repeatability arise when laboratory synthesis is scaled up to clinical-grade manufacturing. Although they are being investigated, cost-effective substitutes like continuous-flow chemical reactors or green synthesis employing biological agents have not yet attained the reliability criteria necessary for regulatory certification. Thus, the broad use of nanomaterials in biomedical AM is still limited by their cost feasibility.

9.8.2 Print Resolution Limits and Layer Adhesion Challenges in Nanoscale AM

Achieving genuine nanoscale resolution is still a technological challenge, even though additive printing allows more fine geometric control. Many AM methods, including selective laser sintering (SLS) and fused deposition modeling (FDM), function at the microscale, with minimum feature sizes usually exceeding 50–100 μm. Even cutting-edge methods like nanolithography-based bioprinting and two-photon polymerization (2PP) must balance material compatibility, printing speed, and precision. The performance and structural integrity of printed structures are further diminished by poor surface roughness and interlayer adhesion. Controlling heat transport, curing rate, and layer fusion at the nanoscale becomes extremely sensitive to the ambience and composition of the material. Excessive heat or photonic energy in bioprinting can denature proteins or harm implanted cells, making attempts to integrate nanostructures with living systems more challenging.

There is potential for overcoming resolution limits through research into hybrid fabrication techniques, such as combining AM with electrospinning or inkjet nanoparticle deposition. These methods are still expensive, though, and need for complex process coordination. It is therefore a continuous engineering challenge to increase nanoscale precision while preserving scalability and biological compatibility.

9.8.3 Cytotoxicity and Environmental Concerns Related to Nanoparticle Exposure

Major issues impeding the clinical and industrial adoption of nanomaterials are their cytotoxicity and environmental impact. Because of oxidative stress, membrane rupture, and DNA damage in cells, many nanoparticles, including silver, zinc oxide, and carbon-based nanostructures, demonstrate dose-dependent toxicity [66]. These impacts may impair tissue compatibility, cause inflammation, or change immunological responses in biological applications. When nanoparticles are released during production, handling, or disposal, there is a chance that they will bioaccumulate and disturb the ecosystem. Nanoparticles could penetrate biological membranes and get into soil or water systems, where they may disrupt trophic chains and microbial communities.

Although surface functionalization and biodegradable nanocomposites have advanced, there is still disagreement on acceptable exposure levels and uniform toxicity evaluation procedures. Public acceptance and regulatory approval are made more difficult by this ambiguity. For additive manufacturing to be integrated sustainably, eco-safe nanomaterials must be developed using green chemistry and thorough life-cycle assessment.

9.8.4 Lack of Standardization in Testing and Regulatory Approval

The lack of standardized testing procedures and regulatory frameworks is a major obstacle to the clinical translation of nanomaterial–AM products. For evaluating nanoscale properties including particle size distribution, surface charge, and quantum effects, conventional evaluation techniques such as those specified by ISO or ASTM for bulk materials are insufficient. Additionally, the performance of the finished item is impacted by the complexity that additive manufacturing adds in relation to digital design parameters, printing accuracy, and post-processing unpredictability. Preliminary guidelines for AM medical devices have started to be released by regulatory agencies like the FDA and EMA, however they frequently ignore nanospecific interactions in favor of macroscopic aspects.

The absence of uniform certification requirements makes it difficult for producers and labs to replicate results consistently. Establishing metrology frameworks, risk assessment models, and validation techniques that consider the special characteristics of nanostructured AM materials requires interdisciplinary cooperation between material scientists, engineers, and legislators in order to close this gap.

9.8.5 Reproducibility and Reliability of Mechanical and Biological Performance

Consistent mechanical strength and biological performance in AM products based on nanomaterials are still very difficult to achieve. Mechanical properties including stiffness, fatigue resistance, and toughness can be significantly changed by slight changes in particle size, dispersion, or interfacial bonding. Comparably, variations in surface chemistry at the nanoscale affect cell adhesion, proliferation, and differentiation, resulting in a range of biological outcomes. Porosity and interlayer bonding are further impacted by AM's process-dependent inconsistencies with regard to layer thickness, print orientation, and heat gradients. Therefore, depending on ambient factors and equipment calibration, similar digital designs might produce different physical and functional features.

For implantable devices, where variations in mechanical or biological response can jeopardize safety and effectiveness, reproducibility problems are especially troublesome. Although AI-driven process optimization, closed-loop feedback control, and advanced in situ monitoring are showing promise as remedies, their incorporation into biomedical manufacturing workflows is still lacking.

9.8.6 Integration Challenges in Combining Nanostructures with Living Cells (Bioprinting)

In bioprinting, combining nanostructures with living cells presents special challenges from a scientific and practical standpoint. Nanomaterials can improve cellular activity by supplying mechanical and biochemical cues, but if they are not properly regulated, they can potentially impair cell viability. It is still technically difficult to disperse nanoparticles uniformly within bioinks without causing toxicity or agglomeration. Furthermore, shear stress, crosslinking kinetics, and environmental factors like pH and temperature must all be balanced to preserve cell viability during printing. Through modifications to viscosity, gelation behavior, and nutrient diffusion, nanostructures can tamper with these properties.

The dynamic mismatch between biological and synthetic components is another drawback. Over time, integration or degradation incompatibilities may arise because nanostructured scaffolds frequently stay static while living tissues expand and remodel. The development of intelligent, bioresponsive nanocomposites that dynamically adjust to cellular and physiological cues during tissue maturation is necessary to address these issues.

9.8.7 Data, Software, and Hardware Interoperability Limitations in AM Workflows

Digital workflows comprising computer-aided design, simulation, and machine control software are essential to additive manufacturing. Interoperability between these systems is still restricted, though. Data loss and incompatibility during design transfer result from the proprietary file formats, toolpaths, and calibration standards used by various AM systems. Precision manufacture at the nanoscale necessitates real-time feedback loops that integrate design, process, and metrology data; yet, this integration is rarely supported by the hardware and software infrastructure now in use [67]. Innovation is slowed down and reproducibility is hampered by this divergence. Although open-source AM software and efforts like ISO/ASTM52900 to define digital manufacturing protocols are increasing transparency, complete interoperability across design, simulation, and fabrication platforms is still a way off. The efficient use of digital twins and AI-driven optimization for the predictive modeling of nanostructured AM systems is further restricted by the absence of consistent data architecture.

There is enormous potential for improving regenerative medicines and customized medicine at the nexus of nanotechnology and additive manufacturing. However, achieving this promise necessitates overcoming formidable obstacles in the areas of digital integration, affordability, reproducibility, and biocompatibility. An interdisciplinary strategy combining materials science, biomedical engineering, regulatory science, and computational modeling is needed to address these problems. The creation of interoperable digital manufacturing ecosystems, uniform regulatory frameworks, and scalable green synthesis techniques will be essential to future advancement. Nanomaterial-AM technologies can progress from experimental prototypes to clinically dependable, financially viable, and morally sound biomedical solutions by methodically resolving these constraints [68, 69].

9.9 Future Directions

There is enormous potential for improving regenerative medicines and customized medicine at the nexus of nanotechnology and additive manufacturing. However, achieving this promise necessitates overcoming formidable obstacles in the areas of digital integration, affordability, reproducibility, and biocompatibility. An interdisciplinary strategy combining materials science, biomedical engineering, regulatory science, and computational modeling is needed to address these problems. The creation of interoperable digital manufacturing ecosystems, uniform regulatory frameworks, and scalable green synthesis techniques will be essential to future advancement. Nanomaterial-AM technologies can progress from experimental prototypes to clinically dependable, financially viable, and morally sound biomedical solutions by methodically resolving these constraints. AI-assisted AM is moving toward autonomous and self-optimising manufacturing, where machine learning, reinforcement learning, physics-informed models and digital twins can improve lattice design, process control and multifunctional smart-material fabrication [70].

9.9.1 Integration of Nanomaterials with 4D Bioprinting for Adaptive and Self-Healing Biomedical Systems

A revolutionary step toward the development of biological systems that are adaptive and self-healing is the combination of nanomaterials and 4D bioprinting. With 4D bioprinting, as opposed to traditional 3D printing, printed structures can gradually alter their mechanical characteristics, shape, or bioactivity in response to physiological stimuli like pH, temperature, or magnetic fields. The responsiveness and functionality of these systems are improved by the addition of nanomaterials, such as graphene, carbon nanotubes, or magneto-responsive nanoparticles. For example, conductive nanocomposites allow for dynamic electrical stimulation in cardiac or brain tissues, and self-healing hydrogels with nanoscale reinforcements can repair structural integrity following mechanical injury. This method has the potential to create scaffolds and implants that actively contribute to tissue regeneration and repair while also adjusting to the changing physiological environment.

9.9.2 Development of AI-Guided Manufacturing Ecosystems for Precision and Personalization

In the context of biomaterials enabled by nanomaterials, artificial intelligence (AI) will be crucial to the transformation of additive manufacturing processes. Real-time sensing, predictive modeling, and autonomous decision-making are all integrated into AI-guided manufacturing ecosystems to maximize print quality, minimize defects, and customize material qualities to meet the demands of specific patients. The ability of machine learning algorithms to interpret data at several scales, ranging from macroscopic mechanical behavior to nanoscale particle dispersion, allows for process modification during production. AI can also suggest new topologies that are optimal for biological response, porosity, and stress distribution using generative design techniques. These systems may simulate every stage of a biomedical device's lifespan, from virtual design to clinical performance prediction, when paired with digital twin technology [71]. This improves repeatability and speeds up regulatory approval. In the end, AI-powered personalization will close the gap between patient-specific manufacturing and computational modeling.

9.9.3 Use of Biodegradable Nanocomposites for Transient Implants and Regenerative Scaffolds

The development of biodegradable nanocomposites is a significant step toward the development of temporary medicinal implants that serve their purpose before safely dissolving inside the body. To improve mechanical strength and bioactivity, these materials which are based on polymers like poly(lactic-co-glycolic acid), polylactic acid, and polycaprolactone (PCL) can be supplemented with inorganic nanoparticles like magnesium oxide, silica, or hydroxyapatite. At the nanoscale, tissue responsiveness and degradation kinetics can be precisely controlled by adjusting particle dispersion and interfacial bonding. A parallel development for transient monitoring or stimulation devices that decompose after therapeutic use are transient electronics, which are constructed from biodegradable conductive nanomaterials [72, 73]. Such materials significantly reduce the need for secondary surgeries and minimize long-term immune complications, advancing the field of regenerative and minimally invasive medicine.

9.9.4 Advances in Multi-Material Additive Manufacturing for Functional Gradient Designs and Hybrid Devices

Future biomedical systems will depend more on multi-material additive manufacturing platforms that can create objects with functional gradients, or spatially variable qualities. This feature makes it possible to design intricate biomimetic structures in which biochemical cues, stiffness, and porosity all smoothly adapt to the environment of the original tissue. For instance, gradient scaffolds that support both soft tissue and mineralized properties are necessary for the interfaces between bone and tendon and bone and cartilage. By adding nanoparticles to these systems, it is possible to locally adjust the electrical conductivity, medication release profiles, or mechanical reinforcement. In order to create integrated devices with electronics, sensors, and microfluidic networks, hybrid additive manufacturing processes which include methods such as direct ink writing (DIW), selective laser sintering (SLS), and stereolithography (SLA) are being investigated. These multipurpose structures open the door for next-generation implants that can transport drugs, stimulate tissue, and monitor in real time.

9.9.5 Expansion of Nanosafety Research and Standardized Bioevaluation Frameworks

Strong nanosafety evaluation and regulatory harmonization are becoming increasingly important as the usage of nanomaterials in biomedical manufacturing grows. Because of their high reactivity and surface area, nanoparticles can interact with biological systems in unpredictable ways, possibly causing genotoxicity, inflammation, or oxidative stress. Nanoscale impacts are frequently missed by current safety evaluation techniques, which were created for bulk materials. Standardized testing protocols covering nanoparticle characterization, biodistribution analysis, and long-term biocompatibility studies must be the main emphasis of future research. Establishing internationally accepted standards for medical devices based on nanomaterials will require cooperation between regulatory organizations like the OECD, ASTM, and ISO. Simultaneously, AI-driven predictive models and computational toxicology can help detect any risks early in the design stage, guaranteeing the ethical and safe development of nanobiomaterials.

9.9.6 Merging Quantum and Nanoscale Phenomena for Ultra-Sensitive Diagnostics and Therapies

Using quantum effects for biomedical innovation is one of the most innovative areas of nanomaterials research. The potential of plasmonic nanoparticles, nitrogen-vacancy nanodiamonds, and quantum dots as ultra-sensitive diagnostic probes that can identify molecular interactions with previously unheard-of accuracy is being investigated. The creation of implantable biosensors that continuously track cerebral activity or cellular metabolism may be made possible by the combination of quantum sensing with AM platforms. Additionally, targeted cancer treatments with less off-target harm are provided by quantum-enhanced photothermal and photodynamic therapies. Advances in bioelectronic interfaces, where quantum tunneling and entanglement events may enhance signal transmission between synthetic electrodes and biological tissues, are another area where the convergence of quantum mechanics and nanotechnology holds promise. Precision medicine's therapeutic specificity and diagnostic sensitivity will be redefined by such technologies.

9.9.7 Global Collaboration in Digital Manufacturing and Open-Source Biomaterial Design

AM and nanomaterials have a collaborative, global future by nature. High-performance technologies are becoming more widely accessible because to open-source platforms for digital manufacturing and biomaterial design, which are encouraging interdisciplinary innovation in academia, business, and healthcare [74]. Researchers from all over the world can effectively expand on current knowledge thanks to shared databases of printed biomaterials, nanoscale characterization data, and simulation models. This trend toward data transparency and collaborative fabrication is best illustrated by global projects like the National Institutes of Health (NIH) 3D Print Exchange and the European Open Science Cloud (EOSC). Decentralized AM facilities with standardized nanomaterial libraries have the potential to transform local healthcare manufacturing into low- and middle-income areas by creating patient-specific, reasonably priced implants on demand. The transition of nanomaterial-based technologies from the lab to international clinical practice will be accelerated by this communal ecosystem.

Convergence across disciplines, technologies, and scales defines the future course of additive manufacturing and nanomaterials. Biodegradable nanocomposites will bring about sustainable, temporary medical devices; AI-driven production will guarantee accuracy and customization; and the incorporation of nanomaterials into 4D bioprinting will allow for responsive, self-healing systems. Quantum-enabled devices will transform molecular-level diagnosis and treatment, while multi-material AM and nanosafety research will increase functionality while maintaining ethical responsibility. In the end, open-source innovation and international cooperation will be the cornerstones of rapid and equitable biomedical progress. As AM and nanotechnology develop together, they have the potential to change healthcare into a regenerative, intelligent, and adaptable industry where materials actively contribute to human health and healing [75, 76].

9.10 Conclusion

One of the most revolutionary advances in modern biomaterials science is the combination of nanomaterials and additive manufacturing (AM). Once separated, these two technological frontiers now work together to create next-generation biomedical systems that combine biological functionality and precision engineering. Researchers and physicians are gaining unprecedented control over mechanical behavior, regenerative potential, and biological interactions as materials are formed through digital manufacturing and nanoscale engineering. A paradigm change from static, passive implants to intelligent, adaptive, and patient-specific biomedical systems is represented by this fusion of nanoscale science and macroscale production.

9.10.1 *Summary of Nanomaterials and Additive Manufacturing as Converging Frontiers in Biomaterials Science*

Nanomaterials have transformed biomaterials research during the last 20 years by providing control over cellular and molecular responses through surface chemistry, size, and quantum-level effects. The design and creation of intricate, hierarchical structures that replicate the architecture of native tissues has also changed as a result of additive manufacturing. The development of hierarchically constructed scaffolds, implants, and devices that perform over many length scales is made possible by their convergence, which closes the gap between molecular functionality and structural accuracy.

While AM guarantees geometric integrity, porosity control, and patient-specific tailoring, nanomaterials such as nanoparticles, nanotubes, and nanofibers provide bioactivity, conductivity, and mechanical reinforcement. When combined, they make it possible to create multipurpose systems with directed tissue regeneration, real-time sensing, and controlled medication release. This combined capability of structural design and biological performance is demonstrated by applications in brain interfaces, cardiovascular stenting, bone regeneration, and dental restoration. By incorporating nanoparticles into AM inks, powders, or resins, features like conductivity, degradation rate, and cellular affinity can be customized, further increasing the adaptability of materials. A new class of "smart" biomaterials that can react dynamically to environmental changes and physiological stimuli is the end product, signaling a significant advancement in biomedical device engineering and regenerative medicine.

9.10.2 *Emphasis on Precision, Functionality, and Customization as Design Imperatives*

Precision, utility, and customisation are the three main design requirements that result from the integration of nanomaterials with AM. In addition to geometric accuracy, precision also relates to molecular control, which defines surface topography, chemical composition, and microstructural gradients that determine interactions between cells and materials. Through surface modification, lithography, and self-assembly, nanotechnology makes this kind of accuracy possible, and AM converts these characteristics into repeatable macroscale structures. Functionality includes biological and electronic reactivity in addition to mechanical support. AM constructions loaded with nanomaterials can resist bacterial colonization through nanostructured surfaces, convey electrical signals for neuronal interfacing, or release medicinal compounds as needed. Hierarchical design allows for this multifunctionality, with each level from bulk shape to nanoscale texture contributing in a synergistic way to total performance.

Perhaps the biggest change in the idea of biomedical design is customization. Implants and scaffolds can be customized to match the anatomy, pathologies, and genetic profile of each patient using digital manufacturing that is guided by medical imaging and computational modeling. Personalized implants, such as biodegradable scaffolds, dental crowns, or titanium hip joints, can now be made quickly and with material compositions tailored for certain therapeutic settings. The ability to customize precision manufacturing is changing the parameters for patient outcomes, safety, and efficacy.

9.10.3 *Recognition of Interdisciplinary Integration*

Multidisciplinary integration is key to the success of AM enabled by nanomaterials. Biomaterials research currently relies on the integration of materials science, data engineering, nanotechnology, and clinical translation; it is no longer adequate for the area to function just within the confines of chemistry or biology. While engineers tune AM settings and computer models for performance prediction, materials scientists offer the fundamental knowledge of the correlations between nanostructure and properties. The functional requirements and safety standards required for human application are simultaneously defined by doctors and biomedical researchers. This cooperation is strengthened by the incorporation of data-driven technologies like artificial intelligence (AI) and machine learning, which make it possible to forecast print results, degradation kinetics, and host reactions.

By connecting laboratory innovation with patient-specific application, this convergence also speeds up the clinical translation pipeline. Interdisciplinary teams can create systems that not only satisfy performance requirements but also dynamically change within live tissues by fusing digital design with biological knowledge. In the end, combining these fields promotes a more comprehensive and systems-based method of designing biomaterials.

9.10.4 Outlook toward Sustainable, Adaptive, and Patient-Specific Manufacturing Paradigms

In the future, it is anticipated that the combination of AM and nanotechnology will support a flexible and sustainable biomaterials production paradigm. The adoption of circular material cycles, green synthesis techniques, and biodegradable nanocomposites will be fueled by growing concerns about environmental and economic sustainability. The digital flexibility of additive manufacturing will enable localized fabrication, on-demand production, and effective resource usage, lowering waste and transportation-related emissions. The next generation of nanomanufactured biomaterials will also be characterized by their adaptability. Real-time monitoring and feedback systems will be incorporated into future scaffolds and implants, allowing for the autonomous modification of characteristics like stiffness, rate of degradation, or medication release in response to the advancement of tissue regeneration. With the help of AI and embedded biosensors, these intelligent systems will make it harder to distinguish between live tissue and devices.

Furthermore, developments in imaging and computer modeling will support the shift toward patient-specific fabrication. Personalized regeneration systems can be created directly from patient data using AI-based optimization and bioprinting, launching a new era of precision medicine where each patient's care is as distinct as they are.

9.10.5 Final Reflection: The Evolution Toward Intelligent and Regenerative Nanomanufactured Biomedical Systems

More than just technical advancement, the development of biomaterials research toward intelligent and regenerative nanomanufactured systems represents a conceptual change in the way medicine interacts with the human body. The new paradigm sees biomaterials as active contributors to adaptation and healing, able to sense, react, and change with biological tissues rather than as passive replacements. In this regard, additive manufacturing gives architectural flexibility and customization, while nanotechnology offers the means of molecular signaling and cell-level communication. Together, they lay the groundwork for a future in which scaffolds actively remodel, implants regenerate tissue, and biosensors provide real-time therapeutic guidance.

The lines between biology and technology will continue to blur as interdisciplinary cooperation expands and digital manufacturing advances. Therefore, the combination of AM and nanomaterials is a defining feature of the shift to patient-centered, data-driven, and adaptive healthcare, where intelligent design and regenerative capabilities come together to improve integration, restore function, and reshape the future of human health. The progression from nanoscale discovery to clinical translation essentially embodies the core of biomaterials science in the twenty-first century a smooth fusion of accuracy, flexibility, and regeneration that fundamentally alters the notion of what biomedical systems are capable of.

References

1. Chakraborty, A., Ravi, S.P., Shamiya, Y., Cui, C., Paul, A.: Harnessing the physicochemical properties of DNA as a multifunctional biomaterial for biomedical and other applications. Chem. Soc. Rev. **50**(13), 7779–7819 (2021)
2. Tripathi, G.K.: Engineered nanomaterials and their properties: a review. Biosci. Biotechnol. Res. Commun. **12**, 764–771 (2019)
3. Aflori, M.: Smart nanomaterials for biomedical applications—a review. Nano. **11**(2), 396 (2021)
4. Mabrouk, M., Das, D.B., Salem, Z.A., Beherei, H.H.: Nanomaterials for biomedical applications: production, characterisations, recent trends and difficulties. Molecules. **26**(4), 1077 (2021)
5. Cardoso, R.V., Pereira, P.R., Freitas, C.S., Paschoalin, V.M.F.: Trends in drug delivery systems for natural bioactive molecules to treat health disorders: the importance of nano-liposomes. Pharmaceutics. **14**(12), 2808 (2022)
6. Yetisgin, A.A., Cetinel, S., Zuvin, M., Kosar, A., Kutlu, O.: Therapeutic nanoparticles and their targeted delivery applications. Molecules. **25**(9), 2193 (2020)
7. Bhatti, S.S., Singh, J.: 3D printing of biomaterials for biomedical applications: a review. Int. J. Interact. Des. Manuf. (IJIDeM), 1–22 (2023)
8. Kafle, A., Luis, E., Silwal, R., Pan, H.M., Shrestha, P.L., Bastola, A.K.: 3D/4D printing of polymers: fused deposition modelling (FDM), selective laser sintering (SLS), and stereolithography (SLA). Polymers. **13**(18), 3101 (2021)
9. Rehman, M., Yanen, W., Mushtaq, R.T., Ishfaq, K., Zahoor, S., Ahmed, A., Kumar, M.S., Gueyee, T., Rahman, M.M., Sultana, J.: Additive manufacturing for biomedical applications: a review on classification, energy consumption, and its appreciable role since COVID-19 pandemic. Prog. Addit. Manuf. **8**(5), 1007–1041 (2023)
10. Zhao, W., Wang, Z., Zhang, J., Wang, X., Xu, Y., Ding, N., Peng, Z.: Vat photopolymerization 3D printing of advanced soft sensors and actuators: from architecture to function. Adv. Mater. Technol. **6**(8), 2001218 (2021)
11. Fidan, I., Huseynov, O., Ali, M.A., Alkunte, S., Rajeshirke, M., Gupta, A., Hasanov, S., Tantawi, K., Yasa, E., Yilmaz, O., Loy, J.: Recent inventions in additive manufacturing: holistic review. Inventions. **8**(4), 103 (2023)

12. Ghomi, E.R., Khosravi, F., Neisiany, R.E., Singh, S., Ramakrishna, S.: Future of additive manufacturing in healthcare. Current Opinion in Biomedical Engineering. **17**, 100255 (2021)
13. Amani, H., Arzaghi, H., Bayandori, M., Dezfuli, A.S., Pazoki-Toroudi, H., Shafiee, A., Moradi, L.: Controlling cell behavior through the design of biomaterial surfaces: a focus on surface modification techniques. Adv. Mater. Interfaces. **6**(13), 1900572 (2019)
14. Cai, S., Wu, C., Yang, W., Liang, W., Yu, H., Liu, L.: Recent advance in surface modification for regulating cell adhesion and behaviors. Nanotechnol. Rev. **9**(1), 971–989 (2020)
15. Gaspar, V.M., Lavrador, P., Borges, J., Oliveira, M.B., Mano, J.F.: Advanced bottom-up engineering of living architectures. Adv. Mater. **32**(6), 1903975 (2020)
16. Sahebalzamani, M., Ziminska, M., McCarthy, H.O., Levingstone, T.J., Dunne, N.J., Hamilton, A.R.: Advancing bone tissue engineering one layer at a time: a layer-by-layer assembly approach to 3D bone scaffold materials. Biomater. Sci. **10**(11), 2734–2758 (2022)
17. Lee, C.Y., Hu, S.M., Christy, J., Chou, F.Y., Ramli, T.C., Chen, H.Y.: Biointerface coatings with structural and biochemical properties modifications of biomaterials. Adv. Mater. Interfaces. **10**(10), 2202286 (2023)
18. Billings, C., Cai, C., Liu, Y.: Utilization of antibacterial nanoparticles in photocurable additive manufacturing of advanced composites for improved public health. Polymers. **13**(16), 2616 (2021)
19. Man, K., Brunet, M.Y., Jones, M.C., Cox, S.C.: Engineered extracellular vesicles: tailored-made nanomaterials for medical applications. Nano. **10**(9), 1838 (2020)
20. Chansoria, P., Schuchard, K., Shirwaiker, R.A.: Process hybridization schemes for multiscale engineered tissue biofabrication. Wiley Interdiscip. Rev. Nanomed. Nanobiotechnol. **13**(2), e1673 (2021)
21. Wang, Q., Zhou, P., Liu, S., Attarilar, S., Ma, R.L.W., Zhong, Y., Wang, L.: Multi-scale surface treatments of titanium implants for rapid osseointegration: a review. Nano. **10**(6), 1244 (2020)
22. Zhu, G., Wang, G., Li, J.J.: Advances in implant surface modifications to improve osseointegration. Mater. Adv. **2**(21), 6901–6927 (2021)
23. Harish, V., Tewari, D., Gaur, M., Yadav, A.B., Swaroop, S., Bechelany, M., Barhoum, A.: Review on nanoparticles and nanostructured materials: bioimaging, biosensing, drug delivery, tissue engineering, antimicrobial, and agro-food applications. Nano. **12**(3), 457 (2022)
24. Sanità, G., Carrese, B., Lamberti, A.: Nanoparticle surface functionalization: how to improve biocompatibility and cellular internalization. Front. Mol. Biosci. **7**, 587012 (2020)
25. Jana, S., Bandyopadhyay, A., Datta, S., Bhattacharya, D., Jana, D.: Emerging properties of carbon based 2D material beyond graphene. J. Phys. Condens. Matter. **34**(5), 053001 (2021)
26. Sahudin, M.R., Zourob, M., Noor Akashah, M.H., Abdul Rani, R., Makhsin, S.R.: Physical properties of graphene. J. Mech. Eng. **12**(1), 225–267 (2023)
27. Hadidi, N., Mohebbi, M.: Anti-infective and toxicity properties of carbon based materials: graphene and functionalized carbon nanotubes. Microorganisms. **10**(12), 2439 (2022)
28. Liu, W., Speranza, G.: Functionalization of carbon nanomaterials for biomedical applications. C. **5**(4), 72 (2019)
29. Guzzi, E.A., Tibbitt, M.W.: Additive manufacturing of precision biomaterials. Adv. Mater. **32**(13), 1901994 (2020)
30. Khalilov, R.: A comprehensive review of advanced nano-biomaterials in regenerative medicine and drug delivery. Adv. Biol. Earth Sci. **8**(1), 5–18 (2023)
31. Abdelkawi, A., Slim, A., Zinoune, Z., Pathak, Y.: Surface modification of metallic nanoparticles for targeting drugs. Coatings. **13**(9), 1660 (2023)
32. DiNoro, J.N., Paxton, N.C., Skewes, J., Yue, Z., Lewis, P.M., Thompson, R.G., Beirne, S., Woodruff, M.A., Wallace, G.G.: Laser sintering approaches for bone tissue engineering. Polymers. **14**(12), 2336 (2022)
33. Sadeghi, B., Cavaliere, P.D.: Reviewing the integrated design approach for augmenting strength and toughness at macro-and micro-scale in high-performance advanced composites. Materials. **16**(17), 5745 (2023)

34. Verma, A., Kapil, A., Klobčar, D., Sharma, A.: A review on multiplicity in multi-material additive manufacturing: process, capability, scale, and structure. Materials. **16**(15), 5246 (2023)
35. Challagulla, N.V., Rohatgi, V., Sharma, D., Kumar, R.: Recent developments of nanomaterial applications in additive manufacturing: a brief review. Curr. Opin. Chem. Eng. **28**, 75–82 (2020)
36. Singh, J., Singh, G., Pandey, P.M.: Additive manufacturing of functionalized nanomaterials for the modern health care industry. In: Additive Manufacturing with Functionalized Nanomaterials, pp. 55–85. Elsevier (2021)
37. Alghamdi, H., Nair, S.A., Neithalath, N.: Insights into material design, extrusion rheology, and properties of 3D-printable alkali-activated fly ash-based binders. Mater. Des. **167**, 107634 (2019)
38. Ma, S., Fu, S., Yang, T., Li, K., Chen, G., Dong, Q., He, P., Sun, Z., Duan, X., Jia, D., Colombo, P.: Unveiling the critical role of rheology modifiers in additive manufacturing of geopolymers and their mechanical properties. Addit. Manuf. **78**, 103826 (2023)
39. Jooken, S., Deschaume, O., Bartic, C.: Nanocomposite hydrogels as functional extracellular matrices. Gels. **9**(2), 153 (2023)
40. Lemos, R., Maia, F.R., Reis, R.L., Oliveira, J.M.: Engineering of extracellular matrix-like biomaterials at nano-and macroscale toward fabrication of hierarchical scaffolds for bone tissue engineering. Adv. NanoBiom. Res. **2**(2), 2100116 (2022)
41. Kruk, T., Bzowska, M., Hinz, A., Szuwarzyński, M., Szczepanowicz, K.: Control of specific/nonspecific protein adsorption: functionalization of polyelectrolyte multilayer films as a potential coating for biosensors. Materials. **14**(24), 7629 (2021)
42. Fua, Y., Downeya, A., Yuana, L., Prattc, A., Balogunc, Y.: In situ monitoring for fused filament fabrication process: a review. Laser. ***97***, 103–110. This is an author-created, un-copyedited version of an article published in additive manufacturing (2021). https://doi.org/10.1016/j.addma.2020.101749
43. Martakis, P., Movsessian, A., Reuland, Y., Pai, S.G., Quqa, S., Garcia Cava, D., Tcherniak, D., Chatzi, E.: A semi-supervised interpretable machine learning framework for sensor fault detection. Smart Struct. Syst. Int. J. **29**, 251–266 (2022)
44. Liu, J., Jeevanandam, J., Danquah, M.K.: Enhancing biomedical metal 3D printing with AI and nanomaterials integration. Meta. **15**(10), 1163 (2025). https://doi.org/10.3390/met15101163
45. Shajari, S., Kuruvinashetti, K., Komeili, A., Sundararaj, U.: The emergence of AI-based wearable sensors for digital health technology: a review. Sensors. **23**(23), 9498 (2023)
46. Yilmaz, N.D.: Smart nanotextiles applications: a general overview. In: Smart Nanotextiles: Wearable and Technical Applications, pp. 1–85. Wiley (2022)
47. Hou, C., An, J., Zhao, D., Ma, X., Zhang, W., Zhao, W., Wu, M., Zhang, Z., Yuan, F.: Surface modification techniques to produce micro/nano-scale topographies on Ti-based implant surfaces for improved osseointegration. Front. Bioeng. Biotechnol. **10**, 835008 (2022)
48. Stich, T., Alagboso, F., Křenek, T., Kovářík, T., Alt, V., Docheva, D.: Implant-bone-interface: reviewing the impact of titanium surface modifications on osteogenic processes in vitro and in vivo. Bioeng. Trans. Med. **7**(1), e10239 (2022)
49. Vyas, J., Raytthatha, N., Vyas, P., Prajapati, B.G., Uttayarat, P., Singh, S., Chittasupho, C.: Biomaterial-based additive manufactured composite/scaffolds for tissue engineering and regenerative medicine: a comprehensive review. Polymers. **17**(8), 1090 (2025). https://doi.org/10.3390/polym17081090
50. Ullah, M.W., Ul-Islam, M., Shehzad, A., Manan, S., Islam, S.U., Fatima, A., Al-Saidi, A.K., El Nokab, M.E.H., Sanchez, J.Q., Sebakhy, K.O.: From bioinks to functional tissues and organs: advances, challenges, and the promise of 3D bioprinting. Macromol. Mater. Eng. **310**(12), e00251 (2025). https://doi.org/10.1002/mame.202500251
51. Alanazi, B.N.: Exploring 4D printing of smart materials for regenerative medicine applications. RSC Adv. **15**(39), 32155–32171 (2025). https://doi.org/10.1039/D5RA04410C

52. Ahmad, A., Imran, M., Sharma, N.: Precision nanotoxicology in drug development: current trends and challenges in safety and toxicity implications of customized multifunctional nanocarriers for drug-delivery applications. Pharmaceutics. **14**(11), 2463 (2022)
53. Tirumala, M.G., Anchi, P., Raja, S., Rachamalla, M., Godugu, C.: Novel methods and approaches for safety evaluation of nanoparticle formulations: a focus towards in vitro models and adverse outcome pathways. Front. Pharmacol. **12**, 612659 (2021)
54. Chen, Z., Lin, Y.T., Salehi, H., Che, Z., Zhu, Y., Ding, J., Sheng, B., Zhu, R., Jiao, P.: Advanced fabrication of mechanical metamaterials based on micro/nanoscale technology. Adv. Eng. Mater. **25**(22), p.2300750 (2023)
55. Sonkaria, S., Khare, V.: Exploring the landscape between synthetic and biosynthetic materials discovery: important considerations via systems connectivity, cooperation and scale-driven convergence in biomanufacturing. Biomanuf. Rev. **5**(1), 1 (2020)
56. Bertassoni, L.E.: Bioprinting of complex multicellular organs with advanced functionality—recent progress and challenges ahead. Adv. Mater. **34**(3), 2101321 (2022)
57. Gao, Q., Kim, B.S., Gao, G.: Advanced strategies for 3D bioprinting of tissue and organ analogs using alginate hydrogel bioinks. Mar. Drugs. **19**(12), 708 (2021)
58. Okiye, S.E., Nwokediegwu, Z.S., Bankole, A.O.: Simulation-driven design of 3D printed public infrastructure: from bus stops to benches. Shodhshauryam, Int. Sci. Ref. Res. J. **6**(4), 285–320 (2023)
59. Chesnais, F., Joel, J., Hue, J., Shakib, S., Di Silvio, L., Grigoriadis, A.E., Coward, T., Veschini, L.: Continuously perfusable, customisable, and matrix-free vasculature on a chip platform. Lab Chip. **23**(4), 761–772 (2023)
60. Chliara, M.A., Elezoglou, S., Zergioti, I.: Bioprinting on organ-on-chip: development and applications. Biosensors. **12**(12), 1135 (2022)
61. Wang, Y., 2022. Design for Circular Cosmetics: a Smart and Green Device for Circular Cosmetic
62. Alshangiti, D.M., El-Damhougy, T.K., Zaher, A., Madani, M.: Revolutionizing biomedicine: advancements, applications, and prospects of nanocomposite macromolecular carbohydrate-based hydrogel biomaterials: a review. RSC Adv. **13**(50), 35251–35291 (2023)
63. Kantaros, A., Ganetsos, T.: From static to dynamic: smart materials pioneering additive manufacturing in regenerative medicine. Int. J. Mol. Sci. **24**(21), 15748 (2023)
64. Peng, Y., Yang, W.: 2D metal-organic framework materials for membrane-based separation. Adv. Mater. Interfaces. **7**(1), 1901514 (2020)
65. Phillips, J.W., Prominski, A., Tian, B.: Recent advances in materials and applications for bioelectronic and biorobotic systems. View. **3**(3), 20200157 (2022)
66. Abbasi, R., Shineh, G., Mobaraki, M., Doughty, S., Tayebi, L.: Structural parameters of nanoparticles affecting their toxicity for biomedical applications: a review. J. Nanopart. Res. **25**(3), 43 (2023)
67. Amici, J., Asinari, P., Ayerbe, E., Barboux, P., Bayle-Guillemaud, P., Behm, R.J., Berecibar, M., Berg, E., Bhowmik, A., Bodoardo, S., Castelli, I.E.: A roadmap for transforming research to invent the batteries of the future designed within the European large scale research initiative BATTERY 2030+. Adv. Energy Mater. **12**(17), 2102785 (2022)
68. Velu, R., Calais, T., Jayakumar, A., Raspall, F.: A comprehensive review on bio-nanomaterials for medical implants and feasibility studies on fabrication of such implants by additive manufacturing technique. Materials. **13**(1), 92 (2019)
69. Zhang, Y., Poon, K., Masonsong, G.S.P., Ramaswamy, Y., Singh, G.: Sustainable nanomaterials for biomedical applications. Pharmaceutics. **15**(3), 922 (2023)
70. Zaman, S., Mahmud, M.S., Mollick, A.A., Lhaden, T., Dantzler, J., Arroyo, S., Goona, N.K., Mesbah, M., Ahsan, M.A., Lin, Y.: Artificial intelligence in additive manufacturing: advances in smart materials, lattice optimization, and process intelligence. Int. J. Adv. Manuf. Technol., 1–15 (2026). https://doi.org/10.1007/s00170-026-18072-y
71. Sahal, R., Alsamhi, S.H., Brown, K.N.: Personal digital twin: a close look into the present and a step towards the future of personalised healthcare industry. Sensors. **22**(15), 5918 (2022)

72. Dutta, A., Cheng, H.: Pathway of transient electronics towards connected biomedical applications. Nanoscale. **15**(9), 4236–4249 (2023)
73. Jamshidi, R., Taghavimehr, M., Chen, Y., Hashemi, N., Montazami, R.: Transient electronics as sustainable systems: from fundamentals to applications. Adv. Sustainable Syst. **6**(2), 2100057 (2022)
74. Mazzolai, B., Mondini, A., Del Dottore, E., Margheri, L., Carpi, F., Suzumori, K., Cianchetti, M., Speck, T., Smoukov, S.K., Burgert, I., Keplinger, T.: Roadmap on soft robotics: multifunctionality, adaptability and growth without borders. Multifunct. Mater. **5**(3), 032001 (2022)
75. Bhatia, R.: Emerging health technologies and how they can transform healthcare delivery. J. Health Manag. **23**(1), 63–73 (2021)
76. Kuo, C.L.: Revolutionizing healthcare paradigms: the integral role of artificial intelligence in advancing diagnostic and treatment modalities. Int. Microsurg. J. (IMJ). **7**, 4 (2023)

Chapter 10
Regulatory, Ethical, and Future Perspectives Introduction

Abstract Modern medicine has changed because of the quick development of biomaterials, which has made advances in precision medication delivery, implantable technology, and regenerative therapy possible. However, the need for strong regulatory, moral, and forward-looking frameworks grows more pressing as the complexity of biomaterial systems increases incorporating nanotechnology, artificial intelligence (AI), and biofabrication. In the changing field of biomaterials research and clinical translation, this chapter examines the relationship between scientific innovation, societal responsibility, and governance. Advanced biomaterials research and approval at the regulatory level provide difficulties about long-term biocompatibility evaluation, safety validation, and classification. Conventional criteria for pharmaceuticals and medical devices frequently do not consider hybrid systems that include digital, synthetic, and biological components. Redefining testing procedures with a focus on openness, reproducibility, and patient safety across the preclinical and post-market stages is the goal of emerging standards from global organizations including the FDA, EMA, and ISO. Innovation in biomaterials ethically brings up important issues related to data ownership, patient autonomy, and fair access. Issues with informed consent, algorithmic bias, and socioeconomic disparities in adoption are brought about by the combination of AI-driven diagnostics, bioprinting, and customized implants. Furthermore, environmental effect and sustainability are increasingly important factors in the moral assessment of the creation and disposal of biomaterials. To shape responsible innovation ecosystems, scientists, doctors, ethicists, and politicians must work together globally and practice anticipatory governance. To promote flexible, patient-centered solutions, it is anticipated that digital twins, predictive modeling, and open-source design frameworks will bridge the gap between laboratory research and regulatory scrutiny. In the end, how biomaterials are manufactured, trusted, and maintained within society's larger vision of environmental stewardship and human health will depend on the convergence of regulatory science, ethical consideration, and technical foresight.

M. Adeoba, T. Pandelani, *Application of Biomaterials in Biomedical Engineering*, Series in BioEngineering,
https://doi.org/10.1007/978-3-032-34477-9_10

10.1 Introduction

By combining materials engineering, biology, and clinical medicine, the discipline of biomaterials research is at the forefront of biomedical innovation, developing solutions that improve, replace, or restore the function of human tissue and organs. As the field develops incorporating additive manufacturing, regenerative medicine, artificial intelligence (AI), and nanotechnology its social, ethical, and regulatory aspects have grown in importance for responsible innovation. Biomaterials are dynamic, bioactive, and frequently intelligent systems that may interact with cellular and molecular processes; they are no longer passive structural supports [1, 2]. Although revolutionary, these developments also put into question accepted standards for patient consent, safety evaluation, intellectual property, and public trust. Therefore, understanding the regulatory, ethical, and societal dimensions shaping biomaterials research and application is essential for ensuring that technological progress aligns with patient welfare and global health priorities.

10.1.1 Overview of the Regulatory, Ethical, and Societal Dimensions Shaping Biomaterial Research and Application

A complicated area of healthcare governance is occupied by biomaterials, which combine the characteristics of biological systems, medications, and medical devices. Concerns like long-term biocompatibility, clinical testing, performance validation, and safety are all part of their development and implementation. Although international standardization organizations (ISO, ASTM), the European Medicines Agency (EMA), and the U.S. Food and Drug Administration (FDA) offer frameworks for testing and certifying biomaterials, new hybrid systems like bioelectronic implants and living scaffolds frequently defy established classifications. The use of biomaterials raises ethical questions about fairness, autonomy, and informed permission, especially when the products are customized or come from biological origins. Access to cutting-edge biomaterials and their fair distribution continue to be major social issues, particularly in healthcare settings with limited resources [3].

10.1.2 The Need for Safety, Accountability, and Patient Welfare in Emerging Biomedical Technologies

The foundations of biomaterials research and translation continue to be safety and patient welfare. Materials must exhibit both functionality and predictability under physiological circumstances since they are either implanted into the human body or employed to control cellular activities. For instance, nanomaterials have remarkable surface control and therapeutic potential, but they can also cause cytotoxicity, accumulation, or unexpected immunological reactions. Similarly, to avoid issues linked to degradation, bioresorbable scaffolds and drug-releasing implants need to be carefully regulated. Beyond laboratory validation, biomaterials accountability includes open reporting, moral clinical trial design, and post-market monitoring to monitor long-term results. Furthermore, additional accountability layers are introduced by the use of AI and machine learning in design and testing, necessitating oversight procedures that guarantee algorithmic transparency, bias reduction, and patient data security [4, 5].

10.1.3 Interconnection Between Innovation, Ethics, and Policy in the Lifecycle of Biomaterials from Design to Clinical Use

Biomaterials innovation is closely linked to regulatory policy and ethical considerations; it does not happen in a vacuum. Researchers, regulators, doctors, and end users provide iterative feedback throughout the biomaterial lifecycle, from conception to clinical application. Choosing between synthetic and biological materials during the design stage presents moral dilemmas pertaining to sustainability and sources that are sourced from humans or animals. Adherence to Good Laboratory Practice (GLP) and Good Manufacturing Practice (GMP) during the manufacturing and testing phases guarantees safety and reproducibility. Adherence to ethical concepts like beneficence, non-maleficence, and fairness is also necessary for clinical translation. Policymakers must strike a balance between safeguarding against unfair access or early commercialization and promoting innovation. Thus, governance of biomaterials represents a dynamic co-evolution of technology, ethics, and policy a triad essential to maintaining public trust while fostering scientific advancement [6].

10.1.4 Global Landscape of Regulation and Governance Across Medical Devices, Implants, and Regenerative Materials

Different legal, cultural, and economic circumstances are reflected in the regulation of biomaterials worldwide. In the US, the FDA mostly classifies biomaterials under the medical device category, assigning them a risk classification (Class I–III) and requiring premarket clearance or approval. While they also use a risk-based methodology, the European Medicines Agency (EMA) and the European Union's Medical Device Regulation (MDR) place more emphasis on clinical evidence and post-market vigilance. With nations like China, South Korea, and Japan enforcing standardized standards through the International Medical Device Regulators Forum

(IMDRF), regulatory frameworks in Asia are changing quickly. However, there are still issues with maintaining intellectual property, assuring cross-border data interoperability, and standardizing international testing standards. The distinction between devices and biologics is becoming more hazy for regenerative biomaterials, like stem cell-based scaffolds and bioactive implants, necessitating the creation of new regulatory classifications [7, 8]. In this setting, ethical governance goes beyond compliance and include promoting accountability, inclusion, and openness in global partnerships.

10.1.5 Objectives and Organization of the Chapter Bridging Materials Science, Clinical Translation, and Societal Responsibility

The goal of this chapter is to present a thorough examination of the ethical, regulatory, and future viewpoints that guide the development and application of biomaterials. It places biomaterials in the larger context of biological innovation, where ethical responsibility, public trust, and scientific advancement must coexist. The first section of the debate looks at the fundamental regulatory concepts that control the creation of materials and their clinical usage, highlighting both accomplishments and existing supervision gaps. After that, it looks at ethical issues such patient autonomy, consent, data governance, and sustainability as well as how social justice contributes to fair access to technology. The chapter concludes by outlining potential future paths for biomaterial governance, with a focus on global harmonization initiatives, AI-enabled risk assessment, and adaptive regulatory approaches.

However, there are still issues with maintaining intellectual property, assuring cross-border data interoperability, and standardizing international testing standards. The distinction between devices and biologics is becoming hazier for regenerative biomaterials, like stem cell-based scaffolds and bioactive implants, necessitating the creation of new regulatory classifications [7, 8]. In this setting, ethical governance goes beyond compliance and includes promoting accountability, inclusion, and openness in global partnerships.

10.2 Key Concepts and Definitions

At the nexus of technology, medicine, and society, biomaterials research necessitates strong frameworks to guarantee that innovation is carried out in a responsible and secure manner. Concerns about safety, effectiveness, ethics, and governance become crucial to the development and application of new materials and biomedical technologies that are intended to interact closely with human tissues. Therefore, it is essential to comprehend the fundamental ideas and terms that underpin regulatory science, bioethics, and policy in order to direct the responsible development of the biomaterials industry. From laboratory inception to clinical translation and post-market surveillance, this section outlines the fundamental concepts, terms, and regulatory routes that support the moral and scientific management of biomaterials.

10.2.1 Definition of Regulatory Science Frameworks Ensuring Safety, Efficacy, and Quality of Biomaterials

The systematic body of knowledge and procedures that enable the creation, assessment, and approval of medical products including biomaterials to guarantee their efficacy, safety, and quality is known as regulatory science [9, 10]. It includes the scientific instruments, procedures, and criteria needed to evaluate the performance of novel materials in clinical and environmental settings as well as their interactions with biological systems. By converting scientific discoveries into regulatory evidence that can be used by agencies like the UK Medicines and Healthcare Products Regulatory Agency (MHRA), the European Medicines Agency (EMA), and the U.S. Food and Drug Administration (FDA) to make decisions, regulatory science serves as a link between innovation and public protection.

Regulatory science establishes important validation criteria for biomaterials, including toxicity, mechanical dependability, sterilization stability, degradation kinetics, and biocompatibility. Additionally, it directs the classification of biomaterial-based products according to their intended use and invasiveness, ranging from Class I (low-risk) to Class III (high-risk) medical devices. Crucially, regulatory science is dynamic, changing in response to new technologies that challenge established evaluation frameworks, such as smart implants, nanomaterials, and 3D printing. As a result, using risk-based regulatory models and adaptive pathways, regulatory science not only protects public safety but also fosters innovation.

10.2.2 Definition of Bioethics

The study of moral dilemmas brought about by developments in biology and medicine is known as bioethics, and it offers the moral foundation for ethical innovation, respect for human dignity, and the welfare of society. Bioethics regulates the development, testing, and application of novel materials and technology in human settings in biomaterials research. It makes sure that the advancement of technology doesn't come at the expense of public health and individual liberties. From laboratory studies using human tissues and animal models to clinical trials evaluating the performance and safety of devices, bioethics is practiced on many levels. It highlights risk-benefit analysis, openness, and informed consent as essential components of studies involving human subjects. Furthermore, bioethics tackles new problems brought up by technologies like gene-activated scaffolds, brain implants, and nanomedicine, where interventions conflate the lines between therapeutic augmentation and restoration [11]. Ultimately, bioethics ensures that scientific ambition remains aligned with human welfare, guiding researchers and policymakers toward equitable, just, and humane technological progress.

10.2.3 Concepts of Risk Assessment, Clinical Validation, and Post-Market Surveillance

The operational foundation of regulatory and ethical monitoring is made up of three interrelated procedures: risk assessment, clinical validation, and post-market surveillance.

The methodical identification, measurement, and mitigation of possible risks related to the use of biomaterials constitute risk assessment. This includes assessing the possibility of infection, mechanical failure, degradation byproducts, and toxicological hazards. Clinical performance under real-world circumstances can be predicted with the use of methods like in vitro–in vivo correlation, failure mode analysis, and probabilistic modeling. Clinical validation guarantees the safe and efficient translation of laboratory results into patient treatment. Preclinical testing, clinical trials, and comparative studies are among the methods used to evaluate how well biomaterials work in comparison to current treatments or standards. Thorough validation guarantees that novel materials fulfill therapeutic objectives without sacrificing functionality or safety.

The ongoing observation of biomaterials after they are used in clinical practice is known as post-market surveillance [12, 13]. It includes gathering information on adverse events, device recalls, and long-term outcome evaluations, all of which provide input for product redesign and regulatory revisions. When combined, these procedures create an ongoing feedback loop that promotes evidence-based innovation and preserves patient safety.

10.2.4 Ethical Pillars in Biomedical Innovation

Autonomy, beneficence, non-maleficence, and justice are the four guiding principles of bioethical decision-making in the study and use of biomaterials. The concept of autonomy emphasizes people's right to make knowledgeable decisions regarding their medical care, including the use of innovative biomaterials or implanted technologies. Its practical expression is informed consent, which guarantees that patients are aware of the advantages as well as any possible hazards [14]. Researchers and clinicians are required by beneficence to act in ways that advance the welfare of their patients. In the case of biomaterials, this entails making certain that the materials not only function technically but also enhance health and quality of life. The principle of non-maleficence, which is summed up in the phrase "do no harm," requires that biomaterials not cause toxicity, immunogenicity, or unanticipated problems. The thorough preclinical investigation of material safety and biocompatibility is guided by this idea. Fair distribution of risks and rewards as well as equal access to innovations are necessary for justice. It addresses inequalities in access to healthcare, especially in low-resource environments where cutting-edge biomaterials might not be available or be too expensive. These pillars work together to form a moral framework that upholds ethical integrity throughout the biomaterials lifecycle, from development and testing to marketing and clinical application.

10.2.5 Distinction Between Regulatory Compliance, Ethical Responsibility, and Social Accountability

Despite their frequent overlap, social accountability, ethical responsibility, and regulatory compliance are different but connected aspects of responsible biomaterial innovation.

Adherence to institutionalized standards, laws, and guidelines such as those established by the FDA or ISO that guarantee the safety, effectiveness, and quality of products is known as regulatory compliance. It is a prerequisite that ensures procedural and legal legitimacy. However, ethical obligation goes beyond mere compliance. It entails exercising moral discernment and actively weighing the effects of innovation on society. For instance, even when a neural implant satisfies legal requirements, ethical duty necessitates concerns about identity, privacy, and autonomy.

The wider societal effects of biomaterials research and application are included in the concept of social responsibility. It places a strong emphasis on environmental stewardship, public participation, and openness. Both regulators and the public hold researchers and industries accountable, especially when it comes to sustainability, accessibility, and risk communication. Essentially, gaining compliance, acting morally, and staying accountable to the common good are the three elements that must be harmoniously navigated for biomaterials to make real development [15, 16].

10.2.6 Terminology in Policy and Governance

A sophisticated architecture of international standards and regulatory routes that guarantee uniformity and dependability across jurisdictions forms the foundation of biomaterials governance. The processes and records required for reliable manufacture and quality assurance of biomedical materials and devices are outlined in Good

Manufacturing Practice (GMP). Traceability, reproducibility, and contamination prevention during manufacturing are guaranteed by GMP compliance. Globally accepted standards for biocompatibility testing, sterilization validation, and material performance evaluation are provided by ISO standards, especially ISO 10993 (biological evaluation of medical equipment) and ISO 13485 (quality management systems for medical devices).

Biomaterial-based product approval and monitoring are supervised by regulatory agencies including the FDA (United States), EMA (European Union), and MHRA (United Kingdom). To make sure that materials fulfill specified safety and performance requirements, each uses organized regulatory processes, such as the FDA's 510(k) clearance and Premarket Approval (PMA) or the EMA's CE marking process. These methods are being updated by emerging frameworks, such as adaptive licensing and real-world evidence evaluation, to consider the quick advancement of technology. Regulatory governance is shifting toward dynamic and integrative models that evaluate not just physical properties but also digital and biological activities as biomaterials increasingly integrate AI algorithms, nanotechnology, and bioelectronics.

The conceptual and practical underpinnings of responsible biomaterials innovation are comprised of the fundamental ideas and definitions of both bioethics and regulatory science. While maintaining public trust, they make sure that technical advancements are in line with society standards of safety, justice, and transparency. The concepts of regulation, ethics, and responsibility will continue to change as biomaterials become more complex integrating nanostructures, live cells, and digital intelligence [17, 18]. Comprehending these frameworks is crucial for both compliance and constructing a future where integrity, inclusion, and the uncompromising protection of human welfare serve as the guiding principles for biomedical advancement.

10.3 Material Types and Properties

The biological and mechanical performance of implants and medical devices, as well as their regulatory classification, ethical acceptability, and quality assurance across international healthcare systems, are all determined by the material basis of biomaterials research. From inert metals to bioactive composites and nanostructured polymers, contemporary biomaterials are used for a variety of clinical applications, including medication delivery, tissue regeneration, biosensing, and structural replacement. However, safety assessment, ethical sourcing, and regulatory classification have become extremely difficult due to the growing complexity of material formulas and production processes. Examining the relationship between material type, ethical governance, and regulatory frameworks, this highlights how composition, origin, and reproducibility influence therapeutic results and public confidence in new biomedical innovations.

10.3.1 Regulatory Classification of Biomaterials Based on Risk and Intended Use

The foundation of biomaterial governance is regulatory classification, which directs the level of supervision needed for clinical trials, post-market surveillance, and preclinical research. Most international frameworks classify biomaterials based on their intended use and degree of risk, including those of the European Medicines Agency (EMA), the U.S. Food and Drug Administration (FDA), and the International Medical Device Regulators Forum (IMDRF).

Class I materials, which only need little clinical evidence and simple manufacturing controls, are used in low-risk applications such surgical gloves, sutures, and dental impression compounds. Class II materials are moderately risky and require performance testing, biocompatibility assessment, and adherence to certain standards (e.g., ISO 10993 for biological evaluation of medical devices). Examples of these materials include bone plates, dental fillings, and contact lenses. Heart valves, orthopedic implants, and tissue-engineered scaffolds are examples of class III materials, which are high-risk goods that have direct contact with vital bodily systems [19]. Clinical trials, stringent premarket approval, and frequently ongoing post-implantation monitoring are also necessary.

The conventional device classification approach is under increasing pressure due to the development of regenerative and hybrid systems, including scaffolds loaded with stem cells, drug-eluting implants, and bioelectronic interfaces. The creation of combination product frameworks that address their composite nature is prompted by the fact that these goods frequently fall under several regulatory categories (device, medication, biologic) [20, 21]. As a result, the area of risk-based classification is still evolving and constantly adjusting to new developments that conflate biology and materials.

10.3.2 Influence of Material Composition (Metallic, Polymeric, Ceramic, and Composite) on Safety Evaluation

A biomaterial's inherent chemical and structural makeup has a significant impact on its safety profile and regulatory assessment. Because of their mechanical strength and resistance to corrosion, metallic materials including titanium, stainless steel, and cobalt-chromium alloys are frequently employed in orthopedic, dental, and cardiovascular devices. Strict testing for cytotoxicity, ion leaching, and wear resistance is necessary since metal ion release, galvanic corrosion, and hypersensitivity reactions are still issues in long-term usage. For soft tissue and drug delivery applications, polymeric materials both natural (like collagen and chitosan) and synthetic (such polyethylene glycol (PEG) and polylactic-co-glycolic acid (PLGA)) offer flexibility, degradability, and adjustable qualities. Degradation kinetics, residual monomer toxicity, and possible immunological responses are the main concerns of polymer safety assessments.

Although they are valued for their osteoconductivity and chemical stability in bone regeneration, ceramic biomaterials like hydroxyapatite and bioactive glasses are mechanically fragile and need to be handled carefully during design validation. Because impurities might result in unanticipated in vivo behavior, their purity and crystallinity affect both biological response and regulatory approval routes. Composites add more layers of complexity by integrating ceramic, polymer, or metal components. Strength, elasticity, and bioactivity are all improved by their multiphasic nature, but safety evaluations are made more difficult by the possibility of interfacial degradation and mismatched mechanical or chemical responses [22, 23]. Surface characterisation and compositional mapping are becoming more necessary for regulatory bodies to guarantee consistency and stability among production batches.

10.3.3 Ethical Considerations of Sourcing

One of the most important ethical considerations in the development of biomaterials is material sourcing. Collagen, silk fibroin, and hyaluronic acid are examples of natural biomaterials that are frequently made from human or animal tissues [24]. Concerns about zoonotic contamination dangers, religious acceptability, and sustainability are raised by their use. Collagen obtained from cows or pigs, for example, needs to be thoroughly sterilized and subjected to traceability checks to prevent the spread of illness, and its use in some cultural or religious contexts (such as Islam or Hinduism) may raise ethical concerns. To ensure adherence to bioethical norms, human-derived materials such as decellularized matrices or allografts need ethical supervision and specific donor consent as shown in Fig. 10.1. On the other hand, while synthetic substitutes reduce ethical debate and enhance reproducibility, they could not have the inherent bioactivity of their natural counterparts. As a result, choosing an ethical source frequently requires balancing sustainability, societal ideals, and biological performance.

Global raw material supply chains complicate ethical certification and traceability. Regulatory frameworks and funding organizations are increasingly mandating compliance with responsible sourcing criteria, akin to "ethical mining" or "biomanufacturing stewardship," to guarantee that biomaterials are produced without environmental harm or human rights violations.

10.3.4 Material Traceability and Reproducibility in Manufacturing and Clinical Applications

Every biomaterial component must be traceable, from the acquisition of raw materials to clinical deployment, to comply with basic ethical and regulatory requirements. Strong records of supplier sources, batch numbers, sterilization protocols, and process parameters are required by regulatory systems. This traceability improves post-market surveillance activities and enables the quick detection and recall of faulty batches.

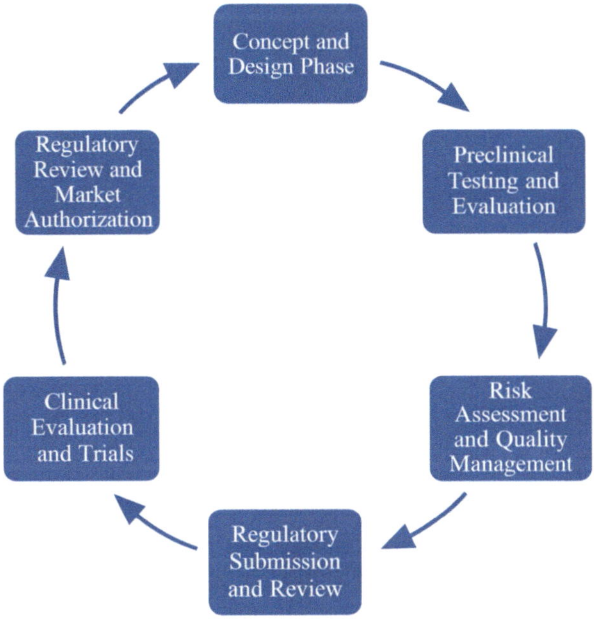

Fig. 10.1 Flowchart outlining the steps involved in regulatory approval of biomaterials, from preclinical testing to market authorization

In biomaterial science, reproducibility is equally important, especially for cutting-edge materials like nanocomposites and 3D-printed implants. Clinical results can be directly impacted by variations in mechanical strength, surface roughness, or degradation rate caused by synthesis or processing variability. Regulatory bodies mandate adherence to ISO 13485 quality management systems and Good Manufacturing Practice (GMP) in order to address this. In order to preserve uniformity between research prototypes and clinical-grade goods, these frameworks standardize the manufacturing, quality assurance, and validation procedures.

Traceability extends to biological reagents and sterilizing techniques as biomaterials increasingly incorporate biological components, such as cells, proteins, or growth hormones. Biological resources are sourced ethically, checked for contamination, and documented at every stage of their lifecycle thanks to ethical oversight [25, 26].

10.3.5 Documentation Requirements for Quality Assurance, Batch Consistency, and Bioequivalence

The procedure of obtaining regulatory approval for biomaterials is supported by extensive documentation. From the examination of raw materials to the testing of the finished product, quality assurance (QA) systems demand thorough documentation of every step of production [27]. It is necessary to show batch consistency through repeatable mechanical, biological, and physicochemical characteristics. Even small deviations have the potential to invalidate clinical data or lead to a reassessment of the safety of the product. Documentation of bioequivalence becomes crucial when altering already-existing materials or procedures. For example, equivalency studies must verify that a manufacturer's modification of a sterilizing procedure or a polymer's molecular weight does not jeopardize safety or efficacy. New and reference batches are compared using methods like mechanical testing, differential scanning calorimetry (DSC), and Fourier-transform infrared spectroscopy (FTIR).

Data integrity verification, risk tracking, and real-time documentation are now made easier by electronic quality management systems (eQMS). Digital traceability, which guarantees openness and auditability throughout the product lifecycle, is becoming more and more necessary for regulatory filings.

10.3.6 Emerging Concerns with Nanomaterials and 3D-Printed Constructs in Regulatory Classification

The science of biomaterials has been transformed by nanomaterials and additive manufacturing (AM), but these technologies also pose challenges to establish regulatory frameworks. Because of their large surface area, high reactivity, and capacity to pass through biological barriers, nanoparticles behave differently from their bulk counterparts. Nanoscale interactions including oxidative stress, genotoxicity, and long-term bioaccumulation might not be adequately captured by conventional toxicity and biocompatibility studies. Thus, regulators are creating testing procedures tailored to nanomaterials that take aggregation tendencies, surface charge, and particle size distribution into account.

In a similar vein, the customizable nature of 3D-printed structures makes classification difficult. An on-demand 3D-printed implant made for a single patient could not cleanly fall within one of the traditional regulatory categories. Variability is introduced by the use of digital design files, patient imaging data, and localized manufacturing, making quality control and validation more difficult. In response, organizations such as the FDA have started to release guidelines on additive manufacturing, with a focus on post-processing, sterilization, and printing parameter validation. Since customized implants and nanostructured devices may have distinct risk profiles, new consent frameworks are ethically required. To promote worldwide harmonization and guarantee patient safety, global standards for reproducibility in 3D printing and nanomaterial safety testing must also be established.

Biomaterials are classified, evaluated, and ethically supervised based on their source, manufacturing process, and material composition. As biomaterials transform from inert substances to multifunctional and nanoscale systems, regulatory frameworks need to grow to include new aspects of responsibility, safety, and reproducibility. This developing field's moral and practical foundation is made up of ethical sourcing, thorough documentation, and open traceability. Adaptive, data-driven strategies that integrate blockchain-enabled traceability, AI-based risk assessment, and computer simulations are anticipated to be used by future regulatory models to handle the increasing complexity of biomaterial innovation [28, 29]. Biomaterials will ultimately improve human health in a responsible, equitable, and sustainable manner if the delicate balance between innovation, ethics, and regulation is maintained.

10.4 Mechanisms and Processes

In a similar vein, the customizable nature of 3D-printed structures makes classification difficult. An on-demand 3D-printed implant made for a single patient could not cleanly fall within one of the traditional regulatory categories. Variability is introduced by the use of digital design files, patient imaging data, and localized manufacturing, making quality control and validation more difficult. In response, organizations such as the FDA have started to release guidelines on additive manufacturing, with a focus on post-processing, sterilization, and printing parameter validation as shown in Table 10.1.

Since customized implants and nanostructured devices may have distinct risk profiles, new consent frameworks are ethically required. To promote worldwide harmonization and guarantee patient safety, global standards for reproducibility in 3D printing and nanomaterial safety testing must also be established.

Table 10.1 Guidelines on additive manufacturing, with a focus on post-processing, sterilization, and printing parameter validation

Regulatory Body/ Organization	Jurisdiction/ Region	Primary responsibilities	Key regulatory frameworks/ guidelines	Relevance to Biomaterials and emerging technologies
U.S. Food and Drug Administration (FDA)	United States	Regulates medical devices, drugs, and combination products; evaluates safety, efficacy, and quality before market approval	*21 CFR Parts 800–898 (Medical Devices)*; *FDA Premarket Approval (PMA)*; *510(k) clearance*; *QSR/ISO 13485 compliance*	Oversee preclinical and clinical validation of biomaterials, implants, and nanomedicine products; enforces post-market surveillance and recalls

(continued)

Table 10.1 (continued)

Regulatory Body/ Organization	Jurisdiction/ Region	Primary responsibilities	Key regulatory frameworks/ guidelines	Relevance to Biomaterials and emerging technologies
European medicines agency (EMA)	European Union	Coordinates evaluation of medicinal products across EU member states; focuses on benefit–risk assessment and pharmacovigilance	*EU MDR 2017/745*; *ISO 10993 (Biocompatibility Testing)*; *Good Manufacturing Practice (GMP)*	Harmonizes biomaterial and device standards under MDR; encourages transparency and traceability of implants
European Directorate for the Quality of medicines (EDQM)	Council of Europe	Establishes standards for materials used in medical and pharmaceutical applications	*European Pharmacopoeia (Ph. Eur.)*	Ensures consistency, purity, and performance standards for biomaterial-based drugs and excipients
International Organization for Standardization (ISO)	Global	Develops consensus-based international standards for quality management and safety	*ISO 10993 Series (Biological Evaluation)*; *ISO 13485 (Medical Devices QMS)*; *ISO/TR 10993–22 (Nanomaterials)*	Defines global benchmarks for testing, certification, and risk management of biomaterials
World Health Organization (WHO)	Global	Promotes international harmonization, ethical oversight, and equitable access to medical technologies	*Global model regulatory framework for medical devices*; *WHO guidelines for ethical review*	Supports developing nations in establishing biomaterial governance, focusing on safety and ethics in low-resource settings
National Institute for health and care excellence (NICE)	United Kingdom	Evaluates health technologies for cost-effectiveness and clinical value	*Medical technologies evaluation Programme (MTEP)*	Ensures that biomaterial-based devices and regenerative products provide measurable patient benefit
Health Canada (HC)	Canada	Regulates medical devices and biomaterials through risk classification and market authorization	*Medical Devices Regulations (SOR/98–282)*; *ISO 14971 (Risk Management)*	Monitors nanomaterial and polymer-based medical technologies for compliance and patient safety

(continued)

Table 10.1 (continued)

Regulatory Body/ Organization	Jurisdiction/ Region	Primary responsibilities	Key regulatory frameworks/ guidelines	Relevance to Biomaterials and emerging technologies
Pharmaceuticals and medical devices agency (PMDA)	Japan	Reviews and approves medical devices and regenerative medicine products; ensures safety monitoring	*Pharmaceutical and medical device act (PMD act)*	Pioneers expedited pathways for advanced regenerative biomaterials and 3D-printed implants
China National Medical Products Administration (NMPA)	China	Oversees premarket approval, quality control, and post-market supervision	*Medical device supervision and administration regulations*	Expanding regulatory infrastructure for nanomedicine, smart implants, and bioprinted products
Australian therapeutic goods administration (TGA)	Australia	Regulates therapeutic goods, including medical devices and biomaterials	*Therapeutic Goods (Medical Devices) Regulations 2002*	Adopts ISO and IMDRF guidelines for evaluating innovative biomaterials and combination products
International medical device regulators forum (IMDRF)	Global	Fosters global regulatory harmonization and convergence	*IMDRF essential principles and GHTF guidelines*	Develops unified frameworks for clinical evaluation, post-market monitoring, and device traceability
Organisation for economic co-operation and development (OECD)	Global	Oversees responsible development of emerging technologies including nanotechnology	*OECD working party on manufactured nanomaterials (WPMN)*	Promotes safety testing protocols and ethical governance for nanobiomaterials
Institutional review boards (IRBs) / ethics committees	Local / institutional	Oversee ethical conduct of human subject research involving biomaterials and devices	*Declaration of Helsinki*; *good clinical practice (GCP)*	Safeguard participants' rights, informed consent, and data privacy during clinical trials

10.4.1 Regulatory Approval Process from Preclinical Testing to Clinical Trials and Post-Market Monitoring

A multistage framework is used in the regulatory approval process for biomaterials to assess their performance, safety, and efficacy in biological, mechanical, and clinical domains. To guarantee ongoing safety and efficacy, this procedure usually starts with preclinical testing, moves forward through clinical trials, and continues into post-market surveillance.

In vitro and in vivo experiments are used to characterize material qualities during the foundational phase of preclinical testing. Cytotoxicity, genotoxicity, hemocompatibility, and degradation behavior are important factors that are assessed in accordance with international standards like ISO 10993. The durability, compatibility with sterilization, and possibility of negative interactions within the body are further determined by mechanical and physicochemical investigations [30, 31].

The material or device moves on to clinical trials, which take place in phases I through III after successful preclinical validation. Phase I trials evaluate biocompatibility and initial safety in small groups of patients or volunteers who are in good health. Phase II concentrates on possible adverse effects, dose optimization, and therapeutic efficacy in the targeted groups. In order to verify efficacy and track infrequent side effects, phase III extends to bigger patient groups and compares the biomaterial or gadget to placebo or conventional treatments.

Marketing permission is given after regulatory agencies, such as the UK MHRA, European Medicines Agency (EMA), or U.S. FDA, conclude that the product satisfies predetermined standards. Post-market monitoring (Phase IV), which records long-term performance statistics, practical efficacy, and any late-emerging issues, is how regulatory scrutiny continues after approval. Biomaterials are kept safe throughout their lifecycle by mechanisms like risk management strategies, required adverse event reporting, and medical device registries.

This cyclical process emphasizes evidence-based governance, where each stage builds upon the previous one to maintain a continuous chain of accountability from design to clinical application.

10.4.2 Mechanisms of Ethical Oversight

The moral and procedural foundation of biomedical research is ethical oversight, which guarantees that both human and animal subjects are treated fairly and with dignity. Institutional Review Boards (IRBs) in the US and Research Ethics Committees (RECs) in Europe and other countries are the main bodies responsible for this oversight. The independent organizations in charge of evaluating research proposals involving human subjects are IRBs and RECs. Their main goals are to evaluate the risk-benefit ratio, make sure informed consent practices are morally sound, and confirm that protocols adhere to pertinent ethical and legal requirements. To reduce potential harm, maintain privacy, and protect vulnerable groups like children, the elderly, or people with cognitive disabilities, they carefully examine research designs [32].

IRBs and RECs monitor ongoing trials after initial protocol clearance to make sure that unanticipated risks are quickly discovered and reduced. This involves making sure that nanostructured materials or implanted devices don't cause unforeseen medical or psychological problems in the setting of biomaterials. By forcing investigators to reveal funding sources, conflicts of interest, and procedures for dealing with unfavorable outcomes, these ethical frameworks also encourage accountability and transparency. IRBs and RECs preserve the integrity of the research process and safeguard the confidence between science and society by serving as both ethical gatekeepers and advisory bodies.

10.4.3 International Harmonization of Standards

International standardization is essential for maintaining uniformity, interoperability, and cross-border safety in the development and production of biomaterials because biomedical innovation is a worldwide endeavor. Key players in creating common frameworks are the World Health Organization (WHO), the American Society for Testing and Materials (ASTM International), and the International Organization for Standardization (ISO). The ISO creates internationally accepted standards that direct testing procedures and production techniques, such as ISO 10993 (biological evaluation of medical equipment) and ISO 13485 (quality management systems for medical devices). With material-specific standards like ASTM F2450 for polymeric biomaterials and ASTM F2043 for resorbable orthopedic implants, ASTM International supports these initiatives. These guidelines guarantee compatibility between items created in various locations, reproducibility, and comparability of outcomes.

In the meanwhile, the WHO offers guidelines for global health policy alignment, clinical trial registration, and ethical behavior. In low-and middle-income nations, its programs, such the Global Benchmarking Tool (GBT) for national regulatory bodies, improve regulatory capacity and standardize approval procedures. Together, harmonization initiatives decrease duplication, spur innovation, and improve access to safe and efficient biomaterials worldwide. In order to expedite international product approval and shorten time-to-market, they also encourage mutual recognition agreements (MRAs) among regulatory agencies, which permit data collected under one jurisdiction to be accepted in another [33, 34].

10.4.4 Data Transparency and Reproducibility in Preclinical and Clinical Research

Particularly in biomaterials research, where intricate biological interactions can make interpretation difficult, transparency and reproducibility serve as the epistemic cornerstones of scientific credibility. In order to facilitate independent verification and replication, data transparency entails the open sharing of experimental procedures, datasets, and results. Journals and regulators alike are increasingly requiring this to address problems including selective reporting, publishing bias, and irreproducible findings. When experiments are repeated under similar circumstances, reproducibility guarantees that independent researchers can get consistent results. Reproducible synthesis techniques, standardized mechanical and biological property testing, and open reporting of unfavorable or ambiguous results are all part of biomaterials science.

Open access to data is made possible by international programs like the EU Clinical Trials Register and ClinicalTrials.gov, as well as the FAIR data principles (Findable, Accessible, Interoperable, Reusable). Data integrity and accountability are further improved along the research-to-market continuum by integrating digital lab notebooks, blockchain-based traceability, and artificial intelligence (AI)-driven audit tools. In addition to bolstering scientific validity, transparent data governance also increases public confidence in the security and dependability of biomaterial advances ([35, 36].

10.4.5 Ethical Processes in Informed Consent, Patient Participation, and Data Protection (GDPR, HIPAA)

The ethical cornerstone of research involving human subjects is informed consent, which guarantees that study participants willingly participate after being fully informed of the risks, advantages, and available options. Consent in the context of biomaterials, especially implanted or regenerative devices, goes beyond simple physical intervention to encompass data collecting and ongoing monitoring. Additionally, patient engagement is emphasized by ethical frameworks as a developing paradigm that transforms patients from passive subjects into active participants in scientific innovation. This participatory approach increases openness and gives people the ability to have a say in how clinical interventions are developed and carried out.

At the same time, personal data is protected by data protection laws like the Health Insurance Portability and Accountability Act (HIPAA) in the US and the General Data Protection Regulation (GDPR) in Europe. Strict rules for data collection, storage, and transfer are established under these laws, especially when it comes to private health and genetic data. Adherence to data privacy rules is essential since biomaterials research frequently incorporates big data analytics, digital health records, and AI-assisted decision-making. Techniques like safe encryption, pseudonymization, and anonymization preserve patient identities while facilitating important scientific discoveries. These procedures promote a more secure and equitable research environment by striking a balance between ethical transparency and privacy protection.

10.4.6 Mechanisms for Recall, Adverse Event Reporting, and Continuous Safety Evaluation

Biomaterials are continuously assessed to identify and reduce any hazards that may arise during extensive clinical usage, even after receiving regulatory approval. Device failures or problems can be reported by patients, manufacturers, and healthcare professionals using adverse event reporting systems like the FDA's MedWatch and the EMA's EudraVigilance. Recall processes are triggered when data indicates that a product may present a serious health risk. Manufacturers may choose to conduct voluntary recalls, or regulators may mandate them. Depending on how serious the problem is, they can range from small corrective measures to a complete market withdrawal.

Device registries, real-world performance monitoring, and post-market clinical follow-up (PMCF) studies all contribute to ongoing safety evaluation. Predictive analytics and AI-based signal detection are two examples of advanced surveillance technologies that enable early danger identification and promote proactive rather than reactive efforts. Together, these techniques provide a learning health system in which feedback from post-market data continuously guides regulatory adaptation and product development. This iterative process guarantees that biomaterial innovation is resilient, adaptable, patient-centered, and progressive.

In order to protect public health and promote innovation, the systems and procedures controlling biomaterials combine scientific rigor, ethical purity, and international cooperation. Every layer adds to a thorough system of accountability, from data governance and worldwide harmonization to ethical supervision and regulatory approval. These frameworks will need to be continuously improved as biomaterials develop toward intelligent, adaptable, and regenerative functions embracing digital transparency, ethical engagement, and global inclusivity [37, 38]. In the end, the robustness and morality of the systems guiding biomaterial research from discovery to treatment are just as important as its technological complexity.

10.5 Design Considerations

Biomaterials design sits at the nexus of ethical duty, legal compliance, and scientific innovation. The demands on biomedical technologies' safety, dependability, and societal alignment rise as they become more complicated, integrating nanomaterials, bioelectronics, and regenerative scaffolds. Therefore, performance optimization, strict risk management, fair access, and environmental sustainability must all be balanced in the design of modern biomaterials. These design concerns span the materials' whole lifecycle, from idea and validation to manufacture, clinical deployment, and end-of-life management, and are not just restricted to the engineering of the materials themselves [39, 40]. Considering ethical, legal, and environmental requirements, this examines the basic ideas and developing paradigms that direct the responsible design of biomaterials.

10.5.1 Designing for Safety, Reliability, and Reproducibility under Regulatory Constraints

The design of biomaterials continues to be based on safety and dependability. Strict regulatory requirements, such as those set forth by the European Medicines Agency (EMA), the U.S. Food and Drug Administration (FDA), and ISO standards (e.g., ISO 13485 for quality management and ISO 10993 for biocompatibility), must be followed at every stage, from material selection to fabrication and clinical testing. Recent biocompatibility literature suggests that classical cytotoxicity and implantation tests should increasingly be complemented by high-throughput functional proteomics to capture molecular-level responses such as apoptosis, adhesion, proliferation and inflammatory signalling [41]. Early incorporation of compliance pathways into the research process is necessary when designing under regulatory constraints. This ensures that every material parameter, surface treatment, and manufacturing step can be verified and replicated.

Performance dependability is especially important for long-term implants and devices like pacemaker electrodes, stents, and prosthesis. Predicting longevity and stability under physiological settings is aided by corrosion analysis, fatigue testing, and accelerated aging research. Conversely, reproducibility guarantees that materials produced in various batches or locations retain the same biological and structural characteristics. Strict process control, verified measurement techniques, and thorough data documenting are necessary for this reproducibility. Because of their enormous potential for customization, emerging fabrication techniques like 3D printing and nanostructuring provide additional regulatory hurdles. Designers are depending more on closed-loop quality systems that continuously monitor all parameters in order to stay in compliance with regulations. These systems demonstrate process consistency and regulatory conformance by combining data-driven monitoring with traceability technologies, frequently using blockchain or digital record-keeping.

10.5.2 Ethical Design Imperatives

Beyond technical compliance, biomaterial design is bound by ethical imperatives that reflect the broader goals of medicine: to alleviate suffering, protect patients, and promote social justice. Ethical design in biomaterials emphasizes three interlinked principles: minimizing harm, ensuring accessibility, and promoting inclusivity.

Predicting and reducing all possible risks related to material toxicity, degradation byproducts, and long-term biological interactions is necessary to minimize injury. Prioritizing patient safety before commercial or technological expediency, ethical design frameworks like the precautionary principle promote proactive risk evaluation even in the absence of complete evidence. Accessibility refers to the fair distribution of biomedical advancements. The high development costs of advanced materials, especially those utilizing nanotechnology or bioprinting, restrict their availability in low-and middle-income areas. Therefore, cost-effective fabrication routes, modular technologies, and scalable production techniques that allow for worldwide distribution are all considered in ethical design.

Biomaterial design must take into consideration the diversity of human biology and experience to be inclusive. The way that materials interact with the body and how patients view medical interventions can be affected by differences in age, sex, genetic background, and cultural setting. Gender-sensitive testing, culturally responsive design frameworks, and co-design with varied user groups guarantee that biomaterials benefit all populations equally. In order to ensure that implants and gadgets meet a broad range of physical and sensory needs, the ethical duty of inclusion also applies to disability representation [42].

10.5.3 Lifecycle Management

As awareness of the environmental costs of raw material extraction, manufacture, and disposal has grown, sustainability has emerged as a crucial design criterion in biomaterials research. Assessing the environmental impact of resource sourcing, energy use, sterilizing, packing, and post-use biodegradation is the task of lifecycle management. Two methods to reduce the environmental impact include biodegradability and recycling. Medical waste can be decreased by using biodegradable polymers, such as polylactic acid (PLA) or polycaprolactone (PCL), which naturally break down in the environment or within the body. In a similar manner, petrochemical-derived materials can be substituted with bio-based polymers produced from renewable feedstocks (such as cellulose, chitosan, and alginate) without compromising functional performance.

Sustainable design also heavily relies on energy efficiency in nanomaterial synthesis and additive manufacturing (AM). Designers can minimize production emissions and material waste by optimizing fabrication processes with sophisticated computer models. In order to ensure ecological safety, regulatory bodies require environmental risk assessments, which analyze possible nanoparticle release or harmful degrading by-products. Circular economic ideas, which call for biomaterials to be recovered, reprocessed, or upcycled after use, are being embraced by designers more and more. Implant-grade titanium and cobalt alloys, for instance, can be extracted from faulty parts and recycled in a controlled environment without sacrificing quality [43]. Regulatory filings that include sustainability indicators strengthen accountability and match the development of biomaterials with more general global sustainability objectives, such the Sustainable Development Goals (SDGs) of the UN.

10.5.4 Risk–Benefit Assessment During Preclinical Validation and Clinical Trials

Any biomaterial's ethical and legal basis rests on how well its possible advantages and disadvantages are balanced. Beginning with pre-clinical testing and continuing through clinical trials and post-market monitoring, risk-benefit analysis is an ongoing process. Materials are thoroughly tested in vitro and in vivo during the preclinical phase to determine their mechanical integrity, biocompatibility, toxicity, and degradation behavior. Standardized procedures for cytotoxicity, sensitization, and implantation tests are provided by ISO 10993 and ASTM F748. The use of predictive toxicology and computational modeling to model long-term biological interactions is growing, which lessens the need for animal testing and promotes moral research methods.

The evaluation broadens to encompass device dependability, performance results, and human safety throughout clinical trials. Regulatory agencies demand thorough records of adverse events, with safety limits determined by comparing them to items that are considered standard-of-care. In high-risk applications like brain implants, tissue-engineered constructions, or drug-eluting systems, where unexpected immunological or inflammatory reactions may occur, striking a balance between innovation and caution is especially important [44, 45]. Transparency, informed permission, and moral justification for patient exposure are guaranteed by a strict risk-benefit framework. Additionally, without sacrificing patient welfare or regulatory compliance, this approach permits adaptive decision-making, which permits materials or devices to be improved in response to real-world performance data [46, 47].

10.5.5 Use of Digital Twins, AI, and Simulation Tools in Compliant and Transparent Design Workflows

The design and validation of biomaterials have been significantly impacted by digital revolution. Design efficiency and regulatory compliance are improved by the predictive and adaptive capabilities offered by digital twins, artificial intelligence (AI), and simulation tools. A digital twin combines real-time data from sensors, images, and experimental research to create a virtual version of a biomaterial, apparatus, or system. It makes it possible to simulate biological interactions, mechanical pressures, and degradation dynamics under varied circumstances. Digital twins are becoming more widely accepted by regulatory bodies as a component of in silico validation frameworks, which lessens the need for expensive and morally dubious animal or human testing.

By employing machine learning algorithms trained on extensive experimental datasets to determine ideal material compositions and geometries, AI-driven design spurs innovation. These systems can find relationships between biological outcomes and nanoscale properties, forecast failure modes, and optimize additive manufacturing parameters. Importantly, AI solutions also improve compliance by generating transparent, auditable design workflows by automatically recording design decisions, identifying abnormalities, and guaranteeing traceability [48]. Multiphysics modeling of heat transport, fluid dynamics, and electrochemical interactions are examples of simulation methods that go beyond mechanical analysis and are especially pertinent to devices like biosensors and neural implants. Combining these computational techniques not only increases dependability but also facilitates flexible regulatory filings, bringing digital innovation into compliance with moral and safety requirements.

10.5.6 Co-Design and Participatory Approaches

A major paradigm shift in the development of biomaterials is represented by the shift toward patient-centered design and co-creation. In the past, engineers and scientists dominated the design of biomaterials, with little involvement from end users. However, human experience is just as important to clinical efficacy and user pleasure as technical performance. Early in the development process, co-design approaches involve patients, clinicians, and caregivers as active participants. In addition to improving usability and patient compliance, this participative strategy guarantees that the design accurately represents actual clinical demands. For instance, compared to designs that are only driven by laboratories, prosthetic materials created with direct input from amputees can achieve higher comfort, aesthetics, and functionality.

Involving clinicians guarantees that biomaterials are compatible with sterilization techniques, surgical workflows, and regulatory documentation procedures. Additionally, by bringing innovation into line with ethical standards and societal ideals, participatory design encourages social accountability. Researchers can find unexpected usability problems, improve safety, and increase public confidence in future technologies by including stakeholder feedback loops into development pipelines. Real-time co-design is now made possible by digital collaboration systems, which let distant teams of engineers, doctors, and patients test virtual prototypes, examine performance simulations, and quickly iterate [49]. By combining materials science and human aspects engineering, this method guarantees that biomaterials are not only practical but also compassionately made for people just as much as for physiology.

More than just technical expertise is needed to design biomaterials within ethical and regulatory frameworks; a comprehensive grasp of the ways in which materials affect society, the environment, and human health is also necessary. Design that is safe, dependable, and repeatable guarantees regulatory compliance, while the moral requirements of sustainability, inclusivity, and accessibility protect public confidence. While participatory methods democratize innovation through patient and physician participation, advanced digital tools like artificial intelligence (AI) and digital twins improve predictive design and transparency.

Designing biomaterials in the future will depend more and more on integrated ecosystems that incorporate ethical governance, computational intelligence, and the concepts of the circular economy. A safer, more just, and sustainable era of biomedical innovation is made possible by such a framework, which guarantees that every biomaterial whether it be an implant, scaffold, or nanocomposite embodies both technological brilliance and moral responsibility [50, 51].

10.6 Applications and Case Studies

Diverse clinical and technological case studies demonstrate the actual application of ethical and regulatory principles in biomaterials science, highlighting the intricacy and dynamic nature of contemporary biomedical governance. As biomaterials and associated technologies from AI-assisted treatment systems to orthopedic implants move closer to clinical translation, they must negotiate a variety of regulatory paths and moral conundrums influenced by the nature of the innovation, local laws, and cultural norms. This section highlights both advancements and ongoing difficulties by looking at key application areas and case studies that show how regulatory science and bioethics interact in real-world settings.

10.6.1 Regulatory Pathways for Orthopedic and Cardiovascular Implants

The 510(k) clearance and the Premarket Approval (PMA) process are the two main routes that the U.S. Food and Drug Administration (FDA) offer for the approval of medical devices, such as orthopedic and cardiovascular implants. Devices that exhibit significant equivalency to an already-approved, lawfully sold device (predicate) are subject to the 510(k) process. Faster market entrance is possible through this technique, which is usually utilized for orthopedic screws, joint replacements, and stents with well-established designs. However, it necessitates thorough documentation to ensure that the material composition, mechanical performance, and safety profiles are equal to those of current technologies.

On the other hand, Class III devices that maintain or support life, including heart valves or sophisticated neurostimulation implants are exempt from the PMA procedure. Comprehensive clinical evidence proving safety and effectiveness through controlled trials is required by PMA. Although it requires a lot of resources, this procedure is necessary for new biomaterials or designs without a corresponding equipment [52]. The FDA requires adherence to Quality System Regulations (21 CFR Part 820) and Good Manufacturing Practices (GMP) in both situations.

Continuous safety assessment is informed by real-world performance data thanks to post-market surveillance systems like the Medical Device Reporting (MDR) system. Globally, similar frameworks are mirrored, such as CE certification under the Medical Device Regulation (MDR 2017/745) of the European Union, underscoring the increasing convergence of device regulation worldwide.

Orthopedic and cardiovascular implants are among the most strictly regulated biomaterial applications due to their vital mechanical and biological roles. These routes show how regulatory science strikes a balance between patient safety and innovation, making sure that advancements in technology are in line with strict safety and moral guidelines.

10.6.2 Ethical and Regulatory Challenges in Tissue-Engineered and Stem-Cell-Based Therapies

Although tissue-engineered and stem-cell-based treatments are at the forefront of regenerative medicine, their biological complexity and propensity for unpredictable behavior in vivo create serious ethical and regulatory issues. These treatments are challenging to categorize under current regulatory frameworks because they incorporate biomaterial scaffolds, bioactive chemicals, and living cells, unlike conventional implants or medications. Under the Center for Biologics Evaluation and Research (CBER), the FDA classifies these goods as Human Cells, Tissues, and Cellular and Tissue-Based goods (HCT/Ps). Products that are "more than minimally manipulated" or meant for non-homologous usage must be submitted as Biologics License Applications (BLAs) or Investigational New Drugs (INDs), backed by substantial preclinical and clinical data. Similarly, these are categorized as Advanced Therapy Medicinal Products by the European Medicines Agency (EMA), which includes tissue-, somatic-, and gene-engineered medicines. Recent analysis of European SoHO and ATMP consultations shows that governance of human-derived biomaterials and advanced therapies remains institutionally fragmented, reinforcing the need for stronger links between tissue-collection systems, therapy developers, regulators and patient stakeholders [53].

Stem-cell treatments ethically put into question long-term patient monitoring, donor anonymity, and informed permission. Constant attention is necessary because to the possibility of tumorigenicity, immunological rejection, and genetic instability. Furthermore, organizations like the WHO are calling for stricter international regulation because the marketing of untested stem-cell treatments in deregulated markets is a global problem [54, 55]. The ethical and regulatory environments around these treatments serve as an example of the conflict between moral obligation and scientific advancement, underscoring the necessity of flexible frameworks that develop in tandem with regenerative medicine.

10.6.3 Case Study: Nanomedicine and the Evolving Regulatory Paradigm for Nanoscale Safety

Nanomedicine's distinct physicochemical characteristics and size-dependent biological interactions make it a challenge to conventional regulatory paradigms. This includes nanoparticles, nanocomposites, and nanosensors. Although nanoparticles' small size (less than 100 nm) allows for improved bioavailability, controlled release potential, and precise targeting, it also presents questions of toxicity, biodistribution, and long-term organ buildup. Instead of developing completely new categories, regulatory bodies have responded by improving already existing frameworks. Although it requires nano-specific characterization, including surface chemistry, aggregation behavior, and stability, the FDA evaluates nanomedicine items using the current drug or device processes. Similarly, risk assessment methods and test procedures tailored to nanotechnology have been introduced by the European Commission and the OECD Working Party on Manufactured Nanomaterials [56].

One notable example is the first FDA-approved nanodrug, liposomal doxorubicin (Doxil®), which showed better pharmacokinetics and less cardiotoxicity than traditional formulations. Its creation did, however, highlight the necessity of interdisciplinary cooperation between toxicologists and materials scientists as well as standardized nano-characterization. The case study on nanomedicine demonstrates how regulatory science is changing from a static to a dynamic model that can handle new hazards without limiting innovation. This change is becoming more and more significant in the larger biomaterials industry.

10.6.4 Case Study: 3D-Printed Medical Devices

Patient-specific implants and anatomical models are now possible thanks to the development of additive manufacturing (AM), also known as 3D printing, in the production of medical devices. It does, however, provide difficult validation and regulatory issues. The FDA must assess manufacturing repeatability, digital file integrity, and material consistency in addition to classifying 3D-printed medical devices into three risk-based categories: Class I (low risk), Class II (moderate risk), and Class III (high risk). Ensuring process control and traceability is a major concern because AM devices are frequently produced in decentralized or hospital-based settings. Recent regulatory analysis of bioprinted constructs highlights that cell-laden, bioactive and patient-specific printed products challenge conventional device categories because their safety depends not only on material properties, but also on bioink composition, cell source, maturation, reproducibility and post-print handling [57].

Verifying mechanical strength, interlayer adhesion, and biocompatibility across production batches are validation challenges. Preclinical mechanical testing, sterilization validation, and digital workflow management are highlighted in the FDA's

2017 guideline document, Technical Considerations for Additive Manufactured Medical Devices. One prominent example is the 510(k) pathway-approved 3D-printed titanium cranial implants, which were shown to be equivalent to traditional implants. In clinical translation, these gadgets demonstrate the potential of digital manufacturing as well as its regulatory difficulty. To guarantee reproducibility and patient safety, harmonizing international standards for 3D-printed biomaterials is still a top goal.

10.6.5 Case Study: Clinical Translation of AI-Assisted Biomaterials

Data governance, algorithmic transparency, and accountability present new ethical and regulatory challenges when AI is included into the design of biomaterials and clinical decision-making [58, 59]. Though their black-box nature makes regulatory evaluation more difficult, AI-assisted systems enhance biomaterial characteristics, forecast patient-specific results, and even automate diagnostic procedures. Frameworks for Software as a Medical Device (SaMD) have been created by regulators such as the FDA, with an emphasis on algorithm validation, bias mitigation, and continuous learning capabilities. Additionally, risk-based categorization and explainability requirements for medical AI systems are mandated by the European Union's AI Act (2024).

The application of AI-driven predictive modeling for orthopedic implant performance serves as a prime illustration. These technologies improve surgical precision by evaluating material stress profiles and patient imaging data, but they also bring up moral concerns of data ownership, consent, and culpability in the event of computational errors. As AI is included in biomaterial innovation pipelines, it is crucial to guarantee algorithmic fairness and cybersecurity resilience. This case study opens the door for responsible digital transformation in biomedicine by highlighting the need to combine data ethics with regulatory compliance.

10.6.6 Comparative Analysis of Regulatory Frameworks across Regions

Regulatory governance of biomaterials varies across regions, reflecting distinct legislative traditions, technological capacities, and healthcare priorities.

The FDA in the US uses risk-based classification and places a high priority on post-market surveillance through its product-centered divisions (CDRH, CDER, and CBER). Its flexible foundations allow for high-impact inventions to be approved more quickly. Traceability, clinical evaluation, and post-market performance studies are prioritized by the European Union, the MDR (2017/745), and the In Vitro

Diagnostic Regulation (IVDR). Although CE marking requires strict documentation and conformance examinations, it guarantees free market movement inside the EU. China, South Korea, Japan, and other Asia-Pacific nations are becoming leaders in the regulation of biomaterials. China's NMPA is harmonizing with ISO and WHO standards to improve global compatibility, while Japan's PMDA promotes industry-academic cooperation. Though programs like the African Medicines Agency (AMA) seek to standardize standards, especially for medical devices and tissue-based therapies, regulatory frameworks throughout Africa are still evolving.

These regional differences highlight the necessity of harmonizing regulations globally to promote fair access and the spread of innovation. In order to match safety standards and expedite international approvals, collaborative networks like the International Medical Device Regulators Forum (IMDRF) are essential. Applications of ethical and regulatory frameworks in biomaterials science show how innovation, governance, and moral responsibility must coexist in a fast-changing ecosystem. Every example, from the FDA's device paths to AI-assisted clinical translation, highlights both advancements and conflicts in striking a balance between human safety and technology potential. The future of safe, transparent, and socially responsible biomedical innovation will be determined by regulatory and ethical adaptation as biomaterial frontiers extend into nanotechnology, regenerative medicine, and intelligent systems [60, 61].

10.7 Recent Advances and Innovations

Emerging technologies like digital manufacturing, bioprinting, nanotechnology, and artificial intelligence (AI) are drastically changing the ethical and regulatory environment around biomaterials. These developments put current frameworks for safety, governance, and accountability to the test in addition to redefining the possibilities of contemporary biomedical systems. Regulators, ethicists, and technologists are developing new approaches to inclusive decision-making, transparent data management, and adaptive oversight to guarantee the responsible translation of scientific advancement into clinical benefit. This section examines seven significant advancements that define the current state of biomaterials ethics and regulation, ranging from worldwide open scientific movements to experimental governance frameworks.

10.7.1 Development of Regulatory Sandboxes for Rapid Testing of Emerging Biomedical Technologies

The emergence of regulatory sandboxes-controlled settings where novel biomedical goods can be evaluated in real-world settings with temporary regulatory flexibility is one of the most revolutionary developments in biomaterial governance. This methodology, which is derived from financial technology (fintech), enables researchers and developers to investigate cutting-edge applications like bioprinted tissues or AI guided implants while preserving oversight through regulatory bodies' iterative input. Recent work on implantable neurotechnologies argues that regulatory sandboxes can support high-risk emerging biomedical devices, but only when they include clear entry criteria, participatory decision-making, adaptive supervision and long-term risk management [62].

Regulatory sandboxes facilitate the expeditious assessment of safety and efficacy data for intricate systems that defy conventional classification, such as gene-edited scaffolds or hybrid biological-electronic implants, in biomedical contexts. To evaluate these mechanisms, organizations like the FDA, EMA, and Japan's PMDA have started trial projects. Sandboxes lessen the "regulatory lag" that frequently postpones clinical translation by encouraging communication between innovators and regulators early in the research process. Additionally, they support risk-proportionate regulation, which matches the level of control to technological uncertainty rather than strict device classifications. In order to detect possible societal hazards before to widespread implementation, the sandbox approach also encourages interdisciplinary cooperation by combining knowledge from materials science, bioethics, and data security [63]. Such adaptive governance frameworks will be essential when biomedical innovation picks up speed in order to guarantee that moral and legal issues develop alongside scientific advancements.

10.7.2 Integration of AI and Predictive Analytics in Risk Assessment and Quality Management

Regulatory science and quality assurance are becoming more and more dependent on artificial intelligence (AI) and predictive analytics. AI models can analyze large datasets, ranging from clinical outcomes to molecular simulations and microstructural imaging, to forecast material performance and risk profiles in the production and validation of biomaterials. By lowering ambiguity and boosting regulatory trust in new products, these technologies aid in evidence-based decision-making. Machine learning techniques are used in risk assessment to find correlations between biological reactions and nanoscale properties, predict degradation paths, and spot anomalies in manufacturing data. For example, preclinical safety evaluations can be conducted without the need for lengthy animal testing thanks to AI-driven toxicology models that can mimic biological interactions with nanoparticles. Predictive analytics can also identify early departures from quality control thresholds, improving adherence to Good Manufacturing Practice (GMP) and lowering the number of product recalls. Current regulatory scholarship emphasises that AI-enabled therapeutic development requires robust oversight, transparent validation, and adaptive guardrails to ensure that AI-supported discovery, manufacturing and clinical translation remain safe, effective and high quality [64].

AI integration also makes adaptive regulation possible, where dynamic modifications to regulatory approval are informed by real-time performance data from linked implants or biosensors. This method changes static compliance into an ongoing, data-driven procedure that is in line with the future of responsive, individualized healthcare. To preserve confidence in automated regulatory judgments, explainable models and established validation procedures must be used to address the ethical issues raised by AI use, such as algorithmic bias and transparency [65, 66].

10.7.3 Blockchain-Based Traceability Systems for Material Origin, Production, and Patient Tracking

With the globalization of supply chains and industry, transparency and traceability have become top issues in the regulation of biomaterials. A decentralized digital ledger called blockchain technology provides a strong way to guarantee unchangeable, end-to-end tracking of supplies, procedures, and patient results. Real-time material provenance verification is made possible by blockchain-based systems, which record each stage of the process, from the synthesis and sourcing of raw materials to sterilization, packing, and clinical deployment. The cryptographic security of each transaction prevents manipulation and allows regulators to audit compliance in the past. Blockchain can connect distinct material IDs to patient information for implants and tissue-engineered items, facilitating recall management and post-market surveillance.

Blockchain promotes ethical transparency in addition to technical traceability, giving patients peace of mind that biomaterials are procured ethically and produced in a humane and sustainable manner [67]. By making interoperable records available to several regulatory agencies, academic institutions, and clinical facilities, it also promotes global harmonization. Blockchain is currently being tested for regenerative medicine supply chains in pilot projects in Europe and Asia, showing promise for increasing public trust and accountability in cutting-edge biomaterials.

10.7.4 Ethical Innovation in Bioprinting and Gene-Edited Biomaterials

Synthetic biology, gene editing, and bioprinting come together to form a new biological frontier and a previously unheard-of ethical dilemma. These technologies raise difficult challenges of identity, consent, and what constitutes "life" in engineered tissues by obfuscating the distinction between artificial materials and living systems. The production of scaffolds and organs tailored to each patient through bioprinting presents a potential remedy for the ongoing organ scarcity. However, strict control over cell procurement is necessary for ethical design, especially when using genetically modified lines or human stem cells. Transparent governance structures are necessary to address issues including donor permission, intellectual property rights, and long-term monitoring of implanted living constructions.

In a similar vein, gene-edited biomaterials that modify cellular or extracellular matrix components using CRISPR provide a challenge to established regulatory classifications. The necessity of thorough preclinical testing and moral risk-benefit analysis is highlighted by the possibility of unexpected genetic effects. Organizations that support responsible innovation frameworks, such as UNESCO and the International Society for Stem Cell Research (ISSCR), place a strong emphasis on the precautionary principle and fair access to new treatments. Therefore, ethical innovation entails a dual commitment: maintaining public trust via inclusion, transparency, and international discourse while progressing gene editing and bioprinting toward clinical benefit.

10.7.5 Global Initiatives for Open Science, Data Sharing, and Reproducible Research Practices

Open science has emerged as a key component of ethical biomaterials research in the age of large data and distributed collaboration. Standardized reporting systems, common digital archives, and open-access databases guarantee that scientific knowledge is visible, reproducible, and available everywhere. Uniform data standards are promoted by initiatives like the FAIR principles (Findable, Accessible, Interoperable, Reusable), which enable regulatory bodies and labs around the world to validate results and reuse datasets for meta-analysis. Global safety benchmarking is improved, duplication is decreased, and innovation is accelerated when experimental techniques are freely shared, especially when it comes to additive manufacturing parameters or nanomaterial toxicity testing.

International initiatives that demonstrate how cooperative data sharing can improve regulatory research include the Human Cell Atlas and the OECD Working Party on Manufactured Nanomaterials. Furthermore, by democratizing access to scientific knowledge, open science supports the ethical imperatives of equity, particularly for researchers working in low-resource environments. Data openness must, however, strike a balance between protecting intellectual property and patient privacy, necessitating safe infrastructures that maintain confidentiality while permitting transparency.

10.7.6 Expansion of Digital Regulatory Ecosystems for Adaptive Compliance and Post-Market Surveillance

Beyond blockchain and artificial intelligence, the digital transformation of regulation includes entire digital regulatory ecosystems. Throughout the biomaterial lifespan, these ecosystems facilitate adaptive, evidence-based oversight by integrating databases, monitoring tools, and predictive models [68]. Adaptive compliance is the ongoing process of matching changing product data with regulatory requirements. For instance, performance indicators can be sent straight to regulatory databases by implantable biosensors, enabling the automatic detection of abnormalities or unfavorable occurrences. Similarly, automated audits are made possible by machine-readable documentation and established ontologies, which lessen administrative load and improve accuracy.

Digital solutions that aggregate data in real-time from wearable technology, patient feedback platforms, and electronic health records improve vigilance in post-market surveillance. EUDAMED and the FDA's Sentinel Initiative are prime examples of early digital supervision initiatives. To enable preventive interventions rather than reactive recalls, future systems are probably going to incorporate AI-driven analytics for early detection of material failure patterns and bad bioreactivity. The idea of regulation as a learning system one that constantly adjusts to advancements in technology and empirical data is supported by these digital ecosystems, which guarantee that biomaterial innovation stays flexible and responsible.

10.7.7 Role of Public Engagement and Education in Shaping Bioethical and Policy Frameworks

Scientific validity is simply one aspect of technological legitimacy; another is public acceptance. Therefore, public involvement and education are essential to forming the biomaterial ethical and policy landscape. Building trust and promoting informed involvement in biological decision-making are two benefits of open and honest communication regarding risks, uncertainties, and advantages. For delicate technologies where acceptability is influenced by ethical intuitions and cultural norms, such as neural implants, gene-edited scaffolds, and nanomaterials, public discussion is particularly important. Initiatives for engagement, such as deliberate forums, patient advocacy groups, and citizen panels, give communities a voice and help shape policy. In addition to improving democratic accountability, this participatory governance keeps moral disputes from turning into popular opposition.

On the other hand, education guarantees that medical professionals, engineers, and legislators have the multidisciplinary literacy required to handle moral conundrums and complicated regulations. The next generation of researchers is prepared to design responsibly within global frameworks by curricula that incorporate data governance, materials science, and ethics [69]. In the end, public involvement grounds scientific advancement in common principles of sustainability, justice, and safety, transforming ethics from a reactive limitation into a proactive catalyst for innovation.

The future of biomaterials regulation is changing because of the convergence of sophisticated materials, digital technologies, and ethical governance. While open research and public participation guarantee inclusion and accountability, innovations like blockchain traceability, AI-assisted risk analysis, and regulatory sandboxes are improving transparency and efficiency. Collectively, these advancements signal a move toward data-driven, ethically informed, and flexible regulation that can strike a balance between short-term innovation and long-term social well-being. Thus, the next era of biomaterials will rely on both technological advancements and a shared commitment to the fair and responsible administration of biomedical advancement.

10.8 Challenges and Limitations

Even though biomaterials science has made great strides, the ethical and regulatory frameworks that oversee their creation are still disjointed, uneven, and frequently unprepared to keep up with the rate of innovation. Novel kinds of biomaterials, like neural interfaces, nanobiotechnologies, and adaptive 4D scaffolds, have emerged faster than conventional supervision methods, creating ambiguity in safety assessment, moral behavior, and global harmonization. Furthermore, new worries around privacy, cybersecurity, and informed consent have surfaced as biomaterials become more digitalized, integrating artificial intelligence, linked sensors, and patient data streams [70, 71]. The main obstacles and constraints that influence the governance of biomaterials research and use both now and in the future are critically examined in this section.

10.8.1 Fragmentation of Regulatory Frameworks across Jurisdictions

The disarray of legal and regulatory frameworks across national and regional borders is one of the most enduring problems in the regulation of biomaterials. Significant differences still exist between jurisdictions despite efforts by international organizations like the World Health Organization (WHO), the International Organization for Standardization (ISO), and the International Medical Device Regulators Forum (IMDRF) to standardize safety and quality standards. For instance, the European Union's Medical Device Regulation (MDR 2017/745) and the U.S. FDA's risk-based classification scheme diverge significantly, especially in terms of preclinical data requirements and conformance evaluation pathways. Similarly, nations in Africa and Asia-Pacific frequently use hybrid frameworks or depend on outside validation, which results in inefficiencies, redundant trials, and patient access delays.

Multinational clinical trials are further complicated by this lack of consistency, as disparate paperwork and ethical requirements can cause delays in approvals and inconsistent patient protections. This fragmentation impedes regulatory interoperability, raising costs and compliance requirements for innovators and decreasing fairness in access to healthcare globally as biomaterials increasingly transcend borders through digital manufacturing and global supply chains.

10.8.2 Limited Guidance for Emerging Fields like Nanobiotechnology, Neural Interfaces, and 4D Biomaterials

New fields like 4D biomaterials, brain interfaces, and nanobiotechnology show how inadequate the current regulatory advice is. Conventional frameworks are not well adapted to technologies that are dynamic, responsive, and biologically integrated because they were created for static, well-characterized materials. For example, surface reactivities and quantum-scale phenomena in nanobiomaterials contradict traditional toxicological models. However, the lack of a commonly recognized set of testing procedures or defined terminology for nanotechnology makes risk assessment and repeatability more difficult. Similar to this, new safety and ethical concerns around cognitive privacy, ownership of brain data, and long-term biocompatibility are brought up by neural interfaces devices that combine electronic circuits with living neural tissue [72, 73].

Traditional mechanical and biological evaluation standards are challenged by 4D biomaterials, which can change over time in response to stimuli. This is because static testing methods are unable to adequately capture the time-dependent transformations of these materials. The absence of regulations in these new areas puts patients at risk for either underregulation, which exposes them to unknown risks, or overregulation, which inhibits innovation. To create flexible, principle-based rules that may change with emerging technologies, international cooperation is desperately needed.

10.8.3 Ethical Tensions Between Innovation Speed and Patient Safety

The ethical need to guarantee patient safety and evidence-based validation frequently clashes with the push to speed up medical innovation, which is fueled by market competition, public demand, and acute health problems [74]. In biomaterials research, where promising innovations like gene-edited tissues or nanotherapeutics can quickly go from bench to bedside, this tension is especially noticeable. Though they run the risk of lowering evidential criteria, regulatory procedures like the FDA's Breakthrough Devices Program and the European Union's accelerated paths are designed to expedite approval for transformational innovations. Small clinical sample sizes or a lack of long-term follow-up data, for instance, may make it difficult to identify uncommon side effects, especially for implanted or biodegradable materials that interact with host tissues over time.

This calls into question the ethical distinction between the responsibility of beneficence (promoting prospective benefit) and the duty of nonmaleficence (avoidance of harm). The professional duty to shield human subjects from early exposure to unknown hazards must be weighed against the public's expectation of quick access to innovation. By guaranteeing continuous assessment following initial approval, strengthening post-market surveillance and adaptable licensing models may aid in balancing these conflicting demands.

10.8.4 Data Privacy, Cybersecurity, and Informed Consent Challenges in Digital Biomaterial Systems

Concerns around data privacy, cybersecurity, and informed consent have become crucial as biomaterials become more and more integrated with digital technology, such as wearable biosensors, AI-powered implants, and connected prosthetics. Large volumes of physiological and personal data are produced by these hybrid systems, making them susceptible to hacking, abuse, and illegal analysis. A foundation for data governance is provided by laws like the Health Insurance Portability and Accountability Act (HIPAA) in the US and the General Data Protection Regulation (GDPR) in Europe. However, continuous, real-time medical devices that transmit behavioral and biological data were not initially intended to be covered by these rules. Furthermore, vulnerabilities are made worse by worldwide differences in digital literacy and enforcement, particularly in environments with little resources.

Additionally, dynamic data use and algorithmic opacity put pressure on informed consent models. Patients may give their agreement for the initial gathering of data, but they may not be informed about the use of secondary data for commercial purposes or algorithmic retraining that follows. Creating dynamic consent frameworks that permit continuous, transparent engagement in digital biomaterial ecosystems while incorporating strong cybersecurity measures to stop data manipulation or exploitation is the difficult part [75, 76].

10.8.5 Inadequate Global Capacity for Oversight in Low-and Middle-Income Countries (LMICs)

The unequal ability of regulatory monitoring around the world, especially in low- and middle-income countries (LMICs), is another significant barrier. Many countries lack the laboratory capacity, skilled workers, and technical infrastructure necessary to assess sophisticated medical devices or complicated biomaterials. Because of this, these nations frequently depend on approvals from outside regulatory bodies (such the FDA or EMA), which could not accurately represent the diversity of the local population, the characteristics of diseases, or the limitations of available resources.

This dependence keeps access and safety disparities alive since items tested in different socioeconomic or environmental contexts may not work as well among LMIC communities. Furthermore, early adverse event detection is hampered by a lack of post-market surveillance infrastructure. To ensure fair and efficient oversight, consistent investment in local regulatory science, bioethics training, and technology infrastructure is still necessary, even though international collaborations like the African Medicines Agency (AMA) initiative are significant steps toward capacity building.

10.8.6 Lack of Standardized Testing Methods for Novel Hybrid and Multifunctional Materials

Significant analytical and methodological hurdles arise from the diversification of biomaterials into hybrid, multifunctional, and bioinspired systems. These materials challenge current test procedures based on single-material standards because they combine metals, ceramics, polymers, biological components, and occasionally living cells. ISO 10993, for instance, offers a thorough framework for biological evaluation of medical devices, but it falls short in capturing emergent or synergistic activities in composite materials. Similar to this, physiological microenvironments like changing pH, enzyme activity, or biomechanical loads are frequently not replicated by mechanical and degradation testing techniques [77]. In addition to making regulatory submission more difficult, the lack of defined test protocols compromises study comparability and reproducibility.

Preclinical evaluation efficiency and reliability could be increased by creating modular, consensus-based testing frameworks, possibly with the use of digital twins and predictive modeling. Novel biomaterials might experience variable performance results or protracted regulatory uncertainty in the absence of such standards.

10.8.7 Public Trust and Perception Barriers Affecting Adoption of Advanced Biomaterials

Lastly, a crucial but sometimes disregarded obstacle to the effective adoption of biomaterials breakthroughs is public trust. Even for technologies that have been scientifically confirmed, negative public perception fueled by past ethical transgressions, media sensationalism, or a lack of transparency can impede acceptance and deployment. For instance, public mistrust of regenerative biomaterials has been influenced by debates over gene editing and stem-cell treatments, while worries about bias in AI and data misuse have an impact on trust in digital health systems. Unfair access or feelings of exploitation, especially in clinical trials involving vulnerable people, can also be the source of public skepticism.

Building trust requires transparent communication, patient engagement, and community-based ethical governance. Stakeholder participation from patients to civil society organizations should be embedded throughout the innovation process. Ethical innovation is not only about compliance but about fostering social legitimacy and shared responsibility in biomedical progress. The difficulties and constraints facing the governance of biomaterials reflect the larger battle in contemporary science to balance the advancement of technology with moral rectitude and universal justice. The gap between innovation and societal readiness could grow because of fragmented legislation, insufficient guidance for developing sectors, data governance issues, and capacity differences. International cooperation, flexible regulatory science, and inclusive ethical frameworks that change in step with material complexity are all necessary to overcome these obstacles [78]. Biomaterials have the potential to become safe, equitable, and transformational agents in the future of medicine, but only with persistent cooperation and public trust.

10.9 Future Directions

The future of biomaterials regulation, ethics, and innovation is entering a phase of transformative convergence where adaptive governance, digital intelligence, and global collaboration redefine how technologies are evaluated, approved, and integrated into healthcare. As biomaterials evolve toward dynamic, intelligent, and regenerative systems, the frameworks that govern them must likewise adapt balancing innovation with responsibility, efficiency with safety, and progress with social trust.

10.9.1 Toward Adaptive and Dynamic Regulation that Evolves with Scientific Innovation

The speed of biomaterial innovation is too fast for traditional regulatory frameworks, which are frequently inflexible and retroactive. An innovative approach is adaptive regulation, which is defined by risk-proportionate supervision, data-driven monitoring, and iterative adjustments. Emerging technologies like nanorobotic systems, AI-driven implants, and 4D biomaterials can be accompanied by dynamic regulatory frameworks. This involves incorporating post-market data analytics and "real-world evidence" to continuously improve safety profiles. Piloting adaptable pathways for early access while guaranteeing continuous evaluation is already being done by regulatory bodies such as the FDA, EMA, and PMDA. These methods foster innovation without sacrificing patient care, particularly in fields where long-term biocompatibility develops gradually, like neuroprosthetics and bioresorbable implants [79].

10.9.2 Establishing Global Harmonization and Mutual Recognition of Biomaterial Standards

The fragmentation of regulations among jurisdictions is one of the most important issues that lie ahead. Harmonization can greatly speed up clinical translation and safe biomaterials' introduction into the market by establishing similar standards, testing procedures, and mutual recognition agreements. Universal standards for additive manufacturing, nanomaterial characterization, and biocompatibility testing are being advanced by initiatives like the International Medical Device Regulators Forum (IMDRF) and ISO technical committees. Additionally, global harmonization improves openness in global supply chains, expedites cross-border approval procedures, and decreases unnecessary animal testing. Digital standardizing platforms, where blockchain-based registries and interoperable databases enable traceable and comparable regulatory filings globally, are anticipated to become more prevalent over the next 10 years.

10.9.3 Integration of Ethical AI Frameworks for Decision-Making in Biomedical Design and Oversight

Strong ethical AI frameworks are required due to the growing use of AI in biomaterial research, which includes predictive modeling, clinical risk assessment, and regulatory reporting. Transparency, explainability, and the absence of algorithmic bias that can disfavor patient groups are essential for AI systems. Automated compliance verification, anomaly identification in manufacturing, and predictive safety evaluation are made possible by incorporating ethical AI into regulatory procedures. In addition to legislation, AI-powered ethical platforms may offer real-time notifications of possible threats to patient safety or privacy. To guarantee that computational intelligence continues to be an instrument of ethical governance rather than a source of opacity, it will be crucial to develop international rules for "AI accountability in biomedicine."

10.9.4 Development of Sustainable and Circular Biomaterial Economies

The next generation of biomaterials and manufacturing environments will be more defined by sustainability. Reducing waste, recovering valuable materials, and ensuring product lifetime traceability from design to disposal are all priorities of a circular biomaterial economy. Non-biodegradable or resource-intensive materials will be replaced with recyclable nanocomposites, biodegradable polymers, and renewable feedstocks. In order to guarantee environmental responsibility, regulatory submissions are also incorporating life-cycle assessment (LCA) and carbon accounting systems. Sustainability and clinical safety are further aligned by policies that support solvent-free synthesis, green chemistry, and localized additive manufacturing. A larger cultural trend toward regenerative sustainability, in which repairing human bodies does not compromise the health of the earth, is reflected in the convergence of environmental and biomedical ethics [80, 81].

10.9.5 Expansion of Participatory Governance

Participatory governance is necessary for the democratization of biomaterial innovation, where a range of stakeholders impact the design and decision-making procedures. It is becoming more widely acknowledged that patients, ethicists, and legislators are not merely passive consumers of biomedical innovations, but rather co-creators. Early in the development cycle, citizen assemblies, ethical review committees, and public discourse forums can all aid in foreseeing societal issues. In addition to addressing access inequities and ensuring inclusivity, this participatory methodology raises public confidence in cutting-edge treatments like gene-edited scaffolds and brain biomaterials. A generation of researchers who are sensitive to the social ramifications of their discoveries will also be produced by integrating ethical literacy and regulatory awareness into scientific education.

10.9.6 Leveraging Digital Twins and Virtual Clinical Trials for Predictive Evaluation and Faster Approval

Preclinical and clinical testing are about to undergo a transformation thanks to digital twins, which are virtual replicas of biomaterials, devices, or even specific patients. Digital twins allow for non-invasive prediction modeling of immunological compatibility, device–tissue interactions, and degradation kinetics by mimicking intricate biological reactions. Regulatory bodies are starting to acknowledge silico models as supplementary evidence in approval processes, which can drastically cut down on development expenses and time. With the help of machine learning algorithms and real-world data, virtual clinical trials can expedite regulatory decisions while maintaining trial population variety. These digital strategies complement iterative optimization and ongoing post-market monitoring, which is exactly in line with adaptive regulatory theories.

10.9.7 Building Resilient Regulatory Ecosystems through Interdisciplinary Education and International Cooperation

An ecosystem that combines ethics, politics, and research via interdisciplinary cooperation is essential to biomaterial governance resilience. To increase institutional capacity for adaptive supervision, training programs that include materials science, regulatory affairs, and bioethics are crucial. International collaboration will promote shared learning and quick responses to new issues including data sovereignty, AI responsibility, and nanotoxicology through academic consortia, policy networks, and international think tanks. With the help of automated compliance engines, real-time transparency dashboards, and interoperable data infrastructures, future regulatory ecosystems are probably going to operate as dispersed networks [82]. These kinds of systems will guarantee that innovation stays responsible and flexible, able to react to both public expectations and scientific disruption.

There will be a confluence of disciplines, countries, and technology in the regulation and ethics of biomaterials in the future. Static rulebooks will be replaced by flexible and standardized frameworks, allowing for ongoing learning and development throughout the innovative lifecycle. As biomedical systems become more digital, ethical AI will be used as a tool for both design and oversight, guaranteeing accountability and transparency. The ethical underpinnings of biomaterial science will be reshaped by sustainability, inclusivity, and participatory governance, guaranteeing that advancement stays ecologically mindful and human centered. In addition to speeding up innovation, digital twins, virtual trials, and circular manufacturing models will help us better grasp the intricate relationship between matter, biology, and society.

Ultimately, the vision for the next era of biomaterial governance is that of a living regulatory ecosystem dynamic, predictive, and global where ethical responsibility evolves in tandem with technological possibility. By embedding adaptability, sustainability, and cooperation at its core, the field will continue to advance safe, effective, and equitable biomedical solutions for an interconnected world.

10.10 Conclusion

The development of biomaterials has drastically changed how biology, technology, and medicine interact, making it possible to replace, repair, and improve human tissues with previously unheard-of accuracy. However, the interaction of innovation, ethics, and regulation has become the defining axis of biomaterials' responsible growth as they become more intelligent, hybridized, and digitally integrated. The strength of governance structures that guarantee safety, equity, and public trust is just as important to the future of biomaterials as developments in material science or technical skills. This conclusion summarizes the interrelated aspects of ethical reflection and regulatory monitoring, reaffirming the principles that support sustainable biomedical advancement and pointing the way toward a more unified and responsible future for the industry.

10.10.1 Summary of the Interplay Between Regulation, Ethics, and Innovation in Biomaterials

A careful balance between innovation and protection governs the creation and application of biomaterials, where moral and legal obligations must coexist with scientific progress. While bioethics provides the normative framework directing the right use of knowledge and technology, regulatory science provides the structural backbone that guarantees safety, efficacy, and quality. They work together to create a dual axis of conscience and control that influences the direction of biomaterials innovation.

By creating uniform protocols for preclinical testing, clinical trials, and post-market surveillance, regulation operationalizes trust and turns scientific innovation into therapeutic utility. But ethics puts that trust in perspective by tackling issues of justice, autonomy, and human wellbeing. By combining the two fields, biomaterials are guaranteed to serve human dignity and the welfare of society in addition to performing as planned. In actuality, this interaction is demonstrated by global regulatory organizations, data protection frameworks, and ethical review boards that strive to balance technical advancement with moral acceptability.

Innovation in biomaterials, particularly in areas such as nanotechnology, neural interfaces, and AI-integrated implants, continually tests the boundaries of existing frameworks. The speed of discovery often outpaces regulatory adaptation, revealing gaps in oversight and ethical guidance. Thus, the field's future depends on regulatory agility and ethical foresight, ensuring that new technologies advance without compromising the fundamental principles of patient safety and social justice.

10.10.2 Reinforcement of Safety, Transparency, and Responsibility as Pillars of Sustainable Progress

The three most important pillars supporting biomaterial innovation are safety, transparency, and responsibility, among other guiding principles. Clinical translation is still primarily determined by safety; all biomaterials must exhibit mechanical integrity, long-term biocompatibility, and predictable breakdown in the human body. This dedication goes beyond preclinical validation to ongoing post-market surveillance, where watchfulness guarantees that unanticipated risks are quickly recognized and reduced. Transparency is equally important for preserving scientific credibility and public trust. Clear communication of risk-benefit profiles, replicable procedures, and open data sharing facilitate group analysis and well-informed decision-making. Transparency must also include algorithmic processes in a time when biomaterials are increasingly interacting with digital systems and personal data. This will guarantee that AI-driven designs and predictive models are still comprehensible and accountable.

By encouraging academics, engineers, physicians, and legislators to acknowledge their collective involvement in determining the societal impact of technology, responsibility helps to close the gap between innovation and ethics. This entails avoiding abuse, lowering disparities in access to cutting-edge treatments, and reducing environmental impacts by using circular and sustainable material solutions. In the end, responsible biomaterial research evaluates success based on its impact on ecological and human well-being in addition to technical performance.

10.10.3 Recognition of Interdisciplinary Collaboration as Key to Ethical Translation and Adoption

Modern biomaterials are complicated and cross discipline boundaries. Materials scientists, bioengineers, ethicists, doctors, and data specialists must collaborate to create, test, and integrate them clinically. Thus, it becomes clear that interdisciplinary cooperation is the key to achieving both social acceptance and ethical translation. It is impossible to address ethical and regulatory issues in a single field, such as those pertaining to neural implants, scaffolds made of stem cells, or AI-assisted diagnostics. Rather, they call for an ecosystemic approach in which ethical considerations and policy insights are incorporated into engineering innovation from the very beginning of research. Transnational advisory networks and multidisciplinary regulatory committees are examples of collaborative governance structures that are essential for making sure that ethical reflection develops in tandem with technology innovation.

Moreover, involving patients, caregivers, and community representatives in the design and evaluation process strengthens legitimacy and inclusiveness. This participatory model ensures that biomaterial innovation aligns with real-world needs and diverse cultural values, reinforcing the ethical foundation of its translation into practice.

10.10.4 Outlook Toward Globally Harmonized, Digitally Integrated, and Ethically Conscious Biomaterials Governance

Global harmonization and digital integration are key to the governance of biomaterials in the future. Regionally fair access to safe and efficient biomaterials would be made possible by streamlined approval processes, less duplication, and unified regulatory frameworks supported by mutual recognition agreements and common standards. Though ongoing institutional and political cooperation is necessary to address jurisdictional fragmentation, international initiatives spearheaded by the WHO, ISO, and IMDRF already indicate progress toward such alignment. Governance structures that are digitally integrated will also be essential for handling the complexity of next-generation biomaterials. Throughout product lifecycles, the integration of blockchain, AI, and big data analytics can improve traceability, transparency, and predictive risk assessment. By automating compliance documentation, enhancing post-market surveillance, and enabling real-time implant performance monitoring, such solutions could make the regulatory environment more flexible and responsive.

At the same time, ethical consciousness must remain central to these digital transformations. As automation and data-driven decision-making become embedded in regulation, human oversight and moral reasoning must not be displaced. Future governance must combine technological precision with ethical empathy, ensuring that the pursuit of efficiency does not erode patient autonomy or accountability.

10.10.5 Final Reflection: The Future of Biomaterials Lies in Innovation Guided by Integrity and Social Accountability

The goal for biomaterials is not simply scientific superiority but also human-centered advancement a meeting point of justice, ethics, and creativity. Biomaterials of the future will probably be responsive, regenerative, and intelligent, able to blend in perfectly with the human body and mind. However, whether these developments are driven by honesty, openness, and a dedication to general welfare will determine their actual success. As science advances, ethical and regulatory stewardship must also advance. Every phase of development, from lab testing to market launch, should be anchored by integrity, and social responsibility should guarantee that advantages are shared fairly and possible risks are appropriately reduced. Future biomaterial science's moral framework will be determined by its ethical obligation to strike a balance between creativity and empathy, ambition and caution, and advancement and inclusivity.

The path forward demands a synergistic alliance between science, governance, and humanity. Only by embedding integrity and accountability within the fabric of innovation can biomaterials achieve their transformative potential restoring function, enhancing life, and strengthening the bond between human values and technological possibility.

References

1. Anju, M.S., Raj, D.K., Madathil, B.K., Kasoju, N., Anil Kumar, P.R.: Intelligent biomaterials for tissue engineering and biomedical applications: Current landscape and future prospects. In: Biomaterials in Tissue Engineering and Regenerative Medicine: From Basic Concepts to State of the Art Approaches, pp. 535–560. Springer Singapore, Singapore (2021)
2. Iqbal, S., Sohail, M., Fang, S., Ding, J., Shen, L., Chen, M., Shu, G., Du, Y.Z., Ji, J.: Biomaterials evolution: from inert to instructive. Biomater. Sci. **11**(18), 6109–6115 (2023)
3. Lantada, A.D., De Maria, C.: Sustainable open-source medical devices manufactured with green biomaterials and accessible resources. Curr. Opin. Biomed. Eng. **28**, 100500 (2023)
4. Chen, R.J., Wang, J.J., Williamson, D.F., Chen, T.Y., Lipkova, J., Lu, M.Y., Sahai, S., Mahmood, F.: Algorithmic fairness in artificial intelligence for medicine and healthcare. Nat. Biomed. Eng. **7**(6), 719–742 (2023)
5. Mensah, G.B.: Artificial intelligence and ethics: a comprehensive review of bias mitigation, transparency, and accountability in AI Systems. Preprint, November, **10**(1), 1 (2023)
6. Kousoulas, S., Perera, D. (eds.): All is in Formation: Architecture, Cybernetics, Ecology. JAP SAM Books (2021)
7. Sawarkar, S., Bapat, A.: Global regulatory frameworks and quality standards for stem cells therapy and regenerative medicines. In: Stem Cell Production: Processes, Practices and Regulations, pp. 69–111. Springer Singapore, Singapore (2022)
8. Shanmugam, D.K., Anitha, S.C., Souresh, V., Madhavan, Y., Sampath, S., Catakapatri Venugopal, D., Saravanan, M.: Current advancements in the development of bionic organs using regenerative medicine and 3D tissue engineering. Mater. Technol. **38**(1), 2242732 (2023)

9. Schuh, J.C., Funk, K.A.: Compilation of international standards and regulatory guidance documents for evaluation of biomaterials, medical devices, and 3-D printed and regenerative medicine products. Toxicol. Pathol. **47**(3), 344–357 (2019)
10. Song, X., Tang, Z., Liu, W., Chen, K., Liang, J., Yuan, B., Lin, H., Zhu, X., Fan, Y., Shi, X., Zhao, P.: Biomaterials and regulatory science. J. Mater. Sci. Technol. **128**, 221–227 (2022)
11. Callanan, A., Hay, D., Bagnaninchi, P. and Paxton, J., 2021. Anthony Callanan TCES Organising Chair The University of Edinburgh
12. Badnjević, A., Pokvić, L.G., Deumić, A., Bećirović, L.S.: Post-market surveillance of medical devices: A review. Technol. Health Care. **30**(6), 1315–1329 (2022)
13. Cioeta, R., Cossu, A., Giovagnoni, E., Rigoni, M., Muti, P.: A new platform for post-marketing surveillance and real-world evidence data collection for substance-based medical devices. Front. Drug Saf. Regul. **2**, 992359 (2022)
14. Gesualdo, F., Daverio, M., Palazzani, L., Dimitriou, D., Diez-Domingo, J., Fons-Martinez, J., Jackson, S., Vignally, P., Rizzo, C., Tozzi, A.E.: Digital tools in the informed consent process: a systematic review. BMC Med. Ethics. **22**(1), 18 (2021)
15. Gruber, H.E., 2022Portal to the New Earth: Sound, Sacred Geometry & Grid Energies for Personal & Planetary Transfromation
16. Hunckler, M.D., Levine, A.D.: Navigating ethical challenges in the development and translation of biomaterials research. Front. Bioeng. Biotechnol. **10**, 949280 (2022)
17. Malsch, I.: Ethics of nanomedicine. In: Nanobiomaterials: Perspectives for Medical Applications in the Diagnosis and Treatment of Diseases, vol. 145, pp. 311–325. Materials Research Forum LLC (2023)
18. Vasoya, N.H.: Revolutionizing nano materials processing through IoT-AI integration: opportunities and challenges. J. Mater. Sci. Res. Rev. **6**(3), 294–328 (2023)
19. Ornaghi Jr., H.L., Monticeli, F.M., Agnol, L.D.: A review on polymers for biomedical applications on hard and soft tissues and prosthetic limbs. Polymers. **15**(19), 4034 (2023)
20. Goebel, S., Verna, V., Marty, C., Neadle, S.W.: General overview of global combination product regulatory landscape. In: The Combination Products Handbook, pp. 441–504. CRC Press (2023)
21. Wasnik, S.: Premarket review and postmarket regulation of combination drug products. In: Combination Drug Delivery Approach as an Effective Therapy for Various Diseases, pp. 331–352. Academic Press (2022)
22. Anavadya, K.K., Vijayalakshmi, U.: A comprehensive review of fabrication techniques and their impact on mechanical behaviour and osteoregenerative applications of bioactive inorganic substituents. Mater. Res. Lett. **11**(10), 821–855 (2023)
23. Sharma, S., Sudhakara, P., Singh, J., Ilyas, R.A., Asyraf, M.R.M., Razman, M.R.: Critical review of biodegradable and bioactive polymer composites for bone tissue engineering and drug delivery applications. Polymers. **13**(16), 2623 (2021)
24. Sun, W., Gregory, D.A., Tomeh, M.A., Zhao, X.: Silk fibroin as a functional biomaterial for tissue engineering. Int. J. Mol. Sci. **22**(3), 1499 (2021)
25. Cornish, N.E., Anderson, N.L., Arambula, D.G., Arduino, M.J., Bryan, A., Burton, N.C., Chen, B., Dickson, B.A., Giri, J.G., Griffith, N.K.a., Pentella, M.A.: Clinical laboratory biosafety gaps: lessons learned from past outbreaks reveal a path to a safer future. Clin. Microbiol. Rev. **34**(3), 10–1128 (2021)
26. Jacobs, M.N., Versteegen, R.J., Treasure, C.a., Murray, J.: Addressing potential ethical issues regarding the supply of human-derived products or reagents in in vitro OECD Test Guidelines. ALTEX-Altern. Anim. Exp. **36**(2), 163–176 (2019)
27. Fan, G., Wang, Q.: Quality control and quality assurance. In: Clinical Molecular Diagnostics, pp. 97–113. Springer Singapore, Singapore (2021)
28. Adebowale, A.M., Akinnagbe, O.B.: Leveraging AI-driven data integration for predictive risk assessment in decentralized financial markets. Int J Eng Technol Res Manag. **5**(12), 295 (2021)

29. Alonge, E.O., Eyo-Udo, N.L., Chibunna, B., Ubanadu, A.I.D., Balogun, E.D., Ogunsola, K.O.: Data-driven risk management in US financial institutions: A theoretical perspective on process optimization. Icon. Res. Eng. J. (2023)
30. Harrington, R.E., Guda, T., Lambert, B., Martin, J.: Sterilization and disinfection of biomaterials for medical devices. In: Biomaterials Science, pp. 1431–1446. Academic Press (2020)
31. Jildeh, Z.B., Wagner, P.H., Schöning, M.J.: Sterilization of objects, products, and packaging surfaces and their characterization in different fields of industry: The status in 2020. Physica status solidi (a). **218**(13), 2000732 (2021)
32. Sheehan, A., O'Sullivan, R.: Ethical Issues in Research With Vulnerable People: A Case Study. In: Ethics and Integrity in Research with Older People and Service Users: Moving Beyond the Rhetoric, pp. 83–109. Emerald Publishing Limited (2023)
33. Ankit, T., Shrikalp, D., Maitreyi, Z., Kumar, J.P., Kiran, K.: Transition of Pharmaceutical Regulations: The New Regulatory Era after Brexit. J. Pharm. Res. Int. **33**(47A), 804–817 (2021)
34. Davidson, P., Kauffmann, C., De Liedekerke, M.G.: How do laws and regulations affect competitiveness. In: OECD Regulatory Policy Working Papers (2021)
35. Norori, N., Hu, Q., Aellen, F.M., Faraci, F.D., Tzovara, A.: Addressing bias in big data and AI for health care: A call for open science. Patterns. **2**(10) (2021)
36. Morrison, M., Prainsack, B.: Responsible personalised medicine: Exploring the ethical, legal, social, political and economic issues of manufacturing, distribution, access and reimbursement. In: A Report by the Future Targeted Healthcare Manufacturing Hub (2022)
37. Alzoubi, L., Aljabali, A.A., Tambuwala, M.M.: Empowering precision medicine: the impact of 3D printing on personalized therapeutic. Aaps Pharmscitech. **24**(8), 228 (2023)
38. Çetin, S., De Wolf, C., Bocken, N.: Circular digital built environment: An emerging framework. Sustainability. **13**(11), 6348 (2021)
39. Jiao, R., Commuri, S., Panchal, J., Milisavljevic-Syed, J., Allen, J.K., Mistree, F., Schaefer, D.: Design engineering in the age of industry 4.0. J. Mech. Design. **143**(7), 070801 (2021)
40. Sauerwein, M., Doubrovski, E., Balkenende, R., Bakker, C.: Exploring the potential of additive manufacturing for product design in a circular economy. J. Clean. Product. **226**, 1138–1149 (2019)
41. Nuño-Soriano, A., Arias-Hidalgo, C., Montalvillo, E., Góngora, R., Hernández, Á.P., Juanes-Velasco, P., Fuentes, M.: Evaluating biocompatibility: From classical techniques to state-of-the-art functional proteomics. Nanomaterials. **15**(13), 1032 (2025)
42. Zdravkova, K., Krasniqi, V., Dalipi, F., Ferati, M.: Cutting-edge communication and learning assistive technologies for disabled children: An artificial intelligence perspective. Front. Artific. Intell. **5**, 970430 (2022)
43. Shi, X., Zhang, G., Lu, Y., Pang, H.: Applications of machine learning in electrochemistry. Renewables. **1**(6), 668–693 (2023)
44. Palazzani, L.: Innovation in Scientific Research and Emerging Technologies. A Challenge to Ethics and Law, p. 150. Springer–Giappicheli, Cham (2019)
45. Stocco, E., Barbon, S., Mammana, M., Zambello, G., Contran, M., Parnigotto, P.P., Macchi, V., Conconi, M.T., Rea, F., De Caro, R., Porzionato, A.: Preclinical and clinical orthotopic transplantation of decellularized/engineered tracheal scaffolds: a systematic literature review. J. Tissue Eng. **14**, 20417314231151826 (2023)
46. Burns, L., Le Roux, N., Kalesnik-Orszulak, R., Christian, J., Hukkelhoven, M., Rockhold, F., O'Donnell, J.: Real-world evidence for regulatory decision-making: guidance from around the world. Clin. Ther. **44**(3), 420–437 (2022)
47. Valla, V., Tzelepi, K., Charitou, P., Lewis, A., Polatidis, B., Koukoura, A., Karapatsia, A., Antonopoulou, K., Prodromidou, K., Papadaki, E., Vassiliadis, E.: Use of real-world evidence for international regulatory decision making in medical devices. Int. J. Digit. Heal. **3**(1), 1 (2023)
48. Owobu, W.O., Abieba, O.A., Gbenle, P., Onoja, J.P., Daraojimba, A.I., Adepoju, A.H., Ubamadu, B.C.: Review of enterprise communication security architectures for improving confidentiality, integrity, and availability in digital workflows. IRE J. **5**(5), 370–372 (2021)

49. Tim, Y., Chiew, T.K., Lim, H.M., Teo, C.H., Ng, C.J.: Design process knowledge for crisis-driven information systems solutions: Insights on building digital resilience from an action design research study. Inform. Syst. J. **33**(6), 1343–1369 (2023)
50. Alshangiti, D.M., El-Damhougy, T.K., Zaher, A., Madani, M.: Revolutionizing biomedicine: advancements, applications, and prospects of nanocomposite macromolecular carbohydrate-based hydrogel biomaterials: a review. RSC Adv. **13**(50), 35251–35291 (2023)
51. Goyal, A.S.: Biomaterials in Biomedical Engineering. Aditya Sandeep Goyal (2023)
52. Dhandapani, V., Saseedharan, P., Groleau, D., Vermette, P.: Overview of approval procedures for bioadhesives in the United States of America and Canada. J. Biomed. Mater. Res. Part B. Appl. Biomater. **110**(4), 950–966 (2022)
53. Morrison, M., Brunel, V., Mahalatchimy, A.: Participation in SoHO and ATMP public consultations: a fragmented institutional landscape. Human. Soc. Sci. Commun. **12**(1), 1–14 (2025)
54. Foong, P.: Unproven Stem Cell Industry in the US: Regulatory Challenges and Enforcement Issues. Biotechnol. Law Rep. **42**(4), 184–198 (2023)
55. Ikonomou, L., Cuende, N., Forte, M., Grilley, B.J., Levine, A.D., Munsie, M., Rasko, J.E., Turner, L., Bidkhori, H.R., Ciccocioppo, R., Grignon, F.: International Society for Cell & Gene Therapy Position Paper: Key considerations to support evidence-based cell and gene therapies and oppose marketing of unproven products. Cytotherapy. **25**(9), 920–929 (2023)
56. Doak, S.H., Andreoli, C., Burgum, M.J., Chaudhry, Q., Bleeker, E.A., Bossa, C., Domenech, J., Drobne, D., Fessard, V., Jeliazkova, N. and Longhin, E: Current Status and Future Challenges of Genotoxicity OECD Test Guidelines for Nanomaterials: A Workshop Report (2023)
57. Perin, F., Ouyang, L., Lim, K.S., Motta, A., Maniglio, D., Moroni, L., Mota, C.: Bioprinted Constructs in the Regulatory Landscape: Current State and Future Perspectives. Adv. Mater. **38**(4), e04037 (2026)
58. Awad, E., Levine, S., Anderson, M., Anderson, S.L., Conitzer, V., Crockett, M.J., Everett, J.A., Evgeniou, T., Gopnik, A., Jamison, J.C., Kim, T.W.: Computational ethics. Trend. Cog. Sci. **26**(5), 388–405 (2022)
59. Hassan, S., Dhali, M., Zaman, F., Tanveer, M.: Big data and predictive analytics in healthcare in Bangladesh: regulatory challenges. Heliyon. **7**(6), e07179 (2021)
60. Anurogo, D., Hidayat, N.A.: The Art Of Televasculobiomedicine 5.0. Nas Media Pustaka (2023)
61. Martínez, S.: Innovations in biotechnology: Bridging the gap between science and medicine. Austra & Lian J. Basic Sci. **3**(1), 11–19 (2022)
62. Chiti, E., Micera, S., Palmerini, E.: Making the case for sandboxes in implantable neurotechnologies. Nat. Commun. **16**(1), 9783 (2025). https://doi.org/10.1038/s41467-025-65584-4
63. Engelmann, W.: Governance and Sandbox: Building self-regulation models for nanotechnologies. J. Entrepr. Res. **1**(1), 13–20 (2023)
64. Singh, R., Paxton, M., Auclair, J.: Regulating the AI-enabled ecosystem for human therapeutics. Commun. Med. **5**(1), 181 (2025)
65. McDermid, J.A., Jia, Y., Porter, Z., Habli, I.: Artificial intelligence explainability: the technical and ethical dimensions. Philos. Trans. R. Soc. A. **379**(2207), 20200363 (2021)
66. Oyasiji, O., Okesiji, A., Imediegwu, C.C., Elebe, O., Filani, O.M.: Ethical AI in financial decision-making: Transparency, bias, and regulation. Int. J. Sci. Res. Comput. Sci. Eng. Inform. Technol. **9**(5), 453–471 (2023)
67. Gross, M.S., Hood, A.J., Miller Jr., R.C.: Nonfungible tokens as a blockchain solution to ethical challenges for the secondary use of biospecimens. JMIR Bioinform. Biotechnol. **2**(1), e29905 (2021)
68. Rehm, H.L., Page, A.J., Smith, L., Adams, J.B., Alterovitz, G., Babb, L.J., Barkley, M.P., Baudis, M., Beauvais, M.J., Beck, T., Beckmann, J.S.: GA4GH: International policies and standards for data sharing across genomic research and healthcare. Cell Genom. **1**(2) (2021)
69. Bates, J., Cameron, D., Checco, A., Clough, P., Hopfgartner, F., Mazumdar, S., Sbaffi, L., Stordy, P., de la Vega de León, A.: Integrating FATE/critical data studies into data science cur-

ricula: where are we going and how do we get there? In: Proceedings of the 2020 Conference on Fairness, Accountability, and Transparency, pp. 425–435 (2020)
70. Jaime, F.J., Muñoz, A., Rodríguez-Gómez, F., Jerez-Calero, A.: Strengthening privacy and data security in biomedical microelectromechanical systems by IoT communication security and protection in smart healthcare. Sensors. **23**(21), 8944 (2023)
71. Popov, V.V., Kudryavtseva, E.V., Katiyar, N.K., Shishkin, A., Stepanov, S.I., Goel, S.: Industry 4.0 and digitalisation in healthcare. Materials. **15**, 2140 (2022)
72. Cho, Y., Park, S., Lee, J., Yu, K.J.: Emerging materials and technologies with applications in flexible neural implants: a comprehensive review of current issues with neural devices. Adv. Mater. **33**(47), 2005786 (2021)
73. Valeriani, D., Santoro, F., Ienca, M.: The present and future of neural interfaces. Front. Neurorobot. **16**, 953968 (2022)
74. Khan, F.: Regulating the revolution: a legal roadmap to optimizing AI in healthcare. Minn. JL Sci. & Tech. **25**, 49 (2023)
75. Affia, A.A.O., Finch, H., Jung, W., Samori, I.A., Potter, L., Palmer, X.L.: IoT health devices: exploring security risks in the connected landscape. IoT. **4**(2), 150–182 (2023)
76. Karamifar, F., Tabibian, S., Rezaei, S.A.: Legal and ethical challenges in digital public health systems: Data privacy, consent, and security. Legal Stud. Digit. Age. **2**(4), 13–25 (2023)
77. Filippi, M., Buchner, T., Yasa, O., Weirich, S., Katzschmann, R.K.: Microfluidic tissue engineering and bio-actuation. Adv. Mater. **34**(23), 2108427 (2022)
78. Lescrauwaet, L., Wagner, H., Yoon, C., Shukla, S.: Adaptive legal frameworks and economic dynamics in emerging tech-nologies: Navigating the intersection for responsible innovation. Law. Econom. **16**(3), 202–220 (2022)
79. Magisetty, R., Park, S.M.: New era of electroceuticals: clinically driven smart implantable electronic devices moving towards precision therapy. Micromachines. **13**(2), 161 (2022)
80. Prescott, S.L., Wegienka, G., Kort, R., Nelson, D.H., Gabrysch, S., Hancock, T., Kozyrskyj, A., Lowry, C.A., Redvers, N., Poland, B. Robinson, J.: Project Earthrise: Proceedings of the Ninth Annual Conference of in Vivo Planetary Health (2021)
81. Upreti, G.: Ecosociocentrism: The Earth First Paradigm for Sustainable Living, pp. 307–367. Springer Nature Switzerland, Cham (2023)
82. Adekunle, B.I., Chukwuma-Eke, E.C., Balogun, E.D., Ogunsola, K.O.: Developing a digital operations dashboard for real-time financial compliance monitoring in multinational corporations. Int. J. Sci. Res. Comput. Sci. Eng. Inform. Technol. **9**(3), 728–746 (2023)

GPSR Compliance

The European Union's (EU) General Product Safety Regulation (GPSR) is a set of rules that requires consumer products to be safe and our obligations to ensure this.

If you have any concerns about our products, you can contact us on ProductSafety@springernature.com

In case Publisher is established outside the EU, the EU authorized representative is:

Springer Nature Customer Service Center GmbH
Europaplatz 3
69115 Heidelberg, Germany

Batch number: 10799746

Printed by Printforce, the Netherlands